Emergency Dysrhythmias ECG Injury Patterns

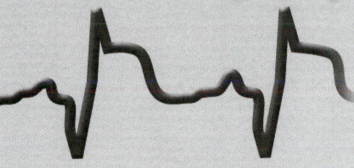

Kevin Brown, MD

THOMSON ™

DELMAR LEARNING

Australia Canada Mexico Singapore Spain United Kingdom United States

Dedication

To my wife Freda, for her encouragement,
support, and advice;
to my children
Nicholas, Arianna, and Maddalena,
whose arrivals
opened a new and cherished world for me;
and to my Aunt Helen,
who was an early supporter.

Special dedication

To all the heroes
involved in the September 11th attack,
especially those emergency medical
service (EMS) rescuers
who gave their lives to save others.

Emergency Dysrhythmias & ECG Injury Patterns

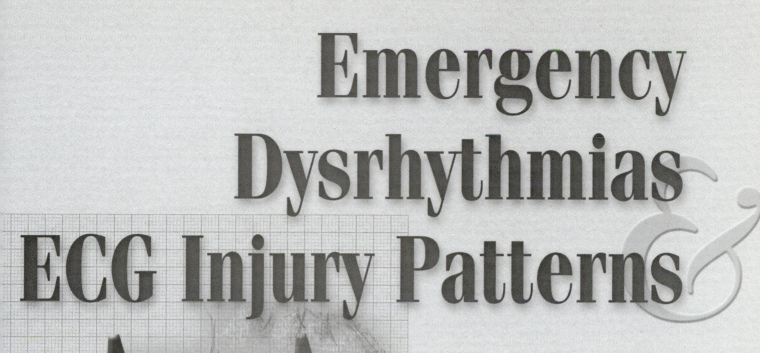

Kevin Brown, MD

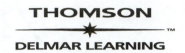

THOMSON
————★————™
DELMAR LEARNING

Emergency Dysrhythmias & ECG Injury Patterns
by
Kevin R. Brown

Executive Director,
Health Care Business Unit:
William Brottmiller

Executive Editor:
Cathy L. Esperti

Acquisitions Editor:
Maureen Rosener

Development Editor:
Darcy M. Scelsi

Editorial Assistant:
Matthew Thouin

Executive Marketing Manager:
Dawn F. Gerrain

Channel Manager:
Jennifer McAvey

Production Editor:
Mary Colleen Liburdi

Cover Illustration:
Mary Colleen Liburdi

COPYRIGHT © 2003 by Delmar Learning, a division of Thomson Learning, Inc. Thomson Learning™ is a trademark used herein under license

Printed in the United States
  2 3 4 5 XXX 06 05 04 03

For more information contact
Delmar Learning,
Executive Woods, 5 Maxwell Drive,
Clifton Park, NY 12065-2919
Or find us on the World Wide Web at
http://www.delmar.com

ALL RIGHTS RESERVED. No part of this work covered by the copyright hereon may be reproduced or used in any form or by any means—graphic, electronic, or mechanical, including photocopying, recording, taping, Web distribution or information storage and retrieval systems—without written permission of the publisher.

For permission to use material from this text or product, contact us by
Tel   (800) 730-2214
Fax   (800) 730-2215
www.thomsonrights.com

Library of Congress Cataloging-in-Publication Data on file

ISBN 0-7668-1988-4

NOTICE TO THE READER

Publisher does not warrant or guarantee any of the products described herein or perform any independent analysis in connection with any of the product information contained herein. Publisher does not assume, and expressly disclaims, any obligation to obtain and include information other than that provided to it by the manufacturer.

The reader is expressly warned to consider and adopt all safety precautions that might be indicated by the activities herein and to avoid all potential hazards. By following the instructions contained herein, the reader willingly assumes all risks in connection with such instructions.

The Publisher makes no representation or warranties of any kind, including but not limited to, the warranties of fitness for particular purpose or merchantability, nor are any such representations implied with respect to the material set forth herein, and the publisher takes no responsibility with respect to such material. The publisher shall not be liable for any special, consequential, or exemplary damages resulting, in whole or part, from the readers' use of, or reliance upon, this material.

Contents

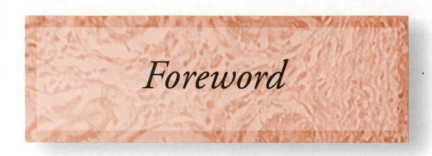

Foreword

Experience may be the best teacher, but it also makes the best teacher. *Emergency Dysrhythmias and ECG Injury Patterns* has been written by a physician educator who is strong in both suits: long experience as a clinician who understands the need for rapid decisions in emergency situations beginning with his work "on the streets" in a busy EMS system; and long experience as an educator who instinctively understands the way to make ECG learning come to life.

This text begins with a simple and systematic presentation on ECG interpretation that guides students seemingly effortlessly to an understanding of basic concepts while giving them a method that will be useful forever after for diagnosing dysrhythmias. There are hundreds of examples and ECG tracings—gathered from actual emergency 9-1-1 calls and emergency department encounters—for both learners and teachers to ground basic concepts through real-life examples.

A special feature of *Emergency Dysrhythmias and ECG Injury Patterns* and one that distinguishes it from all others, are the chapters emphasizing the interpretation of ECGs in the acute phase of cardiac emergencies—the vital time both pre-hospital and in the emergency/critical care units where decisions will be made regarding diagnosis, resuscitation, rate control, reducing ischemia, and establishing reperfusion. As the effort to save myocardium concentrates more and more cardiac care in the first hours of symptom presentation, recognition of ischemia and infarction on the ECG are a vital skill not just for physicians but also for EMTs, paramedic, nurses, nurse practitioners, and physician assistants.

Whether you are a first-time student who is approaching the subject of ECG interpretation feeling your own heart sinking, or as a teacher who is puzzling how to make the difficult subject easier for your students, you are holding the textbook that will make all the difference for rapid and enjoyable mastery of this important area of emergency care.

Diane M. Sixsmith, MD, MPH, FACEP
Chairman, Department of Emergency Medicine
The New York Hospital Medical Center for Queens

Assistant Clinical Professor of Medicine,
Weill Medical College of Cornell University
New York, NY

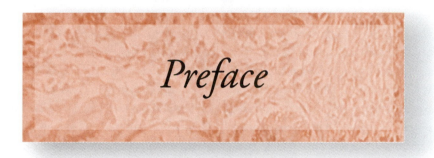

Preface

There has been an explosion of new diagnostic tools and treatment techniques for patients experiencing acute coronary syndromes, yet twelve-lead ECG interpretation and dysrhythmia recognition remain the basic tools for evaluating patients with suspected myocardial ischemia. It is essential that everyone caring for such patients be able to quickly and accurately interpret the ECG tracing and recognize abnormalities.

Emergency Dysrhythmias and ECG Injury Patterns is intended to be used by the entire cardiac care team, including emergency medical technicians (EMTs), paramedics, emergency department and critical care unit nurses, medical students, physician assistants, nurse practitioners, and emergency medicine residents.

It is amazing to realize that only a short time ago, thrombolytic therapy was considered experimental, and that only cardiologists were authorized to administer lytic medication. Today, the focus in treating heart attack patients has shifted to the emergency department in order to medicate as quickly as possible following the onset of chest pain.

In order to achieve the vital "door-to-needle time" 30-minute benchmark for giving this myocardium-sparing drug, every ED triage nurse must be competent at screening twelve-lead ECGs for signs of an acute coronary event. Paramedics also perform twelve-lead ECGs to screen patients with chest pain for acute ST-T wave changes and notify the ED of the imminent arrival of a potential thrombolytic candidate, and in some EMS systems, administer the drug while en-route. Critical care unit nurses have a vital role in evaluating serial ECGs in patients who have received thrombolysis to detect reocclusion as well as being able to evaluate and treat ischemia and reperfusion associated cardiac rhythm disturbances.

Why Another ECG Text?

Since bookshelves are already lined with many well-written electrocardiogram texts, what justifies a new one? As the title illustrates, *Emergency Dysrhythmias and ECG Injury Patterns* is geared toward the initial hours in evaluating acute myocardial infarction (AMI) patients. The early phase after the onset of chest pain is the most dangerous period for patients experiencing an MI—the time associated with the highest mortality rate and the most frequent incidence of life-threatening dysrhythmias. However, many dysrhythmia recognition books fail to even address twelve-lead ECGs, leaving the topic for optional future study. Other ECG books have an inadequate number of self-assessment tracings or contain only a single example of each dysrhythmia, yet numerous patterns are common. Also, many books that describe twelve-lead ECGs are geared toward the cardiologist and are either too sophisticated and detailed or devote only brief attention to the signs of acute coronary syndromes. *Emergency Dysrhythmias and ECG Injury Patterns* has been written for, and by, members of the emergency cardiac care team and specifically addresses acute care issues.

Learning any new field requires practice and feedback—dysrhythmia recognition and ECG interpretation are no exceptions. Questions such as "Why do the P waves 'march through' the QRS complexes?" or "What causes the distorted T wave that is seen just before the cardiac pause?" need to be addressed. The type and scope of self-assessment ECG exercises contained in this book sets *Emergency Dysrhythmias and ECG Injury Patterns* apart from most other texts. Every rhythm and conduction disorder, as well as ischemia, injury, and infarction patterns is illustrated using several examples to aid reader learning.

Emergency Dysrhythmias and ECG Injury Patterns was initially conceived of as a workbook and later expanded to a text. In my teaching experience, most ECG books suffer from being either too complex or too simple to suit the practical needs of EMS, emergency, and critical care staff. Acute care of patients with dysrhythmias is based on identifying which abnormal rhythm is present, selecting a therapy, and determining how fast the abnormal rhythm needs to be corrected. For that reason, cellular concepts and action potentials, although interesting, don't have much practical use when treating patients, so the pages devoted to these areas are briefer than in other books. The examples of acute myocardial injury patterns are emphasized. Areas focusing on practical and patient-centered concepts have been specifically emphasized. The aim of the book is to be a useful tool in the ambulance, in the ED, and in the CCU.

Organization of the Text

Written in a clinically relevant, user-friendly manner, Emergency Dysrhythmias and ECG Injury Patterns integrates fundamental principles of cell function, electrical disorders, and recognition of all of the clinically important rhythm disturbances. It is geared toward those new to ECGs but will be a good review tool for those who wish to be challenged by ECG strips that are not commonly encountered. Numerous tables and illustrative ECG tracings clarify and summarize the text.

Four major text sections are divided into 26 chapters. Section I provides information that will serve to acquire a foundation in order to understand how abnormal cardiac impulses develop and how to assess the different components of the tracing: rate, rhythm, complexes, pacemakers, and so forth. An early chapter presents a systematic approach to dysrhythmias, which is the framework followed throughout the remainder of the self-assessment exercises. In Section II, each dysrhythmia's characteristics are described. Self-assessment ECG tracings follow each explanatory chapter. Section III contains important additional topics, such as artificial pacemakers, the approach to fast and slow dysrhythmias, pediatric dysrhythmias, twelve-lead ECGs, and injury, ischemia, and infarction patterns. Numerous examples of abnormal ST segments are used. Section IV consists of comprehensive practice ECG tracings.

Features

- "Clinical Notes" and "ECG Interpretation Tips" are found throughout the chapters and draw attention to patient-related concepts and topics that facilitate ECG interpretation.

- A list of learner's objectives is contained at the beginning of each chapter. This serves to inform the student of what needs to be learned before proceeding to the next chapter.

- Special characteristics shared by different dysrhythmias are identified that permit them to be included in a general dysrhythmia grouping, such as irregular rhythms, fast rhythms, and slow rhythms. Similarities between various supraventricular rhythms are differentiated from those of ventricular rhythms.

- A "Let's Review" section summarizing important concepts is contained at the end of the chapters.

- The chapter titled "Approach to Bradydysrhythmias and Tachydysrhythmias" emphasizes how the clinician must always attend first to the patient and learn to integrate the ECG findings with the patient's history and exam in order to develop an accurate clinical picture. A quick, vectored patient assessment method is discussed along with treatment management.

- A complete chapter detailing the care and identification of children and infants who present with dysrhythmias.

How to Best Use This Book

This book can be adapted for various readers. Some instructional programs will want to focus on basic dysrhythmia recognition and leave the more advanced topics, such as pacemaker devices and twelve-lead ECGs, for future study. Other groups will want to proceed in a direct sequence from the first chapter to the end. The self-assessment exercises can be used throughout to track the reader's progress.

Instructor's Guide to Text

Many instructors have been forced to make photocopy ECGs for class handouts, homework, and testing. The *Emergency Dysrhythmias and ECG Injury Patterns* text and instructor's manual provide plenty of ECG examples for student practice. The Instructor's Guide provides beginning-of-chapter learning objectives, a chapter-by-chapter glossary, and additional material to assist the instructor in preparing instructor plans and student homework exercises.

About the Author

For twenty-six years, the author has worked in emergency care. He started in 1974 as a paramedic in the pilot class of the Emergency Medical Service system in New York City. He later supervised a paramedic training program and then attended medical school. He currently teaches dysrhythmia assessment to nurses, nurse practitioners, physician assistants, medical students, paramedics, and resident physicians in medicine and emergency medicine. He is the director of an emergency department in New York City and serves as a faculty member of an emergency medicine residency program and a physician assistant program.

Kevin R. Brown, MD, MPH, FACEP
Director, Department of Emergency Medicine
Our Lady of Mercy Medical Center
Bronx, New York

Assistant Professor of Emergency Medicine
Albert Einstein College of Medicine
Bronx, New York

Clinical Instructor Physician Assistant Program
Pace University, New York City

Acknowledgments

This book had many parents assisting in its delivery. I developed the initial concept but was dependent on many others to bring it to fruition, particularly Jean Francois Villain and Lynn Borders-Caldwell. Jean Francois launched me into the publishing field with my first book after gambling on someone with an idea but little writing experience. Lynn tried to get me to adhere to deadlines with superhuman patience.

This book would not have happened had it not been for the perseverance of Ms. Crystal Spraggins, who pushed me to create a superior teaching tool. Crystal spent long hours and hundreds of phone calls discussing the reviewers' comments and coordinating the entire process. My children, now 3, 5, and 7 years old, each came along just when I had again promised Crystal that I was going to sit down and devote all my energy to the project.

I owe a tremendous debt to the reviewers who read every word and made numerous suggestions and criticisms. I want to extend my appreciation to Jeffrey Meyers, MS, EMT-P, Terry Devito, RN, MED, EMT-P, CEN, and Richard K. Beck, BBA, NREMT-P, for their reviews. Cris E. Hanna, NREMT, and Toni Glick, deserve special mention for their voluminous notes and constructive criticism.

Ms. Darcy Scelsi, the Developmental Editor at Delmar Thomson Learning, coordinated the transformation of the manuscript into a readable and visually attractive teaching tool. She skillfully guided preparation of the instructor's guide.

Many of the dysrhythmia strips were provided by paramedics in the EMS Division of the Fire Department of New York. Many paramedic programs in New York City and Westchester County, NY, allowed me the honor of teaching in their programs during the last twenty years.

Finally, I want to thank Dr. Sheldon Jacobson who was my paramedic teacher, and got me started in teaching paramedics and interested in emergency medicine. In 1974 he assembled a group of interested ambulance technicians and motor vehicle operators and transformed us into paramedics who were comfortable evaluating dysrhythmias outside of the hospital. His encouragement and guidance over the years are warmly appreciated. Martin Cohen, MD, is appreciated as the cardiologist who first shared with me a logical approach to abnormal cardiac rhythms.

Avenue for Feedback

The author is interested in receiving reader and instructor feedback, especially with suggestions about how to improve the book's usefulness. Please direct comments to the publisher at alliedhealth@delmar.com.

Kevin Brown, MD

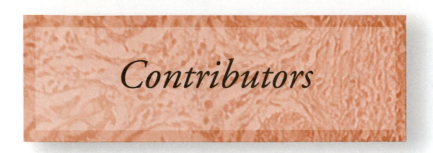

Contributors

Eileen Cafaso NP, RN, FNP
Assistant Professor of Clinical Nursing
Columbia University School of Nursing
Chapter 1: Cardiac Cell Structure and Function

Edward Chu, MD, FACC
Interventional and Consultative Cardiologist
Hampton Roads Cardiovascular Associates
Newport News, Virginia
Chapter 19: Artificial Pacemakers and Automatic Implantable
Defibrillator-Cardiovertors

John Guerriero EMT-P
Paramedic
Lenox Hill Hospital
New York, New York
Chapter 27: Clinical Scenarios in Dysrhythmias Management

Gene Iannuzzi, RN, MPA, CEN, EMT-P
Assistant Director of Nursing
Emergency Department
North Central Bronx Hospital
Bronx, New York

Adjunct Instructor, Allied Health Sciences
Borough of Manhattan Community College
Chapter 27: Clinical Scenarios in Dysrhythmias Management

Artie Romano EMT-P
EMS Training Officer
Greenwich Emergency Medical Services
Greenwich, Connecticut
Chapter 27: Clinical Scenarios in Dysrhythmias Management

Owen Traynor, MD
Emergency Medical Services Director
Saint Clair Hospital
Pittsburgh, Pennsylvania

Associate Medical Director for Paramedic Education
Center for Emergency Medicine of Western Pennsylvania

EMS Attending Physician
UPMC Health System
Pittsburgh, Pennsylvania
Chapter 8: Systematic Interpretation of Dysrhythmias:
Step Six
Chapter 21: Approach to Bradycardias and tachycardias

Lawrence M. Herman, RPA-C
Assistant Professor
Senior Clinical Coordinator, Department of Physician
Assistant Studies
New York Institute of Technology
Old Westbury, New York

Clinical Instructor of Health Sciences
School of Allied Health Technology and Management
The State University of New York at Stony Brook
Stony Brook, New York

Affiliate Clinical Instructor
College of Pharmacy and Allied Health
St. John's University
Jamaica, New York
Chapter 25: Dysrhythmias in Infants and Children

Cardiac Cell Structure and Function

LEARNING OBJECTIVES

Upon completion of this chapter, the reader should be able to:

- *Describe two properties of cardiac conduction cells.*
- *Describe cardiac conductivity and automaticity.*
- *List two functions of the intercalated discs, which connect cardiac cells.*
- *Explain two functions of a cell membrane.*
- *Define the intracellular space and the extracellular space.*
- *Explain the meaning of a cell membrane being semipermeable.*
- *List the function of the ionic channels found in cell membranes.*
- *Explain the electrical process involved in stimulating the heart to contract.*
- *Explain how a polarized cell differs from a repolarizing cell.*
- *Define a cardiac cell's resting membrane potential.*
- *Describe a cell's action potential.*
- *Explain the importance of the plateau phase of a cardiac action potential.*
- *List two benefits that result from the long refractory period of cardiac muscle.*
- *Explain how depolarization differs from contraction.*
- *List the point during the depolarization/repolarization process when cardiac contraction occurs.*
- *Explain how sodium, potassium, chloride, and calcium ions lead to the development and maintenance of the cell membrane potential.*
- *Outline the steps involved in the cardiac muscle excitation-coupling process.*
- *Explain how the electro-mechanical association process unites the action potential and cardiac contraction.*
- *Name the charged salt particles that are released from the sarcoplasmic reticulum during muscle excitation.*
- *List one function of the transverse (T) tubule system and calcium ions during electromechanical association.*

CHAPTER OVERVIEW

The major role of the circulatory system is to provide every body cell with nutrients along with removing cellular waste products. The heart accomplishes these goals by pumping oxygen-rich blood to the cells and transporting blood that contains high levels of carbon dioxide away from the cells to the lungs. Contraction of the heart involves electrical as well as mechanical events. Heart cells will not contract unless they are stimulated by tiny electrical charges. Nerves communicate by transmitting electrical impulses. Nervous impulses result from chemical changes in the cell. Muscles contract in response to the electrical signals generated by nerve cells. Electrophysiology is the study of the changes in the cellular electrical charges. Heart cells are biochemical energy factories that initiate and power the heart's pumping activity. Besides containing muscle cells, the heart is composed of excitatory and conductive cells, which coordinate the contraction and relaxation phases. Disturbances of nerve impulse formation and transmission are major causes of abnormal heart rhythms. Emergency cardiac care is based on stabilizing the mechanical and electrical properties of an injured heart.

INTRODUCTION TO THE HEART AS A PUMP

The heart is a four-chambered pump consisting of two atria and two ventricles (Figure 1–1) . The right side of the heart pumps blood, which has returned from the cells low in oxygen and high in carbon dioxide, to the lungs to be reoxygenated and to release the carbon dioxide. The left side of the heart pumps oxygen-rich blood to every body cell. The ventricles generate the force needed to eject blood through the lungs and into the peripheral circulatory system.

Cells are the fundamental components that make up all body tissues. Two major cell types make up the heart: muscle cells, termed **myocardial cells** or **myocardium** and **conduction cells**, which transmit electrical impulses. Myocardial muscle fibers are able to shorten and stretch, thereby allowing the heart to contract and relax. Before the heart can contract, it first needs to be stimulated by electrical impulses generated by nerves. **Electrocardiography** is the study of the recordings of the electrical activity associated with the beating heart. An **electrocardiogram**, commonly abbreviated as an **ECG**, is the graphic representation of cardiac electrical activity as a series of waves and complexes. It is important to have an understanding of the electrical properties of the heart in order to appreciate the disturbances in the heart's electrical patterns, which are termed **cardiac dysrhythmias**.

Myocardial Cell Properties

Unlike skeletal muscle, which must wait for a nervous signal before contracting, cardiac muscle generates its

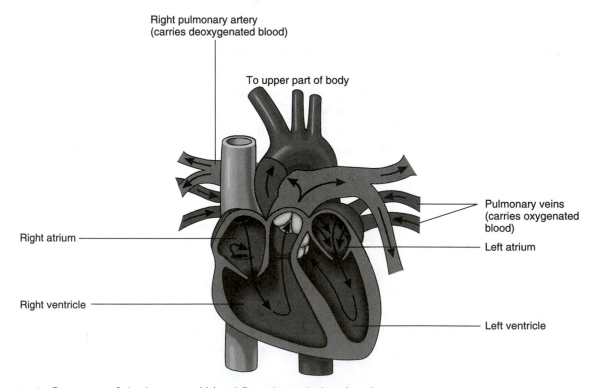

Figure 1-1 Structure of the heart, and blood flow through the chambers.

own activating impulse. For example, the biceps muscle in the upper arm which flexes the elbow is totally dependent on being stimulated by a nervous signal. In contrast to skeletal muscle, the heart initiates its own heartbeat; if a heart is totally severed from surrounding nervous connections, as occurs during a cardiac transplant, it still continues to beat. A special pacemaker mechanism exists within the heart to maintain the cardiac rhythm and will be explained later in this chapter. Cardiac cells share four important characteristics that allow the heart to pump efficiently: (Table 1–1)

- **Automaticity** is the ability of a cell to spontaneously form an electrical impulse. These cells do not need to wait to be activated by other cells.

- **Excitability** is the cell's ability to react to a stimulus. Cardiac cells are able to become excited and respond to a nervous impulse.

- **Conductivity** is the ability of a cell to convey an impulse to adjacent cells in order to excite it. Conductivity permits cells to quickly pass impulses to surrounding cells in order for the heart to become activated.

- **Contractility** is the ability of muscle to react to an electrical stimulus by shortening.

Excitability is analogous to a spark that triggers an instantaneous reaction in surrounding cells. As will be seen in upcoming chapters, disorders of cell excitation and impulse conduction are major causes of cardiac dysrhythmias. For instance, abnormal heart rhythms can result from either increased or depressed excitability, and from depressed or abnormal conduction pathways.

Cardiac Cell Types

There are two types of myocardial cells: one group responsible for impulse initiation and conduction, and the bulk of heart cells responsible for the pumping action.

Myocardial Cells

Heart muscle is composed of individual small fibers termed **myofibrils**. Myofibrils consist of tiny protein filaments, known as **actin** and **myosin**, which interact. When stimulated by an electrical impulse the myofibrils change shape, causing the actin-myosin complex to interact, resulting in shortening of the muscle.

Intercalated discs are unique structures found in the cardiac fibers within the cell membranes at the borders of adjacent cells. The discs offer low resistance to impulse conduction, which permits electrical impulses to travel much faster than possible in skeletal tissue.

Table 1-1 Cellular Properties
■ **Automaticity** is the ability of a cell to initiate an electrical impulse.
■ **Excitability** is the ability of a cell to respond to a stimulus or electrical impulse.
■ **Conductivity** is the ability of a cell to transmit an electrical impulse to other cells.
■ **Contractility** is the ability of a group of cells to shorten their fiber length.

Intercalated discs permit the wave of cardiac excitation to rapidly travel throughout the heart so that the heart chambers can contract simultaneously. Another important feature of cardiac muscle cells depicted in Figure 1–2 that allows them to function as a unit during the pumping action is the branching cell shape pattern, which allows greater cell-to-cell contact. The special branching pattern gives the heart maximal pumping efficiency.

Conduction Cells

The specialized cells making up the electrical conduction system are responsible for initiation and transmission. They do not contain myofibrils and therefore do not contribute to the strength of chamber contraction. These specialized conduction cells are arranged in bundles that form a branching network extending throughout the heart and speed the impulse transmission to all areas of the heart. Myofibrils are never more than a cell

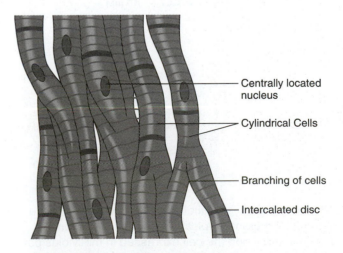

Centrally located nucleus

Cylindrical Cells

Branching of cells

Intercalated disc

Figure 1-2 Cardiac muscle cells.

or two away from the conduction fibers. This close association between electrical cells and the muscle cells allows for almost instantaneous muscle activation and precise coordination of heart activity.

CELLS AND CELL MEMBRANES

Cells are the fundamental structural and functional units of the body. Body tissue is composed of specialized cell groups that carry out different functions. Cell shape and function vary considerably depending on structure and function of the part of the body the cells come from. For instance, nerve cells conduct impulses while the cells associated with the pumping action of heart depend on cardiac muscle cells.

Cell membranes are the walls that enclose cellular material and separates cells from their external environment. The chemical composition within a cell is quite different from the material outside the cell. Cell membranes form a boundary that separates cellular material, such as water, salts, nutrients, proteins, and carbohydrates, from the surrounding environment. For instance, the sodium concentration is much higher out-

side of the cell than within. Cell membranes also play an important role in preventing foreign material such as bacteria from entering, which could harm the cell. The cell membrane does permit certain salts, sugars, and small proteins to enter the cell while blocking entry for others. This selective admission process is referred to as a **semipermeable membrane**.

Intracellular Versus Extracellular Space

The material inside a cell is termed the **intracellular space**, while everything beyond the membrane border is referred to as the **extracellular space**. The concentration of salts on either side of the cell membrane differs considerably. The salt's sodium and calcium particles, which have positive charges, are found in greater concentrations in the extracellular space. In contrast, the positively charged salt potassium and a mixture of negatively charged ions, including phosphate and sulfate, are present in greater amounts within the cell (Figure 1–3). The unequal salt concentrations create an electrical charge across the cell membrane. These cellular electrical charges form the basis of cardiac impulse formation and cardiac conduction.

Electrolytes

Every cell is bathed in a salt solution. **Electrolytes** are salts that become charged particles when dissolved in solution. Major electrolytes include potassium, calcium, sodium, phosphate, and chloride. Electrolytes play a key role in maintaining a cell's electrical charge. Altering the cell membrane's permeability allows different electrolytes to enter and leave. Small changes in the electrolyte concentration result in changes in electrical charge. Electrochemical impulses, which are termed **action potentials**, form the basis for how nerves transmit signals. Nerve and muscle cells communicate by varying the number and intensity of action potentials.

Positively and Negatively Charged Salt Particles

Charged salt particles are termed **ions**. Positively charged ions are called **cations**, while negatively charged ions are termed **anions**. Cations are represented by a (+) symbol while anions are symbolized by a (−) symbol. Major positively charged ions include potassium, calcium, and sodium. Major negatively charged anions include chloride, sulfate, and bicarbonate. **Neutral solutions** have equal positive and negative charges. Cations and anions enter and leave the cell via microscopic openings in the cell membrane termed **ionic channels**. Sodium ions enter through "fast" ionic channels while calcium ions enter through "slow" ionic channels.

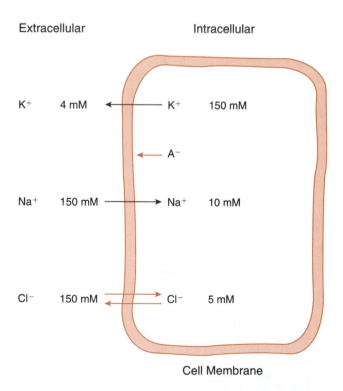

Extracellular   Intracellular

K⁺   4 mM   K⁺   150 mM

               A⁻

Na⁺   150 mM   Na⁺   10 mM

Cl⁻   150 mM   Cl⁻   5 mM

Cell Membrane

Figure 1–3 Distribution of ions contributing to the resting membrane. Typical concentrations of ions inside and outside the cell expressed in milliMoles per liter are shown. (Abbreviations: K⁺ is potassium, A⁻ is anions, Na⁺ is sodium, and Cl⁻ is chloride.)

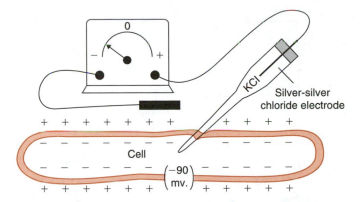

Figure 1-4 Measurement of membrane potential of a cell using a microelectrode and voltmeter.

CELL MEMBRANE CHARGES

The charged particles lined up across the cell membrane result in formation of an electrical charge termed a membrane potential (Figure 1–4). This is similar to the electrical energy that is stored in a battery. The cell membrane shifts from a negative charge to a positive charge, and returns to a negative state during each heartbeat. Cardiac cells continually cycle through ready, active, and recovery phases. Cardiac cells spend very little time at rest; in fact, most time cells are either charging or discharging. Cardiac cells repeatedly go through the cycle: polarization → depolarization → repolarization (Figure 1–5). These phases are similar to the cell's activity phases: ready → active → recovering.

Polarization

A cell at rest is termed **polarized**, which means that it is in the "ready state" waiting to react to a stimulus. The cell membrane charge remains constant during the polarized state. A device that measures energy flow and tests the battery charge is termed a voltmeter. If a voltmeter were equipped with microscopic electrodes that could be attached inside and outside the cell, a net cell charge would be detected (Figure 1–6A). This cell charge is termed the **membrane potential** and during rest has a value -90 mV.

Depolarization

The minimum energy level needed to "trigger" an action potential is termed the **threshold depolarization value**. An action potential is an electrochemical cell signal or impulse. Positively charged sodium ions flowing into the cell cause the membrane potential to become positive. When the threshold depolarization level is reached, ionic channels within the cell membrane spring open, allowing sodium to rush inside (Figure 1–7). Depolarization occurs when enough sodi-

um ions enter the cell and cause the negative resting membrane potential to change to a positive value (Figure 1–6B). When the membrane potential reaches threshold, an action potential fires, stimulating surrounding cells (Figure 1–8).

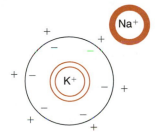

A. Polarization (the ready state)

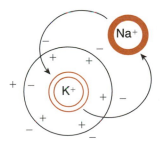

B. Depolarization (the discharge state)

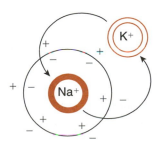

C. Repolarization (the recovery state)

Figure 1-5 The flow of electrolytes across the cell membrane during the various cell phases. (The abbreviation K^+ means potassium and Na^+.)

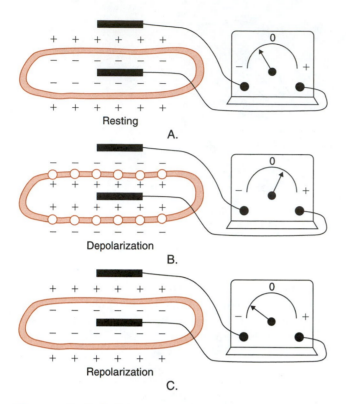

Figure 1-6 Cellular events during an action potential showing: A. Resting negative membrane potential; B. Depolarization with reversed (positive) potential; and C. Reestablishment of resting negative membrane charge during repolarization.

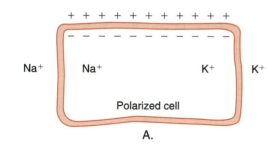

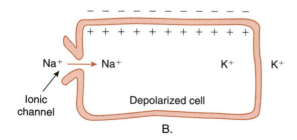

Figure 1-7 A. Electrolyte flow and alignment of membrane charges during cell rest. Ionic channels are closed. B. Sodium flows into the cell via an open ionic channel during depolarization.

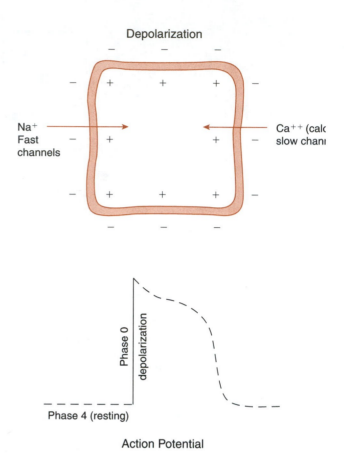

Figure 1-8 A. During depolarization, sodium (Na+) rushes into the cell along with calcium (Ca+). B. As the cell charge changes from negative to positive, depolarization (phase 0) occurs. An action potential forms.

Repolarization

Repolarization is the recovery stage that follows depolarization (Figure 1–6C). During repolarization the cell membrane charge moves from positive back to its resting negative charge (Figure 1–9). As sodium leaves the cell during repolarization, potassium returns inside the intracellular space. Completion of the repolarization phase permits the resting, or "ready-for-action," cell stage. Figure 1–10 illustrates the complete depolarization-repolarization cycle.

ECG AND CARDIAC ACTIVITY

The cardiac depolarization and repolarization phases correspond to cardiac contraction and relaxation (Figure 1–11). The ECG depicts the heart's electrical activity as a series of waves. The ECG tracing reflects atrial depolarization as a P wave. The QRS complex results when both ventricles are depolarized.

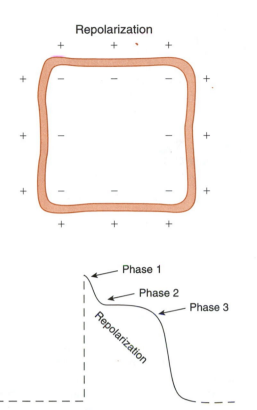

Repolarization

Phase 1

Phase 2

Phase 3

Repolarization

Figure 1-9 A. During repolarization the inside of the cell returns to its original negative charge. B. Repolarization causes phases 1, 2, and 3 of the corresponding action potential.

Repolarization of the ventricles is recorded as a T wave. Atrial repolarization is not seen because the larger ventricular activity overshadows it. A U wave is sometimes seen and it represents late repolarization activity.

Table 1-2 Cellular Electrical Phases

■ **Polarized** = resting cell = cell membrane is *not* permeable = charged state = no current flows

■ **Depolarized** = cell membrane is permeable = discharging state = current flows

■ **Repolarized** = cell membrane is permeable = recharging state = current flow reverses

Cardiac Action Potential

The action potential represents what is happening in a single cell whereas the ECG records activity in the entire heart. During a single cardiac cycle, for instance, some parts of the heart are repolarizing while other areas are depolarizing. Figure 1–12 illustrates the relationship among the action potential, the ECG, and electrolyte activity during the various phases.

The action potential of a single cardiac cell is divided into five phases: 0, 1, 2, 3, and 4. Each of the five cell phases relates to a change in cell membrane permeability to cations, mainly sodium, potassium, and calcium. A cardiac cell's action potential includes:

■ Phase 4: The portion of the action potential when the cell is at rest. Phase 4 has a flat appearance in non-pacemaker cells because current is not flowing.

■ Phase 0: Membrane permeability increases to allow sodium to flow into the cell. Phase 0 consists of a sharp upward spike portion at the explosive start of the action potential (depolarization).

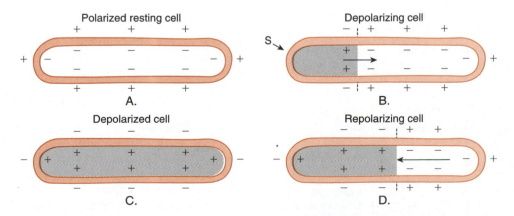

Polarized resting cell

A.

Depolarizing cell

S

B.

Depolarized cell

C.

Repolarizing cell

D.

Figure 1-10 A. Resting heart cell with negative cell membrane charge. B. The cell is stimulated and begins depolarization as the inside of the cell becomes positive. C. A fully depolarized cell. D. Repolarization occurs as the cell regains its negative charge. The arrows show the direction of the depolarization and repolarization charge.

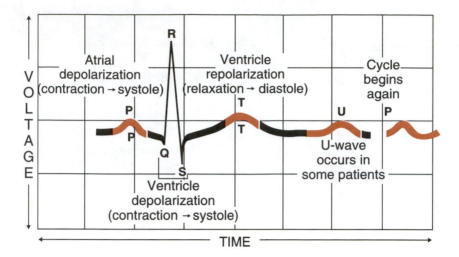

Figure 1–11 Normal ECG waves related to the heart chamber activity.

- Phase 1: The peak portion of the action potential characterized by an abrupt decrease in sodium permeability.

- Phase 2: The action potential reaches a plateau phase due to slow inward movement of calcium ions coupled with some outward potassium zmovement. Phase 2 is the cell's early repolarization phase.

- Phase 3: The late stage of repolarization. Repolarization finishes with an initial sharp increase of potassium permeability, causing potassium to leave the cell.

Pacemaker Cells: Automatic Depolarization

You will recall that automaticity is the ability of a cell to spontaneously generate an action potential. Cells that have the fastest rate of automaticity, meaning that they discharge quicker than other automatic cells, set the

Figure 1–12 Representation of the action potential in relation to the ECG. Arrows indicate the major ionic flow across the cell membrane.

overall heart rate and are termed **pacemaker cells**. Pacemaker cells self-depolarize and start their own cardiac cycle. Automaticity sets pacemaker cells apart from all other heart cells. Cells possessing automaticity do not need to wait until they are stimulated by other cells to depolarize.

The higher the automaticity discharge rate, the faster the pacemaker will stimulate the heart. Automaticity disorders, involving both increased and suppressed automaticity, are a leading cause of the abnormal cardiac rhythms, which will be studied later.

Pacemaker Cell Action Potentials

Even when at rest, pacemaker cells are permeable to sodium ions, causing the membrane potential to slowly develop a more positive cell membrane charge. A pacemaker cell's action potential has a unique shape due to it's sloping phase 4. When the membrane potential gradually reaches the threshold level, an action potential occurs (Figure 1–13).

ELECTRO-MECHANICAL ASSOCIATION

Electro-mechanical association is the process involved in linking a nervous impulse (action potential) to the heartbeat. The electrical and chemical changes that take place on the cellular level have already been described; what remains is to explain how the heart muscle contracts in response to action potentials. Electro-mechanical association, or the **excitation-contraction process**, involves burning fuel for energy, and calcium ions, which is the chemical link between the electrical stimulus and contraction.

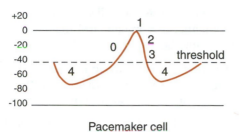

Figure 1–13 Pacemaker cells are capable of spontaneous depolarization. During the resting phase (phase 4) there is a gradual leakage of potassium ions across the cell membrane while sodium enters. When threshold is reached, an action potential "fires."

The following components are important in electro-mechanical association:

- Excitation-contraction coupling. Excitation coupling is the way in which an action potential causes the heart muscle to contract. The end result of changes in the permeability of the cell membrane cause depolarization and cardiac contraction.

- Calcium ions, sarcoplasmic reticulum, and troponin. Calcium ions are an essential component needed for contraction to occur. The cell membrane forms a **sarcoplasmic reticulum**, which is a series of channels extending from the cell membrane. The sarcoplasmic reticulum causes parts of the cell to remain close to the surrounding extracellular environment. When an action potential spreads along the sarcoplasmic reticulum to the interior of the cardiac muscle fiber, calcium ions bathe the myofibrils. Calcium also interacts with the regulatory protein **troponin**. Troponin, in turn, permits actin and myosin filaments to interact. The muscle fibers shorten and muscle contraction follows.

- Transverse tubules. An extensive series of cell channels termed **T tubules** store calcium. When the action potential enters the cardiac muscle via the sarcoplasmic reticulum, the T tubules are signaled to release calcium. When the action potential ends, calcium reenters the T tubules to be stored as the heart relaxes.

- Energy. Cardiac contraction requires a large and steady supply of energy. The electromechanical process is powered by energy in the form of **ATP**, or **adenosine triphosphate**, which is formed from glucose metabolism. The entire electro-mechanical process is shown in Figure 1–14.

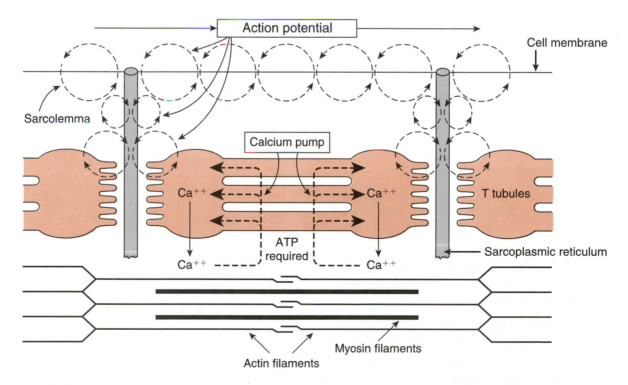

Figure 1–14 Excitation-contraction coupling in muscle, showing an action potential that causes release of calcium ions. There is an interaction between actin and myosin filaments. ATP is the energy source that powers contraction.

Let's Review

1. The heart is able to pump blood because two closely related events become linked: an electrochemical process is united with a mechanical process.

2. Electrical events stimulate mechanical cells. Cells cannot contract without first being stimulated.

3. The rhythmic contraction and relaxation of the heart depends on the specialized cells of the heart's pacemaker and conduction system.

4. Specialized cardiac cells have four properties: automaticity, excitability, conductivity, and contractility.

5. Electrolytes are charged salt particles that are dissolved in solution.

6. A semipermeable membrane separates the electrolytes from different cell regions and permits only certain ions to pass through.

7. Electrolytes enter and leave the cell via different ionic channels located within the cell membrane.

8. Anions are negatively charged electrolytes, which include sulfate, chloride, and bicarbonate.

9. Cations are positively charged electrolytes, which include potassium, sodium, calcium, and magnesium.

10. Myocardial cells consist of tiny myofibrils called actin and myosin.

11. An action potential is an electrical signal that is caused when there is sudden change in a cell's electrical charge.

12. The heart's pacemaker system can form an action potential independent of the nervous system. The nervous system is able to influence the heart rate.

13. Polarized cardiac cells are resting cells. The cell membrane of a polarized resting cell is not permeable to electrolytes.

14. The membrane potential has a charge and during the resting state is negative.

15. The membrane potential returns to a negative value during the recovery or repolarization phase.

16. Automaticity is the cell's ability to spontaneously initiate and maintain a rhythmic beat.

17. Depolarized cells are in the active discharging phase. During depolarization the cell membrane potential becomes more positive.

18. Repolarized cells are in the active, recharging phase. The cell membrane potential returns toward a negative rest during membrane charge.

19. The action potential of cardiac muscle has five phases: Phase 0 represents depolarization and is characterized by the rapid upstroke of the action potential. Phase 1 is represented by a brief period of repolarization, resulting in a quick negative depolarization.

20. Phase 2 of the action potential consists of a plateau (flat) section that serves to prolong repolarization. Phase 3 of the action potential is the late repolarization phase, while phase 4 of the action potential is the resting membrane potential.

21. Electromechanical association is the process that links the membrane charge and energy flow with myocardial contraction-relaxation.

22. Electromechanical association requires energy, which is provided by glucose metabolism. The energy is in the form of adenosine triphosphate (ATP).

23. Cardiac contraction immediately follows depolarization. Cardiac relaxation follows repolarization.

24. Action potentials are carried to the center of cardiac muscle by a system of cell channels called the sarcoplasmic reticulum.

25. Calcium is released from T tubules when an action potential stimulates the muscle and causes the actin and myosin fibers to interact.

26. Each stage of depolarization-repolarization cycle represents hundreds of thousands of individual cell action potentials.

Glossary

Actin Protein filament found in myofibrils that participates in muscle contraction.

Action potential Electrochemical impulses that transmit signals.

Adenosine triphosphate (ATP) Energy formed by glucose metabolism and used to power muscle activity.

Anions Negatively charged ions.

Automaticity The ability of a cell to spontaneously form an electrical impulse.

Cardiac dysrhythmias Disturbances in electrical heart patterns.

Cations Positively charged ions.

Cell membrane Wall enclosing cellular material separating the cell from the external environment.

Conduction cells Type of heart cells that transmit electrical impulses.

Conductivity Ability of a cell to convey an impulse to adjacent cells.

Contractility Ability of a cell to react to an electrical stimulus by shortening the muscle.

Depolarization An electrically active cell as the cell membrane becomes permeable and current flows.

Electrocardiogram (ECG) Graphic tracing that represents the heart's electrical activity.

Electrocardiography Study of the electrical activity associated with the beating heart.

Electrolytes Salts that become charged when dissolved in a solution.

Electromechanical association Chemical and electrical processes that unite an action potential with a cardiac contraction.

Excitability Ability of a cell to react to a stimulus.

Excitation-contraction process Process during which an action potential leads to a cardiac contraction.

Extracellular space All material found outside of the cell membrane.

Intercalated discs Structures found in cardiac fiber within the cell membrane at the border of adjacent cells.

Intracellular space All material contained inside of the cell membrane.

Ionic channel Microscopic openings in the cell membrane that permit cations and anions to enter and leave the cell.

Ions Charged particles in solution.

Myocardial cells Type of heart cells consisting of muscle that allows the heart to contract and relax; also called myocardium.

Myofibrils Small fibers that make up heart muscle.

Myosin Protein filament found in myofibrils.

Neutral solution Solution with an equal amount of positive and negative charges.

Pacemaker cells Cells having the property to spontaneously initiate an action potential, thereby stimulating a heart beat.

Polarized State Cell at rest or in the ready state.

Sarcoplasmic reticulum Series of channels extending from the cell membrane; allows all parts of the cell to remain close to the surrounding extracellular environment.

Semipermeable membrane Property of a cell membrane where certain particles are allowed to pass through while others are blocked.

Threshold depolarization value Minimum energy needed to develop an action potential.

Troponin Regulatory protein that is involved with actin and myosin interaction.

The Pacemaker and Conduction System

LEARNING OBJECTIVES

Upon completion of this chapter, the reader should be able to:

- *Identify the location and function of the SA (sinus) node.*
- *Name the components of the conduction system and the order that the areas are encountered by a sinus impulse after it leaves the sinus node.*
- *Describe the portion of the ECG complex caused by sinus node depolarization.*
- *Describe the portion of the ECG complex caused by atrial repolarization.*
- *Identify the location and function of the atrioventricular (AV) node.*
- *Differentiate between the AV node and the AV junction.*
- *Name the continuation of the AV nodal fibers.*
- *Describe the portion of the ECG complex that is caused by ventricular depolarization.*
- *Describe the portion of the ECG complex that is caused by ventricular repolarization.*
- *Name the AV bundle divisions.*
- *Describe where the Purkinje fibers are located.*
- *Explain what is meant by the term conduction velocity.*
- *List the portion of the conduction system with the fastest conduction velocity.*
- *List the portion of the conduction system with the slowest conduction velocity.*
- *Define a cardiac cell gap junction and list one property of gap junctions that affect conduction velocity.*

CHAPTER OVERVIEW

The heart is stimulated in a rhythmic manner beginning in the sinus node. The cardiac conduction system ensures that the heart becomes stimulated in a swift and efficient manner. Maximal cardiac function is obtained through the coordinated and synchronized conduction system. Stimulation and recovery of different heart areas corresponds to specific ECG waves.

CARDIAC IMPULSE FORMATION AND CONDUCTION SYSTEM

The cardiac conduction system consists of cells that generate and conduct electrical impulses throughout the heart (Figure 2–1). Were it not for the conduction system, stimulation of the heart would take much longer since cell-to-cell spread of the depolarization impulse is quite slow. In order for the heart to contract with greatest efficiency, the cardiac chambers must be primed with just the right amount of blood at exactly the precise moment. The conduction system ensures that the heart is pumping efficiently by coordinating an orderly contraction/relaxation sequence.

Conduction Sequence

The signal for cardiac stimulation starts in the **sinoatrial (SA) or sinus node**, which is located in the posterior wall of the right atrium close to the site where the venae cavae enter (Figure 2–2). The SA node, also known as the sinus node, is the primary pacemaker because it has the fastest spontaneous firing rate. Impulses from the SA node travel through both atria, which then depolarize. Depolarization causes both atria to contract.

The atria and the ventricles are electrically insulated from one another except where the AV node connects the chambers. The **AV node** is located in the base of the right atrium. The conduction impulse travels along the tissues of the **atrioventricular junction**. The AV junction includes the AV node and bundle of His. Within the AV node, atrial fibers join with small junctional fibers of the node (Figure 2–3). The impulse travels through the AV nodal fibers very slowly compared

to the impulse speed in other parts of the conduction system. Slowed AV nodal conduction velocity is beneficial because it allows the atria to finish emptying. As a result, the ventricles contain a maximal amount of blood before contraction occurs, enhancing cardiac output.

The impulse then flows to the **AV bundle**, which is also commonly known as the Bundle of His (Figure 2–4). The AV bundle divides into right and left bundle branches supplying each ventricle.

The **left bundle branch** divides into two parts: the anterior division and the posterior division (also termed fascicles). The **anterior fascicle** supplies the front portion of the left ventricle, while the **posterior fascicle** stimulates the posterior ventricular area. The **Right bundle branch** supplies the right ventricle.

The **Purkinje system** is the final portion of the conduction system. The Purkinje system is made up of many nerve fibers that supply the furthest portion of the ventricles. The Purkinje fibers allow for simultaneous excitation of the right ventricle and much larger left ventricle. The Purkinje fibers subdivide until they form the tiniest network of nerves, forming connections with each of the heart's contractile cells, the **sarcomeres**.

The path that the impulse travels through and the relationship of the ECG to the conduction sequence is illustrated in Figure 2–2.

Conduction Velocity

The electrical impulses travel through the heart at different speeds. **Conduction velocity** refers to the relative transmission speed through different parts of the heart. For instance, conduction is slowest through the AV node and fastest along the Purkinje fibers (Figure

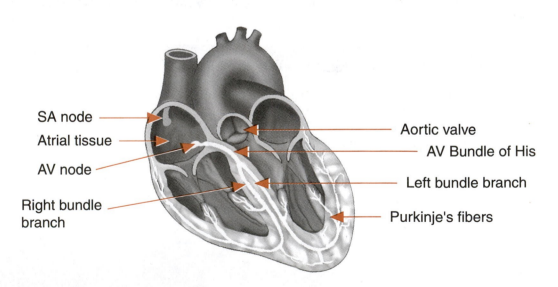

SA node

Atrial tissue

AV node

Right bundle branch

Aortic valve

AV Bundle of His

Left bundle branch

Purkinje's fibers

Figure 2-1 Myocardial conduction system.

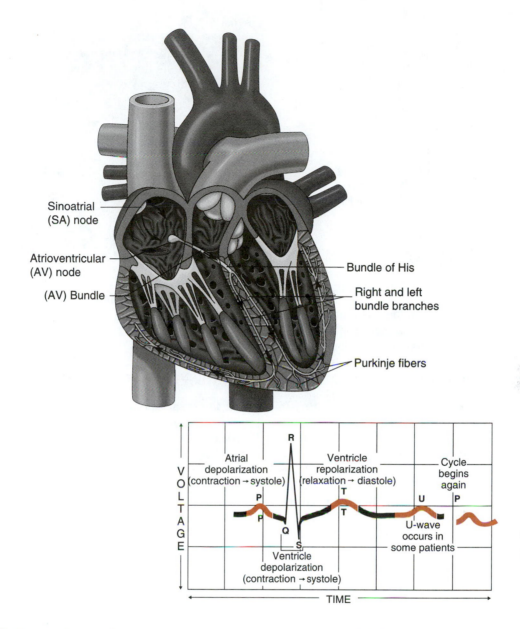

Figure 2-2 The cardiac conduction sequence and its relationship to the ECG.

2–4). The relative transmission speeds in different parts of the heart are listed in Table 2–1. Slowed conduction through the AV node permits the ventricles to fill with blood prior to contraction. Impulse conduction through the ventricles is fastest due to the extensive Purkinje fiber branching pattern needed to activate the thick ventricles.

THE SARCOMERE

The smallest myocardial unit is the sarcomere. The sarcomere contains **cellular gap junctions**, which are made up of intercalated discs that offer very little resist-

Table 2-1 Relative Impulse Conduction Rates	
■ **Atrial:**	0.45–0.6 meter/second
■ **AV node:**	0.1 meter/second
■ **Purkinje/Ventricles:**	1.5–4.0 meters/second (150 times faster than the speed of AV nodal transmission)

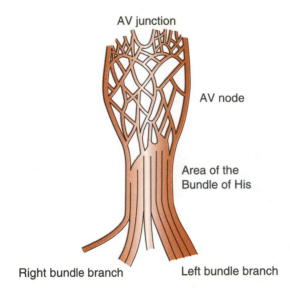

Figure 2-3 At the AV junction there is a gradual transition as the cells from the atria merge with the nodal fibers. The nodal fibers then form the Bundle of His. Note that the fibers are arranged in an interlacing pattern, which slows conduction.

ance to impulse transmission. It is the cellular gap junctions, coupled with the numerous Purkinje fibers that allows for the lightning fast depolarization and repolarization (Figure 2–5). This extensive myocardium branching pattern and close relationship between the conduction fibers and the muscle cells permits the heart to be activated in a rapid, efficient, and coordinated manner.

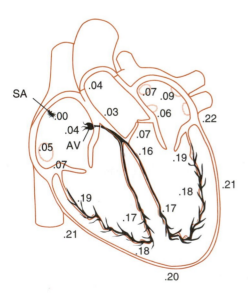

Figure 2-4 The diagram shows how long (in fractions of a second) an impulse takes to activate different heart areas.

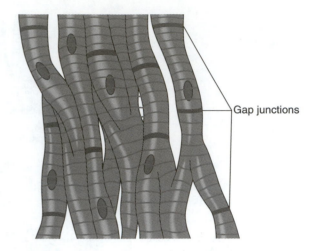

Figure 2-5 Cardiac muscle cell and intimate association of Purkinje fibers lead to rapid spread of depolarization.

ELECTRICAL ACTIVITY AND CORRESPONDING ECG FINDINGS

The ECG machine amplifies the tiny currents associated with cardiac activity and transforms them into a series of waves (Table 2–2 and Figure 2–6). Each cardiac cycle involves the following electrical events linked to their associated ECG findings:

■ Atrial depolarization is represented by the **P wave**.

■ Sinus nodal activity is *not* recorded on the ECG. The SA node is presumed to have depolarized whenever a P wave occurs—but the sinus node actually discharges just before the P wave appears. The sinus node discharge is not seen because in comparison to the size of the atrial tissue being activated, the sinus node is very tiny and does not generate much electrical activity.

Table 2-2 Cardiac Activity Relative to ECG Waves
■ **Sinus node discharge** = no ECG wave
■ **Atrial depolarization** = P wave
■ **Atrial repolarization** = no ECG wave
■ **Ventricular depolarization** = QRS complex
■ **Early ventricular repolarization** = T wave
■ **Late ventricular repolarization** = U wave

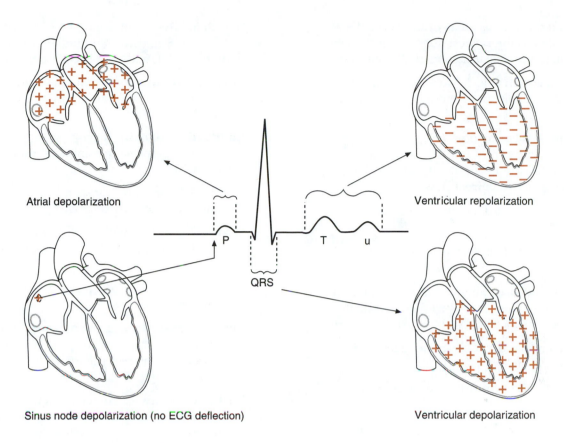

Atrial depolarization

Ventricular repolarization

Sinus node depolarization (no ECG deflection)

Ventricular depolarization

Figure 2-6 Correlation between ECG cycle and cardiac activity.

■ Ventricular activation involves a series of electrical activity and is shown as a group of waves termed the **QRS complex**.

■ Ventricular repolarization causes the **T wave**.

Sometimes another wave, the **U wave**, follows the T wave (Figure 2–7). The U wave is caused by "late" ventricular depolarization events. Certain conditions, including a low serum potassium level, slow heart rates, and ventricular enlargement are associated with prominent U waves.

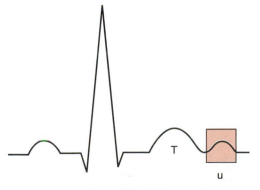

Figure 2-7 The U wave follows the T wave in some cases and represents late repolarization activity.

Let's Review

1. The rhythmic contraction and relaxation of the heart depends on the myocardium first being stimulated to depolarize via cells of the heart's conduction system.

2. The SA node is the cardiac pacemaker because it has the fastest discharge rate. SA nodal impulses travel throughout the atria and into the AV node.

3. The AV node receives the stimulating impulse after the atria are activated.

4. The AV junction includes the AV node and the atrial and ventricular tissue surrounding it. The AV junction connects the atrial and ventricular conduction systems.

5. The AV bundle divides into the right and left bundle branches. The left bundle branch further splits into anterior and posterior divisions, which are termed a fascicles.

6. Conduction velocity is the relative speed of impulse transmission. Conduction velocities

differ in various areas of the heart: the AV node has the slowest conduction velocity while ventricular tissue has the quickest.

7. Conduction velocity refers to the relative transmission speed through different parts of the heart.

8. The smallest myocardial unit is the sarcomere, which have cellular gap junctions that aid in transmission due to its very low resistance to current flow.

9. Sinus nodal activity is not recorded on the ECG.

10. Atrial depolarization is recorded as a P wave.

11. Atrial repolarization is not recorded on the ECG, because it is overshadowed by the QRS complex.

12. Ventricular depolarization is recorded as a QRS complex.

13. Ventricular repolarization is recorded as a T wave.

14. Late ventricular repolarization is sometimes recorded as a U wave.

Glossary

Anterior fascicle Division of the left bundle branch that transmits the depolarization impulse to the front portion of the left ventricle.

Atrioventricular (AV) junction Consists of the the AV node and the bundle of His; carries the electrical impulse to the ventricular muscle cells.

AV bundle See Bundle of His.

AV node Conduction tissue in right atrium where atrial fibers join with junctional fibers.

Bundle branches Divisions of the AV bundle that transmit impulses into the right and left ventricles.

Bundle of His Continuation of AV nodal tissue into the ventricle. The bundle of His divides into the left and right bundle branches.

Cellular gap junctions Cell membrane connections that offer little resistance to current flow.

Conduction velocity Relative speed of an electrical impulse transmission through the heart.

Left bundle branch Transmits depolarization impulse to the left ventricle.

Myocardium The middle layer of heart muscle that provides the bulk of contractile force during systole.

P wave Electrical current formed by atrial depolarization.

Posterior fascicle A division of the left bundle branch that transmits the depolarization impulse to the rear portion of the left ventricle.

Purkinje system Large nerve fibers that form branches in the furthest portion of the ventricles.

QRS complex Sequence of ECG waves formed by ventricular depolarization.

Right bundle branch Continuation of the AV bundle conduction system supplying the right ventricle.

Sarcomere The smallest myocardial unit.

Sinoatrial (SA) node The primary pacemaker of the heart; located in the posterior wall of the right atrium where the venae cavae enter.

T wave Electrical current formed by ventricular repolarization.

U wave Electrical current formed by the late phase of ventricular repolarization.

chapter 3

The Electrocardiogram and Cardiac Complexes

LEARNING OBJECTIVES

Upon completion of this chapter, the reader should be able to:

- *Define the terms electrocardiogram and electrocardiograph.*

- *Describe whether the ECG can provide clinical information concerning cardiac output, blood pressure, or pulse rate.*

- *Describe what an ECG "rhythm strip" is and how a rhythm strip is recorded.*

- *Contrast the purpose of an ECG "rhythm strip" with a twelve-lead ECG tracing.*

- *Compare a single cell's action potential with a P-QRS-T complex.*

- *Label the following areas on sample ECGs:*
  PR interval
  PR segment
  QRS duration
  ST segment
  QT interval
  TP segment
  J point

- *List the normal ECG intervals for the PR interval and the QRS duration.*

- *List the way that myocardial ischemia will alter the J point and the ST segment.*

- *Label the individual components of QRS configurations.*

CHAPTER OVERVIEW

The electrocardiogram (ECG) is the graphic tracing of the heart's electrical forces. The ECG machine, termed the electrocardiograph, detects abnormal cardiac rhythms. The ECG deflections form a series of waves and complexes that represent electrical activity in different areas of the heart. By measuring various intervals and durations in the ECG tracing, information about the flow of cardiac electrical energy can be obtained, which assists in patient assessment and treatment.

INTRODUCTION TO THE ELECTROCARDIOGRAM

The **electrocardiogram**, more commonly referred to simply as the "ECG tracing," is the graphic display of cardiac activity that reflects depolarization and repolarization of the atria and ventricles. While Chapter 1 focuses on a single cardiac cell's action potential, this chapter studies the energy changes occurring in the heart as a whole.

The **electrocardiograph**, commonly known as the "ECG machine," is the device that detects, amplifies, and transforms cardiac electrical activity into the series of waves known as the "P-QRS-T" complex (Figure 3–1). The tiny changes in electrical energy that occur during each heartbeat are displayed on a television-type screen and/ or a written record.

A **cardiac monitor** is an oscilloscope device with a screen that instantaneously displays the heart's rhythm. Cardiac monitors range from relatively simple devices that monitor a single ECG lead from one patient, to complex systems that are able to assess many patients simultaneously employing multiple leads.

ECG Function

The ECG is the major tool for detecting cardiac rhythm abnormalities, especially dysrhythmias that occur during an acute myocardial infarction—some of which are life-threatening. A heart attack, known as an **acute myocardial infarction** and abbreviated "AMI," commonly results in electrical instability that can totally disrupt regular cardiac rhythm. Chaotic electrical activity resulting from an AMI is the leading cause of early sudden cardiac death. The ECG detects abnormalities associated with an AMI.

ECG Limitations

The ECG is only able to assess electrical activity and provides no *direct* information about the heart's mechanical activity such as blood pressure, cardiac output, or the adequacy of myocardial perfusion. Such assessments can only be obtained by evaluating the patient. However, an ECG tracing does provide clinically valuable *indirect* information about cardiac function but this must be inferred by interpreting the recording in the context of the patient's clinical status. Each P-QRS-T cycle corresponds to a complete heart cycle. For instance, in people with normal cardiac function, the rate of ECG cardiac cycles corresponds to the heart rate. However, in some patients with diseased hearts the electrical and mechanical activity are not identical: during pulseless electrical activity, for example, the ECG shows a perfectly normal cardiac rhythm yet the patient is in cardiac arrest.

> ***Clinical Note:*** *The ECG reveals information about cardiac rhythm and pacemaker activity but reveals no data concerning the patient's blood pressure or how well vital body organs are being supplied with blood.*

ECG RHYTHM STRIPS

A standard ECG tracing records twelve different leads. A rhythm strip refers to an ECG tracing that uses fewer leads. See Figure 3–2 for a comparison of the two types of ECG tracings. An **ECG rhythm strip** continuously records one or several leads usually for 10 to 30 seconds or longer. As the name implies, rhythm strips are primarily used to clarify rhythm and conduction disorders (Figure 3–3). Rhythm strips are commonly recorded when drugs are given to convert a dysrhythmia and are recorded during cardiac arrests. Twelve-lead ECGs, in comparison, enable the clinician to localize and detect myocardial damage, and will be studied in a later chapter.

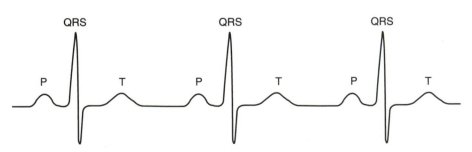

Figure 3–1 Each cardiac cycle is represented by a group of ECG waves termed the P-QRS-T complex.

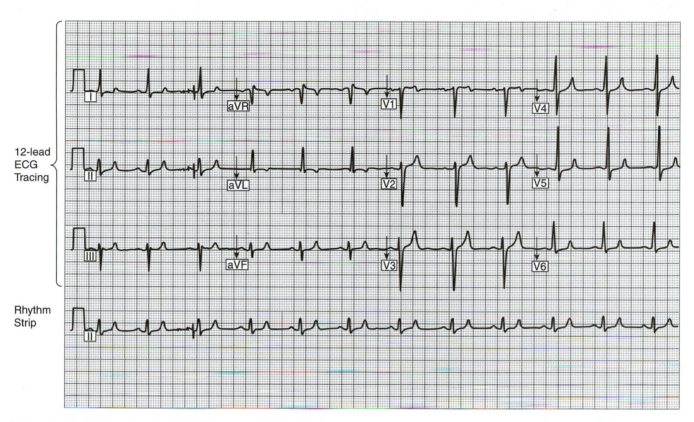

Figure 3–2 A twelve-lead ECG has six limb leads and six chest (precordial) leads. A lead II rhythm tracing is found at the bottom of the ECG.

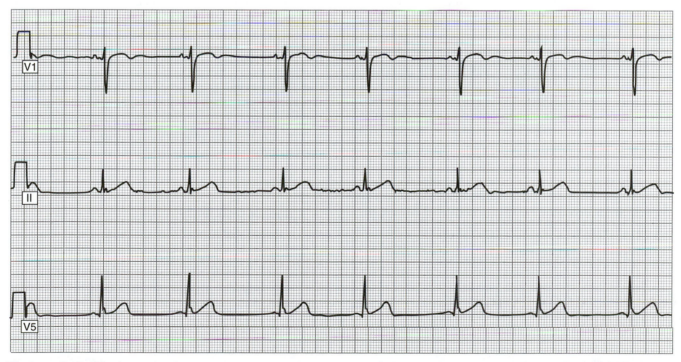

Figure 3–3 Rhythm strip showing three simultaneously recorded leads. Rhythm strips are used to clarify a dysrhythmia.

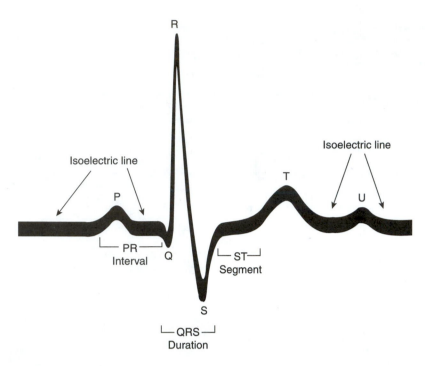

Figure 3-4 ECG intervals, durations, and segments within the cardiac cycle.

ECG "ASSESSMENT" VERSUS ECG "DIAGNOSIS"

ECG assessment describes the process by which an ECG is inspected and the cardiac rhythm is interpreted. ECG assessment should always include consideration of pertinent clinical information, such as the patient's medical history, medications being taken, the patient's present complaint, and most importantly, how the patient is tolerating the dysrhythmia.

It is not accurate to refer to ECG interpretation as ECG "diagnosis," which it is sometimes called. Diagnosis, in contrast, takes place only after a patient's history and physical examination and pertains to the identification of disease. An ECG is analogous to other laboratory or diagnostic tests; they can be interpreted but not actually diagnosed. As an illustration, an ECG may suggest an MI, but an MI can only be diagnosed by assessing the patient. Since several non-ischemic conditions can cause an ECG that mimics an MI, only a clinical assessment can correctly diagnose the condition.

ECG INTERVALS, DURATIONS, AND SEGMENTS

The typical ECG tracing displays a series of P-QRS-T complexes. The P-QRS-T complex is composed of waves and the ECG baseline areas between the waves. These areas are termed intervals, durations, and segments (Figure 3-4). **Intervals** are the distances between two waves or complexes, such as the PR interval. **Duration** is the time it takes for an ECG complex to be recorded, such as the P wave, QRS complex, or T wave. **Segments** are the ECG baselines occurring between waves or complexes. Segments are compared to a normal isoelectric baseline, such as the ST segment.

The PR Interval

The **PR interval** is an important time period that is measured from when the P wave begins until the QRS complex starts (Figure 3-5). The PR interval indicates how much time was required for a depolarization wave to pass through both atria and the AV node, and activate the ventricles.

> **ECG Interpretation Tip:** *Normal PR intervals should not exceed 0.20 second. A prolonged PR interval (greater than 0.20 second) signifies delayed conduction through the AV node (Figure 3-6).*

The QT Interval

The **QT interval** is another important measurement that depends on the total time needed for ventricular activation and recovery (Figures 3-7 and 3-8). Normal

PR Interval

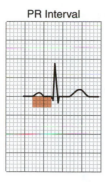

Figure 3–5 PR interval. The PR interval is measured from the beginning of the P wave until the start of the QRS complex.

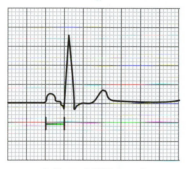

A. Normal PR interval

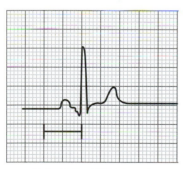

B. Prolonged PR interval

Figure 3–6 A. Normal PR interval is 0.12 to 0.20 second. B. Prolonged PR intervals are greater than 0.20 second and indicate a delay in atrioventricular conduction.

Table 3-1 Normal QT Intervals and Heart Rate		
Measured R-R interval (second)	Heart rate (per minute)	QT interval upper normal limits (second)
1.50	40	0.50
1.20	50	0.45
1.00	60	0.42
0.86	70	0.40
0.80	75	0.38
0.75	80	0.37
0.67	90	0.35
0.60	100	0.34
0.50	120	0.31
0.40	150	0.25

QT interval

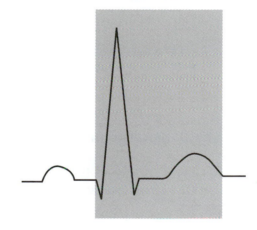

Figure 3–7 QT interval. The QT interval is measured from the beginning of the QRS complex until the end of the T wave. Normal QT intervals vary based on the heart rate.

QT intervals vary based on the heart rate (Table 3–1). Clinically significant prolonged QT intervals are associated with the sudden development of rapid ventricular dysrhythmias. Normal and abnormal QT intervals will be discussed further in a later chapter.

The QRS Duration

The **QRS duration** indicates how long was needed for the ventricles to be activated (Figure 3–9). It provides a measure from the start of the QRS complex to the end of the QRS complex. The **J point** is the junction point where the end of the S wave meets the start of the ST segment (Figure 3–9).

ECG Interpretation Tip: *Normal QRS durations*
are less than 0.12 second. Prolonged QRS
durations, 0.12 second or greater, reflect
delayed ventricular depolarization
(Figure 3–10).

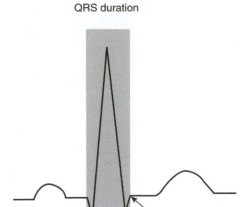

Figure 3–9 QRS duration. The QRS duration is measured from the start of the QRS complex until the end of the QRS complex.

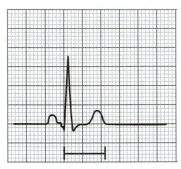

A. Normal Q-T interval

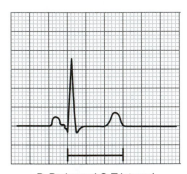

B. Prolonged Q-T interval

Figure 3–8 A. Normal QT interval. B. Prolonged QT interval. Prolonged QT intervals indicate a delay in the repolarization process.

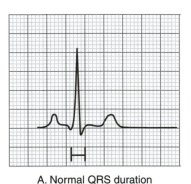

A. Normal QRS duration

B. Prolonged QRS duration

Figure 3–10 A. A normal QRS duration is less than 0.12 second. B. Prolonged QRS durations are 0.12 seconds or greater. and represent delays in ventricular depolarization.

The ST Segment

The ST segment is the portion of the ECG baseline between the end of QRS complex and the start of the T wave (Figure 3–11). Normal ST segments are flat and are compared to a normal isoelectric baseline or PR segment. Ischemia will result in ST segment depression while myocardial injury will elevate the ST segment away from their normally flat appearance (Figure 3–12). The ST segment corresponds to the period following ventricular depolarization until the ventricles start recovering.

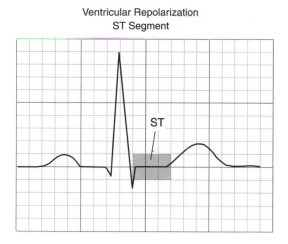

Figure 3–11 ST segment.

The TP Segment

The **TP segment** is the part of the ECG tracing between the end of one complete cardiac cycle and the beginning of the next one. The TP segment is also known as the isoelectric baseline and is an important ECG finding because changes in the ST segment are evaluated in relationship to it.

LABELING QRS COMPLEXES

QRS complex shapes can vary considerably from one ECG tracing to another or even in different leads within the same ECG. It is important to be able to identify and label the various waves making up the QRS complex. Just as the name QRS complex suggests, the classical ventricular activity has three distinct waves. There is an initial small negative wave termed the "Q" wave, after which a large positive wave is written termed the "R" wave, and followed by a small negative "S" wave. Bear in mind that more often than not, ventricular depolarization complexes do not follow this precise sequence. Commonly, the QRS complex is composed of an extra R or S wave, as well as sometimes lacking one component, such as a Q, R, or S wave. However, the ventricular complex is still referred to as a QRS complex although it may lack a Q, R, or S wave or have extra waves. For instance, Figure 3–13 shows a QRS complex that lacks an R wave and several that lack Q waves; still, all are termed QRS complexes.

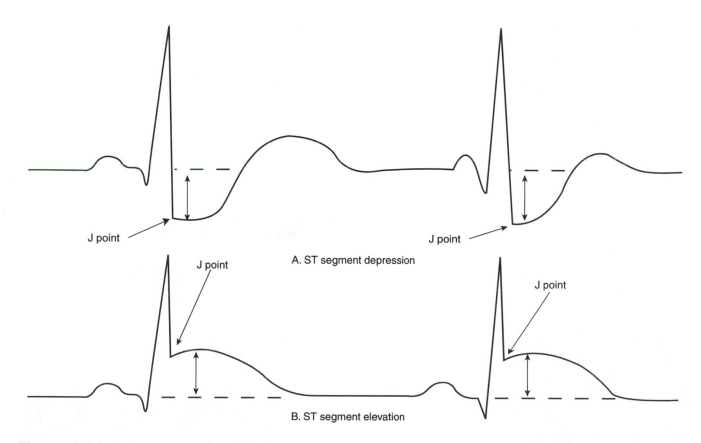

Figure 3–12 A. Depression of the ST segments and J points below the ECG baseline. B. Elevation of the ST segments and J points above the isoelectric baseline.

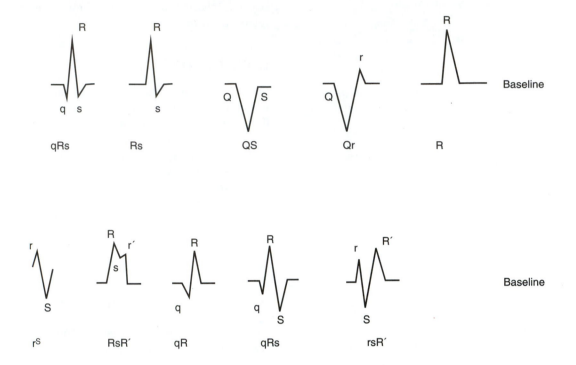

Figure 3–13 Labeling QRS complexes. The configuration and label for each QRS complex is based on the shapes and types of waves present.

QRS Labeling Rules

In order to correctly label or describe waves, some rules about naming ECG complexes must be followed:

■ Following the P wave, if the initial QRS wave is negative it is termed a Q wave.

■ The first upright wave that follows the P wave is designated as an R wave.

■ Any subsequent positive deflections are termed R′ waves.

■ The first downward, or negative, wave that follows the R wave is labeled as an S wave.

■ Any subsequent negative deflections are labeled S′ waves.

■ The uppercase letters R and S are applied when they are the tallest of several types of waves or if they are the only waves of that type found.

■ The lowercase letters s and r are used to designate the smaller wave when more than one type of wave is present, such as two R waves. The largest wave is given a capital letter while the smaller is assigned a lowercase letter (R, r′, respectively).

Figure 3–13 illustrates the application of these rules to some QRS complex examples.

Let's Review

1. The electrocardiogram is the graphic display of cardiac activity that reflects depolarization and repolarization of the atria and ventricles.

2. The electrocardiograph transforms cardiac electrical activity into the series of ECG waves known as the P-QRS-T complex.

3. The ECG assesses only electrical activity while providing no direct information about the heart's mechanical activity.

4.   Each P-QRS-T cycle corresponds to one heart cycle of the contraction-relaxation phases.

5.   Dysrhythmias are abnormal cardiac rhythms.

6.   An ECG rhythm strip records several leads for 10 to 30 seconds or longer and is primarily used to identify specific dysrhythmias and assess the effects of therapy.

7.   An interval is the distance between two waves or complexes. The PR interval is measured from the start of the P wave until the QRS complex is first formed and indicates the speed of atrioventricular conduction. The normal PR interval is from 0.12 to 0.20 second.

8.   Duration is the time it takes for a portion of the ECG tracing to be recorded, such as the P wave, QRS complex, or T wave. The QRS duration indicates the time required for the ventricles to be activated and is normally less than 0.12 second.

9.   Segments are the ECG areas found between waves or complexes.

10.   The ST segment is the ECG area following the QRS complex until the T wave occurs. ST segments are measured from the end of the QRS complex until the T wave starts to be written.

11.   Useful labeling rules can be applied to the QRS complex. The initial wave following the P wave is termed a Q wave if it is negative.

12.   The first upright wave following the P wave is designated an R wave. Any subsequent positive deflections are termed R′ waves.

13.   The first downward, or negative, wave that follows the R wave is labeled an S wave.

14.   Subsequent negative deflections are labeled S′ waves.

15.   Uppercase letters, "R" and "S" are used if they are the only waves of that type found or if they are the tallest of that type.

16.   Lower case letters, "s" and "r" are used when more than one type of wave is present, such as two R waves. The largest wave is designated with a capital letter while the smaller wave is assigned a lowercase letter.

Glossary

Acute myocardial infarction Heart attack involving necrosis of myocardium.

Cardiac monitor Oscilloscope (television type) screen that displays the heart's electrical rhythm.

Duration Time taken for an ECG wave or complex to be recorded.

ECG rhythm strip Continuous recording of a single or multiple leads usually for 10 to 30 seconds, used to identify a dysrhythmia.

Electrocardiogram Graphic display of cardiac depolarization and repolarization commonly abbreviated as ECG or EKG.

Electrocardiograph Device that detects, amplifies, and transforms cardiac electrical energy into a series of waveforms.

Interval Distance between two waves or complexes.

J point Portion of the ECG where the QRS complex ends and the ST segment begins.

PR interval Period of time between the start of the P wave to the beginning of the QRS complex.

QRS duration Period from the start of the QRS complex until the end of the QRS complex. The time period for the ventricles to be activated.

QT interval Period of time from the start of ventricular activation (Q wave) until recovery (T wave).

Segment Portion of the ECG baseline occurring between waves or complexes.

ST segment Portion of the ECG complex from the end of the QRS complex until the beginning of the T wave.

TP segment Portion of the ECG tracing extending from the end of one complete cardiac cycle until the beginning of another; the isoelectric baseline.

ECG Paper and Rate Calculation

LEARNING OBJECTIVES

Upon completion of this chapter, the reader should be able to:

- *State the units of time that the horizontal ECG axis represents.*

- *List the time period represented by one small ECG box and one large ECG box.*

- *List the number of large ECG boxes that make up the following time intervals: one second, three seconds, and six seconds.*

- *State the standard ECG paper speed in terms of the number of large ECG boxes that are found in one minute.*

- *State the voltage units that the vertical ECG axis represents.*

- *List the voltage values along the vertical axis that are represented by one small ECG box, one large ECG box, and two large ECG boxes.*

- *Describe three methods for calculating cardiac rates.*

- *Describe two methods that can be used for calculating rates for an ECG rhythm that is regular.*

- *Specify one method to calculate cardiac rates for an ECG rhythm that is irregular.*

CHAPTER OVERVIEW

No matter which ECG machine is used or where in the world it is used, the paper-speed and height of the calibration signal are the same. ECG paper is standardized using a calibration signal at the start of every ECG tracing to inform the clinician of the relative size that the tracing was recorded. The ECG paper grid markings along the vertical and horizontal planes represent time and voltage increments, respectively. Three methods will be presented for calculating ECG cycle rates; two of which can only be used when the rhythm is regular, while one method is accurate for regular as well as irregular rhythms.

ECG RECORDING PAPER

ECG machines and recording paper are standardized in order for cardiac tracings to appear the same no matter where it is recorded. A standardization test ensures that the size of the waves and time intervals are comparable from one machine to another. Standard ECG paper consists of graphs or grids that allow measurement of different portions of the ECG complexes.

ECG paper consists of large boxes and small boxes. Each small box measures 1 millimeter high by 1 millimeter wide. Each large box measures 5 millimeters high by 5 millimeters wide.

Horizontal ECG Axis

The horizontal grid markings pertain to time frame. When ECG machines were first designed in the early 1900s they were constructed so that the paper speed was 1 inch of paper rolling out of the machine every second. When the metric system measurements were applied, the paper speed was converted so that each inch of paper was equal to 2.5 centimeters (cm). Paper speed is now standardized around the world so that 25 millimeters (mm) of paper is recorded every second. This simple relationship allows the ECG intervals and durations to be measured in thousands of a second. Each small ECG box equals 1 millimeter. Each 1 millimeter box represents 0.04 second or 40 milliseconds. A large ECG box consists of five 1-millimeter boxes. Each large box represents 0.20 second or 200 milliseconds (1/5 of a second). Therefore, five large ECG boxes will be recorded every second.

Vertical ECG Axis

The vertical ECG axis indicates the relative voltage or complex size. Each 1 mm vertical box represents 0.1 millivolt (mV). Ten-millimeter vertical boxes, which is the same as two large 5-mm boxes, equal 1 mV. When an ECG machine is properly calibrated, a 1 mV signal input will cause the stylus to abruptly jump ten small boxes. Figure 4–1 illustrates these values on an ECG strip.

By using these values, the various P-QRS-T components, including the intervals and durations, can be evaluated. Conduction delays and premature ventricular activation can be detected.

> **ECG Interpretation Tip:** *The vertical ECG axis measures voltage. Each 1 millimeter vertical box equals 0.1 mV. The horizontal ECG axis measures time. Each 1 mm box equals 0.04 second or 40 milliseconds, while each large (5 mm) box equals 0.20 second or 200 milliseconds. One second of paper speed will equal five large ECG boxes.*

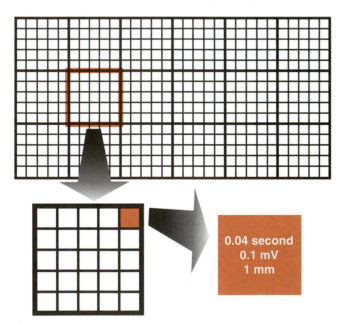

Figure 4–1 ECG monitoring paper with enlarged blocks to illustrate the minimum units of measurement. The small boxes has three values: 0.04 second in duration, 0.1 mV in amplitude, and 1 mm in height. Five small boxes along the horizontal axis measures 0.20 second. Five small boxes equals one large box. Five small boxes on the vertical axis would measure 5 mm and equals 0.5 mV.

0.04 second
0.1 mV
1 mm

CALIBRATION SIGNAL

Electrocardiographs amplify the tiny electrical signals generated by the heart in order to be able to better analyze the waves. ECG machines mark the electrocardiogram with a calibration signal at the start of the recording in order to alert the reader about the standard action or amount of amplification at which the ECG was recorded. The calibration signal alerts the interpreter if the ECG size is nonstandard, that is, if it has been enlarged more than usual or if it has been reduced smaller than usual.

A standard calibration input of 1 mV current raises the recording stylus 10 mm, which is two large, or ten small, ECG boxes (Figure 4–2). This is useful information because an ECG complex that is twice as tall as a corresponding wave represents an electrical charge twice as strong.

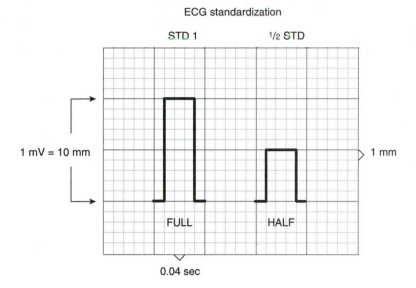

ECG standardization

STD 1   ½ STD

1 mV = 10 mm   1 mm

FULL   HALF

0.04 sec

Figure 4-2 Standardization adjusts the ECG size in order to make the complexes easier to assess. At normal standardization—STD 1—a 1 mV (1 millivolt) calibration signal raises the stylus 10 mm. At half standardization (1/2 standardization or 1/2 STD), a 0.5 mV calibration signal causes the stylus to raise 5 mm. At double standardization—2 STD—a 2 mV calibration signal causes the stylus to raise 20 mm.

Nonstandard ECG Size Recording

ECG machines can be adjusted so that the height of the standardization signal ranges from half to twice the normal size. Being able to alter the standardization is useful in certain cases when the QRS complexes are too large or too small for easy interpretation. For example, in cases involving a pericardial effusion (fluid collection surrounding the heart) or chronic obstructive pulmonary disease, very small P-QRS-T complexes are generated because of the insulating effect caused by the trapped fluid or air surrounding the heart. The ECG can be corrected by recording at twice the usual amplification, which is indicated on the machine as "double" (2X STD), making the enlarged ECG recording is easier to interpret.

ECGs that have very tall QRS complexes, as occurs when there is an enlarged muscle mass size in hypertrophied hearts, can interfere with the interpretation. The large cardiac complexes can be reduced by 50 percent to "half" standardization (1/2 STD), permitting a more accurate assessment (see Figure 4–2).

> *ECG Interpretation Tip: Failure to note a change in standardization could lead to erroneous ECG assessments. Every ECG assessment should begin by noting the standardization signal.*

CALCULATING ECG RATES

Being able to quickly determine cardiac rates is an essential skill. Fortunately, there are several reliable and easy ways to calculate cardiac rates. As the ECG paper in Figure 4–3 shows, time intervals are marked with dots or small vertical lines every one or three seconds. Each 1 second interval on the ECG paper consists of 5 large ECG boxes, or 25 small (1 mm) ECG boxes.

The "Six-Second" or "Times Ten" Counting Technique

The number of P-QRS-T *complexes* noted in a 6-second period is multiplied by 10 to obtain the minute rate.

A variation of the **six-second** or **times ten counting technique** involves counting the number of R-R *intervals* in a six second period. A **cycle length** is the distance between a wave in one complex and the corresponding wave in the next cardiac cycle. For example, the R-R interval is determined and the number of R-R intervals in a 6-second strip is counted and multiplied by 10 to obtain the *rate per minute*. The same method can be used for the atrial rate.

For example, in Figure 4–4 the rate is found to be 80/minute because the 6-second period contains exactly 8 cycle lengths. According to the 6-second counting formula, 8 R-R intervals multiplied by 10 equals a QRS rate of 80/minute.

The "six-second" counting technique's accuracy can be increased by including any fractions of cycle lengths,

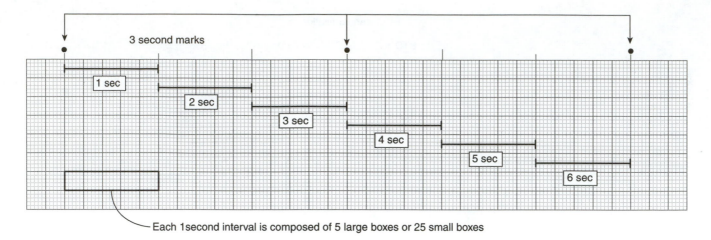

Figure 4–3 ECG intervals.

such as half a cycle, a third of a cycle, a quarter of a cycle, corresponding to 5 beats, 3 beats, or 2 beats, respectively, in your calculations. For instance, when a 6-second interval includes 7 1/2 R-R cycles, the rate is determined by multiplying 7.5 by 10 to equal a cardiac rate of 75/min (Figure 4–5). As an example, what rate would be present if 4 1/3 cycles were counted in a 6-second period as shown in Figure 4–6? This would correspond to a rate of 43/minute because 4.3 is multiplied by 10 to obtain the 60-second rate.

This method can be use for assessing both regular and irregular ECG rhythms.

The "300-Box" Counting Technique

To apply this method, the number of large ECG boxes separating any two consecutive R waves are counted and divided into 300. The number "300" comes from the paper speed of 300 large ECG boxes per minute. One limitation is that the **300-box counting tech-** **nique** is only accurate if the rhythm is regular, that is, when the R-R intervals are constant. Otherwise, the rates would constantly vary as different R-R intervals are measured. The example shown in Figure 4–7 shows approximately 2 1/2 large ECG boxes separating two R waves (a single R-R interval); therefore, the rate is 120 complexes per minute because 300 is divided by 2.5 (300 ÷ 2.5 = 120). Similarly, if there were three large boxes between every two R waves, the rate would be 100/minute because 100 represents 300 divided by 3. Figure 4–8 illustrates the rates that are calculated when there are one, two, or three large ECG boxes between consecutive R waves.

The "Memorization," "Multiple," or "Sequence" Counting Technique

The rates corresponding to multiples for every large ECG box between consecutive R-R intervals are committed to memory. The rates are then called out as each

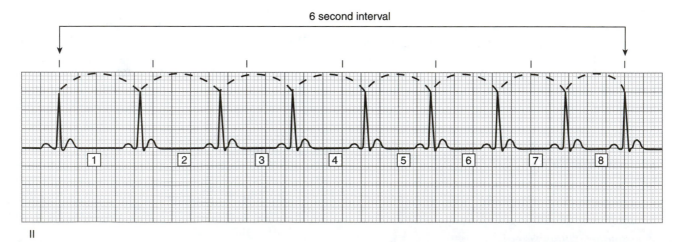

Figure 4–4 Cardiac cycle rate of 80/minute (8 R-R intervals multiplied by 10 equals 80/minute).

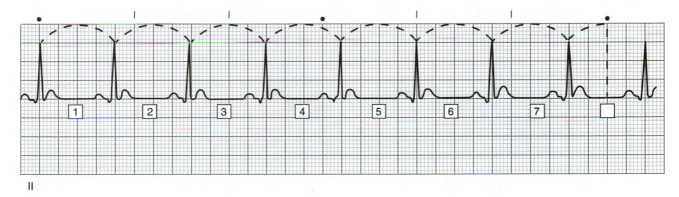

II

Figure 4–5 Cardiac cycle rate of 75/minute (7 1/2 R-R intervals multiplied by 10 equals 75 /minute).

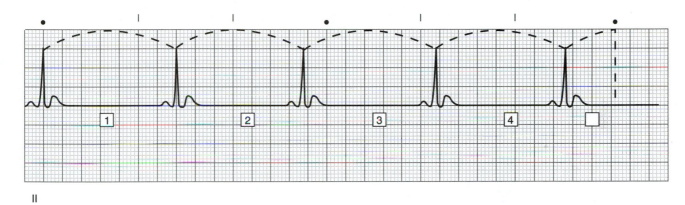

II

Figure 4–6 Cardiac cycle rate of 43/minute (4 1/3 R-R intervals multiplied by 10 equals 43 /minute).

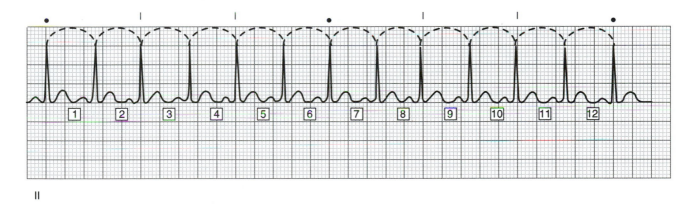

II

Figure 4–7 Cardiac cycle rate of 120/minute (12 R-R intervals multiplied by 10 equals 120 /minute).

large box is counted in the R-R interval. See Figure 4–9. The R-R intervals must be constant in order to use this technique or else the rates would vary greatly as the R-R intervals change. The cardiac rate is based on the number of large ECG boxes between cardiac cycles and corresponds to:

■ 300/minute when there is one large box;

■ 150/minute when there are two large boxes;

■ 100/minute when there are three large boxes;

■ 75/minute when there are four large boxes;

■ 60/minute when there are five large boxes;

Heart rate = 300/min.

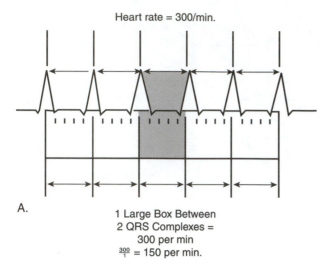

A.

1 Large Box Between
2 QRS Complexes =
300 per min
$\frac{300}{1}$ = 150 per min.

Heart rate = 150/min.

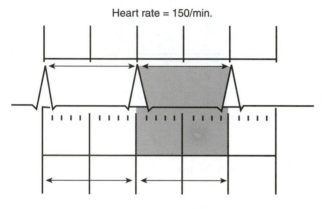

B.

2 Large Boxes Between
2 QRS Complexes =
150 per min
$\frac{300}{2}$ = 150 per min.

Heart rate = 100/min.

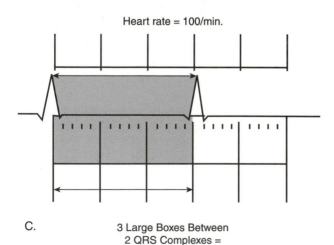

C.

3 Large Boxes Between
2 QRS Complexes =
100 per min
$\frac{300}{3}$ = 100 per min.

Figure 4-8 Calculation using the "300-box" counting technique.

- 50/minute when there are six large boxes;

- 43/minute when there are seven large boxes; and

- 37/minute when eight large boxes are counted.

Let's Review

1. Each small ECG box measures 1 millimeter high by 1 millimeter wide.

2. Each large ECG box measures 5 millimeter high and 5 millimeter wide. Each large ECG box is composed of five small ECG boxes.

3. The standard ECG tracing speed or monitor sweep is 25 mm—5 large ECG boxes or 25 small ECG boxes—per second.

4. Each small ECG box equals 1 mm. Each 1 mm box represents .04 second or 40 milliseconds along the horizontal ECG axis.

5. Each large ECG box is made up of five 1 mm boxes. Each large box is equal to 0.20 second or 200 milliseconds.

6. The vertical ECG axis indicates the relative voltage or complex size.

7. Each 1 mm vertical box represents 0.1 mV. Ten-millimeter vertical boxes (two large 5 mm boxes) are equal to 1 mV.

8. A standard calibration signal causes a 1 mV input, which causes the stylus to rise 10 mm.

9. By adjusting the standardization control to double standardization size (2× STD), ECG tracings with small P-QRS-T complexes will be enlarged two-fold and assessment will be facilitated.

10. By adjusting the ECG to half standardization (1/2 STD), large cardiac complexes can be reduced by 50 percent, permitting a more accurate assessment.

11. Three common rate calculation methods exist: the six second or times ten counting technique, the number of P-QRS-T complexes occurring during a six-second period are counted and multiplied by 10 to obtain the minute rate; the 300-box counting technique, the number of large ECG boxes that separates any two consecutive R waves are divided into 300 (300 represents the paper speed) (This method can only be used for regular rhythms.); the memorization, multiple, or sequence counting technique. The

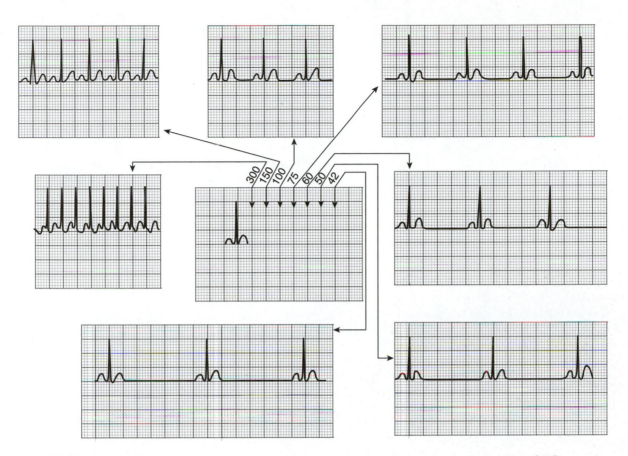

Figure 4–9 Cardiac cycle rates determined by the number of large ECG boxes between two QRS complexes.

rates corresponding to multiples for every large box between consecutive R-R intervals are committed to memory: "300-150-100-75-60-50-43-37" and recalled as the number of large boxes are counted

Glossary

Calibration signal A mark on the ECG tracing to indicate the amount of signal amplification used; standard amplification is 1 mV and causes a stylus deflection of 10 mm.

Cycle length The distance between a wave in one complex and the corresponding wave in the next cardiac cycle.

"Memorization" counting technique The method for calculating a heart rate by memorizing the number of boxes that corresponds to a particular multiple; also called "multiple" or "sequence" counting technique.

Rate per minute The number of QRS complexes in one minute which usually equals the heart beats in one minute.

"Six second" counting technique Method of calculating a heart rate by counting the number of P-QRS-T complexes in a 6-second period and multiplying by 10; also called the "times ten" calculating technique.

"300-box" counting technique The method of calculating a heart rate by counting the number of large ECG boxes between consecutive R waves and dividing that number into 300.

Cardiac Monitors, Lead Systems, and Artifacts

LEARNING OBJECTIVES

Upon completion of this chapter, the reader should be able to:

■ *Describe the basic functional components of an ECG monitor.*

■ *List the six ECG limb lead configurations.*

■ *Define the terms unipolar ECG lead and bipolar ECG lead.*

■ *Identify the chest locations for application of the six precordial ECG leads.*

■ *Explain the functions of the following cardiac monitor controls: (a) gain adjustment; (b) screen sweep (speed) signal; (c) lead selector; (d) rate meter; and (e) alarm limits.*

■ *Explain the function of the ECG monitor's artifact interference filter.*

■ *Describe the function of the "diagnostic mode" display used for cardiac monitoring.*

■ *Explain the effect of a monitor's artifact filter on the ST segment.*

■ *List two limitations of using lead II as the sole monitoring system.*

■ *Describe the advantages of lead V_1 or MCL_1 compared with lead II for continuous monitoring.*

■ *Specify which groups of leads best evaluate cardiac activity in the following heart locations: (a) inferior (diaphragmatic); (b) anterior; (c) lateral; (d) posterior; and (e) right ventricle.*

■ *List six sources of ECG artifact patterns.*

■ *List three actions to reduce ECG artifact.*

CHAPTER OVERVIEW

Cardiac monitoring detects abnormal cardiac rhythms and allows the institution of antidysrhythmic therapy. Small lightweight devices allow cardiac monitoring to begin in the patient's home and during EMS transportation. Certain groups of ECG leads provide more useful information than others; for this reason, leads II and MCL_1 are favored for continuous monitoring.

ECG lead groups provide information about cardiac activity in specific heart regions. Accurate interpretation depends on the knowledge of the area of the heart a lead group is facing. Artifact or man-made electrical disturbances of the cardiac tracing distort the ECG tracing and may mimic dysrhythmias as well as complicate dysrhythmia interpretation. Identification of artifact is critical to proper interpretation.

CARDIAC MONITORS

As described in a previous chapter, the heart emits tiny electrical currents that are detected by electrocardiograph electrodes. The heart's energy flow is amplified by the ECG machine and displayed on a monitor screen and/or printed on ECG grid paper (Figure 5–1). ECG monitoring is routinely used to assess critically ill patients, especially those at risk of cardiac dysrhythmias, such as patients with ischemia or hypoxia, as well as patients who have unstable vital signs. In fact, every year between 350,000 and 400,000 people die during the early phase of a myocardial infarction—either before they arrive at an emergency department or shortly afterward. Early public access defibrillation, public safety first-responder programs, and mobile advanced life support units have focused on preventing and treating patients at risk of sudden cardiac death. Even non-cardiac patients who are at risk of dysrhythmias because they are undergoing medical or surgical procedures, especially if they receive sedation or anesthesia, have their cardiac rhythms routinely monitored. In its simplest form, cardiac monitors include a display monitor screen, or a printout of an ECG tracing, electrode cables, and electrodes that are attached to the patient's skin. Electrodes usually consist of 1 to 2-inch discs that have adhesive backing and contain conductive gel. Most monitors have a **heart rate indicator** that automatically calculates the heart rate based on analysis of the R-R interval, or R waves, which signal each QRS via a beep, click, flash, or via a digital numeric display. ECG monitors can be mounted at the patient's bedside, carried on the stretcher, or be located at a remote central monitoring console.

ECG Monitoring Systems

Several different basic types of monitoring systems are now commonly in use, with models ranging from basic to sophisticated. A basic, "no-frills" version provides single-lead monitoring capability without being able to store rhythm data. Advanced multichannel central recording systems permit continuous monitoring of all twelve leads, including ST segment analysis, and "critical event" summaries (Figure 5–2). They can, for instance, record all premature beats or rapid rhythms during a 24- or 48-hour period, or any ECG tracing event that triggered an alarm, including code summaries that print short tracings of major dysrhythmias that were detected during a resuscitation effort.

Portable Monitors

Monitors for transportation and especially during pre-hospital care need to be compact, lightweight, and battery powered, with filters that eliminate artifact as the patient is moved. Monitors used by EMS usually combine a defibrillator-cardioverter and cardiac pacing module. ECG monitors on hospital code-carts also need to be compact and lightweight enough to be transported quickly to a patient's room or clinic area.

Critical Care Monitors

Monitors that are used in critical care units are fixed location devices that are larger and have more capabilities than portable ones. Hospital based monitor systems usually incorporate multiple display/record channels that can display other physiologic activities including oxygen saturation, respiratory rate, temperature,

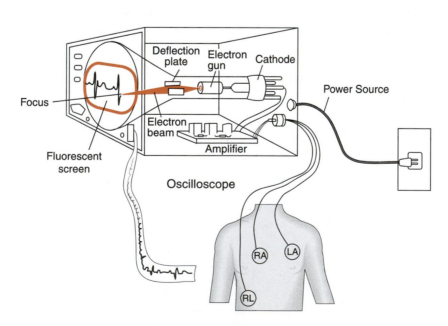

Figure 5–1 The internal components of an ECG monitor.

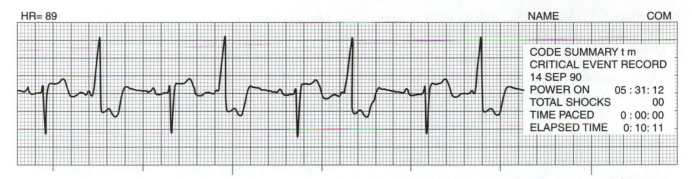

Figure 5–2 Computer-generated critical event record. The code summary indicates the key rhythms and events that occurred during an emergency call. This feature frees staff members to continue providing rather than stop delivering care to document dysrhythmias. The date and time are also printed.

carbon dioxide level, and vital signs in addition to heart rhythm. Monitors employed in operating suites and the postanesthesia care units (PACUs) also monitor arterial and pulmonary artery pressures along with temperature.

Computer-Assisted Rhythm Analysis

By incorporating a computer to track and store monitoring data, comprehensive data and patient condition analysis can be produced. For instance, ECG rhythm trends can easily be detected. Data from hours or days can be stored and presented in graphic or table summaries. Figure 5–3 shows ST segment analysis for a six hour period. This is invaluable in assessing myocardial ischemia and is much more accurate than an observer attempting to visually detect ST segment changes.

Monitor System Features

Standard monitor features include:

- Alarms. Monitors may have graduated warning alarm intensities that are based on the computer-assessed dysrhythmia findings. For instance, a flashing light and soft audible tone can initially be signaled, as when a short series of fast beats is detected, while a loud blaring gong is reserved for critical events such as life-threatening ventricular rhythm disturbances.

- Electrode discs. Self-adhering electrodes that are pre-gelled with conducting jelly that attach to electrode cables.

- A "printout" or "write-out." A written "hard" copy or recorded tracing. This feature can be manually triggered or automatically activated to record whenever an alarm is signaled. Some monitor/recorders automatically print out a summary of critical events, such as when a defibrillation or synchronized cardioversion occurs, printing the information that was recorded two seconds before and after the shock.

- Gain or sensitivity control. Alters the size of the ECG complex. The size can be manually adjusted but most units have an automatic gain control that adjusts the display to the proper height.

- Sweep signal. Regulates the monitor time frame, which is set at the standard "25 mm per second" speed, but can be changed to double-speed to record at "50 mm per second," which can help in the identification of atrial waves when rapid rate dysrhythmias cause them to be hidden or superimposed on each other.

- Lead selector. Chooses the lead(s) to be monitored.

ST Segment Trending

6, 12 or 24 hours

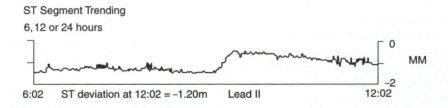

6:02   ST deviation at 12:02 = −1.20m   Lead II   12:02

Figure 5–3 Computer-assisted ST segment trend evaluation is a feature on some cardiac monitors.

■ Rate meter. Digital number display, often in association with an audible or a visual signal for each QRS complex detected.

■ Alarm limits. Sets the desired rates above or below which an alarm is triggered, for instance, heart rates falling below therate set at 50/minute.

■ Alarm device. A visual, audible, or combined warning system that alerts staff that a dysrhythmia has occurred.

■ Recording control. Starts the printout feature.

■ Telemetry capability. Used in some systems because it permits a patient to move freely about the hospital unit while his cardiac rhythm is continuously recorded at a remote base station. The lead information is converted into a radio signal that is received by an antenna, which converts it to an electrical display at a central monitoring station.

> *Clinical Note:* *Being attached to a cardiac monitor for the first time is frightening for most patients. Often, a patient's only experience with cardiac monitors comes from having seen them on television drama shows being applied to critically ill patients. The patient's anxiety can be minimized by discussing the monitor's function with the patient.*

ECG LIMB AND CHEST LEADS

A standard ECG tracing consists of twelve leads, six which are placed on the limbs and six on the chest wall. Continuous rhythm monitoring usually employs less than twelve leads, primarily because most dysrhythmias can be adequately assessed using one or two leads. ("Hospital-based chest pain centers," which monitor patients at risk for ischemia monitor all twelve leads in order to detect the earliest signs of myocardial injury.) From a practical and patient comfort standpoint, using less than twelve leads eliminates cumbersome cables and allows greater patient mobility. Most monitor systems have eliminated placement of limb leads on the extremities, modifying the recordings by applying all leads to the patient's trunk.

Limb Leads

Leads are recorded from electrodes placed on the limbs and chest wall positions. Leads I, II, and III differ from other leads in that they are **bipolar**, meaning that two electrodes are used: one being positive (+) and the other negative (−). **Unipolar** leads employ a single positive electrode and make up the six remaining limb leads. Three limb leads are termed "**augmented**" because their voltage is amplified to match the size of other limb leads. Augmented limb leads are abbreviated "aVR, aVL, aVF." Figure 5–4 illustrates the placement of the limb leads.

Chest or Precordial Leads

Precordial leads consist of a series of leads that are labeled V_1 through V_6 as the electrodes record around the left side of the chest wall (Figure 5–5). Precordial lead placement can be viewed from a point above the heart so that the electrode positions are seen in relation to cardiac chamber location (Figure 5–6). Each chest lead produces a recording from a slightly different van-

Electrode Placement— Limb Electrodes

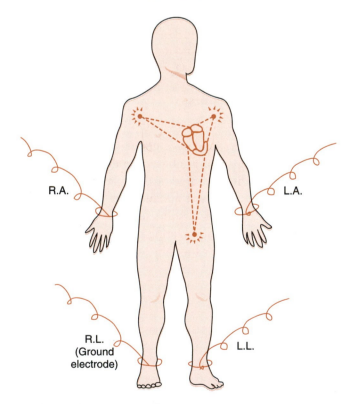

Figure 5–4 Limb electrodes are placed on the wrists and ankles for standard twelve-lead ECGs or on the shoulders and lower abdomen for cardiac monitoring.

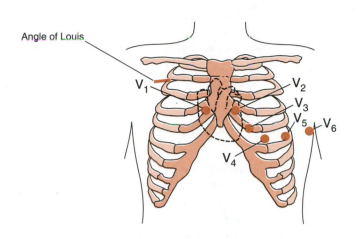

Figure 5-5 Location of the chest electrodes to record precordial leads. The angle of Louis is a landmark marking the junction for the upper and middle portions of the sternum and serves as a reference point for the second intercostal space.

tage point, yielding additional information in order to assess cardiac activity. Further explanation of twelve-lead ECGs will occur in a later chapter.

CONTINUOUS PATIENT MONITORING LEADS

Pre-hospital, emergency department, and critical care units typically employ one or two leads for continuous monitoring. Being able to simultaneously monitor leads II and MCL$_1$ is ideal because they provide the most clinically useful information. Figure 5-7 illustrates the standard chest lead positions for the most commonly monitored leads that utilize a three-cable system:

- Lead I: the positive electrode is placed below the left clavicle and the negative electrode is attached under the right clavicle.

- Lead II: the positive electrode is placed on the left lower chest wall just superior to the rib border, and the negative electrode below the right clavicle.

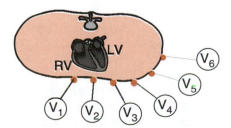

Figure 5-6 Precordial leads shown in the horizontal axis in relation to the surface of the heart.

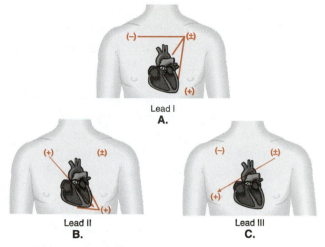

Figure 5-7 The position of the electrodes and the lead systems as they visualize the surfaces of the heart. A. shows lead I. The positive lead is on the left shoulder and visualizes cardiac electrical activity on the left side of the heart. B. shows lead II. The positive lead is on the left side of the chest below the rib cage and visualizes cardiac activity on the left inferior side. C. shows lead III. This lead visualizes electrical activity from the right inferior surface. D. shows MCL$_1$. The positive electrode is over the left intercostal space just left of the sternum. This lead provides the best view of atrial activity.

- Lead III: the positive electrode is attached to the left anterior chest wall just superior to the rib border, and the negative electrode is placed just below the left clavicle.

- MCL$_1$: simulates a precordial V$_1$ position in cable systems that use fewer than four electrodes. The positive electrode is placed just to the right of the sternum in the fourth intercostal space (between the fourth and fifth ribs) while the negative electrode is applied under the left clavicle. Most monitors now employ more than three cables and can obtain a true precordial recording, eliminating the need for modified chest leads.

> **ECG Interpretation Tip:** Leads II and MCL$_1$ are the most useful tracings for detecting dysrhythmias and providing information that complement each other.

> **Clinical Note:** Most electrode cables are color-coded for ease of application: the negative

electrode is usually white, the positive is red, and the ground electrode can be green, brown, or black.

Clinical Note: *When applying electrodes, avoid skin areas with dense hair, which will lead to poor electrode adherence, and avoid placement on muscle. If time permits, the area should be cleansed with an alcohol prep or a soapy gauze pad with brisk rubbing. Diaphoretic skin should be dried and an adhesive solution applied, such as tincture of benzoin, which helps to keep the electrodes in position. Excess hair can be shaved to ensure good contact when several days of monitoring is anticipated.*

Clinical Note: *Chest electrode positions should be applied in a manner that leaves the chest area clear should defibrillation be needed.*

LEAD SELECTION FOR CONTINUOUS MONITORING

Since the advent of coronary care units in the early 1960s, lead II has been used for continuous monitoring because it displays the traditional appearance showing the P-QRS-T waves as upright. The ideal monitoring lead would provide all information which is necessary to identify dysrhythmias. An ideal lead would also make it possible to determine whether a wide and distorted beat originated from a ventricular pacemaker or was due to abnormal ventricular conduction of an atrial impulse. However, no single lead is perfect yet two leads that provide very useful complimentary information for dysrhythmia assessment are leads II and MCL_1. Many ECGs automatically generate rhythm strips containing both of these leads.

ECG Interpretation Tip: *Utilizing a single lead for monitor assessment is usually sufficient for most cases; however, in some cases multiple, simultaneously recorded leads are required to be able to identify a dysrhythmia. What is inconspicuous in one lead sometimes turn out to be obvious in another!*

Simultaneously using leads II and MCL_1 is the best tactic for providing maximal information.

Comparison of Leads MCL_1 and II

In Lead II the positive electrode is placed on the left side of the chest or leg below the heart, which faces the interior surface of the heart. All cardiac activity is sensed as approaching the positive electrode and is recorded as positive deflections. As a result, the P-QRS-T complex in lead II is written as positive.

Lead II has some important limitations, including being unable to distinguish between right and left bundle branch, nor can it differentiate a ventricular ectopic beat from a supraventricular impulse with aberrant conduction. Since these rhythm disturbances are common—and clinically important—many clinicians choose to use MCL_1 if only a single lead can be monitored.

The right precordial lead MCL_1 has been popularized by Henry J. Marriott, M.D., a leader in the field of electrocardiography. In MCL_1 the positive electrode is placed in the right fourth intercostal space—the same site as for V_1—which rests over the left atrium. The vantage point from V_1's electrode position on the left anterior chest detects atrial activity as it comes toward it and as it flows away, resulting in a positive P wave while the QRS complex is negative (Figure 5–8). The P wave—unlike in lead II—can have a variable appearance, often appearing with a sharp, pointed, inverted, or biphasic shape. Table 5–1 summarizes these possibilities.

ECG Interpretation Tip: *The ECG rhythm must be sinus if the P waves are upright and the PR intervals are constant in lead II.*

ECG DEFLECTIONS

When no cardiac current is flowing, such as in between cardiac cycles the ECG displays an isoelectric or flat baseline. *When a depolarization wave flows toward a positive electrode, an upright or positive ECG wave is recorded* (Figure 5–9A) The size of the ECG wave depends on the strength or magnitude of the energy flow. *When a depolarization wave flows away from the positive electrode, a negative ECG wave is recorded* (Figure 5–9B). *When the depolarization wave flows perpendicular to the positive electrode, an isoelectric (flat)*

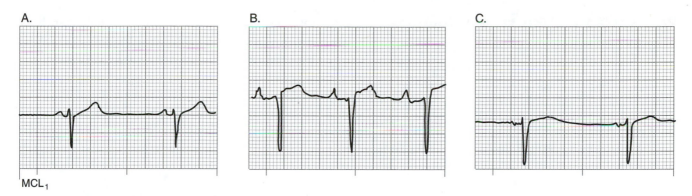

Figure 5–8 Variable P wave shape in lead MCL$_1$. A. The P wave is upright and rounded. B. The P wave is tall and pointy. C. The P wave is positive and negative.

tracing results (Figure 9–5C). *When a depolarization wave initially flows toward a positive electrode and then away from it, a biphasic wave—with an initial positive and later negative component is written (Figure 5–9D).*

Table 5-1 Comparisons of Leads II and MCL$_1$		
Wave	**Lead II**	**Lead MCL$_1$**
P	Positive	Variable: Biphasic (+/– component) or Positive
QRS	Positive	Mainly Negative
T	Positive	Variable

Clinical Note: Experienced ECG interpreters can usually detect dysrhythmias by viewing the monitor screen, but it is often advantageous to print a "hardcopy" of the abnormal rhythm so that the individual waves and duration can be accurately measured and assessed.

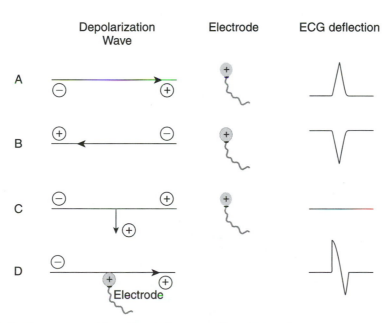

Figure 5–9 ECG deflections caused by electrical current flowing in relation to a positive recording electrode. A. Current flowing toward positive electrode causes positive deflection; B. Wave flowing away from positive electrode causes negative deflection; C. Wave flowing perpendicular to positive electrode causes flat line (currents cancel each other out); D. Wave flowing toward and then away from positive electrode causes a biphasic wave.

OBTAINING AN ADEQUATE ECG TRACING

The following considerations are important for obtaining a technically adequate ECG recording:

- P waves should be prominently displayed because assessment of their relationship to the QRS complexes is key for determining the AV relationship.

- The QRS complex size needs to be tall enough to trigger the monitor's rate detector, especially when performing synchronized cardioversion. The cardioverter automatically designates the tallest wave detected as the QRS complex. A problem occurs when the T wave is the tallest wave, since it will be erroneously selected by the cardioverter synchronizer as the QRS complex. The synchronized shock will be delivered during the wrong phase of the cardiac cycle and could precipitate an unstable rhythm. Another problem happens when the lead being monitored shows T waves that are as tall as, or taller, than the QRS complexes since the rate detector will mistakenly count the heart rate as twice the actual rate.

- Monitor filters are incorporated in portable units to minimize movement artifact and reduce the frequency of false monitor alarms. ECG filters are useful in providing a clear tracing, yet they alter the ST segment appearance rendering the monitor unable to detect myocardial ischemia and injury patterns (Figure 5–10). The problem has been solved by equipping monitors with two display modes: a **"monitoring" mode** in which the filter is operational, and a **"diagnostic" mode** in which the filter has been disabled. The diagnostic mode records an ECG that is equal in quality to a standard ECG. The diagnostic mode is used when the tracing needs to be screened for ST segment analysis, which is essential in detecting acute coronary syndromes. At other times, the filter is used during the monitoring mode to produce a tracing with a more stable baseline by eliminating movement artifact.

HEART REGIONS ASSESSED BY ECG LEAD GROUPS

Certain groups of leads view specific heart regions (Figure 5–11). Clinically important heart regions and the leads that detect activity in these areas include:

- **Inferior heart area**, also known as the **diaphragmatic surface** is best viewed by leads II, III, and aVF.

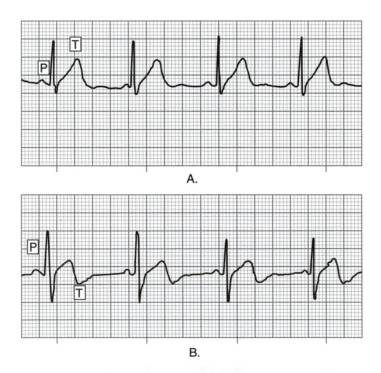

Figure 5–10 Effect of filter on ECG monitor lead display. A and B were recorded a few minutes apart. A. The ECG is displayed without a filter. In B, the electronic filter is activated and this causes the S wave to deepen and the ST-T waves to appear abnormal by mimicking ischemia.

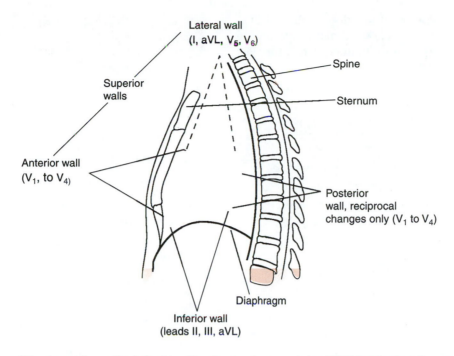

Figure 5–11 View of the heart from the left side. Cardiac regions and the ECG leads that face specific heart areas.

- **Anterior region** is seen best in leads V_1 through V_4.

- **Lateral region** is best seen in leads V_5, V_6, I, and aVL.

- **Posterior surface** can only be assessed indirectly using leads V_1 to V_4.

- **Right ventricle** is assessed using special right-sided precordial leads, which mirror the left-sided precordial positions.

This information is very useful for localizing damaged areas when myocardial injury patterns are studied in a later chapter.

ARTIFACT ECG DISTURBANCES

ECG **Artifact** is an artificial or man-made signal disturbance that distorts the ECG. Artifact commonly distorts an ECG tracing. Being able to distinguish man-made sources of ECG interference from naturally occurring cardiac complexes is important because some artifact patterns resemble dysrhythmias. Artifact is notorious for causing "pseudodysrhythmias," as Figure 5–12 illustrates. In Figure 5–13, the artifact, which is caused by loose or displaced electrodes, mimics grossly chaotic cardiac rhythms. ECG distortion is commonly caused by involuntary patient movement (as with movement disorders such as Parkinson's Disease), from artificial pacemaker spikes, and CPR efforts (Figures 5–14 and 5–15).

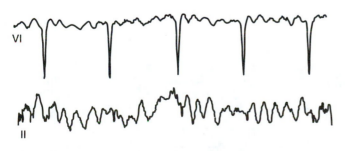
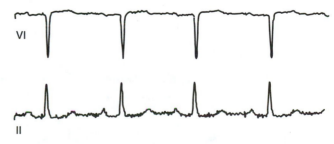

Figure 5–12 "Pseudodysrhythmia" caused by movement artifact. A. Artifact was caused by a patient's extremity tremor. B. The ECG baseline was significantly improved when the electrodes were moved from the extremities to the torso.

The most common type of artifact distorts the flat ECG baseline between cardiac cycles and makes the tracing more difficult to interpret. Common sources of artifact are listed in Table 5-3.

> **ECG Interpretation Tip:** *If the patient has a tremor, the movement artifact can be minimized by moving the electrodes as close to the torso as feasible to avoid artifact. Should respiratory movement cause baseline distortion, moving the electrodes toward the sternum or shoulder area may help avoid the chest movement artifact.*

Table 5-3 Common Sources of ECG Artifact

- Patient or cable movement caused by patient movement, shivering, or seizures is by far the most common source of artifact.

- Dried or inadequate amount of conducting gel.

- Cracked electrode/lead cable.

- Unrecognized standardization/calibration signal.

- Artificial pacemaker or implanted cardioverter-defibrillator discharge signals.

- Improper machine grounding results in stray electrical currents, which create 60 cycles/second interference.

- CPR artifact.

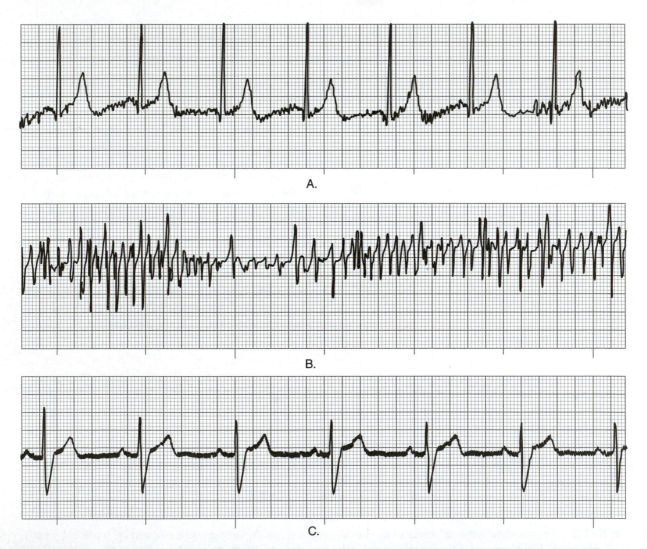

A.

B.

C.

Figure 5-13 A. Movement artifact; B. Seizure induced artifact resembling a tachycardic dysrhythmia; C. Electrical (60 cycle) interference.

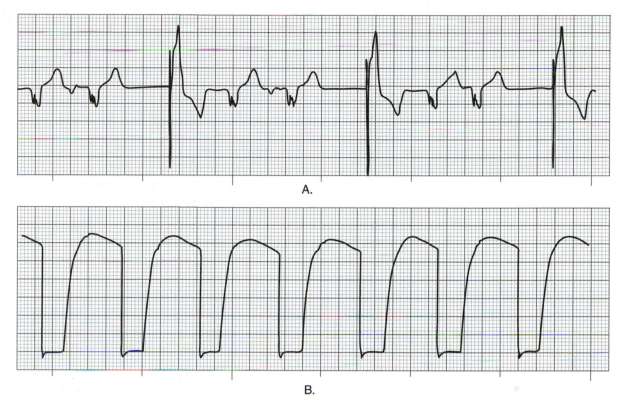

Figure 5–14 A. Artificial pacemaker spikes are seen as the initial part of QRS complexes #3, 6, and 9; B. Pacemaker artifact recorded during a cardiac arrest; no intrinsic cardiac activity is noted.

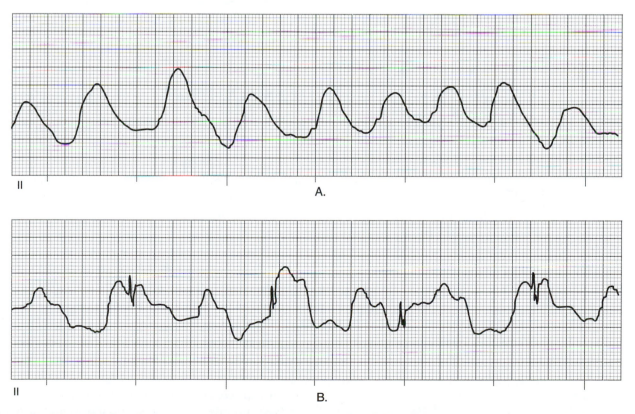

Figure 5–15 A. CPR artifact but no intrinsic cardiac activity; B. CPR artifact superimposed on a pulseless electrical rhythm.

1. Leads I, II, and III are bipolar, using a positive (+) and a negative (−) electrode.

2. In lead II the positive electrode is placed on the left lower leg, which faces the interior surface of the heart. In lead II cardiac activity is seen as approaching the positive electrode and is recorded as positive deflections.

3. Chest or precordial leads consist of positive electrodes, which are labeled V_1 through V_6 as the electrode position shifts along the left side of the chest wall.

4. In MCL_1 the positive electrode is placed in the right fourth intercostal space, which rests over the right atrium.

5. Leads can be grouped according to the areas of the heart recorded and are useful in evaluating cardiac activity in specific cardiac regions. The inferior surface of the heart, also known as the diaphragmatic surface, is best viewed using leads II, III, and aVF. The anterior region is seen best in leads V_1 through V_4, while the lateral region is best seen in leads V_5, V_6, I, and aVL. The posterior heart surface can only be assessed indirectly using leads V_1 to V_3, and the right ventricle is assessed using special right-sided precordial leads.

6. Cardiac monitors have a diagnostic mode that allows accurate ST segment evaluation. Monitors incorporate a filter in the monitor mode, which stabilizes the baseline and minimizes artifact. Accurate ST segment assessment requires that the filter be disabled.

7. Most artifact alters the normally flat baseline between cardiac cycles and makes it difficult to interpret the ECG rhythm.

Anterior leads Leads V_1 through V_4 sense the anterior surface of the heart.

Artifact Man-made ECG disturbances; commonly caused by patient or monitor cable movement.

Augmented lead Amplified voltage of three limb leads (leads aVR, aVL, and aVF).

Bipolar lead Dual lead system using one positive and one negative electrode to monitor cardiac activity (leads I, II, and III).

Diaphragmatic heart surface The inferior surface of the heart is viewed using leads II, III, and aVF.

Diagnostic monitor mode ECG monitor display without the filter activated.

EMS Abbreviation for emergency medical services.

Heart rate indicator ECG monitor display that shows the heart rate based on assessment of the R-R interval.

Inferior leads Leads II, III, and aVF that sense the inferior (diaphragmatic) heart surface.

Intercostal space Chest wall space between two adjacent ribs.

Lateral leads Leads V_5, V_6, I, and aVL sense cardiac activity from the lateral wall of the left ventricle.

MCL_1 lead Unipolar monitor lead with the positive electrode placed in the right fourth intercostal space, that simulates a standard V_1 lead.

Monitor (ECG) filters Incorporated in ECG monitors to eliminate movement and motion artifact. Prevents accurate ST segment analysis

Posterior leads Leads V_1 to V_3 can be used to gather indirect information about the posterior surface of the left ventricle.

Precordial leads Consists of six unipolar leads applied in standard positions on the chest wall.

Right ventricular leads Special right-sided chest leads that mirror the left-sided precordial positions.

Unipolar Lead Single lead system using one positive electrode to monitor cardiac activity.

chapter 6

Systematic Interpretation Approach to Dysrhythmias: Steps One to Four

LEARNING OBJECTIVES

Upon completion of this chapter, the reader should be able to:

- *List the six steps to be followed in the systematic approach to ECG assessment.*

- *State the rationale for following a systematic approach to dysrhythmia interpretation and list two advantages of this approach compared with memorization of dysrhythmia patterns.*

- *Define the terms bradycardia and tachycardia.*

- *List the characteristics needed before an ECG tracing can be classified as a normal sinus rhythm (NSR) in regard to:*
  - *atrial activity*
  - *ventricular activity*
  - *AV conduction*
  - *PR interval*
  - *QRS duration*
  - *QT interval.*

- *Define the upper limit of a normal QRS duration.*

- *Accurately measure QRS durations when shown sample ECG tracings.*

- *Accurately measure QT intervals when shown sample ECG tracings.*

- *Correctly identify prolonged QT intervals when shown sample ECG tracings at various heart rates.*

- *Identify ST segment elevations and depressions when shown sample ECG tracings.*

- *Explain the clinical significance of an ECG displaying ST segment elevation and ST segment depression.*

- *Specify the normal range for a PR interval.*

- *Accurately measure PR intervals when shown sample ECG tracings.*

- *State the normal AV conduction ratio for a normal sinus rhythm.*

- *Correctly determine AV conduction ratios when shown sample ECG tracings.*

- *Explain what is occurring when an ECG tracing has an AV conduction ratio of 3:2 or 2:1.*

- *Describe what is meant by the term supraventricular beat.*

CHAPTER OVERVIEW

In previous chapters, the cellular properties, conduction system, physiologic basis of sinus activity, and cardiac conduction were presented. By using a systematic approach to assessing ECGs, abnormal rhythm patterns can be quickly and accurately identified. Specific ECG abnormalities will be the focus of the remainder of the book. This chapter will describe the initial steps to be used in analyzing ECGs and detecting dysrhythmias. Abnormal ECGs will be presented to illustrate how a rhythm differs from normal sinus rhythm (NSR)—not in order to identify specific disorders. Information about specific rhythm disorders will be acquired in the rest of the book. At this point, it's sufficient to be able to say: "This ECG differs from NSR because the rhythm is irregularly irregular." After completing future chapters, you will be able to identify specific dysrhythmias and choose the correct treatment.

A SYSTEMATIC INTERPRETATION APPROACH

Faced with an unstable patient and a complex dysrhythmia to interpret, novice emergency care providers become as pale, cool, and diaphoretic as the person attached to the ECG. Uncertainty and anxiety can develop because one doesn't know where to begin in analyzing a complex ECG. A good starting place is to compare an abnormal cardiac rhythm to the regular pattern found in **normal sinus rhythm (NSR)**. This helps identify important differences compared with NSR: for instance, if the tracing has wider QRS complexes than NSR, or has more P waves than QRS complexes, or is faster—or slower—than NSR, or is irregular compared with NSR, then it is abnormal and a dysrhythmia exists. Another approach to dysrhythmia interpretation relies on memorization of ECG patterns. Memorization of ECG patterns as a way to identify abnormal rhythms would require sorting through many patterns trying to match the example to a known template. This approach is less effective as Figure 6–1 shows three dysrhythmias exhibiting very different patterns. While the first tracing has a distorted baseline, the second lacks any rhythm or pattern, and the last one shows early beats that disrupt the rhythm. To interpret these strips using a memorization approach, the clinician would have to recall from memory a strip that resembles the one the patient is presenting with. Fortunately, a more interesting and enjoyable way to identify abnormal cardiac rhythms is to develop a systematic approach based on the analysis of common ECG characteristics.

NORMAL SINUS RHYTHM (NSR)

A normal sinus rhythm is produced by an electrical impulse that originated within the sinotrial node at a rate of 60 to 100 bpm. Table 6–1 highlights the key characteristics of NSR. Sinus rhythm occurs when the electrical impulse begins in the normal pacemaker and follows the usual conduction path. This results in a rhythm strip that shows a consistent pattern. In normal sinus rhythm, P waves, QRS complexes, and R-R as well as P-P intervals are uniform in height and duration. AP wave will be present before every QRS complex (Figure 6–2).

SYSTEMATIC APPROACH STEPS

Developing a routine approach to ECG analysis makes the process familiar because the same steps are followed each time an ECG is evaluated. Table 6–2 outlines the steps of the approach that will be followed throughout this book. The assessment order is the same each time: ventricular activity → atrial activity → AV relationship. The reason for beginning with ventricular

Table 6–1 Normal Sinus Rhythm (NSR)

Ventricular rate	60–100 per minute
Ventricular Rhythm	Regular R-R intervals
QRS Configuration	Normal; all QRSs have the same size and shape
QRS Duration	Less than 0.12 second
Atrial rate	Same as ventricular rate, 60–100 per minute
Atrial Rhythm	Regular P-P intervals
Pacemaker	Sinus node
P Wave Configuration	Consistent size and shape; P waves are upright in lead II and biphasic or upright in MCL_1
AV Conduction Ratio	One P wave to each QRS complex (1:1)
PR Interval	0.12 to 0.20 second

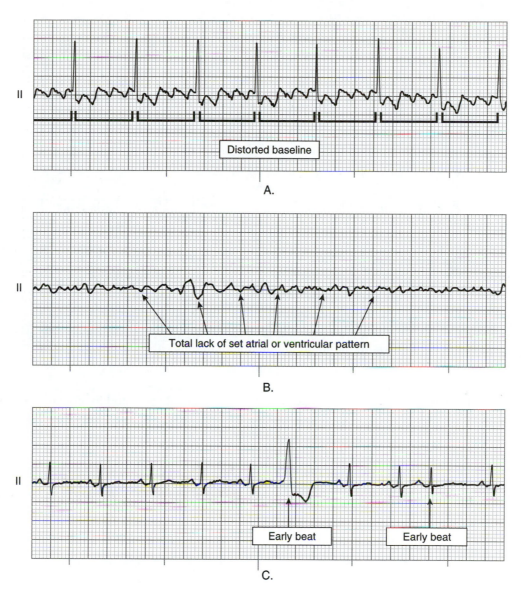

Figure 6–1 Examples of abnormal cardiac rhythms. A. Dysrhythmia with a distorted and irregular baseline. B. ECG tracing lacks any regularity or clear complexes. C. Early beats disrupt the rhythm.

activity is because the QRS complexes are the tallest and easiest waves to identify. Ventricular activity determines the heart rate, which is a major factor contributing to cardiac output. Atrial activity may be rapid, chaotic, and uncoordinated, but as long as the ventricular rate is adequate, the clinical consequences will be minimal. In contrast, should the same chaotic activity affect the ventricles, the pumping action of the heart would cease. The activity of the ventricles is more significant than what is happening to the atria.

In this chapter we will concentrate on steps one through four. Steps five and six will be discussed in detail in the next two chapters.

General Inspection of the ECG Tracing

In step one the rhythm strip is assessed as a whole. Gross ECG abnormalities are noted for later evaluation, such as extra beats, pauses in cardiac activity, distorted complexes, late beats, early beats, or obvious rhythm disturbances. This initial step pinpoints areas that will be returned to later for closer inspection. Next, each wave and complex in several typical complexes is identified. This will usually be easy to do because the QRS complexes are distinguished from the P and T waves without difficulty. Some ECG waves may be hidden in adjacent P-QRS-T complexes as shown in Figure 6–3.

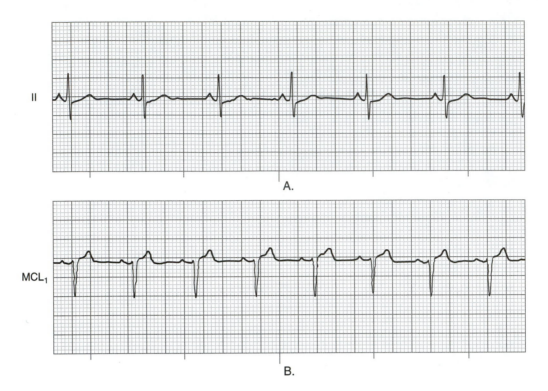

Figure 6–2 Normal sinus rhythm shown in the two leads most commonly selected for continuous monitoring: A. Lead II has upright QRS complexes and strip; B. Lead MCL₁ displays inverted QRS complexes.

During rapid heart rates, for instance, cardiac cycles get squeezed together and the P waves appear to merge with adjacent T waves.

> **ECG Interpretation Tip:** *The ST segments and T waves should be scrutinized for hidden P waves. Tall, peaked T waves often obscure nonconducted P waves. Atrial flutter waves commonly disguise themselves among the ST-T complexes.*

Evaluation of Ventricular Activity

In step two, evaluation of the rate, rhythm, and configuration of the ventricular complexes is important. Does the ECG tracing have a regular rhythm with narrow complexes and a normal rate, or are the QRS complexes rapid or distorted?

Table 6–2 ECG Assessment Steps

Step 1. General tracing inspection

Step 2. Ventricular activity evaluation
- Rate
- Rhythm
- QRS shape
- QT interval
- ST segment

Step 3. Atrial activity evaluation
- Rate
- Rhythm
- P wave shape

Step 4. (AV) atrioventricular relationship evaluation
- PR interval
- AV conduction ratio

Step 5. Comparing the ECG tracing to NSR

Step 6. Evaluation of the dysrhythmia's clinical effect

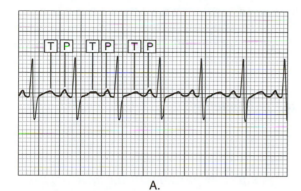

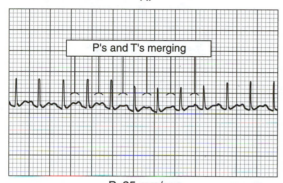

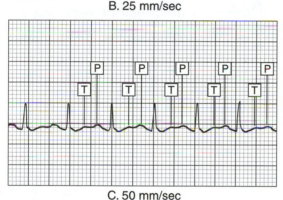

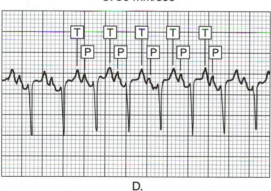

Figure 6–3 Effect of heart rate on the ECG appearance. A. Individual P-QRS-T waves are clearly seen. B. At normal ECG speed (25 mm/second) the P waves and T waves merge together because the rate is faster than 150/minute. C. At twice the normal paper speed (50 mm/second) the individual waves became visible. D. Tall, pointy P waves appear very close to the T waves but can still be identified.

Ventricular Rate

The rate of QRS complexes is counted. This assessment determines if the rate falls within the normal range of 60 to 100/minute for NSR, or if it is below 60/minute, termed **bradycardia** (Figure 6–4), or is faster than 100/minute, termed **tachycardia** (Figure 6–5).

Ventricular Rhythm

The R-R interval regularity is viewed next. Is the ventricular rhythm regular, as expected for NSR, or is it irregular indicating a dysrhythmia is present? If the rhythm is irregular, note whether a pattern exists, and this is useful since many dysrhythmias have recurring cycles. Recognizing such patterns is a useful clue in identifying the dysrhythmia. Typical dysrhythmia patterns are shown in Figure 6–6.

QRS Shape

The shapes of all of the QRS complexes should be identical (refer to Figure 6–2). Normal QRSs have sharp waves, are narrow, and have a constant shape. QRS complexes that are wider than expected or have slurred waves or vary in shape, usually reflect abnormal con-

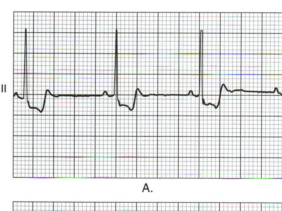

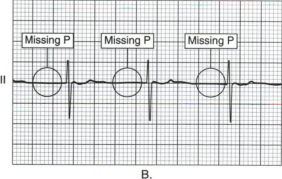

Figure 6–4 Bradycardic rhythms. Two slow tracings have rates below 50/minute. The QRS complexes are narrow in both examples. A. Clear P waves are present. B. P waves are absent so the rhythm cannot be a sinus rhythm. The QRS complexes in strip B arose from the AV junction.

duction or a change in pacemaker location as when the AV junction takes over pacing control when the sinus node fails.

Normal QRS durations should be between 0.06 and 0.11 seconds which corresponds to 1 1/2 to 2 1/2 small ECG boxes (Figure 6–7). The shape and duration of the QRS complex helps to determine where the ventricular depolarization originated. A **supraventricular** beat originates above the point where the AV bundle divides into bundle branches. Supraventricular complexes include sinus, atrial, or AV junctional beats because all have narrow QRS complexes. A QRS complex that is wide and distorted and lacks a P wave likely arose within the ventricles.

> ***ECG Interpretation Tip:*** *If a QRS complex is less than 0.12 second then the beat developed from a supraventricular site. Only supraventricular pacemakers (sinus, atrial, or AV junctional) can stimulate the ventricles in such a quick fashion because they follow normal ventricular conduction pathways. If the QRS complexes are wide (0.12 second or greater), they arose either within the ventricle or from a supraventricular focus but were abnormally conducted.*

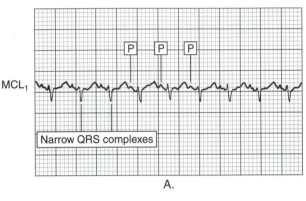

A.

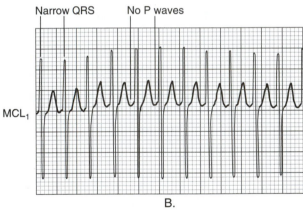

B.

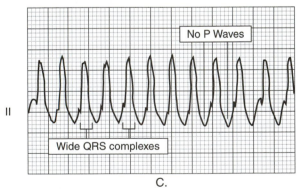

C.

Figure 6–5 Tachycardic rhythms. Three fast tracings have ventricular rates well over 100/minute. A. Shows sinus tachycardia as there are clear P waves and narrow QRS complexes. B. Narrow QRS complexes that lack clear P waves. C. Shows wide QRS complex rhythm without P waves.

QT Interval

The QT interval is the period of ventricular activity beginning when the ventricles are depolarized until the fibers become completely repolarized. The QT interval is measured from the start of the Q wave until the T wave ends. A normal QT interval depends on the heart rate since the repolarization phase decreases as the heart rate increases. A simple guide to normal QT intervals for rates between 50 and 100/minute is 0.40 second +/-0.06 second.

Table 6–3 lists normal QT intervals, which have been corrected based on the heart rate. This is abbreviated at **QTc.** Modern ECG machines automatically calculate the corrected QT intervals and signal prolonged values. Prolonged QT intervals are clinically important because they can precipitate unstable ventricular dysrhythmias leading to cardiovascular collapse.

> ***ECG Interpretation Tip:*** *A normal QT interval for heart rates between 50 and 100/minute is 0.40 second +/− 0.06 second. Prolonged QT intervals alert the clinician to the possibility of rapid unstable dysrhythmias.*

ST Segment

The ST segment is measured from the end of the QRS complex until the beginning of the T wave. Normal ST segments are flat or **isoelectric** (Figure 6–8). It is important to determine if the ST segment is above or

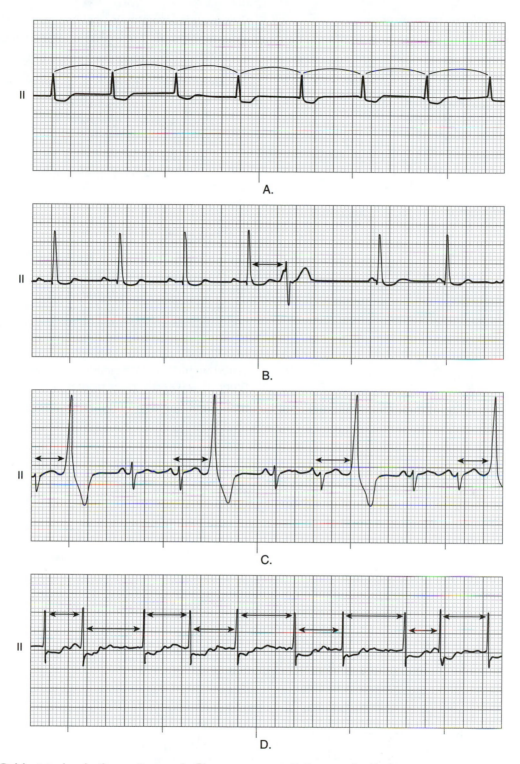

Figure 6–6 Ventricular rhythm patterns. A. Shows constant R-R intervals. B. Shows an intermittently irregular or occasionally irregular variation in R-R intervals. C. Shows regularly irregular intervals—every third R-R interval is premature. D. Irregular intervals in which no pattern exists.

below the ECG baseline because it signifies a disorder in cardiac energy flow that can be associated with ischemia, injury, or caused by medication. The ST segment corresponds to the early phase of ventricular

repolarization. Normally, ST segments may be up to 1 mm above or below the ECG baseline (using the TP segment as a reference mark). Figure 6-9 shows several examples of abnormal ST segments. ST segment

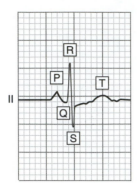

Figure 6–7 QRS duration. This QRS duration is within normal limits.

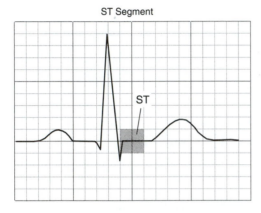

Figure 6–8 ST segments should normally be isoelectric, meaning flat in comparison to the tP interval or PR segment. The J point is where the end of the S wave joins the ST segment.

abnormalities have major patient care implications and will be discussed in considerable detail later in the book.

> **Clinical Note:** *An ST segment abnormality observed in a single rhythm strip lead can raise suspicion of myocardial ischemia or injury—but only a twelve-lead ECG can indicate clinically significant ST findings.*

Evaluation of Atrial Activity

In step three, atrial activity is evaluated in the same way as was done for ventricular activity. First, confirm that atrial activity is present. If P waves are missing, the rhythm must have originated outside of the sinus node such as in the atria or other pacemaker area. If atrial activity is missing entirely, yet the ventricular complexes look normal, the pacemaker must have originated within the AV junction, as shown in Figure 6–10. When P waves are present they are inspected to see if they have a consistent shape within the same lead because changing shapes indicate shifts in the pacemaker's location.

Atrial rate

The normal atrial rate in adults is between 60 and 100/minute and the atrial rate should match the ventricular rate. If this is not the case, some P waves are not being conducted.

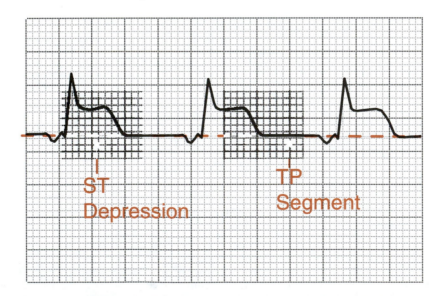

Figure 6–9 ST segment abnormalities. A. Shows 3 mm ST segment elevation. B. Shows 3 mm ST segment depression. The TP segment is used as the reference point to compare the ST segment to the ECG baseline.

Table 6–3 QT Interval: Upper Limits of Normal

Heart rate per minute	Men and Children (Second)	Women (Second)
40	0.49	0.50
45	0.47	0.48
50	0.45	0.46
55	0.43	0.44
60	0.42	0.43
65	0.40	0.42
70	0.39	0.41
75	0.38	0.39
80	0.37	0.38
85	0.36	0.37
90	0.35	0.36
95	0.35	0.36
100	0.34	0.35

Reprinted from Lipman, B. C. and Casclo, T: ECG Assessment and Interpretation: FA Davis Company, Philadelphia, PA, 1994. Table 3-3, p.56.

Atrial Rhythm

In NSR, all P-P intervals will be the same except for a slight beat-to-beat variation due to the influence of the respiratory cycle on sinus node regularity. Irregular rhythms have one of three patterns:

a) *Intermittently irregular pattern.* A generally regular rhythm is occasionally disrupted such as by an early or missing beat. Premature complexes are the most frequent cause of occasionally disrupted P-P intervals.

b) *Regularly irregular pattern.* The P-P intervals change in a recurring pattern. One type of regularly irregular pattern is the waxing-waning rhythm associated with the respiratory cycle. The P-P intervals rhythmically increase and decrease.

c) *Irregularly irregular pattern.* No consistent atrial rhythm exists. Instead, the regular P-P pattern of NSR is replaced by a grossly irregular atrial rhythm. One of the most common causes of an irregularly irregular pattern is caused by a dysrhythmia termed atrial fibrillation that will be explained in a later chapter.

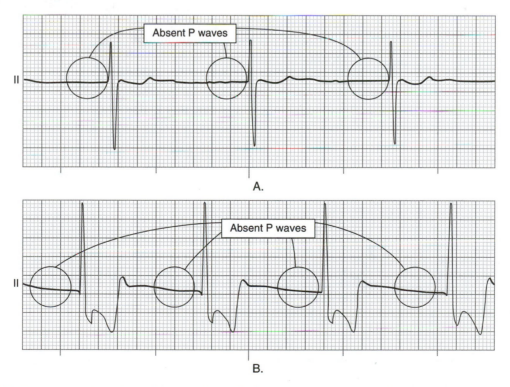

Figure 6–10 AV junctional rhythms. In strips A and B, P waves are absent and the baselines are flat. Atrial activity is lacking.

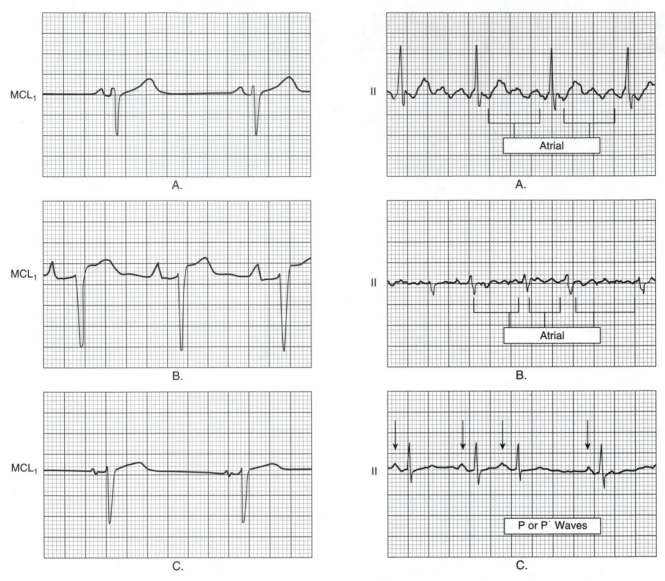

Figure 6-11 P waves in lead MCL₁. The shape of the P wave normally is variable: it may be upright (A), pointed (B), or biphasic (C).

Figure 6-12 Atrial wave shapes. A. P waves have been replaced by rapid, regular atrial ("flutter") waves. B. Rapid, irregular atrial ("fibrillatory") waves. C. The third beat is a notched, ectopic atrial (P′) wave.

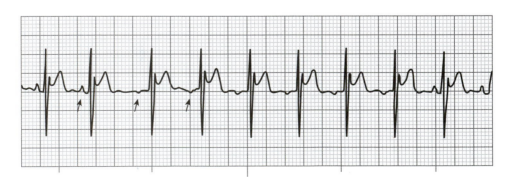

Figure 6-13 Alterations in P wave shapes in the same lead indicates a shift in pacemaker location.

P Wave Shape

In normal sinus rhythm P waves regularly occur and have identical shapes. The P wave appearance varies in different ECG leads but is always the same within a single lead. In lead II, P waves appear as small, positive deflections and usually have a rounded, slightly uneven shape. In lead MCL$_1$, P waves typically have a positive as well as a negative component (Figure 6–11). Abnormal waves, such as **fibrillatory (f) waves**, **flutter (F) waves**, or **P prime (P′) waves**, indicate that the atrial rhythm developed outside the sinus node. Figure 6-12 shows examples of these distorted atrial waves. Sudden changes in the P wave shape in one lead indicates a change in pacemaker location (Figure 6–13).

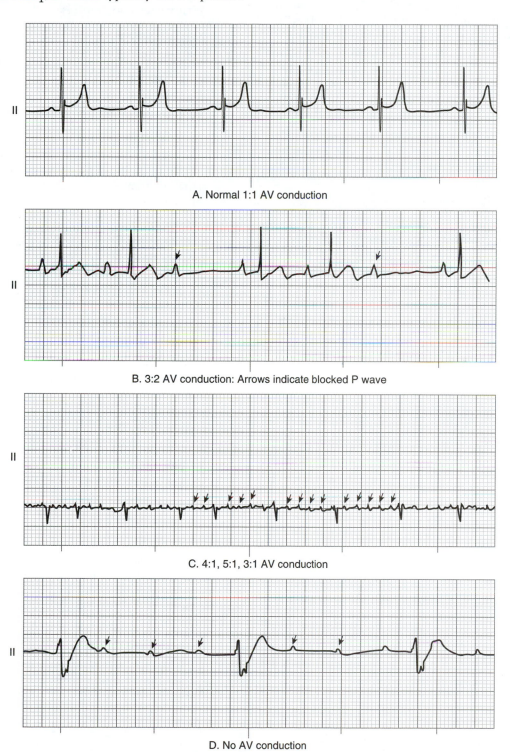

A. Normal 1:1 AV conduction

B. 3:2 AV conduction: Arrows indicate blocked P wave

C. 4:1, 5:1, 3:1 AV conduction

D. No AV conduction

Figure 6–14 Examples of different atrioventricular conduction patterns.

Evaluation of the AV Relationship

In step four, information about AV conduction is determined by evaluating the relationship between the P waves and the QRS complexes.

PR Interval

The PR interval is measured from the start of the P wave until the beginning of the QRS complex. The PR interval records the time required for the sinus impulse to begin activating the atria until the ventricles start becoming stimulated. The PR intervals should be constant from beat-to-beat and should not exceed 0.20 second. A common ECG disturbance occurs when the PR interval is prolonged or greater than 0.20 second. The cause of PR interval prolongation is a delay in the conduction velocity through the AV node which delays the start of ventricular activation.

A-V Conduction Ratios

In normal sinus rhythm, every P wave is quickly followed by a QRS complex. This is termed 1:1 AV conduction ratio and means that a single P wave is associated with each QRS complex. When there are more P waves than QRS complexes, some P waves were not conducted. For instance, AV conduction ratios of 2:1 or 3:1 mean that two P waves exist for each QRS complex, or that three P waves are present for each QRS complex, respectively. Figure 6-14 shows examples of abnormal AV conduction.

Let's Review

1. ECG assessment is easier when an organized plan is followed. The systematic approach presented begins with an overall assessment of the ECG tracing to detect obvious abnormalities, along with identifying waves and complexes. A general inspection identifies areas of the ECG tracing that need closer inspection later.

2. Ventricular activity is assessed in regard to rate, rhythm, shape, duration, QT interval, and ST segment analysis. Normal QRS complexes consist of narrow shapes with sharp waves and a constant shape.

3. Normal QRS durations are less than 0.12 second. Narrow QRS complexes indicate that a supraventricular pacemaker must be present.

4. Wide QRS complexes with durations of 0.12 second or greater indicate that there was a delay in the ventricles. In wide QRS complexes, the beat represents either a supraventricular impulse that followed an abnormal ventricular path, or one that has a ventricular pacemaker.

5. A normal QT interval depends on the heart rate. When the heart rate is between 50 and 100/minute, a normal QT interval is 0.40 +/− 0.06 second.

6. There is no need to memorize normal QT intervals as reference tables are available and most ECG machines automatically calculate the QT interval and correct the value based on the heart rate (QT_C).

7. Prolonged QT intervals may lead to rapid, unstable ventricular dysrhythmias.

8. Ventricular rhythm patterns can be regular or irregular. Irregular rhythms are described as intermittently irregular, regularly irregular, or irregularly irregular. The rhythm pattern often aids in the identification of the dysrhythmia.

9. Abnormal ST segments are commonly caused by myocardial ischemia and injury, but they may also be due to drugs, premature beats, and bundle branch blocks.

10. Some dysrhythmias involve cardiac rate disorders. Bradycardic rhythms have rates less than 60/minute. Tachycardic rhythms have rates above 100/minute.

11. The ST segment is the area of the ECG complex that starts at the end of the QRS complex until the T wave begins. Normal ST segments are generally flat and are within 1 mm above or below the ECG baseline. An abnormal ST segment may be elevated or depressed greater than 1mm from the baseline. The TP segment is used as the baseline reference point.

12. P wave shapes vary depending on the lead being viewed. P waves in lead II are positive, while in lead MCL_1, P waves can be positive, negative, or biphasic (partly negative and positive).

13. Atrial rhythms can be regular or irregular. Irregular rhythms may be regularly irregular, irregularly irregular, or intermittently irregular.

14. AV conduction is assessed by measuring the PR interval and evaluating the AV conduction ratio.

15. The PR interval reflects the time for a sinus impulse to stimulate the atria, exit the AV node, and begin ventricular activation. Normal PR intervals range from 0.12 to 0.20 second and are constant from beat-to-beat.

16. Prolonged PR intervals are greater than 0.20 second and indicate that conduction through the AV node is prolonged.

17. The normal AV conduction ratio is 1:1, which signifies that there is a single P wave for each QRS complex. AV conduction ratios that are greater than 1:1 indicate that one or more atrial impulses have been blocked from reaching the ventricle. AV conduction ratios greater than 1:1 are common findings in AV heart blocks.

Glossary

Atrioventricular conduction ratio Number of P waves relative to the number of QRS complexes.

Bradycardia Rate Cardiac activity that is slower than normal (below 60/minute).

Cardiac output Amount of blood pumped by the heart in one minute.

Fibrillatory (f) waves Abnormal atrial waves occurring in atrial fibrillation.

Flutter (F) waves Abnormal atrial waves occurring in atrial flutter.

Isoelectric baseline Portion of the ECG tracing that is flat and neither elevated or depressed compared with the TP segment.

Normal sinus rhythm (NSR) Regular pattern of the cardiac conduction cycle originating in the sinus node at a rate between 60 and 100 beats per minute.

P prime (p′) waves Abnormal P waves signifying sinus pacemakers.

QTc interval A QT interval that has been corrected based on the heart rate.

ST segment abnormality Abnormally elevated or depressed segment greater than 1 mm from the ECG baseline (compared with the TP segment).

Supraventricular Beat that arises above the ventricles but is not sinus in origin.

Tachycardia Cardiac activity that is faster than normal (above 100/minute).

TP segment Represents the ECG baseline and is the area from the end of the T wave until the following P wave starts. This area is used to judge whether the ST segment is elevated or depressed.

chapter 7

Systematic Interpretation of Dysrhythmias: Step Five

LEARNING OBJECTIVES

Upon completion of this chapter, the reader should be able to:

- *Describe the sequence of assessment steps needed to form dysrhythmia interpretation.*

- *Apply the systematic analysis format to sample ECG tracings that contain dysrhythmias and determine how each rhythm disorder differs from NSR.*

- *Given sample ECG tracings having wide QRS complex rhythms, identify those that developed from a supraventricular pacemaker but have abnormal ventricular conduction.*

- *Given sample ECG tracings having wide QRS complex rhythms, identify those that developed from a ventricular pacemaker site.*

- *Given sample ECG tracings showing narrow QRS complex rhythms, identify whether each developed from a sinus, atrial, or junctional pacemaker site.*

- *Given sample ECG tracings containing extra P waves, assess the AV relationship.*

CHAPTER OVERVIEW

In Chapter 6, the first four steps of a systematic interpretation approach to evaluating ECG tracings was presented. Now the information that was collected in those steps will be analyzed and assembled into an explanation of the type of abnormal cardiac rhythm present. The focus of this chapter is to learn to detect how ECG tracings differ from normal sinus rhythm. Naming the particular dysrhythmia is not important at this point as specific interpretation skills will be developed in the rest of this book. Many examples of abnormal cardiac rhythms will be shown, and the ways in which the dysrhythmia differs from NSR will be discussed.

According to Chapter 6's "Systematic Approach to ECG Interpretation," step one involved a general inspection and identification of individual waves. During step two, ventricular activity was assessed, while atrial activity was evaluated in step three. In step four the AV relationship was studied. This chapter begins with step five: putting the information together to determine how the ECG tracing differs from NSR.

THE NEXT STEP

Chapter 6 showed how the initial steps of the systematic approach aided in gathering information by evaluating all parts of the ECG tracing. Now, the data obtained are used to determine how the tracing compares to NSR. A specific interpretation is not expected at this point, yet many basic concepts about ECG analysis have already been mastered. In later parts of the book, these data will allow a specific interpretation to be formed to account for the rhythm disturbance.

For now, only the general interpretation process will be discussed. The assessment in this section seems too brief, but this material is intended as a general overview. The specifics of dysrhythmia interpretation will be mastered in subsequent chapters.

In steps one through four information is evaluated by looking at different parts of the ECG: inspecting the P waves, QRS complexes, AV conduction ratios, pauses, rates, rhythms, or other abnormalities. Now, in step five, these details need to be assembled to account for the abnormal cardiac rhythm. If there are no ECG variations when compared to NSR—the yardstick by which all tracings are compared—then the ECG tracing must be normal and the assessment is complete. More likely, in emergency cardiac care cases, the rhythm will differ in one or more ways from normal sinus rhythm, so the dysrhythmia needs to be identified. Dysrhythmias mainly differ from NSR in four general ways: the rhythm may be faster than NSR, slower than NSR, the tracing may have more P waves than NSR, or it may be irregular.

> *ECG Interpretation Tip:* *ECG Interpretations need to convey as much pertinent information as possible, including the rate, the mechanism of the cardiac rhythm, the pacemaker site(s), and the conduction*

activity. The description also needs to account for all abnormal findings such as fast rates, slow rates, wide complexes, absent waves, and extra P waves.

Comparing ECG Tracings to NSR

At this point, the reader should be able to calculate cardiac rates, measure PR intervals and QRS durations, determine AV conduction ratios, and identify general deviations from NSR. The first example is Figure 7–1.

Example #1 (Figure 7–1)

■ *Step 1: General Inspection.* The sample ECG tracing looks very different from NSR because the rhythm is irregular, there are extra P waves, and the ventricular rate is slow. During the next three steps additional information will be gained. See Figure 7–1 Answer.

■ *Step 2: Ventricular Activity.* The QRS complexes are narrow (0.10 second) and have an irregular rhythm that is slow (45/minute). The rate is calculated by noting the number of QRS complexes in the six-second strip and multiplying by 10 to obtain the minute rate. (Note that the rate *cannot* be calculated by using the number of ECG boxes separating two P waves—the P-P interval—because the rhythm is irregular.) The ST segment is also noted to be depressed below the baseline.

■ *Step 3: Atrial Activity.* All P waves are upright and have the same shape. The P wave rate is 75 per minute and is obtained by dividing the number of large ECG boxes separating two P waves—the P-P

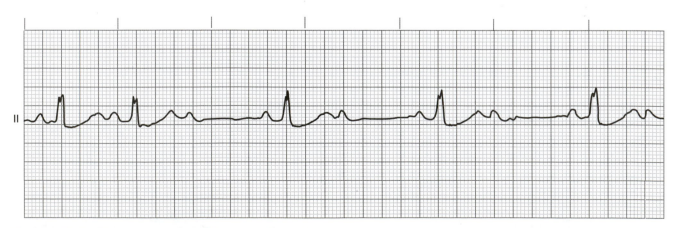

Figure 7-1 The first sample ECG tracing for analysis.

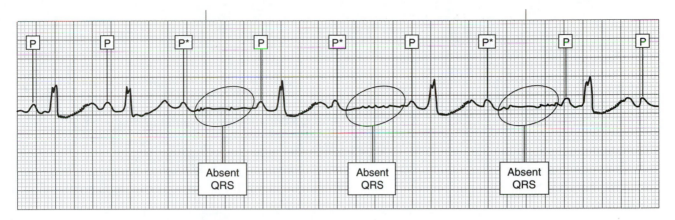

Figure 7–1 Answer (P* indicates nonconducted P waves.)

interval—into 300 (which is the rate of ECG boxes per minute). Since there are four large ECG boxes making up the PR interval, 300 divided by 4 is equal to 75/minute. The rhythm is regular because the P-P intervals are constant.

■ *Step 4: AV Relationship.* The PR interval is 0.24 second—longer than expected if this was NSR (0.20 second). The PR intervals are constant but not every P wave is linked to a QRS complex (Figure 7–1 Answer). During the later half of the tracing there are two P waves for each QRS. The AV conduction ratio for the last three QRS complexes is 2:1, meaning that there were two P waves for each QRS. In contrast, NSR always has an AV conduction ratio of 1:1.

■ *Step 5: Interpretation/ Reasoning.* Let's look at how the tracing differs from NSR: since extra P waves are found without associated QRS complexes, some type of nonconduction exists. Conduction disorders usually occur in, or below, the AV node. The ven-

tricular rate is less than 60 per minute so the term bradycardia is used, yet the atrial rate is normal. The QRS complexes are narrow so the ventricular complexes must have developed from a supraventricular pacemaker. The PR interval is longer than expected for a NSR so a transmission delay of the sinus impulses is present. (This dysrhythmia will be explained in subsequent chapters as a second degree AV heart block.)

Example #2 (Figure 7–2)

■ *Step 1: General Inspection.* The overall rhythm is very irregular and the rate is rapid.

■ *Step 2: Ventricular Activity.* The QRS complexes are narrow (0.06 to 0.08 second) and the rhythm is grossly irregular. No set pattern for the R-R intervals exists—they are grossly irregular. The ST segments are depressed 3 mm below the baseline and have a "scooped out" or rounded appearance. The

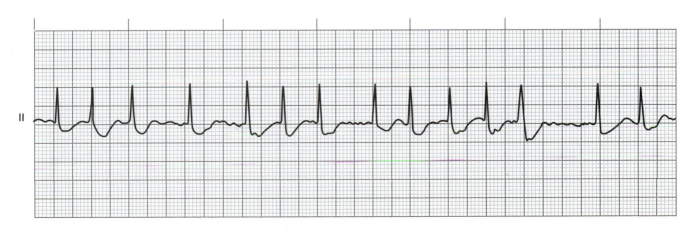

Figure 7–2 The second sample tracing for analysis.

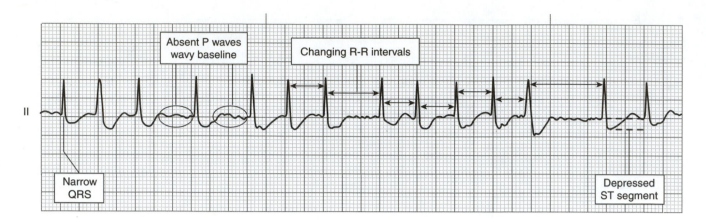

Figure 7–2 Answer The key ECG findings are labeled.

QT interval is 0.34 second, which is normal. (See Figure 7–2 Answer.)

- *Step 3: Atrial Activity.* P waves are absent. Instead, a fine wavy, almost flat (isoelectric) baseline exists.

- *Step 4: AV Relationship.* Neither a PR interval or an AV conduction ratio can be determined because distinct atrial activity cannot be found.

- *Step 5: Interpretation/Reasoning.* The narrow QRS duration indicates that intraventricular conduction is normal. The pacemaker impulse must have originated from a supraventricular focus, that is, from either a sinus, atrial, or AV junctional pacemaker. The absence of P waves rules out the sinus node as the pacemaker. (The grossly irregular ventricular rhythm shown in this example is typical of a dysrhythmia termed atrial fibrillation, which will be studied in a later chapter. Like wise, the ST segment depression is clinically important and may indicate ischemia or be due to medication. These

findings will be explored in later chapters.)

Example #3 (Figure 7–3)

- *Step 1: General Inspection.* The tracing does not have an organized pattern and looks chaotic.

- *Step 2: Ventricular Activity.* No organized ventricular activity exists. Instead, the ECG baseline has an irregular "zigzag" appearance with constantly changing sizes and shapes.

- *Step 3: Atrial Activity.* Organized atrial activity is not seen.

- *Step 4: AV Relationship.* An AV relationship cannot be detected because neither atrial nor ventricular complexes are present.

- *Step 5: Interpretation/Reasoning.* No organized cardiac activity exists. Since NSR displays regular and coordinated cardiac activity, this example repre-

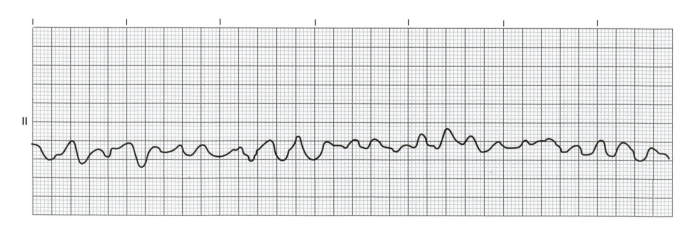

Figure 7–3 The third example for analysis.

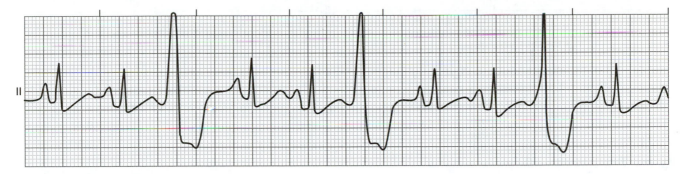

Figure 7–4 The fourth example for analysis.

sents the opposite extreme. (This ECG tracing occurs during cardiac arrests and is termed ventricular fibrillation—the leading cause of sudden cardiac death. Unless the erratic heart activity can be quickly corrected, heart muscle will soon die.)

Example #4 (Figure 7–4)

■ *Step 1: General Inspection.* The rhythm is irregular but a pattern exists. Two different types of ECG beats are present, some of which are narrow and others that are wide and distorted (Figure 7–4 Answer).

■ *Step 2: Ventricular Activity.* The rhythm is regularly irregular and the rate is just over 90/minute. The third beat of each group is early and distorted. The R-R intervals are regular except when the distorted complexes appear. Some of the QRS complexes are tall, wide, and bizarre. No P waves accompany the tall, early beats (beats # 3, 6, 9). All of the other beats have narrow QRS complexes. The ST seg-

ments of the narrow beats are depressed 2–3 mm, while the ST segments of the distorted beats are depressed 10 mm. The T waves of the early, wide beats occur in a direction opposite to the QRS complex.

■ *Step 3: Atrial Activity.* Regular atrial activity is seen before the narrow beats, but P waves are not seen before the early beats (# 3, 6, and 9).

■ *Step 4: AV Relationship.* The AV conduction is 1:1 conduction for the majority of beats—the ones with narrow QRS complexes. The distorted early beats with wide QRS complexes lack P waves, so an AV conduction ratio does not exist.

■ *Step 5: Interpretation/Reasoning.* Aside from the irregular rhythm caused by the early beats, the ECG resembles a normal sinus rhythm. The wide QRS complexes have distorted shapes and lack P waves which is evidence that they arose from a ventricular pacemaker. Since P waves are absent, the sinus node cannot be the pacemaker for the early beats,

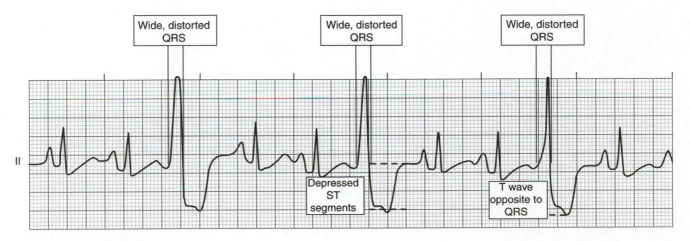

Figure 7–4 Answer

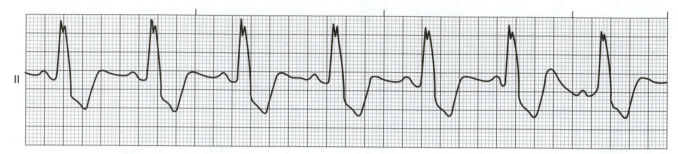

Figure 7–5 The fifth example for analysis.

and further argues in favor of their development within the ventricles. (These early beats are termed premature ventricular complexes, which is a logical description. The early discharge of these beats often results from an irritable pacemaker site within the ventricles.)

Example #5 (Figure 7–6)

■ *Step 1: General Assessment.* The overall pattern is regular with wide, distorted QRS complexes (Figure 7–5 Answer).

■ *Step 2: Ventricular Activity.* The R-R intervals are regular. The QRS complexes are notched and the duration is beyond the normal value of 0.12 second. The ventricular rate is 65/minute and the ST segments are depressed 8–10 mm below the ECG baseline. The T waves are inverted and it is difficult to tell where the QRS complex ends and the ST segment begins. The QRS duration cannot be accurately measured but it is abnormal and well over 0.16 second.

■ *Step 3: Atrial Activity.* The shapes of the P waves

are consistent and upright as expected in lead II. The atrial rate is equal to the ventricular rate. The P-P intervals are regular, indicating that the sinus node is normally discharging.

■ *Step 4: AV Relationship.* The PR interval is normal. Each QRS is preceded by a single P wave and each P wave is followed by one QRS complex, indicating a normal AV relationship.

■ *Step 5: Interpretation/Reasoning.* The sinus pacemaker activates the heart in a normal manner at a rate that is within the normal range (60 to 100/minute) for normal sinus rhythm. The wide and notched QRS complexes indicate that ventricular conduction is abnormal. (This is a common type of intraventricular conduction defect termed a bundle branch block. The significance of a bundle branch block will be described in a later chapter.)

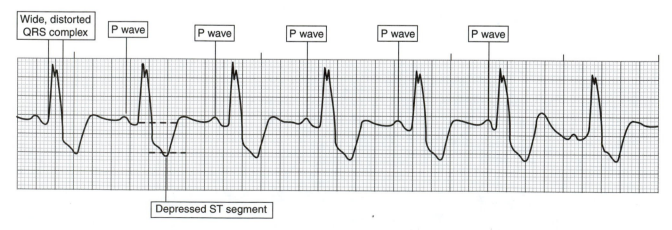

Figure 7–5 Answer The key findings of a wide QRS complex rhythm with associated P waves labelled.

MORE PRACTICE ECG TRACINGS

In the last section of this chapter, the analysis of the ECG tracings was provided; now the reader needs to apply the same steps that were used for the five examples to these practice tracings. The goal is to note the way(s) in which the practice tracings differ from normal sinus rhythm. Specific dysrhythmia interpretations are not expected. Answers are provided in Appendix A.

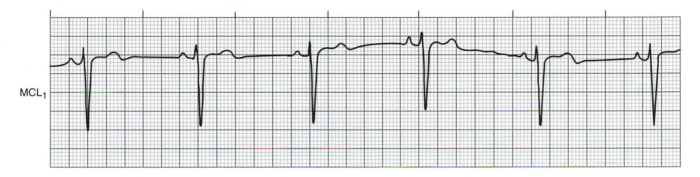

Figure 7-6 The sixth example for analysis.

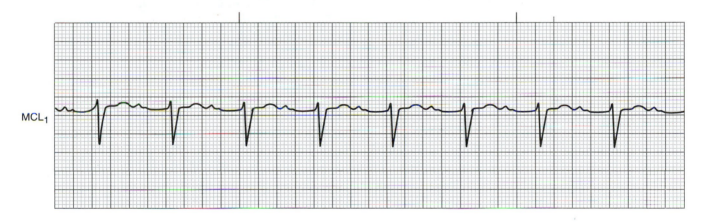

Figure 7-7 Example #7

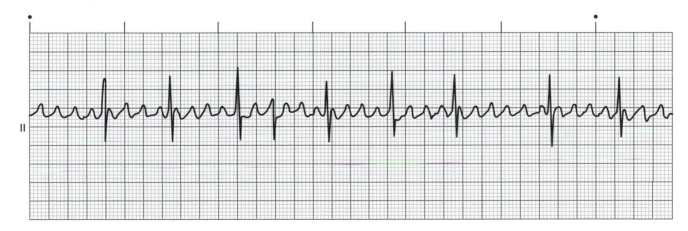

Figure 7-8 Example #8

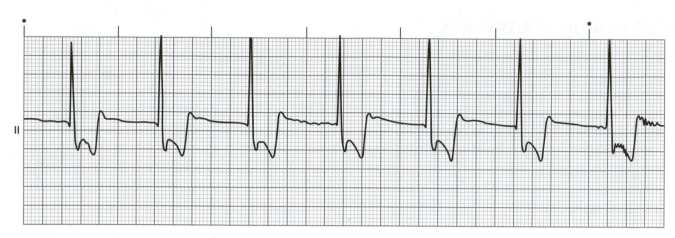

Figure 7-9 Example #9

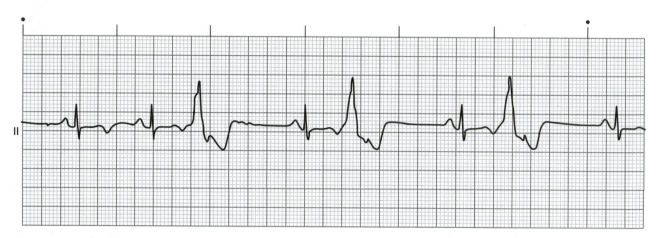

Figure 7-10 Example #10

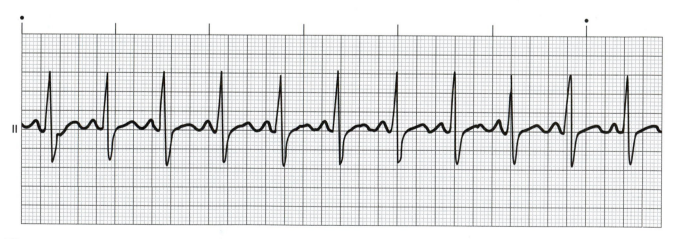

Figure 7-11 Example #11

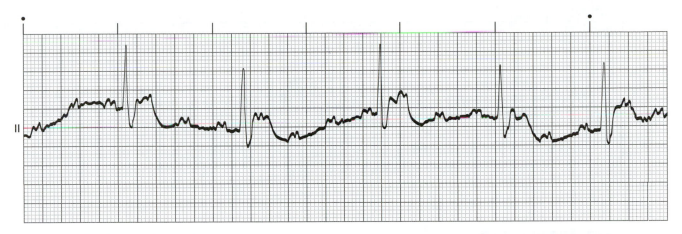

Figure 7–12   Example #12

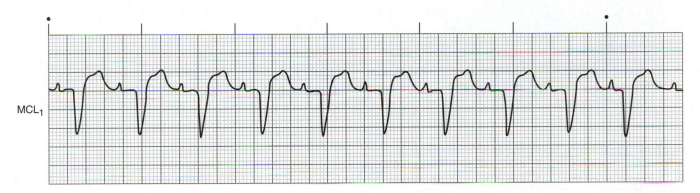

Figure 7–13   Example #13

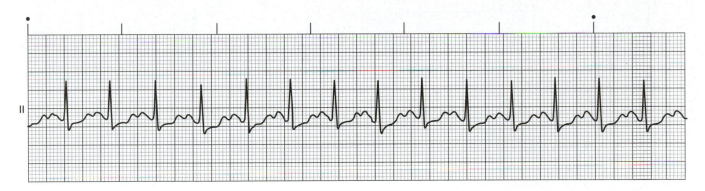

Figure 7–14   Example #14

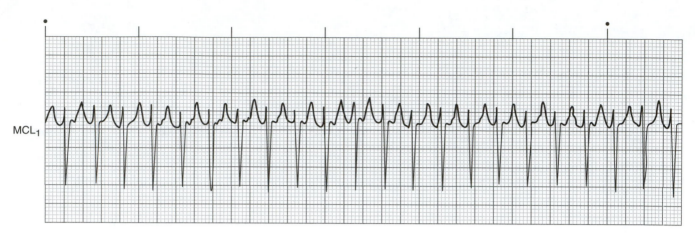

Figure 7–15 Example #15

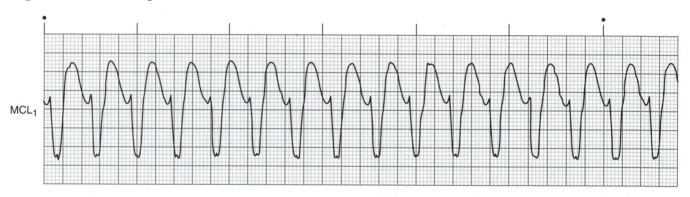

Figure 7–16 Example #16

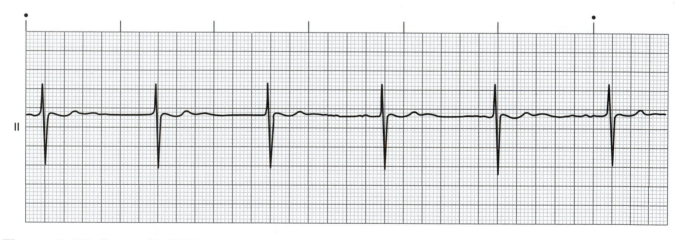

Figure 7–17 Example #17

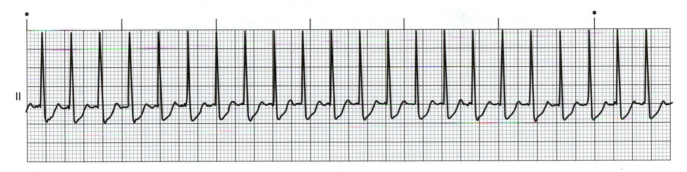

Figure 7–18 Example #18

Let's Review

1. The systematic assessment approach to ECG interpretation helps to develop a consistent technique to follow when faced with any type of rhythm disorder.

2. Abnormal ECG tracings can be analyzed by looking for the ways in which they differ from NSR, including abnormalities in rate, pacemaker sites, P wave shapes, PR intervals, QRS durations, ST segments, and conduction ratios.

3. ECG interpretations are complete if they convey the pacemaker site, conduction activity, atrial and ventricular rates, and the clinical effect of the dysrhythmia on the patient's condition.

4. The last step in our standardized approach involves evaluating the patient in order to evaluate the effect that a dysrhythmia is having on a patient's condition.

Systematic Interpretation of Dysrhythmia: Step Six

LEARNING OBJECTIVES

Upon completion of this chapter, the reader should be able to:

■ *Describe the importance of assessing the clinical effects of a dysrhythmia in addition to identifying the abnormal cardiac rhythm.*

■ *Name the four general patient-types who experience dysrhythmias.*

■ *Discuss the relationship between stroke volume and heart rate.*

■ *List two determinants of cardiac output.*

■ *Explain the term peripheral vascular resistance.*

■ *Discuss how peripheral vascular resistence relates to arterial blood pressure.*

■ *Describe the effect of myocardial ischemia on cardiac contractility.*

■ *Describe the mechanisms by which impaired tissue perfusion can result from the following types of dysrhythmias: slow, fast, and irregular.*

■ *List five clinical findings associated with hemodynamic compromise.*

■ *List three dysrhythmias that are unstable rhythms because they are prone to sudden deterioration.*

■ *Name two dysrhythmias that occur in patients who are not in cardiac arrest but who require immediate treatment to prevent clinical deterioration.*

■ *Name two dysrhythmias that can safely wait up to several hours before therapy becomes effective.*

■ *List three dysrhythmias that are associated with stable vital signs, are not likely to deteriorate, and do not require urgent therapy.*

CHAPTER OVERVIEW

This chapter concentrates on the sixth and final step outlined in the "Systematic Interpretation of Dysrhythmias": determining the clinical significance of the abnormal cardiac rhythm. The earlier steps were described in the chapters 6 and 7. Regardless of where the patient is being assessed, whether in the field, the emergency department, or in a critical care unit, a standard clinical assessment evaluation such as that taught in the American Heart Association's Advanced Cardiac Life Support course is followed. Evaluating the patient with a dysrhythmia entails obtaining a thorough patient history and physical examination. Symptoms and physical findings yield clues to the seriousness of the disordered cardiac rhythm. The clinical significance of each dysrhythmia depends on how a rhythm disturbance affects a patient's well-being. If a dysrhythmia causes clinical consequences, how rapidly treatment must be started will be discussed.

ASSESSING THE CLINICAL EFFECTS OF A DYSRHYTHMIA

Having completed an evaluation of the ECG tracing, the next step is to assess the clinical effects caused by a dysrhythmia.* Once the clinical assessment is completed, treatment options can be considered.

Patients tolerate dysrhythmias in very different ways and display a wide variety of presentations—from being asymptomatic while experiencing a physiologic dysrhythmia such as sinus bradycardia in a marathon runner, to mild distress occurring in the young woman experiencing a supraventricular tachycardia and complaining of palpitations. At the other extreme, a patient can be in a shock owing to a very rapid or irregular dysrhythmia. Identical dysrhythmias are often experienced quite differently by two patients. This explains why there is no simple answer to the question, "How should this dysrhythmia be treated?" The answer is "well..., it depends." It depends primarily on how well the patient is tolerating the dysrhythmia and the inherent stability of the dysrhythmia, that is, how likely is the rhythm disorder to deteriorate. For instance, does the patient appear comfortable with stable vital signs, or is the patient hypotensive and having labored breathing? ECG interpretation must take place simultaneously with patient assessment in order to determine the need for emergency interventions.

*All patient care first begins with assessing the patient, but it is stressed that the patient with a dysrhythmia is continuously evaluated.

> **Clinical Note:** *"Treat the patient, not the monitor" is an important clinical adage. Regardless of the dysrhythmia, the crucial concern is how well the patient is tolerating the abnormal rhythm. The patient's clinical status will largely determine how rapidly the dysrhythmia needs to be treated.*
> *In emergency cardiac care, the answer to this question often determines whether medication or electrical shock therapy is initially used.*

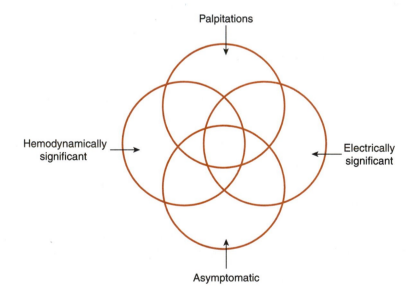

Figure 8-1 Four patient populations with dysrhythmias. The palpitations group includes patients who are aware of their heartbeat. The electrically significant group involves dysrhythmias that have the capability to abruptly deteriorate into life-threatening rhythms. The hemodynamically significant group involves patients who experience a fall in cardiac output or an increase in myocardial oxygen demand. The asymptomatic group feels well and is unaware of their abnormal hearth rhythm. There is an overlap between different groups. (Modified with permission from Ramo, BW, The patient history in Waugh, RA, Wagner GS, Ramo, BW, Gilbert, M (eds.). Cardiac Arrhythmias: A Practical Guide for the Clinician 2nd ed. Philadelphia: FA Davis Publishers. 1994: 34, Figure 2–1.)

HOW PATIENTS EXPERIENCE DYSRHYTHMIAS

The following two sections are based on the excellent discussion presented in Barry Ramo's chapter "The Patient History" in *Cardiac Dysrhythmias: A Practical Guide for the Clinician* (2nd ed. Waugh, R.A., et. al., eds. Philadelphia: FA Davis Publishers, 1994.).

There are four general patient-types who experience dysrhythmias. Three of the patient groups overlap as shown in Figure 8-1—those with palpitations, those who have an electrically significant response, and those who develop a hemodynamically significant response. Patients who are not experiencing symptoms or clinical consequences are generally unaware of their dysrhythmias.

Patients Having Palpitations

This patient group has one of the most common cardiac symptoms and typically occurs with rapid, slow, or irregular heart rhythms. Palpitations may occur with both minor and major dysrhythmias. Patients with **palpitations** become aware of their heart beating. Figure 8-2 illustrates a rhythm abnormality that commonly causes patients to sense "skipped beats."

Patients Having an Electrically Significant Response

The group of patients experiencing **electrically significant responses** to dysrhythmias have the potential to deteriorate into unstable ventricular tachydysrhythmias that may lead to shock or even death. Figure 8–3 is an example of a disrhythmia causing a patient to show signs and symptoms of a serious condition—overlapping with the hemodynamically significant group—as it can abruptly lead to cardiac arrest.

Patients Having a Hemodynamically Significant Responses

The group of patients experiencing **hemodynamically significant responses** to dysrhythmias usually have a decreased cardiac output. Dysrhythmias that cause hemodynamic consequences cause significant signs and symptoms, including shortness of breath, pul-

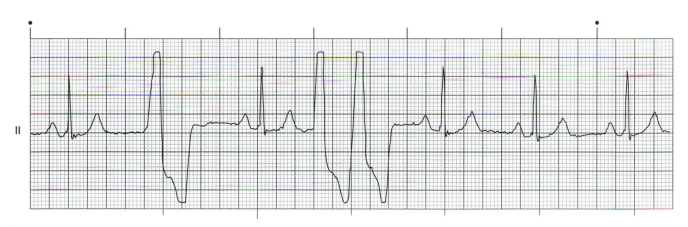

II

Figure 8–2 This irregular rhythm usually causes palpitations, but is electrically and hemodynamically stable.

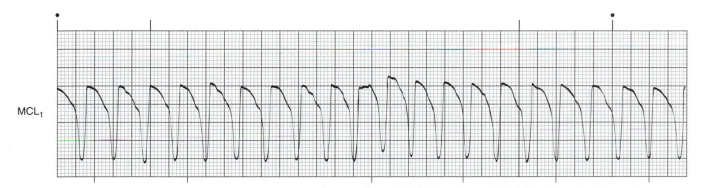

MCL₁

Figure 8–3 Thisvery fast, wide QRS complex rhythm usually belongs in both the electrically and hemodynamically unstable groups.

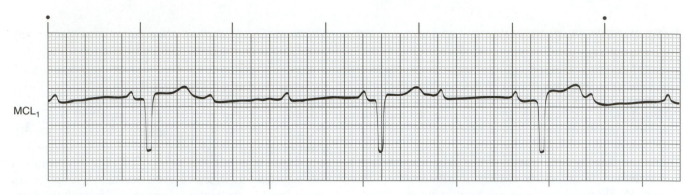

Figure 8–4 This very slow rhythm with missing QRS complexes can cause hemodynamic and electrical instability.

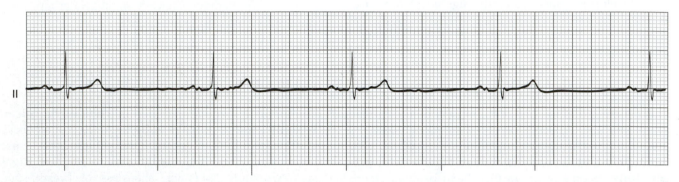

Figure 8–5 This slow, regular, narrow QRS complex tracing may or may not produce hemodynamically unstable symptoms and signs (The notched shape of the P waves is an incidental finding).

monary congestion, ischemic chest pain, near-syncope, pallor, and diaphoresis. Such dysrhythmias may cause an increase in myocardial oxygen demand due to the rapid heart rate. Heart failure, syncope, fatigue, confusion, and angina may also be associated with the hemodynamically significant patient group. Figure 8–4 shows an ECG tracing that is usually associated with a marked fall in cardiac output due to slow ventricular rate and the loss of coordination between the atria and ventricles. Figure 8–5 shows a slow heartbeat that may cause fatigue and weakness but usually does not cause serious hemodynamic compromise. The rate is slower than normal, but the rhythm is usually associated with an adequate cardiac output.

DYSRHYTHMIA MECHANISMS RELATED TO SYMPTOMS

The signs and symptoms caused by a dysrhythmia are determined by the type of dysrhythmia as well as the patient's underlying physical and general medical condition. A dysrhythmia's characteristics involve how fast, slow, or irregular the rhythm is and whether atrioventricular coordination is maintained. Important patient characteristics depend on the **intravascular volume** (whether the patient is dehydrated or fluid overloaded), age, since infants and the elderly have less tolerance to

abnormal rhythms, and the presence of underlying coronary artery disease. If a patient has serious coronary artery disease or congestive heart failure, even a modest increase in heart rate can cause angina and shortness of breath.

Patient characteristics and dysrhythmia characteristics interact to preserve or disturb hemodynamic well being. These factors account for the finding that distinctly different dysrhythmias can cause similar symptoms, while identical dysrhythmias can cause markedly different symptoms. Some patients are able to tolerate a rapid supraventricular dysrhythmia for days while others become acutely short of breath after only a few hours.

Symptoms and physical signs caused by dysrhythmias include:

■ *Near-syncope and fainting.* **Syncope** is a loss of consciousness due to inadequate blood flow to the brain. Slow rhythms and those with prolonged cardiac pauses can cause the patient to feel "lightheaded" or dizzy, and to "almost pass out." Likewise, very rapid dysrhythmias can cause the same effects. This near-syncopal state is much more common than actually fainting. It is important to inquire whether the patient lost consciousness while sitting or lying down since this is characteristic of dysrhythmia-related syncope. In contrast, syncope that develops shortly after standing, is often due to non-cardiac factors. It is also helpful to determine whether the patient experienced palpitations before losing conciousness because this also suggests a dysrhythmia cause.

■ *Palpitations.* Often described variously as "thumping," "flip-flopping," "fluttering," "pounding," "skipping," or any other term suggestive of an irregular chest sensation. Palpations can occur with irregular or tachycardic dysrhythmias.

■ *Anxiety and hyperventilation.* These two common findings are associated with dysrhythmias. Since such complaints are often attributed to a benign "nervous" problem, the possibility of a dysrhythmia should be considered.

■ *Weakness and fatigue.* A loss of exercise tolerance such as being able to walk fewer steps or climb less flights of stairs than usual is typical of a dyshrythmia.

■ *Angina.* Angina is an important symptom related to dysrhythmias. Chest pain or discomfort can be caused by fast, slow, or irregular cardiac dysrhythmias, as well as those dysrhythmias causing a loss of atrioventricular coordination. Angina occurs due to the combination of decreased coronary artery perfusion and increased myocardial oxygen need.

■ *Confusion and altered mental status.* An alteration in mental status does not typically result from dysrhythmias but can theoretically occur in elderly patients who have a limited cardiac reserve and borderline cerebral circulation. Impairment of cardiac function caused by a dysrhythmia can cause confusion or lethargy in older patients.

HOW DYSRHYTHMIAS CAUSE A FALL IN CARDIAC OUTPUT

The following concepts help to understand the way in which dysrhythmias can adversely affect a patient's condition by causing a fall in blood pressure that decreases organ perfusion.

■ **Cardiac output** (CO) is the amount of blood pumped by the heart in one minute. Cardiac output is determined by **stroke volume** (SV), which is the amount of blood ejected from the heart with each heart beat, multiplied by the heart rate (HR). For an average 70 kg person, a typical stroke volume is approximately 70 cc, and the resting heart rate is about 70/minute. Since the cardiac output is determined by multiplying the stroke volume by the heart rate, the average cardiac output is determined from the calculation: 70 cc × 70 bpm, which yields a cardiac output of 4900 cc (approximately 5 liters) per minute. The equation that explains the relationship between the different variables is written as:

$$CO = SV \times HR$$

If the heart rate increased from 50 to 80 bpm, for example, while the stroke volume remained fixed at 70 cc, the cardiac output will increase by 2100 cc/minute (50 bpm × 70 cc = 3500 cc compared with 80 bpm × 70 cc = 5600 cc). The increased cardiac output is 2100 cc per minute due to the heart rate rise of 30 beats/minute. Likewise, a decrease in stroke volume from 70 cc to 50 cc, as a patient in heart failure may experience, while the heart rate remains at 70/minute will cause a significant fall in cardiac output by 1400 cc/minute. (The difference in cardiac output is 70 cc × 70/minute = 4900 cc versus 50 cc × 70 bpm = 3500 cc.)

Generally, an increased heart rate will result in a higher cardiac output. There is a unique combination of heart rate and stroke volume for each patient that will result in a maximal cardiac output. However, at fast heart rates (greater than 150/minute), cardiac output can fall, especially in patients with underlying coronary heart disease because the **ventricular filling period** is significantly decreased. As a result of the shortened diastolic filling time, that is the period of ventricular filling during diastole, stroke volume decreases because the ventricles are not maximally filled before contraction. This can occur even in healthy adults when the heart rate exceeds 180/minute, especially if it lasts for several hours.

In people with atherosclerotic heart disease, rates as low as 120/minute are fast enough to cause a diminished cardiac output. At tachycardic rates, the myocardial oxygen demand significantly increases. Very slow heart rates, below 45 beats per minute, can also result in a decreased cardiac output. Although slow heart rates can have an increased stroke volume due to a longer diastolic filling time, this compensatory mechanism is limited. Therefore, dysrhythmias that decrease either stroke volume or heart rate can cause a marked fall in cardiac output.

■ **Arterial blood pressure (BP)** is determined by the cardiac output and **peripheral vascular resist-**

ance (PVR), which is the resistance to blood flow caused by the precapillary arterioles. When a large group of arterioles constrict, such as the blood vessels in the skin, total peripheral vascular resistance increases. When arterioles dilate, resistance decreases and blood flow increases, while arterial pressure diminishes.

■ **Systolic blood pressure and tissue perfusion.** Tissue perfusion can be maintained across a wide range of arterial blood pressures because blood flow **autoregulates**, meaning that tissue and organ blood flow alter in order to maintain an adequate circulation. Hypotension is a late sign of inadequate perfusion and poor hemodynamic status. One of the earliest signs of decreased perfusion is an alteration in mental functioning because the brain is very sensitive to even a small fall in cerebral blood flow. Altered mental states include confusion, anxiousness, and agitation, as well as near-syncope.

Even as cardiac output decreases, blood pressure tends to be sustained, at least temporarily, by peripheral vasoconstriction. Prolonged vasoconstriction contributes to worsening tissue perfusion. Vasoconstriction initially occurs in peripheral tissue, such as the skin, which appears cool and pale. Eventually, core organs, such as the kidneys, brain, heart, and lungs experience decreased blood flow. Prolonged periods of inadequate perfusion, which is termed **shock**, can lead to irreversible cell damage and tissue death.

Cardiac Ischemia

Myocardial ischemia occurs when the oxygen demand by the heart muscle exceeds the oxygen-rich bloodflow supplied by the coronary arteries. Myocardial ischemia further interferes with cardiac contractility. When a dysrhythmia coexists with ischemia, a moderate fall in cardiac output can have a dramatic affect. The heart's oxygen demand is proportional to the myocardial workload: as the heart rate or stroke volume increases, so does the heart muscle's oxygen needs. A tachycardic dysrhythmia increases both myocardial workload and myocardial oxygen demand, which can lead to cardiovascular collapse.

UNSTABLE DYSRHYTHMIAS THAT MAY ABRUPTLY DETERIORATE

Dysrhythmias that cause hemodynamic instability or produce serious symptoms, such as anginal chest pain, shortness of breath, or syncope are inherently unstable and can suddenly deteriorate into an unreliable ven-

tricular tachydysrhythmia. Certain dysrhythmias, even in the absence of hemodynamic instability, are electrically unstable including:

■ advanced forms of atrioventricular (AV) blocks

■ ventricular tachycardia (VT)

These dysrhythmias can suddenly deteriorate into ventricular fibrillation and will be studied in upcoming chapters. Patients with an advanced AV heart block typically develop less efficient backup pacemakers. They have a limited ability to increase their slow heart rates. If the **escape pacemaker** were to suddenly fail, the patient will develop cardiac arrest. In addition, such dysrhythmias often indicate ongoing cardiac ischemia. Rapid ventricular tachycardias can also abruptly progress to cardiac arrest. As a reference tool for review during the upcoming chapters, Table 8–1 lists the clinical effects that different dysrhythmias may have on cardiac output. For instance, a mild sinus bradycardia with a rate in the 50s is almost always well tolerated as is a sinus rhythm with a simple AV block.

EVALUATING THE URGENCY AND NEED FOR TREATMENT

Answering the following questions can aid in assessing the need for treatment and determining how fast the treatment must begin:

■ Does the patient complain of worrisome symptoms, such as shortness of breath, chest pain, dizziness, feeling faint, or a sense of impending doom?

■ What is the patient's mental status? Is the patient lethargic, agitated, confused, or panicky?

■ Is the dysrhythmia occurring during an acute myocardial infarction?

■ How well are the patient's vital organs being perfused? What is the patient's blood pressure? Are there signs of decreased cardiac output, such as cool, clammy, or mottled skin, or is the capillary refill time prolonged beyond 2 seconds, pulmonary congestion, hypotension, or cyanosis present?

■ What is the likelihood that the rhythm will deteriorate in the near future (refer Table 8–1)? Is the dysrhythmia highly unstable such as ventricular tachycardia which is prone to sudden degeneration into cardiac arrest?

Patients who have positive findings to the above questions need careful monitoring and have an urgent need for treatment. In some cases, such as when patients exhibit signs of shock, or who have an altered mental

Table 8-1 Dysrhythmias Classified by Their Effect on Cardiac Output

- **Dysrhythmias with Normal Hemodynamics that are Stable**
  - Sinus rhythm with premature atrial or junctional complexes
  - Artificial pacemaker rhythm with 1:1 capture
  - Atrial fibrillation with an average ventricular response between 60 and 100/minute
  - Atrial flutter with an average ventricular response between 60 and 100/minute
  - Sinus rhythm with first-degree AV block
  - Sinus rhythm with occasional PVCs
  - Sinus bradycardia averaging 50 to 60/minute
  - Sinus arrhythmia
  - AV junctional rhythm averaging 50 to 60/minute
  - Sinus rhythm with second-degree AV block Mobitz Type I
  - Isorhythmic AV dissociation

- **Dysrhythmias with Normal or Near-Normal Hemodynamics that are Potentially Destabilizing**
  - Sinus rhythm with short episodes of ventricular tachycardia (lasting 30 seconds or less)
  - Sinus rhythm with short episodes of PSVT
  - Accelerated junctional rhythms below 100/minute
  - Artificial pacemaker rhythm with frequent PVCs that are multifocal or occur in couplets
  - Sinus rhythm with second-degree AV block Mobitz Type II
  - Atrial flutter or fibrillation with tachycardic ventricular rates
  - Sinus rhythm with sinus arrest
  - Sinus bradycardia with rates below 40/minute

- **Dysrhythmias with Significantly Altered Hemodynamics that are Generally Unstable**
  - Ventricular tachycardia (with pulses) lasting over 30 seconds
  - Sinus rhythm or atrial fibrillation with complete AV heart block
  - Very slow (below 40/minute) sinus, junctional, or idioventricular rhythms
  - Malfunctioning artificial pacemakers with idioventricular escape rhythms

- **Dysrhythmias with Absent Hemodynamics—Lethal Conditions**
  - Ventricular fibrillation
  - Asystole
  - Pulseless ventricular tachycardia or flutter
  - Agonal idioventricular complexes
  - Pulseless electrical activity (Electromechanical dissociation [EMD])
  - Complete AV heart block with ventricular standstill

Classification devised by Fritz Streuli, M.D.

status, immediate therapy is needed. In other cases, therapy can safely wait hours or days. The next section discusses the timing of therapy.

> ***Clinical Note:*** *The need for immediate treat-ment of a dysrhythmia is based on the clinical judgment that the patient's condition is associated with hemodynamic instability, the patient is exhibiting serious symptoms, or an inherently unstable rhythm is present. Emergent treatment must be started immediately to prevent deterioration of the patient's condition.*

Establishing Treatment Priorities

Advanced cardiac life support (ACLS) measures are directed at stabilizing life-threatening dysrhythmias and preventing serious dysrhythmias from deteriorating. Patients with underlying cardiac disease and the elder-ly do not tolerate dysrhythmias for any length of time. On the other hand, patients who are otherwise healthy can tolerate very rapid atrial dysrhythmias for extended periods. In the pre-hospital setting, a major concern is whether the patient can safely wait until arrival in the ED before treatment is started or must it be done at the scene or en route. Treatment by EMS that stabilizes a patient's condition or prevents deterioration in the field is indicated, whereas nonessential therapy is best avoided because treatment prolongs on-scene time, delays ED arrival, and prevents the paramedic unit from being available for other assignments.

Patients in cardiac arrest obviously receive the highest priority and must be treated at once. Immediate treat-ment of an abnormal cardiac rhythm is also indicated in cases where the patient is in shock and cardiac arrest is imminent, such as in an unconscious patient with weak pulses, hypotension or pulmonary edema. Also, patients having an acute myocardial infarction and unstable ventricular dysrhythmias must be treated with-out delay. Early myocardial reperfusion using throm-bolytic agents will salvage myocardium and improve survival but can paradoxically increase the incidence of transient ventricular dysrhythmias. Thrombolytic-associ-ated dysrhythmias are generally responsive to therapy and are a welcome indicator that coronary blood flow has been reestablished.

Let's Review

1. Evaluating the patient always takes precedence over analyzing the ECG.

2. After the ECG has been analyzed, treatment options can be evaluated, taking into consideration the clinical effects that a dysrhythmia is causing and the electrical stability of the dysrhythmia.

3. Dysrhythmias may have no clinical conse-quences, be an incidental finding, produce palpitations, cause hemodynamic compro-mise, or they can be life-threatening.

4. Regardless of the dysrhythmia, the main clinical concern is how well the patient is tolerating the abnormal cardiac rhythm.

5. Whether a dysrhythmia needs to be treated immediately or urgently is based on the dysrhythmia's likelihood of deteriorating into an unstable rhythm and whether hemodynamic compromise is present.

6. At very fast heart rates, cardiac output falls due to the diminished ventricular filling time. At very slow heart rates, cardiac output can also fall.

7. Very irregular and uncoordinated cardiac rhythms can cause a fall in cardiac output due to the loss of atrioventricular coordination.

8. One of the earliest signs of diminished cerebral blood flow is an alteration in mental status. Cerebral function is depend-ent on a constant supply of glucose and oxygen. Even a temporary decrease will cause confusion, agitation, or a loss of consciousness.

9. An ischemic heart causes a fall in cardiac output due to diminished contractility and leads to ventricular dysrhythmias.

10. Emergent therapy of dysrhythmias is indicated when hemodynamic instability, serious symptoms, such as chest pain or shortness of breath, or an inherently unstable cardiac rhythm exists.

Glossary

Advanced cardiac life support (ACLS) measures Treatment measures aimed at stablizing cardiac dysrhythmias and treating acute cardiac conditions.

Arterial blood pressure Pressure in the circulatory system, determined by the cardiac output and the peripheral vascular resistance.

Autoregulation Tissue and organ blood flow alters in response to energy needs in order to maintain adequate circulation.

Cardiac output Amount of blood pumped by the heart in one minute.

Diastolic filling time Period during diastole when the ventricles fill with blood prior to contraction.

Electrically significant response Patient's response to a dysrhythmia that may involve deterioration into ventricular dysrhythmias that could lead to shock or death.

Escape pacemaker Backup pacemaker site that discharges in the event that the sinus node fails.

Hemodynamically significant response Patient's response to a dysrhythmia that includes significant signs and symptoms, such as, a fall in blood pressure, decreased cardiac output, pulmonary congestion, near-syncope, or a loss of consciousness.

Intravascular volume Assessment of a patient's circulatory fluid status in order to determine whether the patient is dehydrated or fluid overloaded.

Myocardial oxygen demand Heart's oxygen requirement based on it's workload: the more work, the more oxygen (and glucose) that is needed.

Near-syncope Nearly fainting or almost losing consciousness.

Palpitations Sensation of "skipped beats" or "racing heart" in response to a rapid, slow, or irregular cardiac rhythm.

Peripheral vascular resistance Overall resistance to blood flow caused by the precapillary arterioles; a key determinant with cardiac output of arterial blood pressure.

Precapillary arterioles Smallest arteries that cause the overall circulatory resistance which contributes to blood pressure.

Shock Inadequate tissue perfusion. Associated with pale, clammy skin, confusion, and shortness of breath.

Stroke volume Amount of blood ejected from the heart with each beat.

Syncope Fainting or losing consciousness due to inadequate oxygen flow to the brain.

Systolic blood pressure Peak arterial pressure corresponding to cardiac contraction (systole).

Tissue perfusion Adequacy of circulation to the body tissues.

Ventricular filling period Same as diastolic filling time.

Sinus Dysrhythmias

LEARNING OBJECTIVES

Upon completion of this chapter, the reader should be able to:

- *Given sample ECG tracings, identify disorders of sinus activity.*

- *Describe how sinus rhythm disorders differ in appearance from normal sinus rhythm (NSR).*

- *List the primary cause of a sinus arrhythmia.*

- *Describe the ECG characteristics of a sinus arrhythmia.*

- *Describe two ways in which a sinus arrhythmia differs from NSR.*

- *Discuss the clinical significance and treatment of sinus arrhythmia.*

- *State the upper rate limit of a sinus tachycardia in an adult.*

- *Describe the ECG characteristics of a sinus tachycardia.*

- *List five causes of sinus tachycardia.*

- *Discuss the clinical significance and treatment of sinus tachycardia.*

- *Describe how the ECG characteristics of sinus tachycardia differs from NSR.*

- *List the ECG characteristics of sinus bradycardia.*

- *State the upper and lower rate limits for sinus bradycardia.*

- *List five causes of sinus bradycardia.*

- *Describe how the ECG characteristics of sinus bradycardia differs from NSR.*

- *Discuss the clinical significance of sinus bradycardia.*

- *List three options for treating clinically significant sinus bradycardia.*

- *Describe the system of classifying sinus blocks.*

- *Describe two mechanisms by which sinus block occurs.*

- *Describe how the ECG characteristics of sinus block differs from NSR.*

- *Discuss the clinical significance and treatment of sinus block.*

- *Describe what is occuring during AV dissociation.*

- *Explain what is occuring when AV dissociation occurs during very slow sinus bradycardia.*

- *Define an escape beat or rhythm.*

- *List the ECG characteristics of escape beats/rhythms.*

- *List two causes that favor the development of escape beats/rhythms.*

- *Name two higher pacemaker sites that must fail in order for an idioventricular escape pacemaker rhythm to develop.*

- *Describe the characteristics of tachycardia-bradycardia ("tachy-brady") syndrome.*

CHAPTER OVERVIEW

Sinus dysrhythmias are caused by disorders of SA node rhythm and/or rate. Rates are either too fast, too slow or the rhythm is irregular. Infrequently, they are caused by abnormal impulse conduction. Sinus disorders consist of normal cardiac complexes (P-QRS-T) that appear identical to those in normal sinus rhythm. Emergent therapy is hardly ever needed to treat sinus disorders, unless the ventricular rate slows enough to cause hypotension or loss of consciousness. Rapid sinus rates are only treated when they increase the heart's oxygen needs during an acute cardiac event.

SINUS DISORDERS

Disorders of sinus function are usually not serious and almost never life-threatening. They develop in response to an underlying disorder, such as hypovolemia, fever, or pain. Therapy for sinus disorders therefore, is directed at the underlying condition rather than the rhythm disorder itself. However, extremely low cardiac rates, ranging from 30 to 40/minute, and prolonged rapid rates around 150/minute are capable of causing marked symptoms.

Depolarization of the sinus node is abnormal when it becomes accelerated, depressed, or very irregular. Disorders involving the autonomic nervous system are a leading cause of the SA node discharging too slow, too fast, irregularly, or blocking impulse conduction.

SINUS NODE FUNCTION

Normal sinus rhythm exists when the sinus node discharges between 60 and 100 times per minute and has normal AV and ventricular conduction. Examples of NSR for review are found in Figure 9–1.

Pacemaker cells possess automaticity, which is the ability to spontaneously become active (depolarize) without requiring an external stimulus like the cells do. SA node cells rhythmically develop small electrical charges that are transmitted along the specialized cells of the *conduction pathways* to stimulate the heart. Specialized conduction pathways insure that activation quickly spreads throughout the heart in a coordinated pattern. Heart rate control is determined by cells that have the fastest rate of automatic discharge (automaticity). The sinus node is normally the pace-setter or pacemaker for the heart because it has the fastest rate of spontaneous

depolarization. Cells with higher automaticity rates depolarize faster and thereby suppress slower automatic cells. For example, an abnormal pacemaker that develops in the ventricle and discharges faster than the SA node, will take over the pacemaker role and suppress sinus activity. Clinically, this can occur in the event that ischemia causes irritable ventricular tissue to fire rapidly.

> *ECG Interpretation Tip:* If the P wave in lead II is not positive, the rhythm is not sinus (except if the right arm and left arm leads have been mistakenly reversed or in the rare condition of dextrocardia [the heart is on the right side of the chest]).

> *Clinical Note:* Cells that have the fastest discharge rate control the overall heart rate. Normally, heart rate control rests with the sinus node, but not uncommonly, other irritable cells with faster rates of automaticity compete with the SA node.

Escape Pacemakers

Cells other than those within the sinus node do have pacemaker potential under normal conditions because they are suppressed by faster sinus node cells. However, when the sinus node slows, pauses, or even totally ceases firing, these back-up pacemakers fortunately emerge. *Escape pacemakers* include atrial tissue,

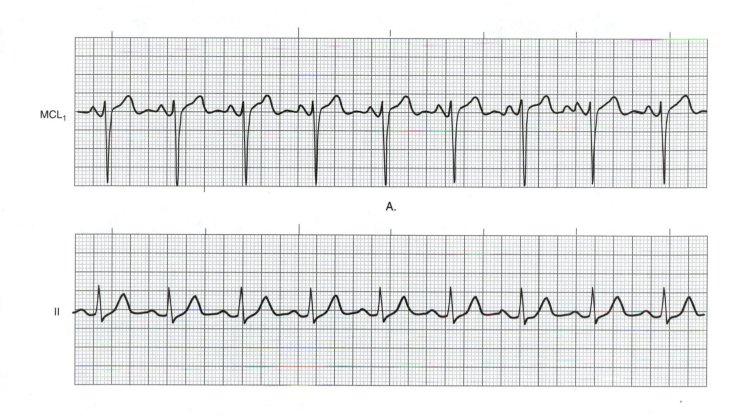

Figure 9–1 Normal sinus rhythm shown in two common monitoring leads. The main difference in P-QRS-T complex shapes in these leads involves the direction of the QRS deflection: in lead MCL$_1$ the QRS complex is mostly negative, while in lead II it is largely positive.

the AV junction and ventricular tissue. Escape rhythms do not compete with the SA node since they only emerge when higher sites fail. An example of escape pacemaker rhythm is seen in Figure 9–2 when the sinus node suddenly stops pacing the heart after the second beat. The

AV junction quickly steps in to stimulate the ventricles and prevent asystole. Figure 9–3 shows two examples where the sinus node fails completely and slower escape rhythms rescue the silent heart. Table 9–1 lists the ECG characteristics of escape pacemaker activity.

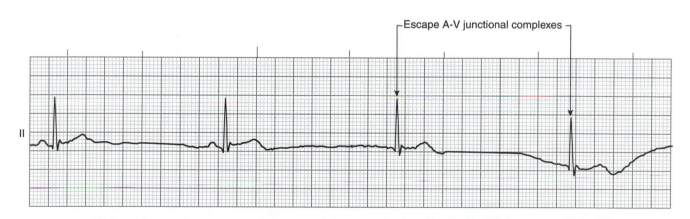

Figure 9–2 Escape pacemaker rhythm. A backup pacemaker in the AV junctional (beats number 3 and 4) develops after the sinus rate slows below 40/minute. The junctional beats lack P waves but are otherwise identical to the first two beats, which are sinus.

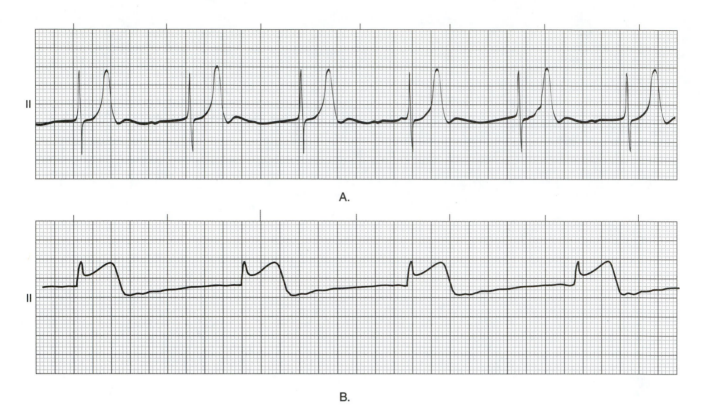

Figure 9-3 Escape pacemaker rhythms. Sinus activity is absent in both ECG tracings. In strip A the rhythm consists of narrow QRS complexes at a rate of 50/minute. In strip B the rhythm consists of wide QRS complexes (at a rate of 30/minute) that have siginificantly elevated ST segments.

Clinical Note: *The sinus node can lose control of the heart rate in two very different ways: (a) if it ceases to discharge or (b) an irritable cell fires more rapidly and takes away control. Escape pacemakers passively discharge to rescue an electrically silent or slow heart. In contrast, irritable groups of cells depolarize and take control of a normally functioning SA node. Escape pacemakers assist the SA node, while irritable fast pacemakers threaten SA function.*

Age-Related Sinus Rates

The average rate that sinus node discharges varies based on the person's age. The SA node discharges between 60 to 100 times per minute or an average of 80 times per minute in adults. Pacemaker tissue is responsive to changing cell needs, depolarizing faster when body tissue needs more blood such as during exercise, while slowing down during rest or sleep. Children's heart rates are considerably faster than adults because of their higher metabolic rate. Newborn heart rates are at least 140/minute and can be as fast as 200/minute. Children up to age two have resting rates above 100/minute. By ten years of age, children's heart rates approach those of an adult, averaging 80/minute with ranges between 60 and 100/minute. Older patients tend to have heart rates in the low 60's and 50's. Although heart rates may be outside the usual NSR range of between 60 to 100/minute, a rate faster or slower may be adequate and normal for an individual. Heart rates also have a cyclical daily variation. Cardiac rates slow during sleep, especially during the very early hours of the day. Heart rates also accelerate during the day when people are the most active.

ECG CHARACTERISTICS OF SINUS DISORDERS

One finding that is shared by every sinus disorder is that the *P-QRS-T complexes appear normal*—just as seen in NSR. For instance, in sinus tachycardia, the rate of P-QRS-T complexes is between 100 and 150/minute, but the rhythm otherwise appears identical to NSR.

Table 9-1	ECG Characteristics of Escape Pacemakers		
Pacemaker	P Waves	PR Interval	QRS Complexes
Sinus	Present	Normal	Narrow
AV junction	Absent or retrograde	Shortened	Narrow
Idioventricular	Absent	Absent	Wide and distorted

Likewise, when the rate is slower than 60/minute as in sinus bradycardia, the cardiac complexes still have normal P-QRS-T shapes. Even in sinus block aside from the irregular cardiac rhythm caused by entire P-QRS-T complexes being dropped, the rest of the conducted beats are normal.

> **ECG Interpretation Tip:** Disorders of sinus rhythm have normal P-QRS-T complexes but differ from NSR in regard to either rate, rhythm, conduction, or all three.

P Wave Shapes

The P wave shapes vary based on the lead being viewed. There is no single "normal" P wave shape, however, the size and shape of the P waves in a single lead should be identical from one beat to the next. In lead II P waves are upright, have a rounded appearance and have a consistent shape from beat-to-beat. In lead MCL_1 there is more variability in the P wave shape and it can appear pointy, upright, asymmetric, or biphasic. Figure 9–4 illustrates various P wave shapes.

SINUS ARRHYTHMIA

Sinus arrhythmia is an irregular cardiac rhythm caused by sinus node rhythm variability (Figure 9–5). Sinus arrhythmia is an exaggeration of the normal respiratory cycle variability, where P-P intervals can vary by as much as 0.16 second or 4 small ECG boxes. Even during NSR, a slight variability in sinus node rhythm due to the respiratory cycle is common. Sinus arrhythmia is not an abnormal cardiac pattern; it is an exaggeration of normal nervous system changes associated with breathing.

> **Clinical Note:** An easy way to remember the ECG findings seen with sinus arrhythmia is the heart rate increases during inspiration. The R-R intervals shorten as the P-QRS-T complexes crowd together. During exhala-

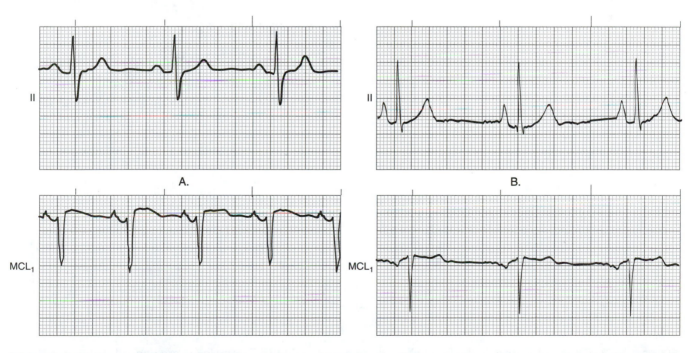

A.

B.

Figure 9–4 Normal P waves with different shapes. Note that the P wave configurations vary considerably in these sinus examples. Some Ps are notched, while others are pointed, inverted, rounded, and tall.

tion the heart rate slows, the R-R intervals lengthen, and the P-QRS-T complexes move apart.

ECG Interpretation Tip: *Sinus arrhythmia differs from NSR only in regard to the variability of sinus activity. Otherwise, the P-QRS-T complexes are identical to NSR but have a varying rhythm (Table 9–2). Sinus arrhythmia can be emphasized by having the patient take a deep breath and watching the ECG rhythm changes.*

Table 9–2 Key ECG Features of Sinus Arrhythmia

■ **P waves:**	Normal
■ **QRS complexes:**	Normal
■ **T waves:**	Normal
■ **AV conduction:**	Normal. A single P wave occurs before each QRS.
■ **Rhythm:**	Varies with respiratory cycle
■ **Rate:**	Normal

Causes of Sinus Arrhythmia

Variation in sinus node discharge is due to the effects of breathing upon the autonomic nervous system.During inhalation the lungs expand, causing a small increase the amount of blood returning to the heart. This causes stretch receptors located in the heart wall to respond by briefly speeding the heart rate to carry the extra blood. As sinus pacemaker activity increases, the P-QRS-T complexes appear closer together. During exhalation, the process is reversed and the blood volume in the lungs slightly decreases. The heart rate then momentarily slows, mediated by the vagal (parasympathetic) nerves, while the ECG complexes spread further apart. The ECG reflects this nervous system variability as a waxing and waning heart pattern. These effects on the cardiac cycle are more noticeable in children and patients with chronic obstructive lung disease.

ECG Interpretation Tip: *The sinus node is the pacemaker in sinus arrhythmia but the impulses develop in a regularly irregular fashion, due to the influence of the central nervous system and the respiratory center.*

Clinical Significance of Sinus Arrhythmia

This is a benign dysrhythmia which is commonly seen in healthy people. Sinus arrhythmia has no effect on a patient's hemodynamic status and is an incidental ECG finding.

Emergency Treatment for Sinus Arrhythmia

No treatment is required.

SINUS TACHYCARDIA

Sinus tachycardia is a rhythm originating in the SA node at a rate over 100/minute (Figure 9–6). The heart rate generally ranges from 101 to 150/minute but it can be even faster. This rhythm disorder is easy to identify because P waves can be seen before each narrow QRS complex. When the rate approaches 140/minute P waves may be difficult to identify because the cardiac

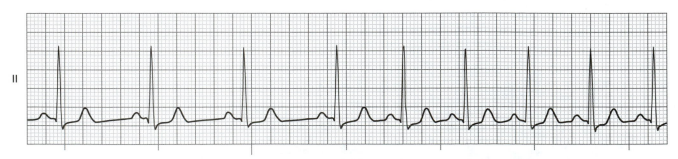

II

Figure 9–5 Sinus arrhythmia. In the first half of the tracing, the P-QRS-T complexes are spaced farther apart, while during the latter half the complexes are close together.

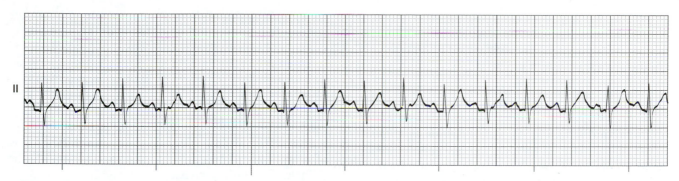

Figure 9–6 Sinus tachycardia with rate of approximately 150/minute. The P waves and the preceding T waves appear close together.

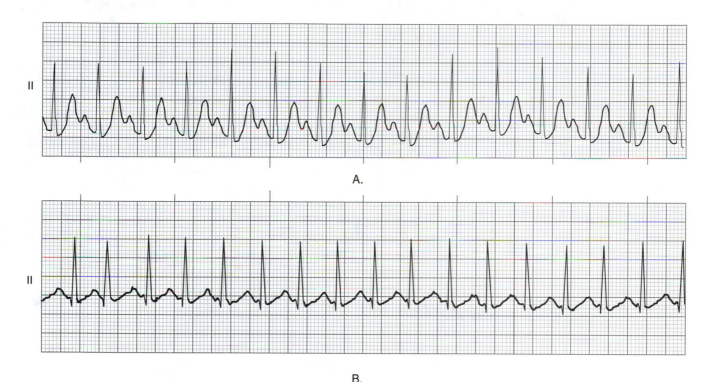

A.

B.

Figure 9–7 Rapid sinus tachycardias with P waves appearing to merge into the T waves. In B it is no longer possible to identify P waves.

complexes appear closer together. P waves merge with the T waves of the preceding complexes when the rate is very rapid (Figure 9–7). Sinus tachycardia looks just like NSR except that the rate is faster than normal. Sinus tachycardia is a normal finding in children less than 2 years of age but is abnormal in adults especially those at rest.

Sinus tachycardia is a *secondary dysrhythmia*, meaning that it develops in response to another condition such as anxiety, dehydration, heart failure, or fever. When the underlying disorder is corrected, the rate slows to normal.

ECG Interpretation Tip: The cardiac rate in sinus tachycardia ranges from 101 to 150/minute, but in some circumstances it may be as high as 180/minute in adults, and as fast as 220/minute in infants.
As the rate exceeds 150/minute in adults, the rhythm becomes much less likely to be originating in the sinus node.

The upper limit for sinus node discharge in adults is about 160 beats per minute (bpm) but may reach as high as 180/minute in severely stressed patients. In unusual cases it can even be faster.

Causes of Sinus Tachycardia

Sinus tachycardia occurs when the SA node is stimulated and reflects an increased degree of automaticity (self-depolarization). Decreased parasympathetic nervous tone as well as increased sympathetic system activity accelerates SA node firing. An increased heart rate reflects the body's response to some physiologic or emotional stress. While an increased heart rate can result from cardiac conditions, such as during *congestive heart failure (CHF)* or an *acute myocardial infarction (AMI)*, it is most often due to non-cardiac conditions (Table 9–4).

Diverse conditions such as anemia, pain, drugs/medications (including cocaine, amphetamines, and albuterol medi-inhalers) exercise, fever, shock, and dehydration cause increased heart rates.

Table 9–3 Key ECG Features of Sinus Tachycardia	
■ **P waves:**	Normal
■ **QRS complexes:**	Normal
■ **T waves:**	Normal
■ **AV conduction:**	Normal. A single P wave occurs before each QRS.
■ **Rhythm:**	Regular
■ **Rate:**	Faster than 100/minute; the upper limit is 150/minute

Table 9-4 Causes of Sinus Tachycardia

- ■ **Normal Variant** (young children, exercise, anxiety)
- ■ **Sympathomimetic Drugs** (drugs that simulate (mimic) sympathetic nervous system stimulation, such as cocaine, epinephrine, albuterol, ephedrine)
- ■ **Vagolytic Drugs** (atropine opposes the actions of the parasympathetic (vagal) system)
- ■ **Pain**
- ■ **Fever, Sepsis**
- ■ **Hypovolemia and Dehydration**
- ■ **Hyperthyroidism, Anemia**
- ■ **Congestive Heart Failure, Cardiogenic Shock, Ischemia**
- ■ **Pulmonary Disorders** (embolism, chronic obstructive lung disease)

Clinical Significance of Sinus Tachycardia

In many situations an increased heart rate is an appropriate and useful compensatory mechanism. Generally, an increased cardiac output is beneficial, as in cases of hemorrhage and hypoxia, because more oxygen and nutrients are available to cells. But at other times, such as in patients with limited cardiac reserve or coronary artery disease—especially in patients experiencing a myocardial infarction—an accelerated heart rate can be detrimental because fast heart rates increase the work of the heart and increases the myocardial oxygen demand. Tachycardia can worsen the ischemia and increase the infarction size.

Elderly patients with underlying heart disease do not tolerate rapid rates for very long, because increased rates have shortened ventricular filling times. Despite the increased heart rate, cardiac output may actually fall because the stroke volume decreases owing to shortened ventricular diastolic filling time. For instance, some elderly patients who present with a rapid heart rate due to dehydration develop ischemia. While the tachycardia is useful because more blood is being pumped, the heart must work harder.

Emergency Treatment for Sinus Tachycardia

There is no specific therapy for sinus tachycardia since treatment must be aimed at the underlying cause. For instance, there is no benefit to giving a drug to slow a sinus tachycardia which is due to a high fever, unless appropriate treatment is also started to lower the fever and treat the underlying infection.

Clinical Note: *Treatment of sinus tachycardia is directed toward the underlying cause. Sinus tachycardia will resolve spontaneously when the underlying problem is corrected.*

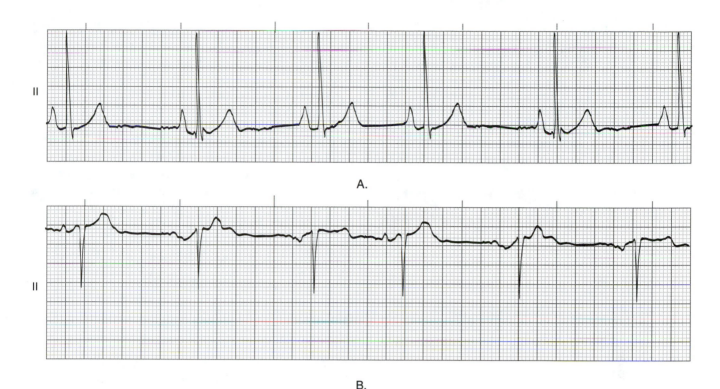

A.

B.

Figure 9–8 Sinus bradycardias. Both ECG tracings show cardiac rates below 60bpm. Otherwise, the pacemaker is the sinus node and the P-QRS-T complexes are identical to NSR.

An exception to the treatment principle concerning sinus tachycardia involves an acute myocardial infarction. Medication is used to slow the heart in order to minimize myocardial damage. Beta-blocking agents, such as metoprolol or atenolol, reduce the heart rate which lessens the heart's workload. The treatment goal during a myocardial infarction is to slow the heart rate to between 55 and 65/minute. Beta blocker treatment during an MI has improved survival and decreased the incidence of unstable ventricular dysrhythmias. In myocardial ischemia, oxygen administration, and analgesics, as well as beta-blocking agents are also effective in slowing the heart.

SINUS BRADYCARDIA

Sinus bradycardia originates in the sinus node at a rate less than 60/minute (Figure 9–8). Apart from the decreased sinus node automaticity, the cardiac complexes appear identical in all ways to NSR (Table 9–5). Moderately slow rates, as in the high 40's and 50's are generally well tolerated. However, during ischemia or in a patient exhibiting signs of inadequate perfusion, bradycardia may require treatment. Heart rates below 45/minute usually result in dizziness, fatigue, weakness, near-syncope or fainting.

Causes of Sinus Bradycardia

As discussed earlier with fast heart rates, the interplay of the sympathetic and vagal nervous system influences the heart rate.

The most common cause of sinus bradycardia is due to increased vagal (parasympathetic) tone. Sinus node depression is common in patients taking calcium channel-blocker medication or beta-blocker drugs that decrease the SA node's depolarization rate. During an MI, bradycardia serves a protective role because a slow rate decreases the heart's oxygen requirement and min-

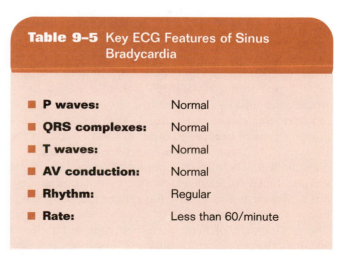

Table 9–5 Key ECG Features of Sinus Bradycardia	
■ **P waves:**	Normal
■ **QRS complexes:**	Normal
■ **T waves:**	Normal
■ **AV conduction:**	Normal
■ **Rhythm:**	Regular
■ **Rate:**	Less than 60/minute

imizes cardiac damage.

Most sinus bradycardias are not pathologic. During sleep, the heart rate slows and well-conditioned athletes typically have slow resting heart rates. Bradycardia in the elderly is usually normal but may be due to atherosclerotic degeneration of the nodal tissue. Enhanced parasympathetic tone as occurs during a **vasovagal fainting** episode is another cause of sinus brachycardia. Table 9–6 lists the common causes of sinus bradycardia.

Table 9-6 Causes of Sinus Bradycardia

- **Normal Variant** (especially in the elderly)
- **Physiologic** (sleep, athletic conditioning)
- **Increased Vagal Tone** (examples: pharyngeal suctioning, vomiting, straining during defacation)
- **Inferior Wall Myocardial Infarction**
- **Hypothyroidism**
- **Drugs** (beta adrenergic-blocking agents, calcium channel blockers, meperidine, digitalis)
- **Hypothermia**
- **Sick Sinus Syndrome** (Tachy-bradycardia Syndrome)
- **Hyperkalemia** (elevated serum potassium)
- **Increased Intracranial Pressure**
- **Intense Visceral Pain**

Clinical Significance of Sinus Brachycardia

A thorough patient evaluation is needed to assess the significance of any dysrhythmia but this is especially important in the setting of a slow heart rate. Slow cardiac rates are normal in many people. If a patient is experiencing abnormal bradycardia without symptoms, immediate therapy is not needed. In fact, accelerating a slow heart during myocardial ischemia would likely worsen the injury.

Most patients can tolerate rates as slow as the mid-40's reasonably well because in order to compensate for the slow rate, the stroke volume increases due to a longer diastolic ventricular filling period. The higher stroke volume helps to maintain cardiac output during slow rates. Should the rate slow too much, the patient will become symptomatic.

The earliest sign of inadequate perfusion is an altered state of consciousness: restlessness, agitation, lethargy,

confusion, and eventually syncope. Patients with slow heart rates commonly complain of weakness, light headedness, dizziness, dyspnea on exertion, fatigue, chest pain, near-syncope, and shortness of breath. Physical signs indicating inadequate cardiac output include hypotension, prolonged capillary refill time, and those due to sympathetic system stimulation include pale, moist, and clammy skin.

Bradycardic rates which are slow enough to decrease cardiac output, commonly result in escape pacemaker firing. As the SA node slows, back-up pacemakers can emerge from the atria, AV junction, or within the ventricles to pace the heart (Figures 9–9 and 9–10). Escape beats differ from sinus beats: they may lack P waves, have altered P waves, or distorted QRS complexes. Bradycardias due to high vagal tone often have prolonged PR intervals as well. The prolonged PR intervals found with bradycardic rates return to normal as the rate increases.

ECG Interpretation Tip: *Escape pacemaker rhythms often accompany symptomatic slow rates. Escape beats/rhythms differ from the sinus beats in appearance and follow prolonged ECG pauses.*

Emergency Treatment for Sinus Bradycardia

Sinus bradycardia does not require treatment unless the rate is less than 45/minute and the patient is symptomatic. Treatment is indicated in the setting of ischemic heart disease when a slow rate allows ventricular escape beats to develop, the patient becomes hemodynamically unstable, or signs of inadequate perfusion exists, such as ischemic chest pain, shortness of breath, confusion, or agitation.

The acute cardiac treatment algorithm for patients with bradycardia is listed in Figure 9–11. *Most cases of sinus bradycardia, however, do not need therapy.*

Clinical Note: *Sinus bradycardia does not require treatment unless the patient is hemodynamically compromised or if escape rhythms develop in the setting of ischemia. Atropine and epinephrine can exacerbate ischemia and must be used with caution.*

Treatments for sinus bradycardia include:

- Transcutaneous artificial pacing is the first choice because it offers more accurate rate control;

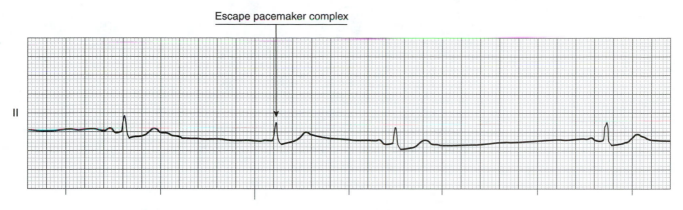

Figure 9-9 Sinus bradycardia allow an escape pacemaker to fire. Sinus activity is very slow.

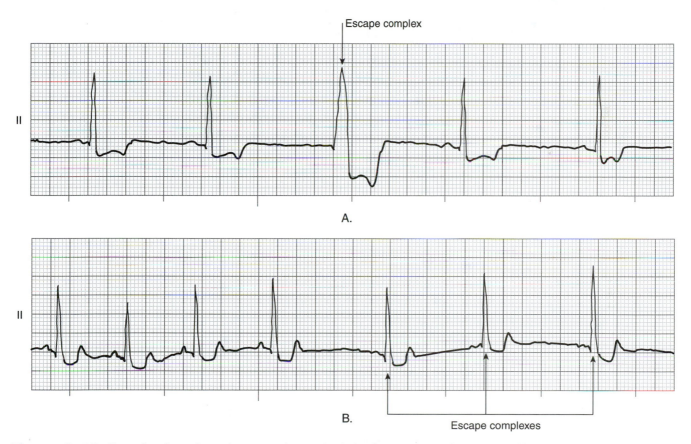

Figure 9-10 Sinus bradycardia with escape beats. In A the first, second, fourth, and fifth beats are sinus beats, while the third is an escape beat that develops due to the long cardiac pause after the second sinus beat. In strip B a pause occurs after the first four sinus beats, leading to the formation of three escape complexes.

- Intravenous boluses of 0.5 to 1 mg atropine every 3 to 5 minutes to a total dose of 0.03 to 0.04 mg/kg;

- Epinephrine IV infusion* at 2 to 10 micrograms per minute

- Dopamine IV infusion* at 5 to 20 microgram/kg per minute

- Isoproterenol IV infusion* at 2 to 10 micrograms per minute (rarely used)

*rarely if ever needed for slow sinus bradycardia

ECG Interpretation Tip: *Sinus arrhythmias appear more pronounced during bradycardic rates.*

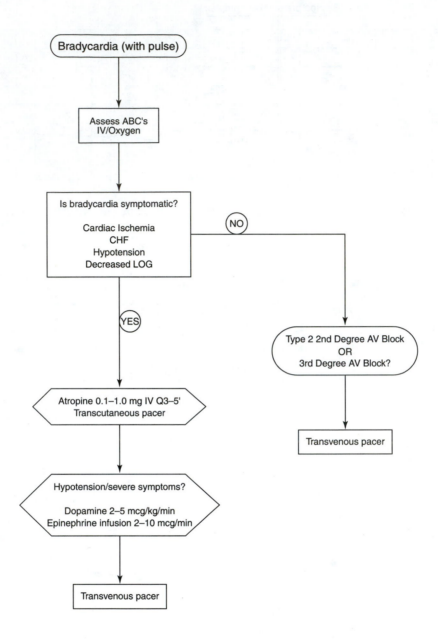

Figure 9-11 ACLS treatment algorithm for adult bradycardic rhythms. (Reprinted with permission EmedHome.com website (http://www.emedhome.com)

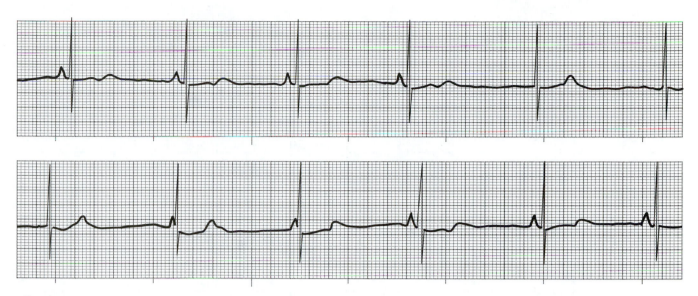

Continuous

Figure 9-12 Atrioventricular dissociation. In this continuous recording, note how the P wave relationship to the QRS complexes changes. Strip A shows sinus bradycardia for the first four beats. Next, the sinus pacemaker further slows, allowing a junctional escape pacemaker to pace the heart for five beats (beats number 5 through 9). Sinus activity then speeds up to recapture the pacemaker role in beats number 10 through 12. There is no anatomic blockage of impulses bwtween the atria and the ventricle.

ISORHYTHMIC AV DISSOCIATION DUE TO SINUS BRADYCARDIA

Slow sinus node discharge may cause periods of AV junctional rhythms, or *isorhythmic AV dissociation*, during which the atria and ventricles beat independently (Figure 9–12). Isorhythmic AV dissociation occurs when SA pacemaker slowing allows AV junctional cells to "escape" suppression and temporarily control the heart rate.

Isorhythmic dissociation occurs when the similar discharge rates of the SA node and AV junction interfere with one another. AV dissociation does not indicate an AV nodal conduction disorder. AV dissociation is commonly mistaken for complete AV heart block but it is actually a benign condition.

SINUS BLOCK

Sinus block occurs when the SA node fails to stimulate the atria, causing ECG pauses where the missing P-QRS-T complexes cycles were expected (Figure 9–13) (Table 9–7).

Sinus block mechanisms can involve either: (a) failure of the SA node to depolarize, or (b) inability of the atrial tissue to respond to a SA node impulse. The first possibility involves failure of the SA node to *generate* an impulse while the second reflects failure of the atria to *conduct* an impulse. Both conditions reflect suppression of SA nodal activity and result in missing cardiac cycles (Figure 9–14). Sinus block may occur: (a) intermittently, resulting in *occasionally missed* cardiac complexes, or (b) completely, causing a *total lack* of sinus functioning in which case it is termed sinus arrest. During sinus arrest, should an escape pacemaker fail to discharge, asystole and cardiac arrest would quickly ensue. Fortunately, this rarely happens because back-up escape rhythms quickly discharge.

Table 9-7 Key ECG Features of Sinus Block	
■ **Atrial activity:**	Irregular due to absent beats
■ **Ventricular activity:**	Irregular due to absent beats
■ **AV conduction:**	Normal
■ **Rhythm:**	Irregular due to absent beats
■ **Key finding:**	Completely absent P-QRS-T complexes

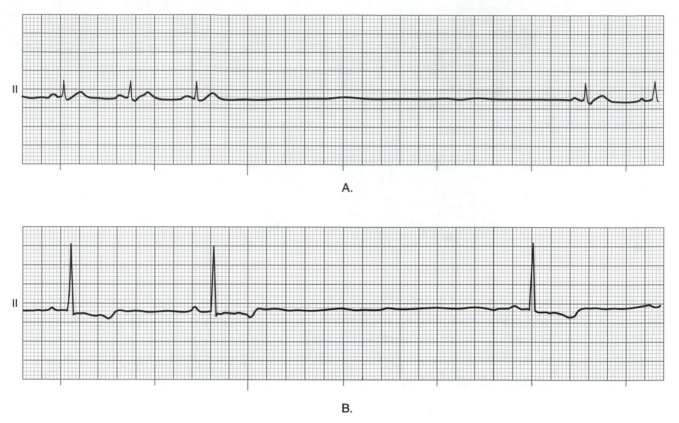

Figure 9–13 Sinus block. There is a very long pause after the third beat in strip A and the second beat in strip B. (The lack of an escape junctional pacemaker signifies widespread pacemaker dysfunction.)

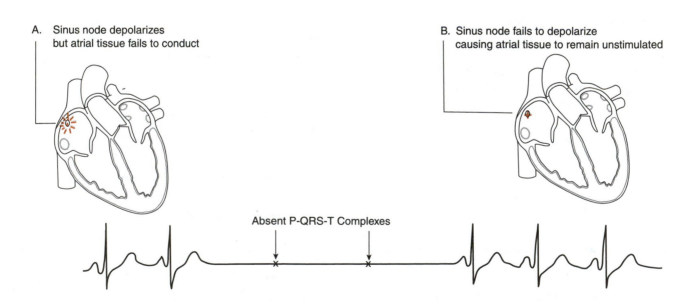

Figure 9–14 Illustration of two mechanisms which are responsible for cardiac pauses. In A the sinus node fires but the impulse is blocked from depolarizing the atrium. In B the SA node fails to depolarize.

Causes of Sinus Block

A common causes of sinus block is gradual degeneration of the SA node. This is associated with aging or drugs that suppress SA nodal function such as digitalis, calcium channel blockers, and beta adrenergic-blockers. Less common causes are found in Table 9–8.

Clinical Significance of Sinus Block

Sinus block can present as a sudden and unexplained loss of consciousness or lightheadedness. *Stokes-Adams Syndrome* is syncope caused by heart block. Some patients complain of a "skipped beat," palpitations, and dizziness. When ECG pauses are seen, the beat terminating the pause should be examined to determine whether it is an escape beat.

ECG Interpretation Tip: *During sinus block, the ECG shows brief asystolic pauses in which entire cardiac cycles (P-QRS-T complexes) are absent. These pauses are often terminated by escape complexes or rhythms.*

Terminology Describing Sinus Node Failure

The terminology applied to sinus dysfunction is imprecise:

- *Sinus block* refers to occasional SA failure in which one or two cardiac cycles are dropped (Figure 9–15B).

Table 9-8 Causes of Sinus Block

- **Drugs that Depress Sinus Function**
- **Fibrotic Degeneration of the SA Node**
- **Hyperkalemia**
- **Myocardial Ischemia**
- **Increased Vagal Tone**
- **Carotid Body Hypersensitivity**
- **Carotid Sinus Massage**
- **Rheumatic (inflammatory) Heart Disease**
- **Myocarditis** (inflammation of heart muscle)
- **Coronary Artery Diseases** (ischemia, injury, and infarction)

- *Sinus arrest* refers to SA node failure that lasts for a prolonged period. In sinus block the prolonged P-P interval pause is usually a multiple of the underlying P-P cycle (Fugre 9–15A). In sinus arrest the pause is not a multiple of the underlying P-P interval. For example, a pause in sinus activity that lasts exactly twice the usual P-P interval is termed a sinus block, while a pause that equals approximately 5 1/2 P-P intervals is referred to as sinus arrest.

For simplicity, this book uses the term sinus block for all failures of sinus function. Sinus block includes sinus arrest.

Emergency Treatment of Sinus Block

Sinus block is rare and a prolonged sinus block that requires acute intervention is even rarer. The need to treat sinus failure depends on the duration of the cardiac pause and how well the patient tolerates the pause. If the sinus block is due to drug toxicity, withholding the offending medication is usually sufficient. If the patient's condition is stable, no further therapy is required. However, for a patient who loses consciousness, develops chest pain, or becomes hypotensive, the bradycardia acute cardiac treatment algorithm in Figure 9–11 is used. The treatment section includes use of an artificial pacemaker, atropine, and epinephrine infusion.

SICK SINUS SYNDROME (S-S-S)

Sick sinus syndrome refers to a group of dysrhythmias that share alternating fast and slow ECG rhythms, including sinus bradycardia, sinus tachycardia, sinus block, along with failure of escape pacemakers (Figure 9–16). Classically, S-S-S describes the patient who abruptly develops sinus arrest that is associated with abrupt loss of consciousness. The temporary asystolic period ends when an escape pacemaker fires.

TACHY-BRADY SYNDROME

Tachy-brady syndrome is a related term that is applied to a similar condition in which a rapidly shifting heart rate involves atrial dysrhythmias, such as atrial fibrillation, which will be presented in the next chapter, along with slow sinus rhythms (Figure 9–17). In a small group of patients this can be caused by a *hypersensitive carotid sinus* caused when pressure applied to the neck over the carotid gland, such as while shaving with an electric razor, or due to a tight necktie causes marked slowing of the sinus node.

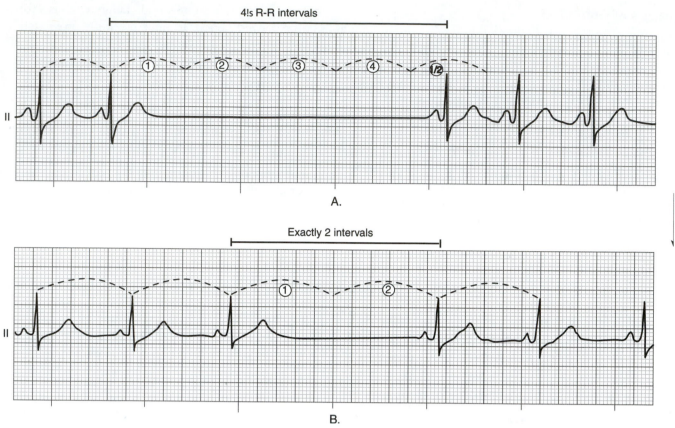

Figure 9–15 Sinus block versus sinus arrest. In strip A the cardiac pause does not equal a multiple of the normal R-R interval. In strip B the pause exactly equals two R-R intervals.

ECG Interpretation Tip: *If an ECG rhythm originates in the sinus node and has a rate between 60 to 100/minute but does not meet the other criteria for NSR, it is described as a sinus rhythm rather than normal sinus rhythm. A rhythm is only described as NSR if it is normal in all respects. Figure 9–18 illustrates this concept since both examples show sinus rhythm but they have wide and bizarre QRS complexes. Although they are examples of sinus rhythms, they are certainly not normal.*

SUMMARY OF SINUS DISORDERS

Sinus disorders refer to abnormalities of SA node rate, rhythm, or conduction. Sinus arrhythmia, sinus brady-cardia, sinus tachycardia, and sinus blocks are examples of dysrhythmias originating in the SA node. While all are rhythm disorders, they are not all pathologic. Disordered cardiac rhythms must be viewed within the clinical settings. For instance, a patient with a fever is expected to have a rapid rate since this helps to dissipate heat. People who are sleeping have a slower heart rate than when awake. Also, patients who have a normal rhythm aside from an irregular sinus rhythm due to respirations are entirely normal. Table 9–9 compares the findings in various types of sinus dysrhythmias. The next chapter will provide practice tracings showing many sinus disorders.

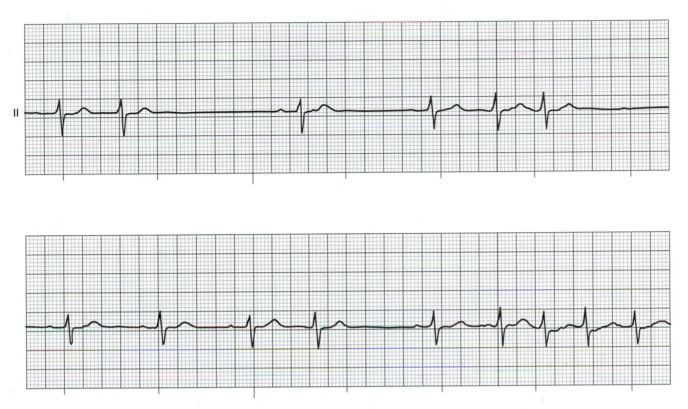

Figure 9-16 Brady-tachy syndrome. This tracing illustrates the striking variation in cardiac rate ranging between a very fast rate alternating with long pauses in electrical activity.

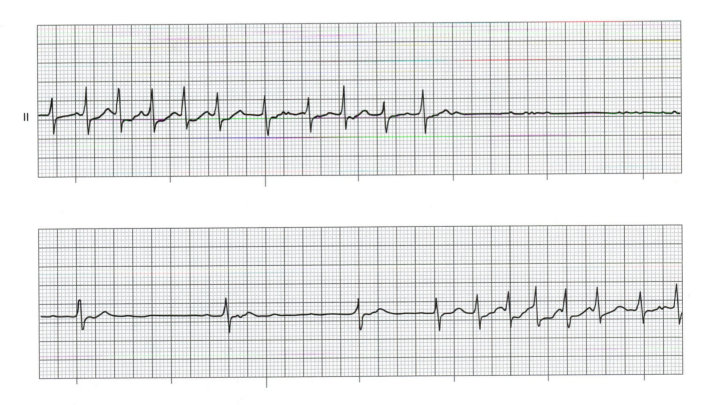

Figure 9-17 Sick sinus syndrome. There are long pauses between sinus beats. The rhythm also shows alteration from bradycardia to tachycardia.

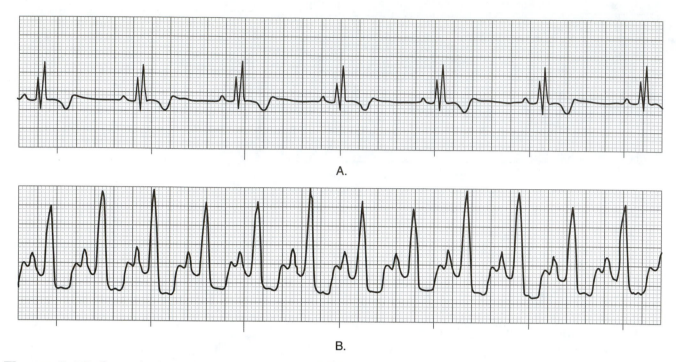

Figure 9-18 Sinus rhythm with wide and distorted QRS complexes. Note that these are not labeled normal sinus rhythm because they deviate from NSR criteria. In both tracings, the pacemaker is the sinus node but the QRS complexes are markedly distorted. Therefore, they are listed as sinus rhythms—not normal sinus rhythm.

Table 9-9 Comparison of Sinus Dysrhythmias

Type	Findings
Normal Sinus Rhythm	Normal; rate 60 to 100/minute
Sinus Bradycardia	Rate <60/minute; otherwise normal
Sinus Tachycardia	Rate >100/minute; otherwise normal
Sinus Block	Pause in sinus discharge; irregular rhythm; otherwise normal

Let's Review

1. Sinus dysrhythmias may be too fast, too slow, irregular, or have blocked conduction.

2. Sinus dysrhythmias share a narrow (less than 0.12 second duration), normal appearing QRS complex because ventricular conduction is normal.

3. Cells within the SA node have the fastest rate of spontaneous depolarization (automaticity), making it the heart's normal pacemaker.

4. The SA node can be replaced as the pacemaker if it fails to discharge, discharges too slowly, or if cells outside of the sinus node fire more rapidly.

5. The normal adult range for the sinus node is 60 to 100 pacemaker impulses per minute. Infants and young children have considerably faster rates, whereas the elderly have slower rates.

6. The shape of the P wave depends on the lead being monitored. Lead II displays upright P waves while the appearance in MCL_1 is more variable—it may look pointed, upright, inverted, or have both positive and negative components.

7. The sympathetic (adrenergic) nervous system increases the heart rate and speeds impulse conduction. The sympathetic nerves initiate the body's response to stress as metabolism increases and prepares the body for increased activity.

8. Increased vagal tone from the parasympathetic nervous system has the opposite effect: as metabolism slows and the body prepares for rest. The heart rate decreases and AV conduction slows.

9. Sinus arrhythmia has marked P-P interval variation that is associated with breathing. During inspiration the cardiac complexes move closer together as the sinus node briefly speeds up. During exhalation, the cardiac complexes spread apart as the sinus node slows down.

10. Sinus tachycardia originates in the sinus node at a rapid rate greater than 100 up to 150/minute. Sinus tachycardia is a secondary dysrhytmia because it occurs in response to some body stresses, such as fever, hypovolemia, anxiety or shock.

11. Sinus tachycardia increases cardiac output up to a certain rate. A prolonged episode of rapid sinus tachycardia can cause a fall in cardiac output secondary to decreased ventricular filling and ischemia-induced contractility dysfunction.

12. Sinus bradycardia originates in the sinus node at rates below 60 per minute.

13. Sinus bradycardia rarely requires immediate treatment except when associated with signs of inadequate tissue perfusion, which usually occurs when rates fall below 40/minute.

14. Sinus block involves failure of the sinus node pacemaker impulse to depolarize the atria.

15. When the sinus node fails to discharge, the ECG shows a pause in cardiac activity. The ECG pause of sinus block is usually ended by an escape beat from a back-up pacemaker.

16. During sinus block the heart remains unstimulated for one or more complete cardiac cycles.

17. Sick sinus syndrome involves a combination of dysrhythmias, including bradycardia, tachycardia, and block.

18. The term tachy-brady syndrome is applied the cardiac rhythm abruptly alternates between tachycardia and bradycardia.

Glossary

Acute myocardial infarction (AMI) Heart attack, involving myocardial necrosis due to a blocked coronary artery.

Adrenergic drugs Medication which stimulates sympathetic nerves.

Adrenergic nervous system Name for the sympathetic system.

Autonomic Nervous System Composed of the sympathetic and parasympathetic systems which have opposing actions; these two systems that work together to maintain a normal heart rate and A-V conduction.

Conduction pathways Route an electrical charge which starts in the sinus node is transmitted via specialized cells.

Congestive heart failure (CHF) Inability of the heart to pump enough blood to meet the body's needs; usually associated with pulmonary congestion and leg edema.

Escape pacemakers Backup pacemakers that become active if the sinus node fails, including atrial tissue, the AV junction, and ventricular tissue.

Hypersensitive carotid sinus Overactive gland in neck that results in marked sinus node slowing due to pressure applied to the neck.

Isorhythmic AV dissociation Condition in which the atria and ventricles beat independently and interfere with sinus activity.

Parasympathetic system Decreases the heart rate and slows AV conduction when active.

Secondary dysrhythmia Rhythm disorder that develops in response to another condition; such as sinus tachycardia in response to a fever.

Sick Sinus syndrome (S-S-S) Group of dysrhythmias that involve alternating fast and slow ECG rhythms, including sinus bradycardia, sinus tachycardia, sinus block, and escape pacemakers.

Sinus arrest Prolonged failure of the sinus node to initiate a heart beat.

Sinus arrhythmia Benign irregular cardiac rhythm caused by sinus node variability due to the respiratory cycle.

Sinus block Failure of the sinus node to generate an impulse or conduct the impulse to atrial tissue.

Sinus bradycardia Slow cardiac rhythm originating in the sinus node at a rate less than 60/minute.

Sinus tachycardia Rapid cardiac rhythm originating in the sinus node at a rate of over 100/minute.

Stokes-Adams Syndrome Syncope due to AV heart block.

Sympathetic nervous system Accelerates the heart rate, speeds AV conduction, and increases the force of contraction when stimulated.

Tachy-Brady syndrome Condition in which the cardiac rhythm alternates between tachycardia and bradycardia.

Vasovagal faint Brief loss of consciousness; "simple faint;" caused by an exaggerated parasympathetic nervous system response to some stimulus.

Sinus Dysrhythmias: Self-Assessment ECG

LEARNING OBJECTIVES

Upon completion of this chapter, the reader should be able to:

■ *Correctly identify sinus disorders when presented with sample ECG tracings.*

■ *Explain the reasoning for selecting a particular dysrhythmia interpretation.*

■ *Correctly assess the PR intervals, QRS durations, AV conduction ratios, and ST segments when presented with sample ECG tracings.*

CHAPTER OVERVIEW

The following twenty-five ECG tracings should be evaluated in regard to ventricular activity, atrial activity, and AV conduction, and an overall ECG interpretation made. All abnormalities shown in these ECG tracings are limited to sinus disorders. Note that both lead II and MCL$_1$ are used. Answers are provided in Appendix A. If any difficulty is encountered, Chapter 9 should be reviewed.

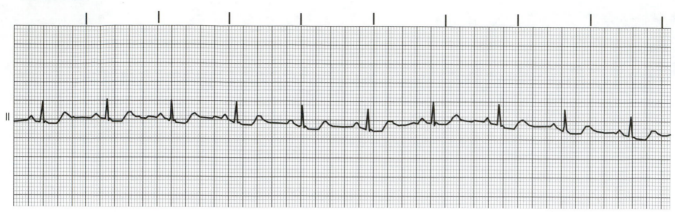

Figure 10-1   Rate _____
Rhythm _____
QRS Duration _____
PR Interval _____
AV Conduction Ratio _____
ST Segment _____
Interpretation _____
Reasoning _____

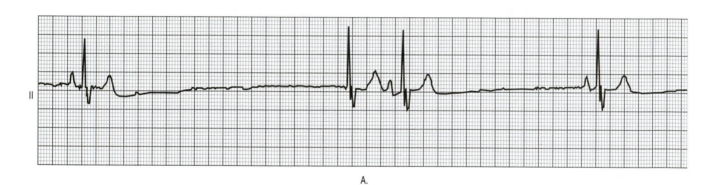

A.

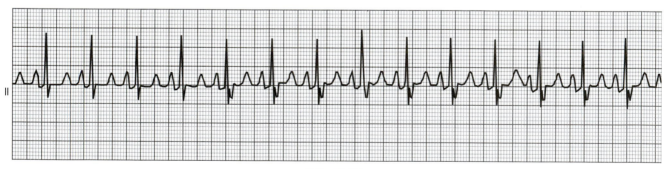

B. Recorded later

Figure 10-2   Rate _____
Rhythm _____
QRS Duration _____
PR Interval _____
AV Conduction Ratio _____
ST Segment _____
Interpretation _____
Reasoning _____

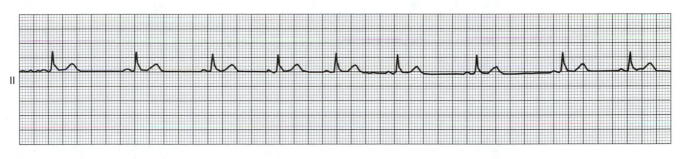

Figure 10–3   Rate _____
Rhythm _____
QRS Duration _____
PR Interval _____
AV Conduction Ratio _____
ST Segment _____
Interpretation _____
Reasoning _____

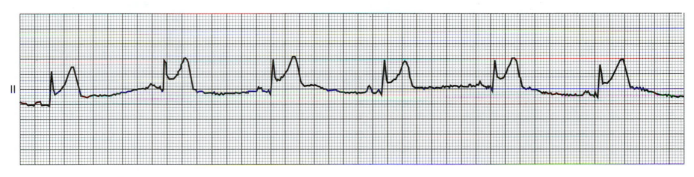

Figure 10–4   Rate _____
Rhythm _____
QRS Duration _____
PR Interval _____
AV Conduction Ratio _____
ST Segment _____
Interpretation _____
Reasoning _____

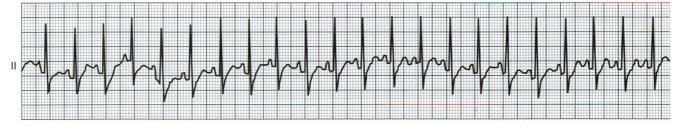

Figure 10–5   Rate _____
Rhythm _____
QRS Duration _____
PR Interval _____
AV Conduction Ratio _____
ST Segment _____
Interpretation _____
Reasoning _____

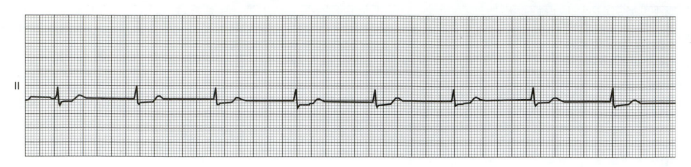

Figure 10-6   Rate _____
Rhythm _____
QRS Duration _____
PR Interval _____
AV Conduction Ratio _____
ST Segment _____
Interpretation _____
Reasoning _____

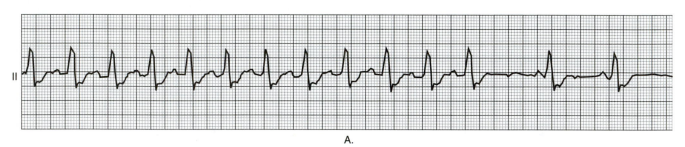

A.

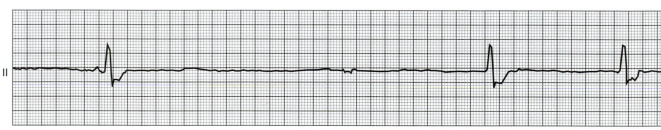

Continuous recording   B.

Figure 10-7   Rate _____
Rhythm _____
QRS Duration _____
PR Interval _____
AV Conduction Ratio _____
ST Segment _____
Interpretation _____
Reasoning _____

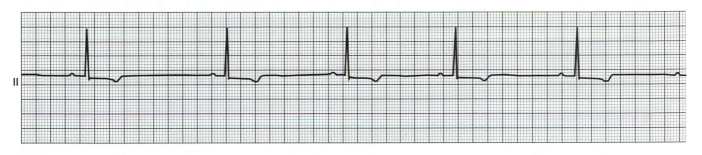

Figure 10-8   Rate _____
Rhythm _____
QRS Duration _____
PR Interval _____
AV Conduction Ratio _____
ST Segment _____
Interpretation _____
Reasoning _____

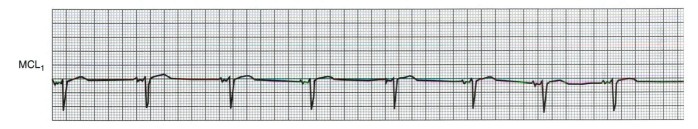

Figure 10-9   Rate _____
Rhythm _____
QRS Duration _____
PR Interval _____
AV Conduction Ratio _____
ST Segment _____
Interpretation _____
Reasoning _____

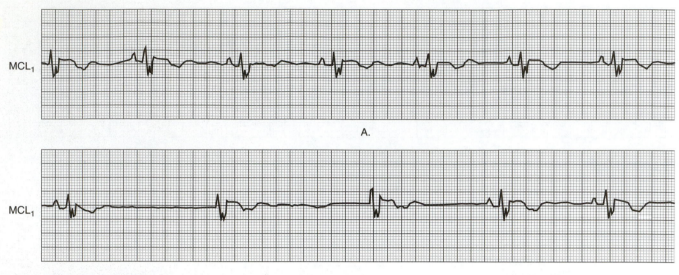

MCL₁

A.

MCL₁

Continuous recording

B.

Figure 10-10　Rate _____
　　　　　　　　　Rhythm _____
　　　　　　　　　QRS Duration _____
　　　　　　　　　PR Interval _____
　　　　　　　　　AV Conduction Ratio _____
　　　　　　　　　ST Segment _____
　　　　　　　　　Interpretation _____
　　　　　　　　　Reasoning _____

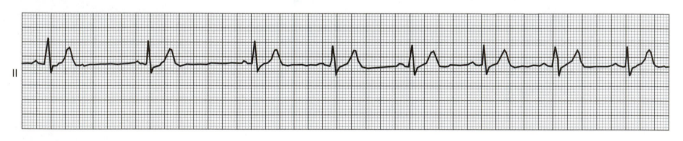

II

Figure 10-11　Rate _____
　　　　　　　　　Rhythm _____
　　　　　　　　　QRS Duration _____
　　　　　　　　　PR Interval _____
　　　　　　　　　AV Conduction Ratio _____
　　　　　　　　　ST Segment _____
　　　　　　　　　Interpretation _____
　　　　　　　　　Reasoning _____

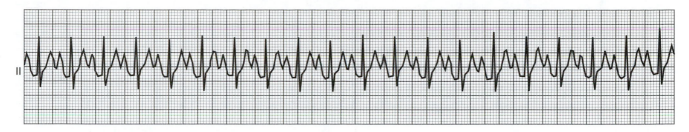

Figure 10–12   Rate _____
Rhythm _____
QRS Duration _____
PR Interval _____
AV Conduction Ratio _____
ST Segment _____
Interpretation _____
Reasoning _____

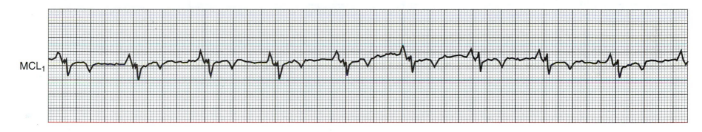

Figure 10–13   Rate _____
Rhythm _____
QRS Duration _____
PR Interval _____
AV Conduction Ratio _____
ST Segment _____
Interpretation _____
Reasoning _____

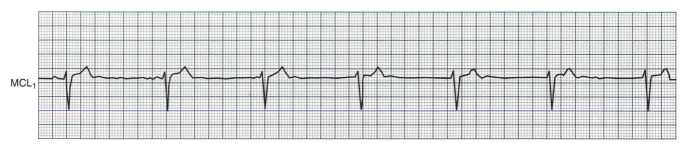

Figure 10–14   Rate _____
Rhythm _____
QRS Duration _____
PR Interval _____
AV Conduction Ratio _____
ST Segment _____
Interpretation _____
Reasoning _____

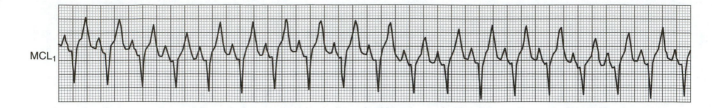

Figure 10–15 Rate _____
Rhythm _____
QRS Duration _____
PR Interval _____
AV Conduction Ratio _____
ST Segment _____
Interpretation _____
Reasoning _____

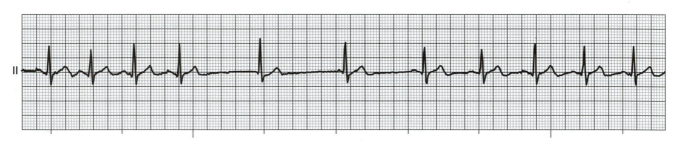

Figure 10–16 Rate _____
Rhythm _____
QRS Duration _____
PR Interval _____
AV Conduction Ratio _____
ST Segment _____
Interpretation _____
Reasoning _____

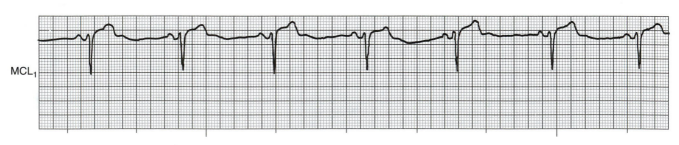

Figure 10–17 Rate _____
Rhythm _____
QRS Duration _____
PR Interval _____
AV Conduction Ratio _____
ST Segment _____
Interpretation _____
Reasoning _____

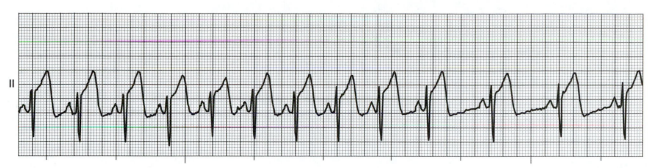

Figure 10–18 Rate _____

Rhythm _____

QRS Duration _____

PR Interval _____

AV Conduction Ratio _____

ST Segment _____

Interpretation _____

Reasoning _____

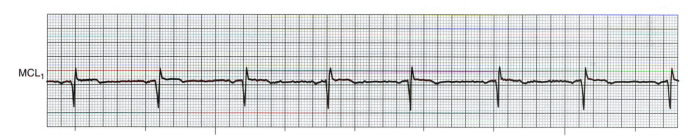

Figure 10–19 Rate _____

Rhythm _____

QRS Duration _____

PR Interval _____

AV Conduction Ratio _____

ST Segment _____

Interpretation _____

Reasoning _____

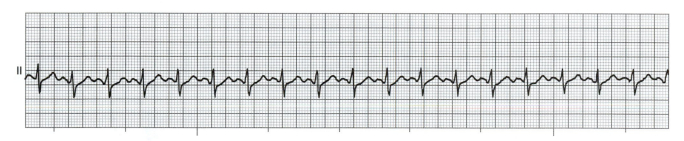

Figure 10–20 Rate _____

Rhythm _____

QRS Duration _____

PR Interval _____

AV Conduction Ratio _____

ST Segment _____

Interpretation _____

Reasoning _____

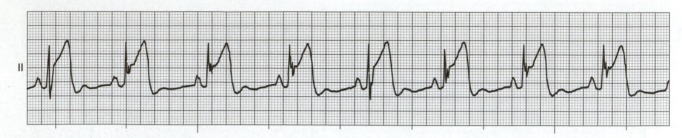

Figure 10–21 Rate _____
Rhythm _____
QRS Duration _____
PR Interval _____
AV Conduction Ratio _____
ST Segment _____
Interpretation _____
Reasoning _____

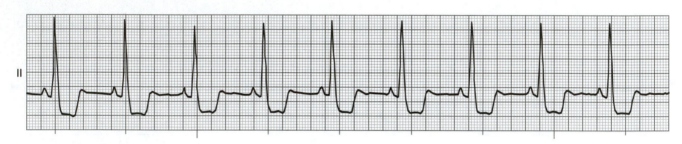

Figure 10–22 Rate _____
Rhythm _____
QRS Duration _____
PR Interval _____
AV Conduction Ratio _____
ST Segment _____
Interpretation _____
Reasoning _____

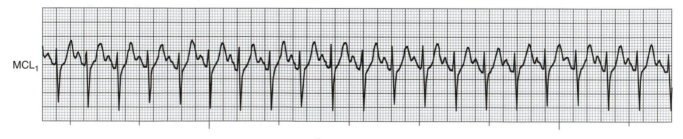

Figure 10–23 Rate _____
Rhythm _____
QRS Duration _____
PR Interval _____
AV Conduction Ratio _____
ST Segment _____
Interpretation _____
Reasoning _____

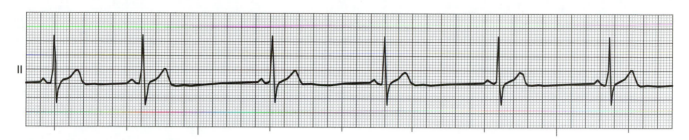

Figure 10–24 Rate _____
Rhythm _____
QRS Duration _____
PR Interval _____
AV Conduction Ratio _____
ST Segment _____
Interpretation _____
Reasoning _____

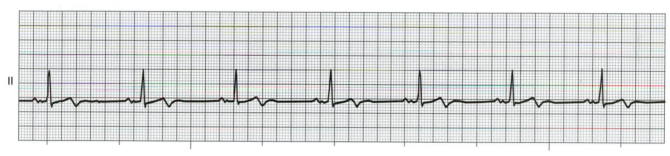

Figure 10–25 Rate _____
Rhythm _____
QRS Duration _____
PR Interval _____
AV Conduction Ratio _____
ST Segment _____
Interpretation _____
Reasoning _____

Supraventricular Dysrhythmias—Part One

Upon completion of this chapter, the reader should be able to:

- *Describe how reentry and increased automaticity cause supraventricular dysrhythmias.*

- *List three major ECG characteristics of supraventricular rhythms.*

- *List the ranges of atrial rates for common supraventricular tachydysrhythmias.*

- *List the ECG characteristics of premature atrial complexes (PACs).*

- *Explain the mechanism by which PACs develop.*

- *Describe three possible atrial wave shapes found in PACs.*

- *Discuss the clinical significance and treatment of PACs.*

- *Describe how a premature junctional complex (PJC) differs from a PAC.*

- *List the ECG characteristics of PJCs.*

- *Define the term multifocal atrial tachycardia (MAT).*

- *List the ECG characteristics of MAT.*

- *Discuss the clinical significance and treatment of MAT.*

- *Define the term wandering atrial pacemaker (WAP).*

- *List the ECG characteristics of a WAP.*

- *List the possible pacemaker sites for a WAP.*

- *Define the terms supraventricular tachycardia (SVT) and paroxysmal supraventricular tachycardia (PSVT).*

- *List the ECG characteristics of a SVT.*

- *Explain the mechanism by which a SVT develops.*

- *Contrast the relative speed with which an episode of SVT starts and ends to that of sinus tachycardia.*

- *List the clinical significance and treatment for SVT.*

CHAPTER OVERVIEW

Supraventricular dysrhythmias originate outside of the sinus node, either in the atria or AV junction. As a result, supraventricular complexes have abnormal P wave shapes or absent P waves. Like sinus beats, supraventricular complexes have narrow QRS complexes because ventricular conduction is normal. Supraventricular dysrhythmias are mainly a problem due to their rapid rates.

SUPRAVENTRICULAR DYSRHYTHMIAS

This chapter begins the study of ECG disorders that develop outside of the normal sinus pacemaker. The term **supraventricular** refers to the area of the heart located above the branch point of the AV bundle (His bundle) and includes the atria and the AV junction. Supraventricular dysrhythmias are grouped together because they arise from sites above the ventricles and have similar ECG characteristics: absent or abnormal P waves with a narrow QRS complex. The QRS complex is normal in supraventricular disorders since conduction beyond the AV junction follows a normal pathway. Figure 11–1 illustrates common supraventricular beat findings. Several dysrhythmia types are grouped under the supraventricular heading including atrial, nodal reentry, and AV junctional rhythms (Figure 11–2).

> ***ECG Interpretation Tip:*** *A useful rule is: all beats with QRS complexes that are less than 0.12 second must have developed in a supraventricular pacemaker: sinus, junctional, or atrial.*

For convenience, the term "supraventricular" is applied to narrow QRS complex rhythms that arise from the atria or AV junction. Often, it is not possible to determine with certainty whether the complex arose in the atria or in the AV junction. While the term supraventricular lacks specificity, it is useful because it differentiates this group of cardiac rhythm disorders from the more serious ventricular dysrhythmias. This broad distinction is useful because there are major treatment differences between supraventricular and ventricular rhythm disturbances.

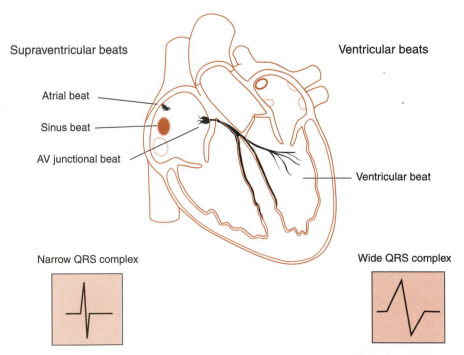

Figure 11-1 Supraventricular compared to ventricular complexes. Supraventricular beats result in narrow QRS complexes, whereas ventricular beats have wide QRS complexes, but there are some exceptions. *(From Lipman BC, Casio T. ECG assessment and interpretation. Philadelphia: FA Davis Publishers; 1994; p 89, Figure II–2.)*

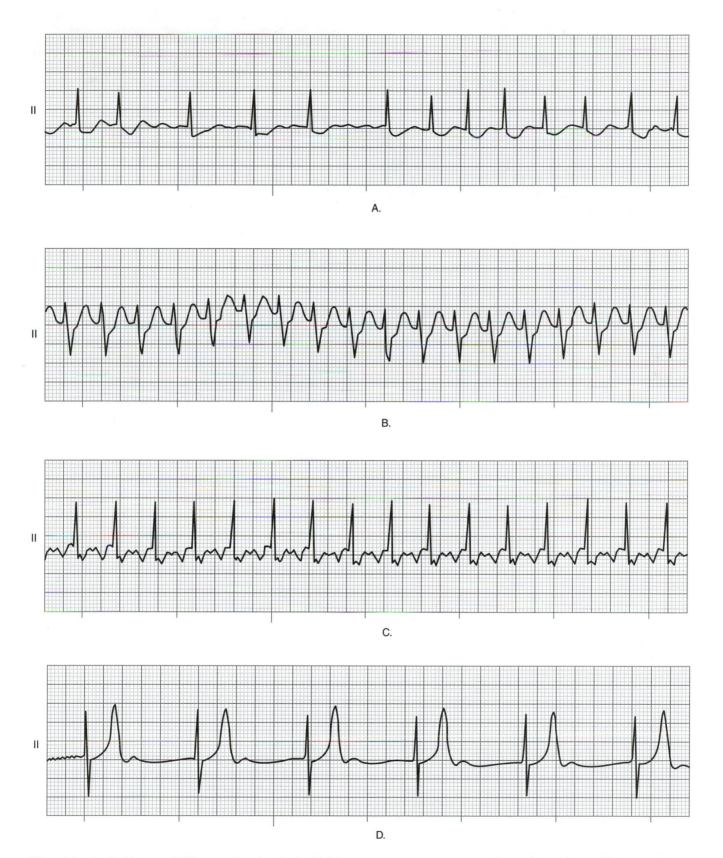

A.

B.

C.

D.

Figure 11–2 Narrow QRS complex dysrhythmias. Tracings A through D show four types of supraventricular dysrhythmias, all of which have narrow QRS complexes with durations of less than 0.12 second.

ECG Characteristics of Supraventricular Dysrhythmias

A key feature of supraventricular complexes is that they have distorted or absent P waves because atrial depolarization is altered (Figure 11–3). The P wave is replaced by an atrial wave which differs from sinus beats. Atrial waves that replace P waves are termed **P′ waves** and have a distorted appearance: tall, pointy, notched, biphasic, flattened, or saw-toothed shapes. P′ waves are often hidden in the preceding T waves and commonly are missing in supraventricular rhythms.

> ***ECG Interpretation Tip:*** *Supraventricular beats or rhythms have altered or absent P waves because they originate outside the sinus node. They have normal QRS-T complexes because ventricular activation and recovery are normal.*

Clinical Significance of Supraventricular Dysrhythmias

Supraventricular dysrhythmias, in general, require treatment when they occur so fast as to cause ischemia and/or hypotension. Older patients and those with compromised cardiac function, such as congestive heart

Table 11-1 Key ECG Features of PACs & PJCs	
Atrial activity:	Irregular with distorted P′ waves in PACs and shortened PR intervals or missing P′ waves in PJCs
AV conduction:	Normal or shorter than normal, especially with PJCs
Ventricular activity:	Irregular with narrow QRS complexes

failure, are the most vulnerable to the loss of sinus activity. Brief episodes of supraventricular dysrhythmias are more of a nuisance than a cause for concern. Most patients seek medical assistance for supraventricular dysrhythmias because they experience palpitations, general weakness, dizziness, shortness of breath, or fatigue.

One of the initial steps in evaluating premature beats and rapid rhythms is distinguishing supraventricular from ventricular dysrhythmias. Patients generally tolerate rapid supraventricular dysrhythmias better than fast ventricular dysrhythmias. Wide QRS complex rhythms usually signify a ventricular rhythm, but there are a

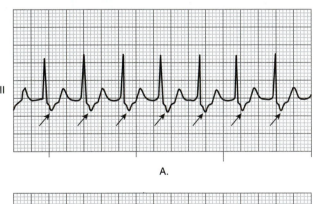

A.

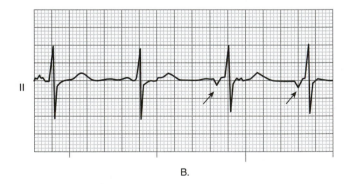

B.

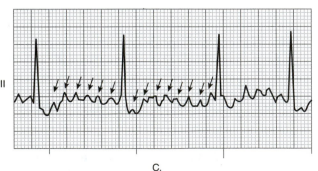

C.

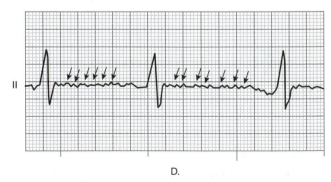

D.

Figure 11-3 Atrial waves. Tracings A through D show how P′ waves (arrows) in various atrial dysrhythmias differ from the P waves of sinus beats.

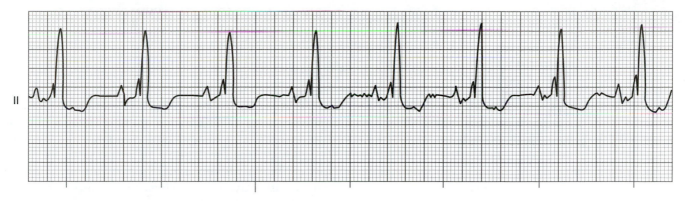

Figure 11–4 Sinus rhythm with wide and distorted QRS complexes due to a bundle branch block. The P waves before each QRS clearly indicate a sinus pacemaker.

few exceptions because *not all supraventricular complexes have narrow QRS complexes* (Figure 11–4). Supraventricular beats can have a wide QRS complex if ventricular conduction is abnormal. For instance, an underlying bundle branch block is a common cause of a wide QRS complex rhythm; this is termed **aberrant conduction**.

> *ECG Interpretation Tip: Not all wide QRS complexes are due to ventricular impulses; some supraventricular complexes are conducted aberrantly, resulting in a prolonged QRS duration. Others are wide because of a preexisting bundle branch conduction block.*

MECHANISMS OF DYSRHYTHMIA FORMATION

There are two ways that abnormal cardiac impulses develop: increased automaticity and via a reentry pathway. (Conduction abnormalities are another leading cause of dysrhythmias and will be discussed in a later chapter.)

- **Decreased automaticity** slows the depolarization rate of the SA node and leads to bradycardic rhythms.

- **Increased automaticity** accelerates the depolarization rate of the SA node and other ectopic pacemakers.

- A **reentry** mechanism involves the development of a recurring depolarization cycle because the conduction pathway cells have different conduction rates.

Automaticity

Automaticity is the ability of pacemaker cells to spontaneously depolarize. The cells of the sinus node produce a heart rate between 60 and 100/minute in adults. Increased automaticity and decreased automaticity can cause dysrhythmias. Some conditions that increase sinus node automaticity such as sympathetic nervous stimulation or adrenergic drugs, will speed the heart rate. Sinus tachycardia is due to increased automaticity while sinus bradycardia indicates decreased automaticity. Ischemia often leads to premature ventricular complexes because ectopic pacemaker sites become irritable from decreased oxygen delivery and respond with increased automaticity.

Reentry

Reentry is the leading mechanism by which most tachydysrhythmias develop. While increased automaticity involves abnormal impulse formation, reentry involves abnormal impulse *conduction*. Reentry can occur in any part of the conduction system, as well as in every heart area including the atria, sinus node, AV node, and the His-Purkinje ventricular tissue, in addition to the cardiac muscle itself.

Myocardial cells normally transmit impulses at a constant speed and in one direction. The conduction system becomes uniformly depolarized and repolarized. The uniform repolarization phase is termed the **refractory period**, which means that the heart cannot be stimulated again until it becomes fully repolarized. Ischemia and abnormal conduction pathways set the stage for a reentry process that is associated with tachydysrhythmias, by delaying the repolarization phase.

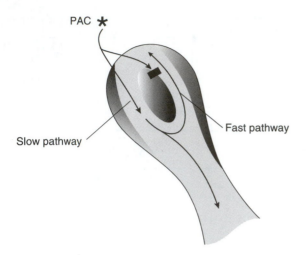

PAC ✱

Slow pathway

Fast pathway

Figure 11–5 The AV node is the site of a reentry circuit. PSVTs often start when a PAC enters the node and travels down two functionally different intranodal pathways. The PAC impulse is blocked in the fast limb but conducts along the slow pathway. The PAC impulse crosses over to the fast limb from the slow path and travels back up to the atria. The impulse circles around to start the cycle over.

SUPRAVENTRICULAR DYSRHYTHMIAS AND REENTRY

Most supraventricular dysrhythmias are caused by a reentry process. While reentry can occur in most areas of the heart, the AV node is the most common (Figure 11–5). Two limbs of a conduction pathway can have different rates of conduction forming a faster and a slower path. A premature atrial complex often initiates a series of abnormal beats by traveling along both paths. The PAC travels down the fast path while transmission is delayed in the slower path since it has not been fully repolarized. Yet the PAC is able to stimulate the second limb by traveling along the slowed path in a backwards direction, thereby establishing a rapid tachydysrhythmia.

PREMATURE SUPRAVENTRICULAR COMPLEXES

Premature beats occur earlier than expected and are common in healthy as well as ill patients. Premature complexes can arise in the atria, AV junction, or in the ventricles. Because they share similar ECG characteristics, premature atrial and junctional complexes will be discussed together.

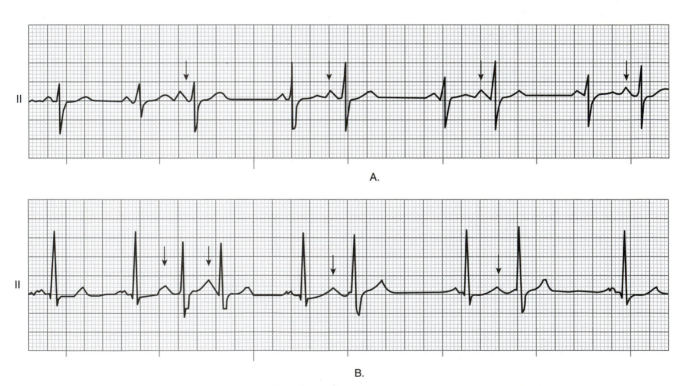

II

A.

II

B.

Figure 11–6 Premature atrial complexes. PACs are marked by arrows. Note that the PACs occur prematurely, have narrow QRS complexes, and the P′ waves differ from the sinus P waves. In strip B the P waves of the sinus beats have a notched shape.

Premature Atrial Complexes (PACs)

Premature atrial complexes (Figures 11–6 and 11–7) are ectopic beats that originate earlier than expected within atrial tissue. They occur early, or prematurely, during the R-R cycle suddenly disrupting an otherwise regular rhythm. Premature atrial complexes usually have a narrow QRS complex since ventricular conduction is normal.

PAC with Aberrant Ventricular Conduction

Sometimes, a PAC occurs so early that the ventricular tissue is still partially refractory from the previous sinus beat, resulting in a distorted QRS-T complex because ventricular conduction is altered (Figure 11–8).

Non-Conducted PACs

An interesting but uncommon event occurs when the PAC forms too early. When the premature complex occurs so early it is not conducted at all. The only ECG evidence is a P′ wave without a QRS-T complex. (Figure 11–9). This occurs when a PAC occurs during the upstroke of the previous sinus beat's T wave while the tissue is still refractory and the QRS is blocked. A blocked PAC appears as a sudden pause in cardiac activity. Inspection of the T wave occurring just ahead of a pause, will identify the hidden premature atrial wave as the true cause of the pause.

> **ECG Interpretation Tip:** *The most common cause of an ECG pause is a blocked PAC— not failure of the sinus node. A tall, peaked T wave occurring just before the ECG pause signals the blocked PAC.*

Premature Junctional Complexes (PJCs)

The junctional area surrounds the AV node and includes the atrial tissue along with the nodal fibers as they exit the node to form the AV bundle (Figure 11–10). In **premature junctional complexes** the junctional area prematurely depolarizes ahead of the next expected sinus impulse disrupting the regular P-P cycle (Figures 11–11 and 11–12).

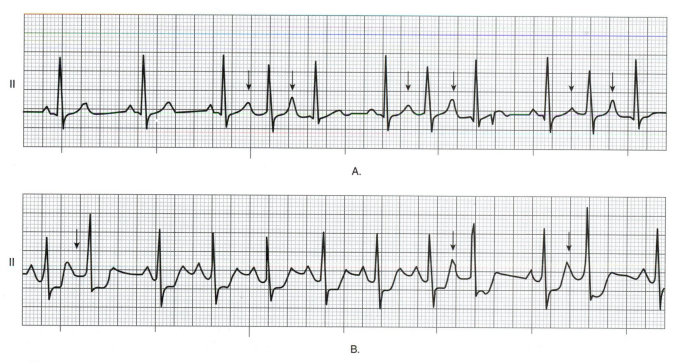

A.

B.

Figure 11–7 The P′ waves of the PACs are indicated by arrows. Note how the P′ waves can only be seen indirectly by the way they distort the preceding T waves. The PACs cause the T waves to have a tall and pointy appearance.

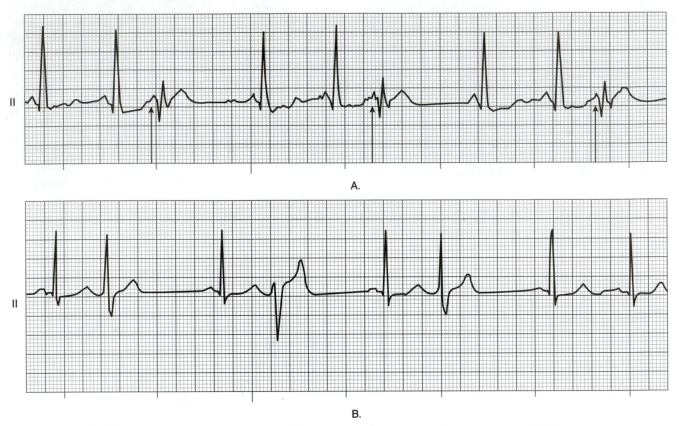

Figure 11–8 PACs with aberrant conduction. The early atrial complexes have distorted QRS complexes because the ventricular conduction is abnormal. In strip A the distorted QRS complexes (beat numbers 3, 6, and 9) are associated with clear P′ waves (indicated by arrows). In strip B the wide, distorted QRS complex (beat number 4) has a P′ wave as part of the preceding T wave (indicated by arrow). Most abnormal conduction of early beats occurs when refractory ventricular tissue is encountered.

P′ Wave in PJCs

The P′ wave appearance of PJCs is variable (Figures 11–13 and 11–14): a) an inverted, or negative, P′ wave deflection in lead II with a shortened PR interval; b) more commonly, a P′ wave is not found because the associated QRS hides the P′ wave; c) the P′ wave sometimes follows the QRS complex due to **retrograde** (backward) conduction.

ECG Patterns of Premature Supraventricular Complexes

Premature complexes commonly occur in a regular patterns, such as after every other sinus beat, termed **atrial bigeminy** (Figure 11–15), or following two sinus beats as **atrial trigeminy** (Figure 11–16). Premature beats can also occur in groups without intervening sinus beats: a pair of early beats is known as a **couplet** (Figure 11–17). Three or more consecutive PACs or PJCs that occur at a rate over 100 per minute is termed supraventricular tachycardia (Figure 11–18).

> *Clinical Note:* PACs are much more common than PJCs. Premature complexes (atrial, junctional, and ventricular) have little clinical consequence.

Causes of Premature Supraventricular Complexes

PACs and PJCs can form by either increased automaticity or a reentry circuit. Ectopic supraventricular pacemaker sites discharge and interrupt the normal sinus rhythm. Premature complexes are often associated with diseases that indirectly dilate and enlarge the atrial muscle, such as cor pulmonale (chronic pulmonary disease causing right-sided heart failure), pulmonary embolism, pneumonia, or rarely, an atrial infarction. A benign cause of increased atrial automaticity is sympathetic nervous system stimulation due to caffeine intake or anxiety (Table 11–2).

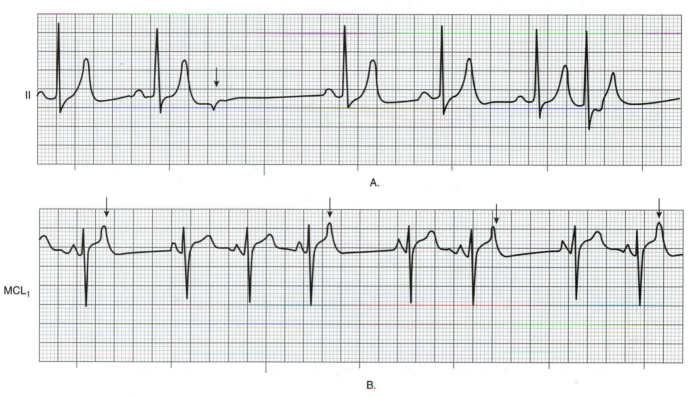

Figure 11-9 Nonconducted PACs. The arrows indicate the nonconducted P′ waves in strips A and B. The pause in strip A after beat number 2 is due to a blocked PAC. In strip B the tall, pointed T waves hide nonconducted P′ waves. Note the pauses in cardiac activity following the nonconducted P′ waves (arrows).

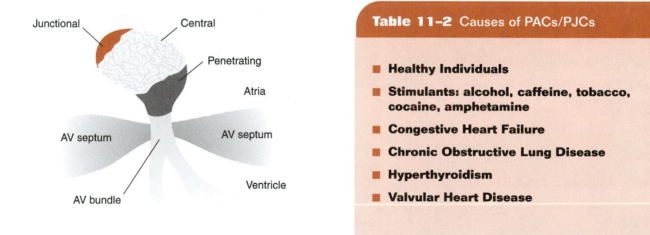

Figure 11-10 Diagram of AV node and junctional tissue. AV nodal tissue consists of several fiber types. Junctional tissue is a transitional area that lies between the atrial tissue and the node. *(Modified with permission from Phillips RE, Feeney MR, The cardiac rhythms, a systematic approach to interpretation. 3rd ed, Philadelphia: WB Saunders; 1990: 275, Figure 5–3.)*

Table 11–2 Causes of PACs/PJCs
■ **Healthy Individuals**
■ **Stimulants: alcohol, caffeine, tobacco, cocaine, amphetamine**
■ **Congestive Heart Failure**
■ **Chronic Obstructive Lung Disease**
■ **Hyperthyroidism**
■ **Valvular Heart Disease**

Clinical Significance of Premature Supraventricular Complexes

Premature supraventricular complexes have only minor clinical significance. Identifying these beats is important mainly to distinguish them from premature ventricular complexes which are more significant. PACs have little effect on cardiac output and patients are usually not aware of them.

Emergency Treatment for Premature Supraventricular Complexes

No emergent treatment is needed. Therapy is directed towards the underlying condition.

ECG Interpretation Tip: *When there are frequent PACs the ECG can be misinterpreted as atrial fibrillation because both rhythms are quite irregular. This can be avoided because only a single P wave or P′ wave is seen before each QRS complex in frequent PAC rhythms. Numerous fibrillatory waves occur before each QRS complex in atrial fibrillation.*

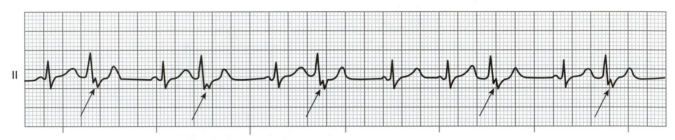

Figure 11–11 PJCs. Frequent premature junctional complexes. PACs lack P waves prior to the QRS complexes. Instead, P′ waves are hidden within the ST segments (arrows).

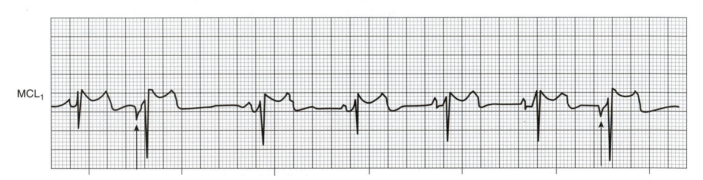

Figure 11–12 PJCs. Beats number 2 and 7 are premature junctional complexes. The inverted P waves are marked with arrows.

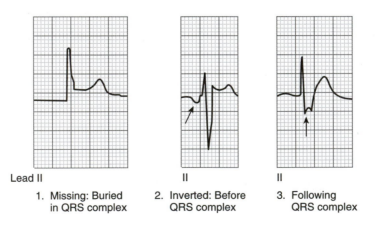

Lead II

1. Missing: Buried in QRS complex

II

2. Inverted: Before QRS complex

II

3. Following QRS complex

Figure 11–13 P′ wave in AV junctional complexes.

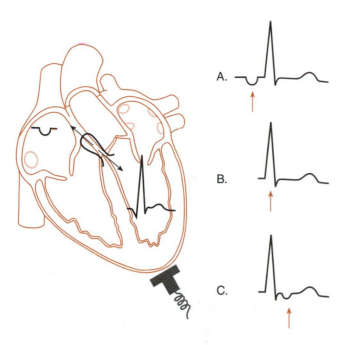

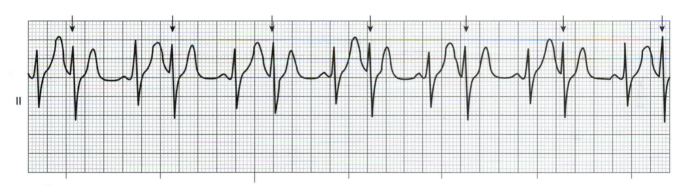

Figure 11–14 P′ wave relationship to the QRS complex in junctional complexes. Of the three possibilities shown, the absent P wave form shown in (B) is the most common. In example A, the P wave is inverted and has a short PR interval while in example C, the P′ wave follows the QRS complex. *(Used with permission from Lipman BC, Casio T. ECG assessment and interpretation. Philadelphia: FA Davis Publishers; 1994; 115, Figure 8–1.)*

II

Figure 11–15 Atrial bigeminy. Every other beat is a PAC, which gives a pattern showing two beats followed by a pause. The PACs are indicated by arrows.

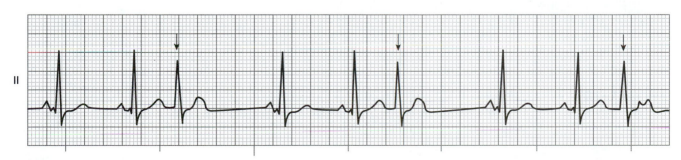

II

Figure 11–16 Atrial trigeminy. Following every two sinus beats is a PAC. Every third beat is a PAC (indicated by arrows).

Continuous recordings

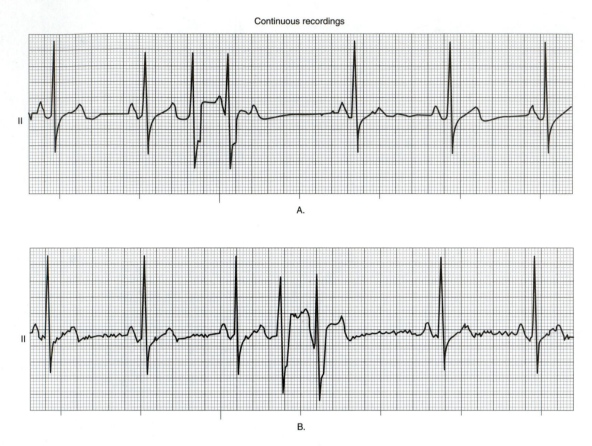

Figure 11-17 Couplets of PACs. The continuous ECG recording shows the development of two groups of consecutive PACs. Beats number 3 and 4 in strip A and beats number 4 and 5 in strip B are consecutive PACs (arrows).

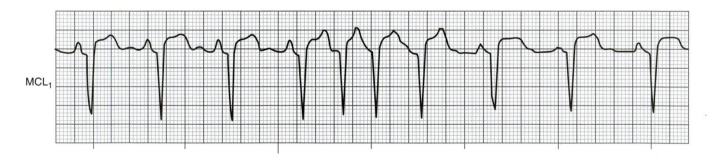

Figure 11-18 Three consecutive PACs. Beats number 5 through 7 (arrows) are successive PACs without intervening sinus beats. Paroxysmal supraventricular tachycardia is defined as three or more consecutive PACs at a rate greater than 100/minute.

MULTIFOCAL ATRIAL TACHYCARDIA (MAT)

The chaotic atrial rhythm in **multifocal atrial tachycardia** has at least three different P′ wave shapes, varying PR intervals, and a rate over 100/minute (Figure 11–19). Untreated MAT usually has a rate between 110 and 130/minute. MAT is actually sinus tachycardia with very frequent PACs (Table 11–3). The term multifocal pertains to multiple pacemaker sites.

Causes of MAT

Multiple ectopic pacemaker sites (foci) depolarize within the atria—as the name MAT implies—due to increased automaticity. The P′ waves in MAT often appear peaked and pointed, which is common with chronic obstructive lung disease that results in right atrial enlargement. In contrast to isolated PACs, MAT is usually found in elderly, seriously ill patients with COPD-induced cor pulmonale (Table 11–4). MAT can also occur with shock, acid-base, and electrolyte disorders.

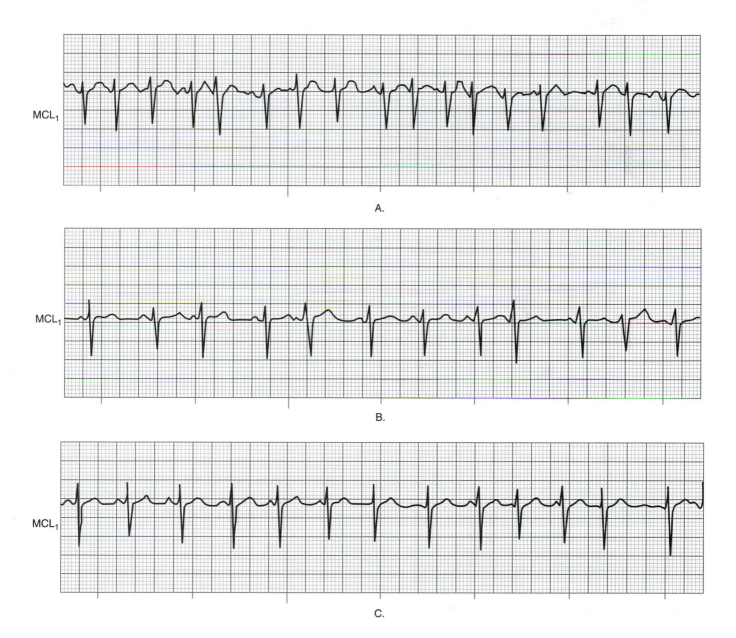

A.

B.

C.

Figure 11–19 Multifocal atrial tachycardia (MAT). In examples A through C the rate of this narrow QRS complex rhythm exceeds 100/minute and the P′ waves have at least three different shapes. The frequent PACs cause a very irregular rhythm as seen in all three examples.

Table 11–4 Causes of Multifocal Atrial Tachycardia

- **Chronic Obstructive Pulmonary Disease (most common cause)**
- **Cor Pulmonale (Heart failure caused by COPD)**
- **Pulmonary Embolism**
- **Hypoxia**
- **Digitalis Toxicity**
- **Hypokalemia (Low serum potassium level)**

Table 11–3 Key ECG Features of Multifocal Atrial Tachycardia

■ **Atrial activity:**	Chaotic rhythm; 3 or more P' wave shapes
■ **AV conduction:**	Normal; 1:1; PR intervals vary from beat to beat
■ **Ventricular activity:**	Narrow QRS complexes; identical shapes
■ **Atrial and Ventricular rate:**	Over 100/minute

Clinical Significance

MAT occurs due to chronic lung disease. The degree of tachycardia and frequency of PACs is related to the severity of the lung disease.

Emergency Treatment for MAT

Therapy is directed at the underlying illness rather than at the rhythm disorder. MAT is a chronic condition and therapy aimed at controlling the dysrhythmia, without modifying the underlying chronic lung disease, will be unsuccessful.

Clinical Note: *Even though the term "multifocal atrial tachycardia" is applied to this uncommon rhythm disorder, it is actually a sinus tachycardia with frequent PACs. Unlike the benign nature of isolated PACs, MAT results from severe chronic obstructive pulmonary disease.*

ECG Interpretation Tip: *MAT is commonly confused with atrial fibrillation since both are narrow QRS complex rhythms that are markedly irregular. Unlike atrial fibrillation, in which organized atrial activity is missing, MAT has distinct but varying ectopic P' wave shapes.*

WANDERING ATRIAL PACEMAKER (WAP)

In **wandering atrial pacemaker** the pacemaker site briefly shifts between the sinus node, an atrial location, a junctional site, and back to the sinus node (Figure 11–20). Unlike the case with PAC/PJCs, there is no competition between the sinus node and other pacemaker sites. Wandering atrial pacemaker occurs because of a brief slowing of sinus function. WAP involves a shift from the SA node to several pacemaker sites until the sinus node resumes control. WAP is an uncommon disorder. Table 11–5 lists the features of WAP.

Causes of WAP

While WAP may be associated with more serious conditions such as myocarditis, pericarditis, or digoxin toxicity, it generally is short-lived and benign. WAP is most often found in healthy people.

Clinical Significance of WAP

While WAP results in an interesting ECG pattern, it is a benign condition that does not interfere with cardiac output.

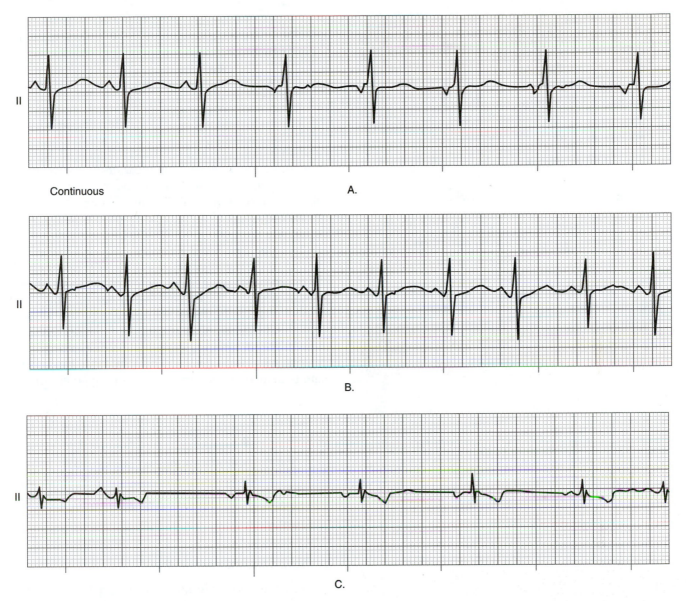

Continuous

A.

B.

C.

Figure 11-20 Wandering atrial pacemaker (WAP). Strips A and B are continuous and illustrate the changes in P wave shapes while the QRS complexes remain the same. In strip A sinus activity is present for the first three beats but after the 4th beat a junctional rhythm occurs for five beats (arrows). Sinus activity resumes in strip B. Strip C shows a similar shift to an atrial rhythm after the second beat (arrows). Sinus activity resumes as beats numbber 6 and 7.

Emergency Treatment for WAP

Emergency treatment is not needed.

> *Clinical Note: WAP is a benign, transient ECG finding seen in the setting of temporary sinus slowing. Unlike MAT, a chronic disorder, there is no competition with the sinus node. WAP subsides when the sinus node accelerates to resume pacemaker control.*

SUPRAVENTRICULAR TACHYCARDIA (SVT)

Supraventricular tachycardia is a narrow QRS complex dysrhythmia with a regular rhythm that originates within the atria at a rate of 150 to 250 bpm (Figure 11–21). Common rates that distinguish supraventricular tachycardias are presented in Table 11–6. In its simplest form, SVT is three or more consecutive PACs occurring at a rate greater than 100/minute (Figure 11–22). Most cases of SVT are due to a reentry pathway within the AV node, which lasts minutes to hours.

SVT occurs at approximately 200/minute, which is considerably faster than sinus tachycardia. There are sever-

Table 11-5 Key ECG Features of Wandering Atrial Pacemaker

■ **Atrial activity:**	Changing P and P' shapes; grossy irregular
■ **AV conduction:**	Normal
■ **Ventricular activity:**	Normal shape; irregular rhythm
■ **Other:**	Pacemaker transiently shifts to atrial and junctional sites when the sinus node slows

Table 11-6 Pacemaker Rates in Various Rapid Supraventricular Disorders

Dysrhythmia	Rate (Range)	Average Rate
Sinus tachycardia	100–150/minute	125/minute
Paroxysmal supraventricular tachycardia (PSVT)	150–250/minute	200/minute
Atrial flutter	250–350/minute	300/minute
Atrial fibrillation	350–600/minute	475/minute

Table 11-7 Key ECG Features of PSVT

■ **Atrial activity:**	Regular; unable to see P' waves
■ **AV conduction:**	1:1 unless digitalis toxicity present
■ **Ventricular activity:**	Regular and narrow.
■ **Rate:**	200/minute (150–250/minute)
■ **Onset/Termination:**	Abrupt

al forms of SVT based on whether the rhythm is transient or sustained and whether the P' waves have the same or different shapes.

Paroxysmal SVT (PSVT)

As the term implies, PSVT occurs in brief sudden bursts referred to as paroxysms (see Figure 11–23). Episodes of PSVT begin and end abruptly. Table 11–7 lists the features of PSVT. PSVT is a recurrent disorder. PSVT episodes can be sporadic or frequent and can last minutes, hours, or days. A PAC strikes during the relative refractory period of a sinus beat and a reentry circuit within the AV node develops. Less commonly, PSVT can be caused by a rapid ectopic atrial pacemaker. The abrupt onset of PSVT is shown in Figure 11–23. PSVT can occur for a short period of time and be self limited, which is typical, but it can last for hours and cause hypotension. PSVT is usually well tolerated in young individuals—and patients without ischemic or valvular heart disease; however, in the elderly and patients with coronary artery disease, PSVT can precipitate ischemia, pulmonary edema, and hypotension.

ECG Interpretation Tip: PSVT is a rapid, regular, narrow QRS complex transient tachydysrhythmia that starts and ends suddenly. PSVT is a common disorder and seldom causes serious symptoms or signs.

P' Waves Appearance in PSVT

P' waves are typically not seen during PSVT because the rapid rate causes the QRS-T complexes to be crammed together. The upright ECG deflections that are commonly seen between QRS complexes—which are commonly mistaken as P' waves—are actually T waves (Figure 11–24).

Causes of PSVT

PSVT mainly occurs in people without heart disease but can complicate other cardiac conditions, especially mitral valve prolapse (Table 11–8).

Emergency Treatment for PSVT

Most PSVT cases can be effectively treated in the emergency setting. Effective long-term therapy is best guided by electrophysiologic studies, during which the reentry pathway can be induced, identified, and eliminated using sound waves.

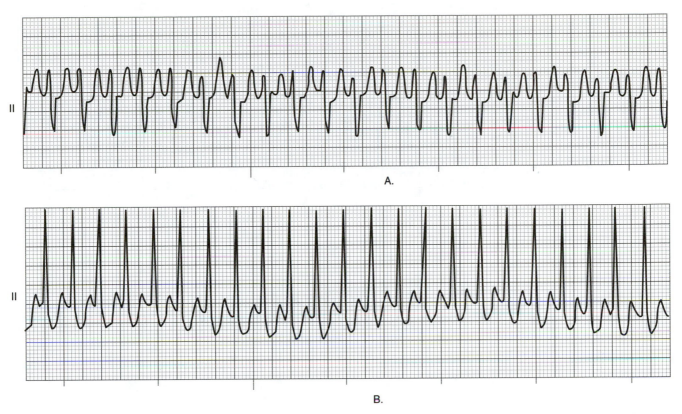

A.

B.

Figure 11–21 Supraventricular tachycardia is a narrow QRS complex dysrhythmia with a regular rhythm that originates within the atria at a rate of 150 to 250 bpm

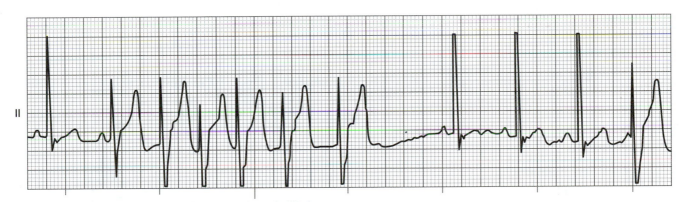

Figure 11–22 Supraventricular tachycardia. Strip shows a 6-beat episode of paroxysmal SVT abruptly disrupting NSR.

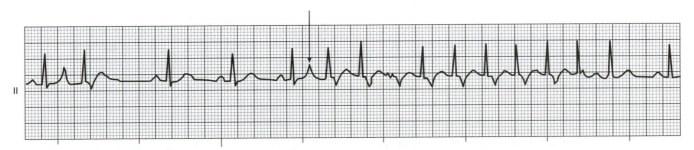

Figure 11–23 Brief episode of PSVT. A short bout of SVT is initiated by a PAC (indicated by an arrow). The 10-beat episode is preceded and followed by sinus complexes.

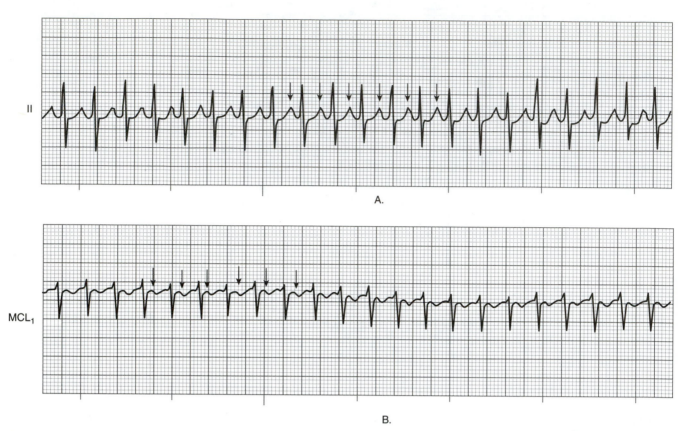

Figure 11–24 Supraventricular tachycardias. The two examples show narrow QRS complex rhythms, absent P waves, at rates 150 bpm and above. The arrows indicate the T waves which are frequently misidentified as P waves. Strips A and B show sustained SVTs at rates approximately 190/minute.

Table 11–8 Causes of PSVT
■ **Otherwise Normal Heart**
■ **Valvular Heart Disease**
■ **Digitalis Toxicity**
■ **Wolff-Parkinson-White Syndrome (Preexcitation disorder)**

Emergent therapy is directed at interrupting the re-entry circuit and restoring NSR. Treatment is based on whether the patient's condition is stable or unstable. See the general approach to the adult tachycardia treatment guideline found in Table 11–9.

In *unstable patients* synchronized electrical cardioversion is the treatment of choice. However, this is rarely needed unless the patient is near collapse. Instead, adenosine works so rapidly and eliminates the need for an electric shock.

In *stable patients* the following techniques and drugs are useful:

■ Adenosine (Adenocard(R)) is the drug of choice for treating PSVT as it interrupts the reentry cycle and terminates the dysrhythmia in 90% of the cases. Adenosine is administered as a 6 mg rapid bolus and, if unsuccessful, the dose can be doubled to 12 mg. Additional doses in refractory cases is not effective.

■ Vagal maneuvers including carotid sinus massage (CSM) and performing a Valsalva maneuver can increase parasympathetic tone (Figure 11–25). (With the availability of adenosine, and lack of side effects compared with vagal maneuvers, many clinicians omit vagal maneuvers altogether.)

Table 11-9 Approach to Narrow QRS Complex Tachycardias

The following steps are helpful when faced with a rapid, narrow-QRS complex dysrhythmia:

■ A 12-lead ECG to identify the specific ECG disorder

■ Oxygen, intravenous access, and monitoring vital signs

■ Assessing the patient and clinical data to determine the need to treat and the urgency of treatment

■ Vagal maneuvers are occasionally effective

Therapy

■ Adenosine is the first-line drug

■ Cases unresponsive to adenosine: further therapy depends on cardiac function:

　■ *Normal cardiac function:* calcium channel blockers or beta-blocker, digoxin, electrical cardioversion, or other antidysrhythmics

　■ *Impaired cardiac function:* electrical cardioversion, digoxin, amiodarone, or diltiazem

Approach to Specific Regular, Narrow-QRS Complex Rhythms

Depending on the results from the above actions, the following therapy can be used for the specific rhythm disorder:

■ **PSVT:** is caused by a reentry circuit, which responds best to adenosine or electrical cardioversion.

　■ Adenosine is highly effective, reverting to sinus rhythm in over 90% cases.

　■ Cardioversion is *rarely* needed but can be useful for unstable PSVT that is associated with impaired cardiac function.

■ **MAT with *normal cardiac* function:** due to an excited automatic ectopic pacemaker, which does not respond to synchronized cardioversion.

　■ Calcium channel blockers, beta-adrenergic blockers, and amiodarone.

■ **MAT with *impaired* cardiac function:** cardioversion should be avoided in favor of amiodarone and/or diltiazem

■ **AV junctional tachycardia** caused by an automatic rapid pacemaker that is treated with:

　■ *Normal cardiac function:* amiodarone or calcium channel blocker or beta-adrenergic blocker. Cardioversion is not recommended.

　■ *Low ejection fraction or CHF:* cardioversion is avoided in favor of amiodarone.

■ **Atrial fibrillation/flutter:** discussed in chapter 12

■ **Ventricular tachycardia:** discussed in chapter 16

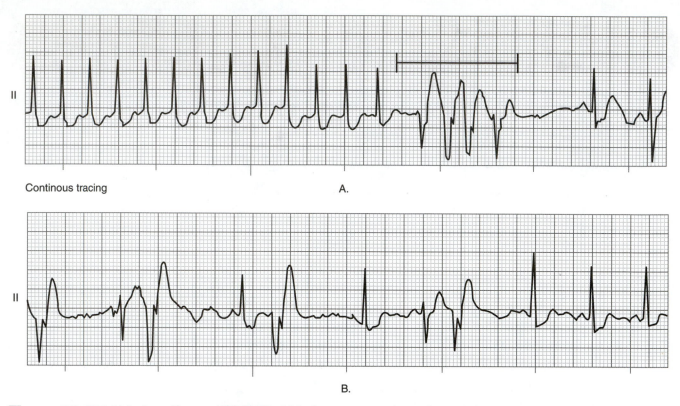

Continous tracing

A.

B.

Figure 11–25 Valsalva effect on PSVT. The Valsalva maneuver is performed during the period marked with a horizontal bar.

- Calcium channel blockers

  - Diltiazem (Cardizem®) is given at 0.25 mg/kg by slow IV administration over 2 minutes. The average dose for a 70 kg patient is 20 mg. If unsuccessful, a 0.35 mg/kg diltiazem dose can be given ten minutes after the initial dose (a 25 mg dose for a 70 kg patient).

  - Verapamil (Isoptin®, Calan®) is administered initially as a 2.5 to 5 mg IV dose that is given over 1 minute. A repeat dose of 5 to 10 mg can be given 15 to 30 minutes later.

- Beta blocking agents

  - Metoprolol (Lopressor®) 5 mg by slow IV administration at 5 minute intervals to a total of 15mg.

  - Atenolol (Tenormin®) 5 mg by slow IV administration over 5 minutes. A second 5 mg dose can be given 10 minutes after the first dose.

- Digoxin 0.5 mg by slow IV administration over 2 minutes. A dose of 0.25 mg can be given 30 minutes later. These agents work by slowing

the ventricular rate by increasing AV nodal refractoriness. In patients with WPW, digitalis is relatively contraindicated because it can paradoxically increase the ventricular rate by favoring conduction along the bypass tract.

Successful cardioversion can be recognized when a sinus rhythm returns at a much slower rate. Note the absent P waves in Figure 11–26A and how P waves become visible after treatment in Figure 11–26B.

Clinical Note: *Beta blockers and calcium channel blockers should not be used together as the incidence of hypotension and bradycardia increases.*

Sustained SVT with 2:1 Conduction

Sustained SVT with 2:1 AV conduction is an uncommon drug-induced dysrhythmia. Digoxin, calcium channel blocking agents, or beta-adrenergic blockers can cause any SVT that does not have 1:1 AV conduction (Figure 11–27).

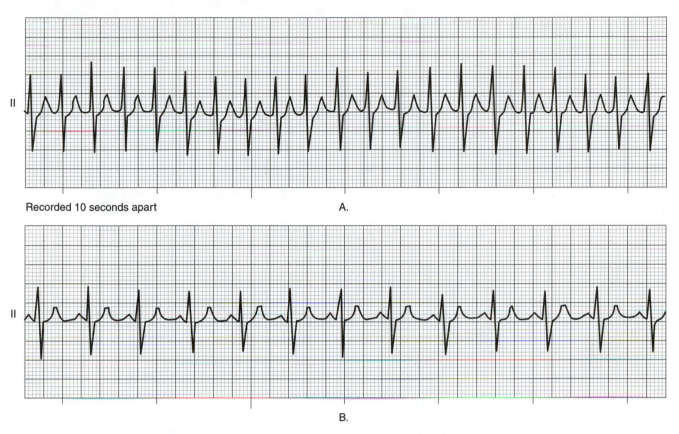

Recorded 10 seconds apart   A.

B.

Figure 11-26 Before and after Adenosine. A shows a typical SVT pattern. B shows the return of sinus rhythm. The QRS complexes are identical.

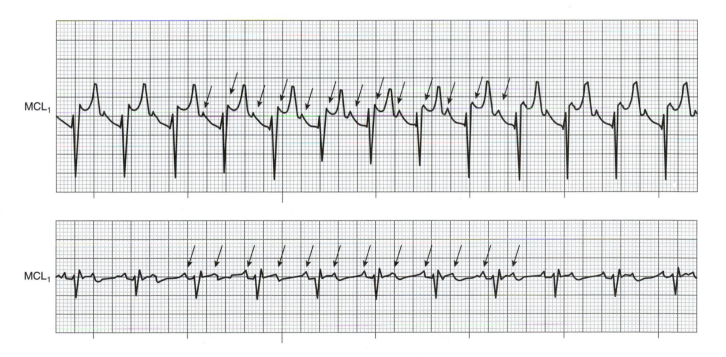

Figure 11-27 Sustained SVT with 2:1 AV conduction. The arrows indicate the P′ waves in both tracings. Every other P′ is blocked. Strip B shows an 8 beat burst of PSVT initiated by a PAC (arrow).

Sustained SVT is much less common than paroxysmal SVT and is usually due to digitalis toxicity. The non-paroxysmal SVT form should be suspected whenever the AV conduction is impaired, having AV conduction ratios of 2:1, 3:1, or 4:1. Standard therapy for paroxysmal SVT form will not be effective for the nonparoxysmal form unless the digitalis or other offending drug is withdrawn. Synchronized electrical cardioversion in digitalis toxicity can cause degeneration into an unstable ventricular dysrhythmia.

General Approach to Adult ACLS Tachycardia Treatment Guideline

The advanced cardiac life support (ACLS) tachycardia treatment guideline is a bit more detailed than earlier editions but it is workable and was developed through an evidence-based approach. An overview of the principles of adult tachycardia treatment will be presented now while the individual components will be introduced when the specific dysrhythmias are presented. For each patient encountered with an abnormal rhythm, the following approach is helpful: assess the patient, identify and evaluate the dysrhythmia, and treat the patient—not just the abnormal ECG tracing. Information that will be helpful in appropriately applying the algorithm includes:

■ *Stable versus unstable patient condition.* Patients who are experiencing tachycardias are classified as having a stable or unstable condition (Figure 11-28). Unstable rapid rhythms need to be treated with immediate electrical cardioversion. Unstable conditions pertain to hypotension, altered mental status, ischemic chest pain, or pulmonary edema that is caused by directly by the rapid ventricular rate, which usually has a ventricular rate greater than 150/min. In general, medication to control the rate or convert the rhythm can be used if the patient is stable; otherwise electrical cardioversion should be performed. However, there are many patients who fit into the "gray zone", not critically unstable but with a marginal systolic blood pressure who needs urgent treatment but who are stable enough to withstand the five minute medication trial.

■ *Make a specific rhythm diagnosis.* The guidelines stress the need to identify specific types of tachydysrhythmias rather than applying a single treatment to every case. The cause and type of disorder need to be identified, if possible, because some therapies are more effective for certain rhythm disorders and less effective for others. For instance, the treatment algorithm has decision branch-points when a SVT, a junctional tachycardia, ventricular tachycardia, or atrial fibrillation/flutter is identified (Figure 11-29). Four general tachycardia types are identified next.

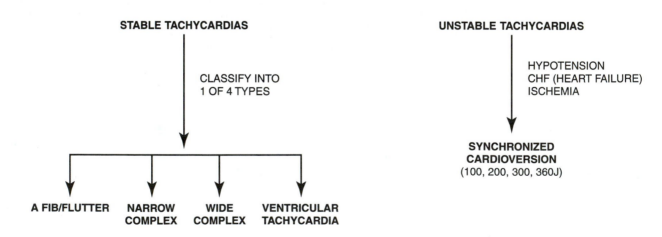

Figure 11-28 Stable versus unstable patient condition.

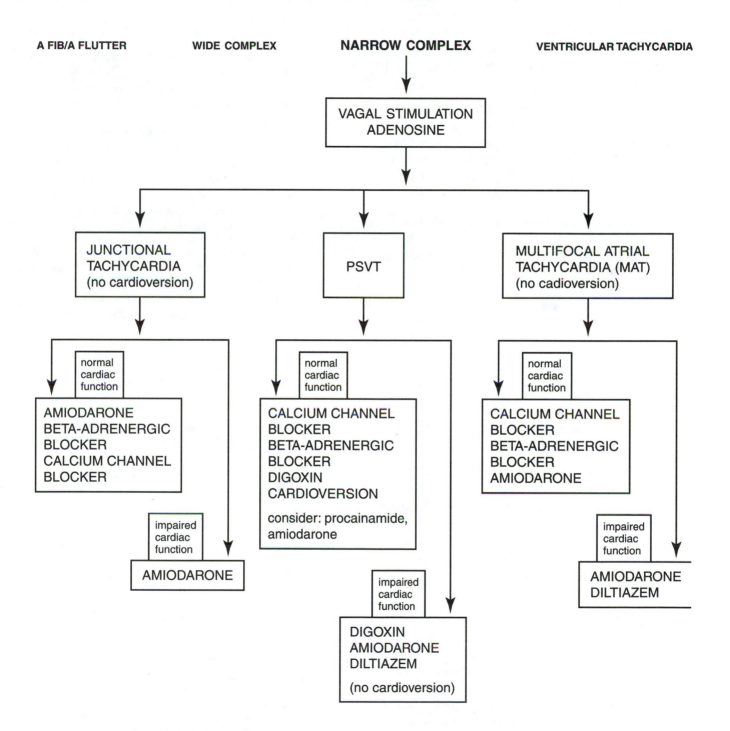

Figure 11–29 Advanced cardiac life support treatment approach to adult bradycardias. (Used with permission of EmedHome.com website (http://www.emedhome.com/)

■ *Assign the dysrhythmia to 1 of 4 tachycardia types.* The initial assessment classifies the rapid disorder into 1 of 4 tachydysrhythmias: narrow-QRS complex tachycardia, atrial fibrillation/flutter, stable wide-QRS complex tachycardia: unknown type, or stable ventricular tachycardia: monomorphic VT &/or polymorphic VT. For each group, a specific treatment pathway is indicated and will be presented later.

■ *Wide or narrow QRS complex?* This information is important in guiding medication choice. Narrow complex tachycardias are supraventricular disorders. Wide complex tachycardias are usually ventricular, but some are actually be SVTs with aberrant ventricular conduction.

■ Duration of rhythm disorder. The duration that a dysrhythmia has lasted is a very important treatment consideration for patients with atrial fibrillation and flutter (which will be presented in chapter 12):

■ Atrial fibrillation/flutter that has lasted *less than 48 hours* can be immediately cardioverted. Early cardioversion is safe and associated with a low risk of embolization.

■ Atrial fibrillation/flutter *lasting over 48hrs or for an unknown period of time*: the best approach is to first control the ventricular rate, start anticoagulation, and plan to cardiovert in two days using either electrical or chemical means.

■ *Impaired cardiac function.* Patients with a history of impaired cardiac function, heart failure, low cardiac ejection fraction, will be treated differently from those with previously normal cardiac function. Most antidysrhythmic agents can lower the blood pressure somewhat but preferred agents can minimize the effect to avoid worsening the already compromised condition.

■ *Use only one antidysrhythmic for a specific rhythm disorder.* Because all antidysrhythmics are proarrhythmic, it is best to use only the preferred drug for a specific rapid rhythm disorder especially in cases of impaired cardiac function. By limiting the use of dysrhythmias to a single agent, additional dysrhythmias will be limited. If one drug is unsuccessful, electrical cardioversion should be considered rather than using multiple medication. This is a distinct change from earlier ACLS protocols and the current guidelines advocate using electrical cardioversion more frequently.

Let's Review

1. Supraventricular dysrhythmias originate outside the sinus node and are characterized by narrow QRS complexes having absent or abnormally shaped P waves.

2. All beats with normal QRS complexes having a duration of less than 0.12 second, must have formed in a supraventricular site: sinus, atrial, or AV junctional.

3. P′ waves are abnormally shaped atrial waves that replace sinus P waves. P′ waves are caused by abnormal supraventricular pacemaker sites. Common P′ waves include: atrial fibrillation waves, flutter waves, premature atrial complexes, or AV junctional complexes.

4. The clinical significance of a particular dysrhythmia depends on the patient's age, the underlying medical condition, the ventricular rate, as well as how long the dysrhythmia has lasted, and the patient's vital signs.

5. Supraventricular dysrhythmias develop via an increased or decreased automaticity, a reentry mechanism, or through conduction disorders.

6. Premature supraventricular complexes include early atrial and junctional beats. PACs and PJCs have abnormally shaped or absent P waves with normal, narrow QRS complexes.

7. Premature supraventricular complexes are benign and do not require therapy unless they lead to frequent episodes of PSVT.

8. Nonconducted PACs disrupt the cardiac rhythm and the only ECG sign of their presence are sudden pauses which are preceded by distorted T waves.

9. Multifocal atrial tachycardia (MAT) is a grossly irregular rhythm characterized by a rate over 100/minute and P waves having at least three different shapes.

10. MAT typically occurs in elderly patients with advanced chronic lung disease (COPD).

11. Wandering atrial pacemaker (WAP) is a benign dysrhythmia characterized by a pacemaker that shifts between the sinus node, atria, and AV junctional sites.

12. Paroxysmal supraventricular tachycardia is a narrow QRS complex rhythm that originates outside the sinus node and lacks P waves.

13. PSVT starts and ends abruptly.

14. PSVT with 2:1 AV conduction is caused by drug toxicity (digitalis, beta-adrenergic blockers, and calcium channel blockers).

15. PSVT occurs in sudden bursts and episodes typically last for less than an hour.

16. The nonparoxysmal form of SVT is uncommon and usually due to digitalis toxicity. SVT with 2:1 AV conduction is indicative of the non-paroxysmal type.

Glossary

Aberrant conduction Abnormal conduction through the ventricles resulting in wide QRS complex rhythms.

Atrial bigeminy Premature complexes that occur after every other sinus beat.

Atrial trigeminy Premature complexes that occur after every two sinus beats.

Carotid sinus massage (CSM) Pressure applied to the carotid sinus in the neck.

Cor pulmonale Right-sided congestive heart failure caused by chronic obstructive pulmonary disease.

Couplets Premature complexes appearing in groups of two.

Decreased automaticity Diminished depolarization rate.

Digoxin Drug that increases the heart's contractility.

Fibrillatory waves Chaotic, uneven atrial waves characteristic of atrial fibrillation.

Flutter waves Atrial waves chracteristic of atrial flutter; having sharp positive and negative components. Also termed saw-toothed atrial waves.

Increased automaticity Accelerated depolarization rate.

Multifocal Multiple pacemaker sites.

Multifocal atrial tachycardia (MAT) A chaotic atrial rhythm consisting of varying P wave shapes, varying PR intervals, and an accelerated heart rate.

Myocarditis Inflammation of the myocardium.

P' waves Abnormal P waves of atrial dysrhythmias that have a distorted appearance; tall, pointy, notched, asymmetric, biphasic, flattened, or saw-toothed.

Paroxysms Brief, sudden episodes.

Paroxysmal supraventricular tachycardia Abrupt episodes of supraventricular tachycardia.

Pericarditis Inflammation of the pericardial sac.

Premature atrial complexes (PACs) An ectopic supraventricular beat that occurs earlier than expected within the atrial tissue.

Premature junctional complexes (PJCs) An ectopic supraventricular complex that occurs earlier than expected within the AV junction.

Pulmonary embolism Blockage of pulmonary artery by a blood clot.

Reentry Development of a recurring depolarization cycle resulting from varying conduction rates of the conduction pathways.

Refractory period Inability of heart muscle to be stimulated again until the tissue is fully repolarized.

Retrograde conduction Conduction which flows in a reversed direcion.

Saw-toothed atrial wave Atrial wave characteristic of atrial flutter; its positive and negative shape resembles the teeth of a hand saw. Also termed flutter waves.

Supraventricular The area of the heart located above the branch point of the bundle of His, including the atria and AV junction.

Supraventricular tachycardia (SVT) Dysrhythmia characterized by an accelerated heart rate that originates in the atria and has a regular rhythm with narrow QRS complexes.

Wandering atrial pacemaker (WAP) An uncommon dysrhythmia involving an alteration in supraventricular pacemaker sites; impulses are generated by differing sites until the sinus node resumes control.

Supraventricular Dysrhythmias—Part Two

LEARNING OBJECTIVES

Upon completion of this chapter, the reader should be able to:

- *Describe the ECG characteristics of atrial flutter.*

- *Discuss the mechanism by which atrial flutter develops.*

- *State the major determinant of ventricular response in atrial flutter.*

- *Discuss the effect that each of the following ventricular responses will have on cardiac output: A) 300/minute; B) 150/minute; C) 75–100/minute; and D) 50/minute*

- *List three treatments for atrial flutter having a tachycardic ventricular rate.*

- *List the ECG characteristics of atrial fibrillation.*

- *Explain the mechanism by which atrial fibrillation develops.*

- *Describe the meaning of the terms "uncontrolled" versus "controlled" ventricular responses in atrial fibrillation.*

- *List three treatments for atrial fibrillation having a tachycardic ventricular response.*

- *Explain the significance and list two causes of a regular ventricular rhythm in atrial fibrillation.*

- *Describe two ECG differences in the appearances of atrial rhythm between atrial flutter and atrial fibrillation.*

- *Explain the term "atrial fib-flutter."*

- *Describe the ECG characteristics of an AV junctional rhythm.*

- *List the average discharge rate for an escape junctional rhythm.*

- *List the range of pacemaker rates for accelerated junctional rhythms.*

- *Define ventricular preexcitation and explain the underlying anatomic disorder.*

- *List the ECG characteristics of Wolff-Parkinson-White (W-P-W) syndrome.*

- *Explain the primary problem when atrial fibrillation occurs in a patient with Wolff-Parkinson-White syndrome.*

- *List the ECG characteristics of Lown-Ganong-Levine (L-G-L) syndrome.*

- *Name two dysrhythmias that patients with ventricular pre-excitation are prone to developing.*

- *List three drugs to avoid when treating W-P-W syndrome and L-G-L syndrome and two drugs that are useful and safe.*

Two important supraventricular tachydysrhythmias are atrial fibrillation and atrial flutter which share the characteristics of being considerably faster then 100/minute and having narrow QRS complexes. Atrial fibrillation is a very common dysrhythmia characterized by a chaotic, unsynchronized atrial rhythm. In contrast, atrial flutter is much less common and has a rapid, coordinated atrial rhythm. Atrial flutter's ventricular rhythm is usually regular unless treatment has been started, which tends to create an irregular AV conduction. The different atrial wave appearances provides the main clue to tell fibrillation and flutter apart.

Junctional dysrhythmias are included in this chapter because they develop in a supraventricular site, that is, they arise before the His bundle splits. An junctional rhythm also has narrow QRS complexes and can occur at rates ranging from bradycardia (common) to tachycardia (uncommon). Escape junctional rhythms can arise due to sinus node depression, whereas accelerated and tachycardic junctional rhythms arise due to a rapid reentry rhythm or fast ectopic junctional pacemaker that competes with the sinus node. The atrial waves of junctional rhythms also vary from the absence of P′ waves (most common) to an inverted position seen just before the QRS or in a position immediately following the QRS complex.

Accessory AV conduction pathways and preexcitation dysrhythmias will be explored in this chapter because they only become a clinical problem when associated with rapid atrial disorders. Accessory pathways involve abnormal conduction that bypass the AV node and can result in some of the fastest ventricular responses because the protective role of the atrioventricular node's long refractory period is lost.

ATRIAL FLUTTER

Atrial flutter is a rapid ectopic tachycardia characterized by an atrial rate between 250 and 350/minute and caused by a reentry mechanism. The SA node is no longer the pacemaker, having been replaced by an atrial pacemaker that results in very rapid atrial and ventricular rates (Figure 12–1 and Table 12–1). The atrial rhythm is regular and the rate averages 300/minute—the ECG has one flutter wave occurring every large ECG box.

The ventricular rate can vary widely depending on AV conduction and whether medication has been administered. Untreated, atrial flutter occurs at a ventricular rate of 150/minute—half the atrial rate since the AV node blocks every other flutter wave. Following treatment, the rate often slows below 100/minute—from 3:1, 4:1, or 6:1 AV conduction. In unusual cases the AV conduction can be 1:1 and the ventricular rate can be as fast as 240 to 300/minute (Figure 12–2).

because the ventricular rate to a large measure determines the patient's clinical condition.

Flutter Wave Appearance

Atrial flutter shows organized P′ waves, which are known as "flutter" waves, giving this dysrhythmia a distinctive ECG pattern and making it relatively easy to identify. Figure 12–3 shows the initial negative deflection and subsequent positive component that are characteristic of flutter waves. The early part of the flutter wave reflects atrial depolarization while the negative portion reflects repolarization and is labeled as "Ta" in Figure 12–3. Flutter waves are regular and so pronounced that they stand out as "sawtooth," "picket fence," or "zigzag" pattern (Figure 12–4).

ECG Interpretation Tip: A complete ECG interpretation should include the AV conduction ratio along with the average ventricular rate. For example, "Atrial flutter with 4:1 AV conduction and a ventricular rate of 75/minute" conveys more useful information than simply "atrial flutter," especially

Table 12-1 Key ECG Features of Atrial Flutter

■ **Atrial activity:**	"Sawtooth/picket-fence" appearance; P′ waves at 300/minute
■ **AV conduction:**	Usually 2:1, 3:1, or 4:1.
■ **Ventricular activity:**	Narrow QRS complexes

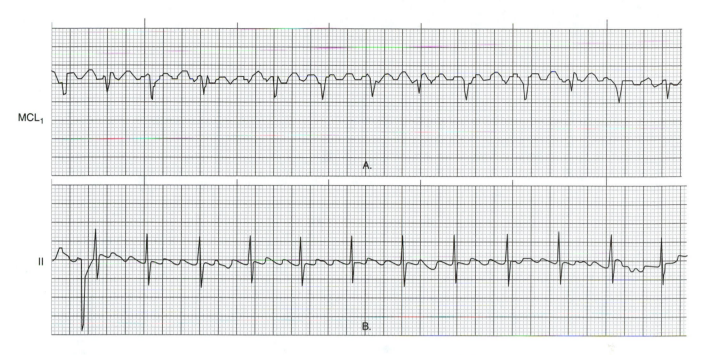

MCL₁

II

A.

B.

Figure 12–1 Atrial flutter. Multiple atrial flutter waves are seen between QRS complexes.

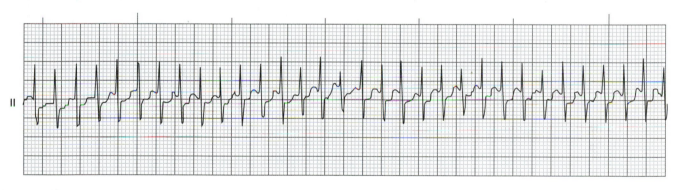

II

Figure 12–2 Atrial flutter with 1:1 AV conduction. The narrow QRS complex tachycardia has a ventricular rate of 240/minute. 1:1 conduction during flutter is rare and happens when the atrial rate is at the slow end of the range for flutter (250–350/minute) or an accessory pathway bypassing the AV node exists such as Wolff-Parkinson-White syndrome.

> *ECG Interpretation Tip* *Lead MCL₁ shows flutter waves best, lead II is adequate, while lead I poorly shows atrial activity. Flutter waves may appear as a flat line in lead I (Figure 12–5).*

Ventricular Response

Conduction of every flutter wave is known as 1:1 conduction and results in a ventricular rate of 300/minute. This is fortunately prevented due to the AV node's long refractory period which prevents overstimulation of the ventricles. AV conduction ratios are usually even-numbered multiples of a ratio such as, 2:1, 4:1, or 6:1 (Figure 12–6). Interestingly, odd-numbered conduction ratio multiples such as 3:1 or 5:1 are unusual, and occurr only after medication (Figure 12–7).

The ventricular response is described as either uncontrolled or controlled based on the ventricular rate.

"Uncontrolled" Atrial Flutter

Atrial flutter that has just recently started ("new onset") has a ventricular rate of 150/minute due to the 2:1 AV conduction.

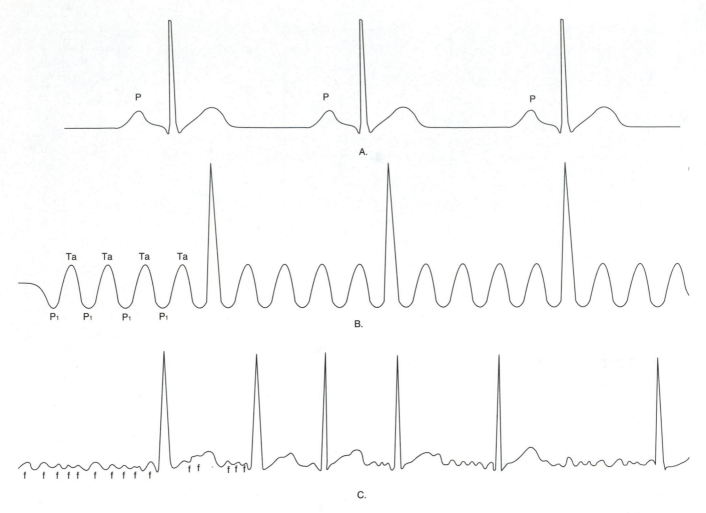

Figure 12-3 Atrial waves compared to P waves. Note that each flutter wave in example B is composed of an initial negative deflection followed by a sharply positive portion which has been marked "Ta" because it is thought to reflect atrial repolarization. The fibrillatory waves (Example C) vary in height, width, and regularity. Sinus activity is presented for comparison in example A.

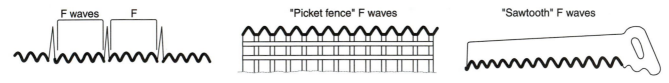

Figure 12-4 Characteristic flutter waves. The atrial waves are regular and uniform in shape—unlike the variable shapes seen with fibrillatory waves.

"Controlled" Atrial Flutter

The ventricular response is "controlled" in atrial flutter when it is less than 100/minute. This represents a form of physiologic "block," which is beneficial, in contrast to the pathologic block found with AV heart block. The AV node's long refractoriness is a safety mechanism that prevents the ventricles from becoming overstimulated.

Figure 12–8 shows the protective function that the AV node serves as it filters out half of the flutter waves. Since the atrial rate in atrial flutter is 300/minute, the ventricular rate will be 150/minute for conduction ratios of 2:1. When flutter is associated with ventricular rates of 150/minute, 100/minute, or 75/minute, the respective AV conduction ratios are 2:1, 3:1, and 4:1.

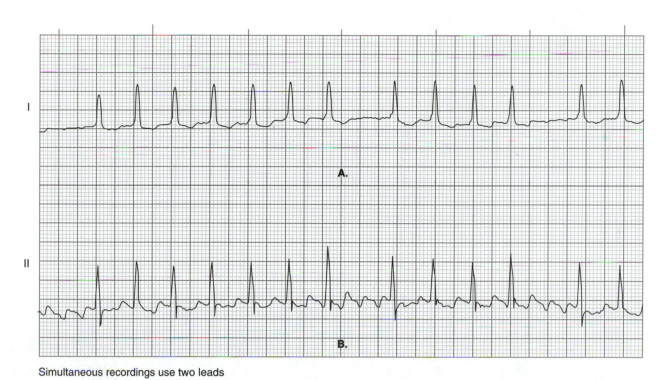

Simultaneous recordings use two leads

Figure 12–5 Flutter wave appearance depends on the recording lead. Atrial flutter waves do not show well in lead I while they are clearly shown in lead II which was simultaneously recorded using two leads.

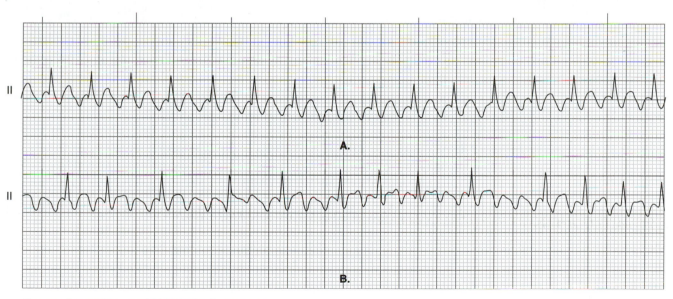

Consecutive tracing recorded several minutes apart

Figure 12–6 Atrial flutter with changing AV conduction. Strips A and B are consecutive tracings recorded several minutes apart. In strip A the AV conduction is 2:1, while in strip B the conduction becomes variable (2:1, 3:1, and 4:1) due to medication.

The AV conduction ratio in atrial flutter also determines the clinical consequences. For example, an atrial rate of 300/minute with a 4:1 AV conduction produces a ventricular rate of 75/minute. which is usually well tolerated. But a 2:1 AV ratio which produces a ventricular rate of 150/minute, commonly causes decreased tissue per-

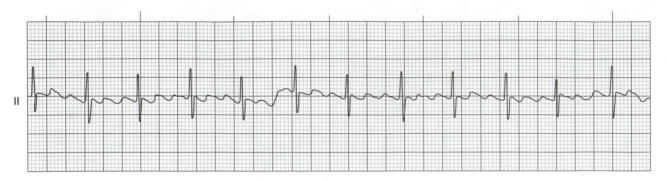

Figure 12-7 Atrial flutter with 3:1 AV conduction. This conduction ratio is unusual and occurs during medication. The conduction ratio will mostly be 2:1, 4:1 or 6:1.

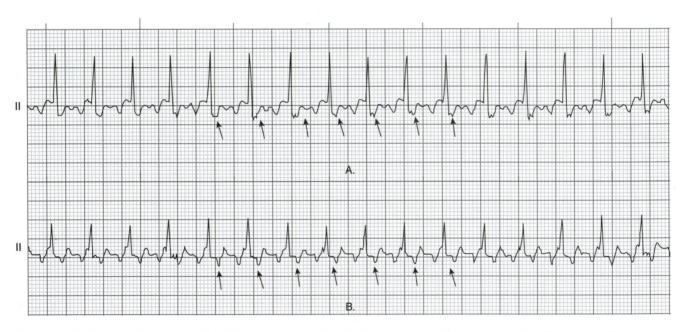

Figure 12-8 Atrial flutter with 2:1 AV conduction. Atrial flutter may be misinterpreted if the 2:1 conduction is not detected. In the two examples, the second F wave for each QRS is hidden in the ST segments (arrows). Flutter should be suspected whenever a regular, narrow QRS complex tachydysrhythmia has a rate of precisely 150/minute.

fusion, myocardial ischemia, and hypotension if it exists untreated for an extended period.

ECG Interpretation Tip: *Atrial flutter with 2:1 AV conduction should be suspected whenever the ECG appears to show a sinus tachycardia at precisely 150 /minute. The T waves often hide a second nonconducted P' wave. A useful diagnostic aid is to administer adenosine or to use vagal maneuvers to uncover hidden flutter waves.*

ECG Interpretation Tip: *The term "block" should be avoided when referring to atrial flutter with conducion other than 1:1. The decreased AV conduction in such cases is a normal protective mechanism, rather than a pathological block. Describing atrial flutter with "4:1 conduction" is preferred to "4:1 block" for that reason.*

STABLE TACHYCARDIAS

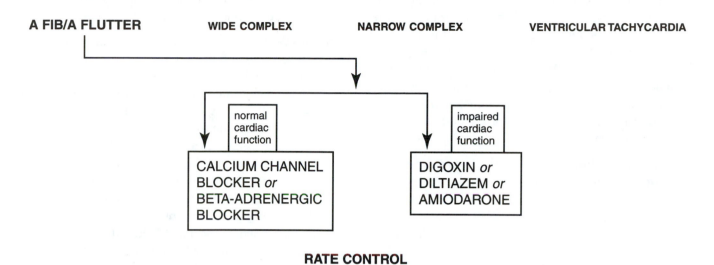

Figure 12–9

Causes of Atrial Flutter

Atrial flutter is usually caused by a reentry circuit within the atria. The flutter impulse is conducted through atrial tissue in a circular fashion, causing continuous atrial stimulation. Atrial flutter is associated with organic heart disease, such as hypertensive disease, but it is not specific for a particular heart disease (Table 12–2). Flutter also occurs in noncardiac-related diseases, such as pulmonary embolism, hypoxia, and lung disease. Flutter can uncommonly exist in a chronic form for months to years.

Clinical Significance of Atrial Flutter

The clinical effects of atrial flutter depend on the AV conduction ratio. If the ratio is 3:1 or 4:1, the ventricular rate is well tolerated. Ratios of 2:1 or 1:1 can cause ischemia or heart failure.

Emergency Treatment of Atrial Flutter

Emergency care treatment focuses on the following three management goals:

1. Treating unstable patients immediately using electrical cardioversion;

2. Controlling the ventricular rate; and

3. Converting the dysrhythmia to a normal sinus rhythm. Conversion can be done using drugs or a synchronized electric shock if anticoagulation is not needed because the dysrhythmia has been present less than 48 hours making the possibility of thrombo-embolic events less of a concern. If the dysrhythmia has lasted for 48 hours or longer or the duration is unknown, adequate anticoagulation must be achieved first.

Table 12–2 Conditions Associated with Atrial Flutter

- **Cor Pulmonale (heart failure resulting from COPD)**
- **Rheumatic Valvular (mitral and tricuspid stenosis) Disease**
- **Coronary Heart Disease**
- **Pulmonary Embolism**
- **Hypertensive Heart Disease**
- **Hyperthyroidism**
- **Pericarditis/Myocarditis (Inflammation of the pericardial sac or heart muscle)**
- **Digitalis Toxicity**

- *Urgent rate control.* In most emergency care settings, whether it involves EMS care in the field, in the ED or in critical care units, the major initial therapy aimed at ventricular rate control as shown in figure 12-9. Once the patient's heart rate is slowed and the condition is stabilized, therapy will usually be guided by a cardiologist who will attempt to convert the dysrhythmia after adequate anticoagulation has occurred (figure 12-10). An echocardiogram can assess for a mural thrombus prior to cardioversion.

- *Chronic AF.* In patients with atrial fibrillation that is long-standing, electrical or chemical cardioversion is not indicated as the dysrhythmia will recur even if cardioversion is temporarily successful. Ventricular rate control is the key in stabilizing such cases.

- *Dysrhythmias lasting for <48 hours or >48 hours.* Episodes of atrial fibrillation or flutter that have been present less than 48 hours can generally be cardioverted without the need for anticoagulation. In cases lasting two days or longer, mural thrombi are common and anticoagulation is needed for several days prior to attempting cardioversion.

- *Impaired Heart Function.* Cardiac failure in the setting of atrial flutter/ fibrillation is a major consideration because many drugs used to slow the ventricular rate have a negative inotropic effect thereby decreasing contractility. Impaired cardiac function limits the types of drugs that can be used. For instance, calcium channel blockers, beta-adrenergic blockers, and procainamide should be avoided in patients with tachydysrhythmias with impaired cardiac functioning. Amiodarone and digoxin are safe in patients with diminished ejection fraction and heart failure. Digoxin actually increases contractility but takes several hours before it becomes effective. Electrical cardioversion can also be used in those situations.

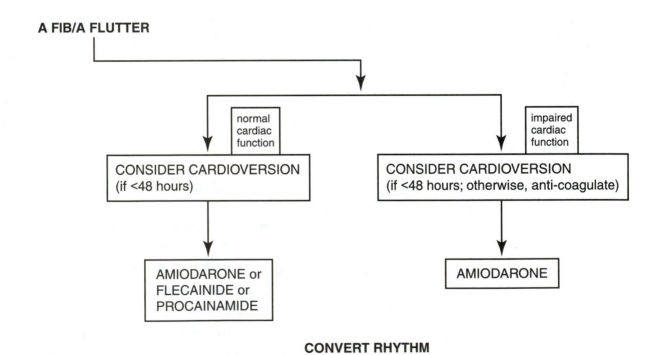

STABLE TACHYCARDIAS

A FIB/A FLUTTER

normal cardiac function

CONSIDER CARDIOVERSION
(if <48 hours)

impaired cardiac function

CONSIDER CARDIOVERSION
(if <48 hours; otherwise, anti-coagulate)

AMIODARONE or FLECAINIDE or PROCAINAMIDE

AMIODARONE

CONVERT RHYTHM

Figure 12–10

Acute treatment is directed at controlling the ventricular response, which improves cardiac output. The fundamental approach depends on whether the patient is stable or unstable:

- *Unstable condition*. Patients with hypotension, congestive heart failure, or in shock can be electrically cardioverted at low energy levels beginning at 50 watts/second. Atrial flutter is one of the easiest tachydysrhythmias to electrically convert.

- *Stable condition*. There are several medication choices to treat stable cases of atrial flutter:

  - A beta-adrenergic blocker such as metoprolol or propranolol can be used to slow the ventricular rate.

  - Calcium channel blockers such as cardizen or verapamil are usually effective. Both types of agents should be used with caution in congestive heart failure. Using a beta-adrenergic blocking drug and a calcium channel blocking agent together has a much greater tendency to depress myocardial contractility and cause hypotension because each can decrease stroke volume. For that reason, beta-blockers and calcium channel blockers should not be used together.

  - Digoxin (Lanoxin®) has a slower onset of effect, taking up to 1 to 2 hours to slow the ventricular rate, but in contrast to beta-blockers and calcium channel blockers, it causes increased contractility. Conversion to NSR occasionally occurs following digital use but spontaneous reversion is also common.

Clinical Note: Distinguishing atrial flutter from ventricular tachycardia may be difficult if abnormal ventricular conduction results in a rapid wide QRS complex rhythm. During emergency cardiac care, it is safer to treat the dysrhythmia as if ventricular tachycardia—the more serious condition—exists. Incorrectly treating ventricular tachycardia incorrectly as if it were an SVT with aberrant ventricular conduction could result in deterioration of the patient's condition.

ATRIAL FLUTTER WITH BRADYCARDIC VENTRICULAR RATES

When atrial fibrillation is overtreated in an attempt to slow the ventricular response, the ECG may display unusually high AV conduction ratios such as 6:1, 7:1, or even higher. Ventricular bradycardia in the face of atrial flutter is pathologic and due to overtreatment. AV conduction can be significantly decreased with digitalis or calcium channel blockers such as diltiazem and verapamil, or with beta-adrenergic blockers such as metoprolol and propranolol.

ATRIAL FLUTTER WITH A VARIABLE VENTRICUALAR RESPONSE

It is unusual to encounter changing AV conduction ratios during atrial flutter (e.g., 2:1, 4:1, and 6:1) but this can occur as the patient is being medicated.

SPECIAL CASE:

ATRIAL FLUTTER WITH AV DISSOCIATION

In atrial flutter with complete AV dissociation, the ECG shows a slow, regular ventricular rhythm lacking a fixed PR interval or a set AV conduction ratio. In Figure 12–11 the "FR" interval (distance from the start of the flutter wave to the start of the QRS complex) constantly changes because medication has completely interrupted conduction. Flutter waves appear to "march" into and through the QRS complexes. For patients in stable condition, the best treatment of overmedication is to observe the patient while the ventricular rate slowly increases as the drugs are metabolized. Very slow ventricular rates can be treated with an artificial pacemaker.

REGULAR NARROW COMPLEX TACHYCARDIAS AT 150/MINUTE

Unrecognized atrial flutter with 2:1 conduction is commonly mistaken for sinus tachycardia. The primary reason is because atrial flutter with 2:1 AV conduction produces a regular, narrow QRS complex tachycardia at a rate between 140 and 160/minute. The second flutter wave contained in the ST-T complex is frequently overlooked (Figure 12–12). Another clue that an ECG tracing is not likely to be sinus tachycardia is the unusual ventricular rate of 150/minute. Sinus tachycardia at 150/minute is considerably faster than the sinus node at rest usually discharges. Although the sinus can go that high, it is more likely to be due to a supraventricular pacemaker.

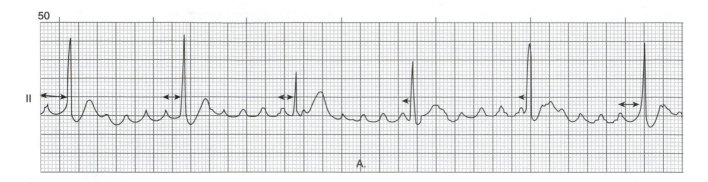

Figure 12-11 Atrial flutter with AV dissociation. Note that the FR intervals (indicated by double arrows) differ widely among the QRS complexes in both examples. Some F waves appear to merge into the R waves. Complete AV dissociation is present.

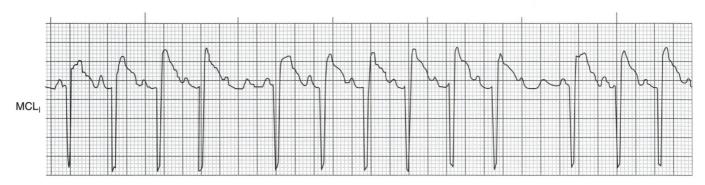

Figure 12-12 Atrial flutter with 2:1 AV conduction and the effects vagal maneuvers. Most of the tracing shows 2:1 conduction which makes it difficult to see the second F waves that are hidden in the ST segments. Carotid sinus massage (marked "CSM") unmasked the flutter waves.

Clinical Note: *Useful techniques to unmask hidden flutter waves include carotid sinus massage and the Valsalva maneuver which increase the parasympathetic nervous system tone. Administering adenosine can briefly reveal flutter waves when the ventricular rate is 150/minute. Vagal maneuvers and adenosine transiently increase AV nodal refractoriness, causing the ventricular response to briefly slow, and aid in the interpretation of flutter cases when the typical flutter waves are not obvious.*

ATRIAL FIBRILLATION (AF)

Atrial fibrillation is a narrow QRS complex tachycardia that arises from multiple atrial pacemaker sites and is characterized by an irregularly irregular ventricular rhythm (Figure 12–13). The atria are stimulated between 350 and 600 times/minute, replacing distinct atrial waves by a chaotic, wavy ECG baseline (Table 12–3). The ventricular rate is highly variable. The ventricular response can be either rapid, controlled (under 100/minute), or even bradycardic. The P′ waves are termed "f," "fib," or fibrillatory waves. Fibrillatory waves are smaller and have a more variable appearance than with flutter waves.

Atrial fibrillation is a very common supraventricular dysrhythmia, which accounts for why it is encountered much more frequently than either atrial flutter or paroxysmal supraventricular tachycardia. *In fact, atrial fibrillation is the most common chronic dysrhythmia and its incidence increases with age.* Fibrillation can occur transiently, lasting for minutes, hours, or days, although it may be chronic, lasting for years.

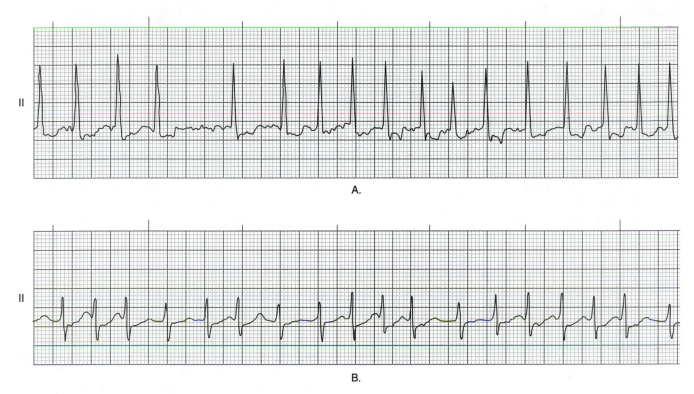

Figure 12-13 Atrial fibrillation with tachycardic ventricular rates. Strips A and B show the hallmark findings of fibrillation: narrow QRS complexes with a chaotic baseline and an irregularly irregular ventricular rhythm. The ventricular response typically ranges between 120 and 140/minute before medication has an effect.

ECG Interpretation Tip: *Common causes of irregular tachycardic dysrhythmias include atrial fibrillation, multiformed atrial tachycardia, and sinus tachycardia with frequent premature complexes.*

ECG Interpretation Tip: *A complete ECG interpretation should include the average ventricular rate because this often determines the clinical significance; for example, "atrial fibrillation with a ventricular rate of about 120/minute" provides more useful information than simply "atrial fibrillation" because the ventricular response could be fast, slow, or within a normal sinus range of 60-100/minute.*

Table 12-3 Key ECG Features of Atrial Fibrillation

■ **Atrial activity:**	Rapid, chaotic, fibrillatory waves
■ **AV conduction:**	Random
■ **Ventricular activity:**	Narrow QRS complex, irregularly irregular rhythm

AV Nodal Function in A-Fib

Although the AV node is being stimulated several hundred times per minute in atrial fibrillation, fortunately only a fraction of the atrial impulses are conducted. Each time a fibrillatory wave reaches the AV node, the node becomes slightly more refractory and less able to transmit impulses. The increasing degree of AV node refractoriness protects the ventricles from being overstimulated, which is why the node is known as the "gatekeeper."

Ventricular Rate

Untreated atrial fibrillation has a ventricular rate between 130 and 150/minute and is termed an **"uncontrolled" or tachycardic ventricular response**. Atrial fibrillation that have been appropriately treated has a ventricular rate below 100/minute and is referred to as **"controlled" ventricular responses** (Figure 12–14).

Clinical Note The pulse in atrial fibrillation is usually diagnostic since the cardiac rhythm is irregularly irregular and the pulse pressures vary because the stroke volume varies from beat to beat. Some pulses are strong while others are weak. Many fibrillatory waves that are seen on the ECG are so weak that they do not generate pulse and are not palpable.

ECG Interpretation Tip Fibrillatory waves may have coarse or fine amplitude. MCL$_1$ is the best lead for viewing atrial activity and detecting atrial fibrillation. In contrast, atrial activity may be barely visible using lead I or appear as a flat line. Fibrillation

should be suspected whenever the ventricular rhythm has narrow QRS complexes and is irregularly irregular.

Causes of Atrial Fibrillation

Fibrillation occurs in patients with and without heart disease (Table 12–4). The most common conditions associated with atrial fibrillation are rheumatic valvular disease, hypertensive heart disease, "binge" and chronic alcohol use, hyperthyroidism, and coronary artery disease.

Clinical Significance of Atrial Fibrillation

The loss of atrial contraction in fibrillation decreases cardiac output because it normally assists in the later phase of ventricular filling. Atrial contraction contributes about 25 percent to ventricular filling. Atrial contraction is referred to as the "atrial kick," since it fills the ventricular volume to its maximum before contraction. In atrial fibrillation, the loss of atrial contraction results in a 20-25 percent decrease in normal stroke volume. Since atrial fibrillation is associated with a diminished filling time and a loss of atrial contraction, cardiac output can fall dramatically which can cause ischemia and congestive heart failure.

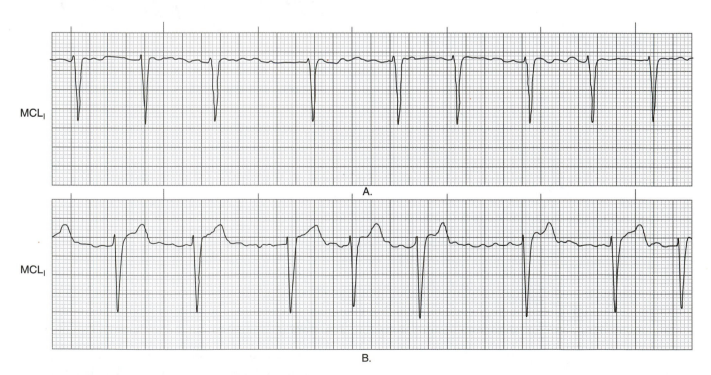

MCL$_1$

A.

MCL$_1$

B.

Figure 12-14 Atrial fibrillation with a controlled ventricular response. After medication is given, the ventricular rates in strips A and B are well below 100/minute.

Clinical Note: *The decreased cardiac output occurring in atrial fibrillation due to the loss of atrial contraction has a greater effect in patients who have underlying cardiac compromise such as congestive heart failure, coronary artery disease, and especially those with valvular heart disease, because cardiac output is already impaired.*

Table 12-4 Conditions Associated with Atrial Fibrillation

- **Hypertensive Heart Disease**
- **Ischemic Heart Disease**
- **Valvular (particularly mitral) Heart Disease**
- **Pericarditis**
- **Pulmonary Embolism**
- **Idiopathic (No Obvious Cause)**
- **Alcohol (Binge Drinking and Chronic Use)**
- **Hyperthyroidism**

Emergency Treatment for Atrial Fibrillation

The treatment guide for atrial fibrillation is identical to that for atrial flutter. Therapy for atrial fibrillation is based on two considerations: (1) how the patient tolerates the rapid rate, and (2) how long the dysrhythmia has lasted. When a patient shows signs of decompensation, or exhibits serious symptoms, such as pulmonary edema or ischemic chest pain, then the dysrhythmia needs rapid treatment often using electrical cardioversion. If the patient is stable, which is the majority of the cases, then medication can be used to control the ventricular rate. If the rate becomes controlled with medication and the dysrhythmia is a new finding, chemical cardioversion to restore NSR can be done during the first few days of hospitalization. Conversion of AF to NSR is generally not part of emergency care unless the patient is critically ill and needs to be electrically cardioverted.

For cases of AF lasting 48 hours or greater, the patient must be anticoagulated prior to cardioversion. Thrombi (clots) typically form in the fibrillating atria and they can be sent into the circulation if a return to NSR occurs before adequate anticoagulation occurs.

The adult acute cardiac care of atrial fibrillation and atrial flutter treament algorithms are found in Figures 12–9 and 12–10. The following general guidelines apply:

- If the patient is *unstable*, that is, with a systolic blood pressure less than 90 mm Hg, experiencing ischemic chest pain, or is in congestive heart failure, then synchronized electrical cardioversion beginning at 200 watt/seconds (joules) is indicated. Medication to reduce anxiety, such as midazolan (Versed®) or an analgesic such as morphine sulfate is often given prior to cardioversion.

- In patients who are in *stable* condition, the following medication can be used:

  - Calcium channel blocker: Diltiazem (Cardizem®) using an initial dose of 0.25 mg/kg, (20 mg for a 70 kg patient) is administered intravenously over 2 to 5 minutes. If the ventricular rate reduction is not adequate, a second IV dose of 0.35 mg/kg (a 25 mg dose for a 70 kg patient) can be administered over 2 to 5 minutes, 15 minutes later. A continuous diltiazem infusion at 5 to 15 mg/hour for maintenance, rate control, can be given for up to 24 hours.

  - Beta-Adrenergic Blocker: Metoprolol (Lopressor®) in mg slow IV doses over 2 minutes can be repeated every 5 to 15 minute intervals up to 3 doses (total of 15 mg).

  - Digoxin has frequently been used in the past to control ventricular rate but has largely been replaced by newer agents. Digoxin has a slow onset and usually takes hours to be effective and is less effective than other agents. An advantage of digoxin is that it does not depress contractility. Therefore, digoxin can be safely used in conjunction with either calcium channel blockers or beta blocker agents.

Clinical Note: *Calcium channel blockers should not be used in combination with beta blockers because significant hypotension and AV heart block can result. Digoxin can be safely used with either calcium channel blockers or beta-blockers because digitalis does not depress contractility.*

CHRONIC ATRIAL FIBRILLATION

Although atrial fibrillation can occur for short periods, it is often a chronic condition that is reasonably well tolerated. After several failed attempts at converting atrial fibrillation to NSR, therapy is directed at maintaining ventricular rate control and preventing strokes. Chronic fibrillation is more frequent in patients with valvular heart disease and dilated atria. A major preventable complication of chronic fibrillation is the development of atrial mural thrombus (clot), which can embolize to the brain and cause a stroke. Long-term anticoagulation using warfarin (Coumadin®) significantly decreases the risk of stroke.

SPECIAL CASE:

BRADYCARDIC AF WITH REGULAR R-R INTERVALS

In atrial fibrillation, the findings of a bradycardic ventricular rate with a regular R-R interval indicate that the patient has been overmedicated in an attempt to slow the ventricular response (Figure 12–15). *Regular R-R intervals in AF only occurs due to complete AV heart block and the devlopment of an escape ventricular pacemaker* (Figure 12-16). Overtreatment with digoxin, beta-blockers, and calcium channel antagonists can "overshoot the mark" and cause bradycardia and AV heart block (Figure 12-17).

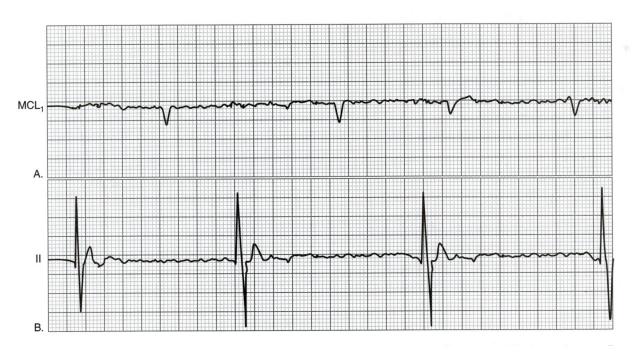

Figure 12–15 Atrial fibrillation with bradycardic rates due to overtreatment. Strip A and B show abnormally slow rates of 40/minute.

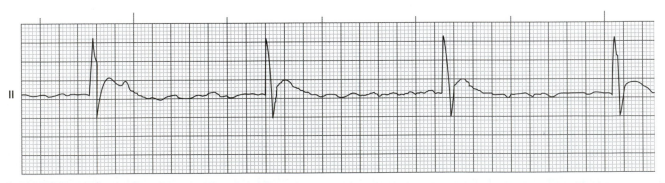

Figure 12–16 Atrial fibrillation with regular R-R intervals (complete AV dissociation). It is abnormal to have a regular ventricular rhythm in atrial fibrillation because random AV conduction results in variable ventricular activity. In this case, there are separate atrial and ventricular pacemakers.

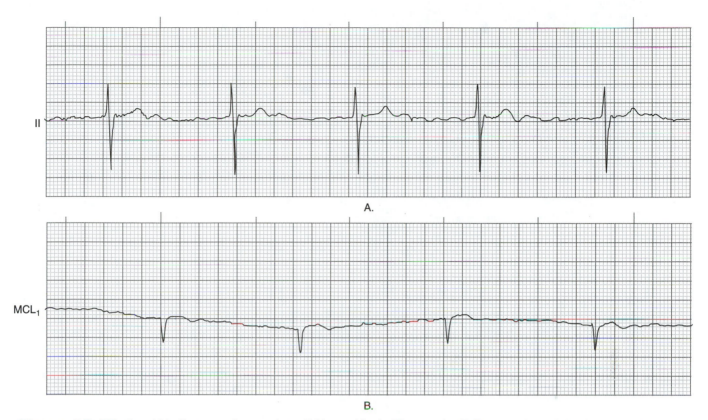

Figure 12–17 Atrial fibrillation with complete AV heart block. The regular R-R intervals and the bradycardic ventricular rate are two clues that these cases of heart block result from overmedication.

ECG Interpretation Tip: *The hallmark finding of a grossly irregular ventricular rhythm in atrial fibrillation is lost when complete AV block also exists. A regular ventricular rhythm in atrial fibrillation is usually due to excess digoxin, beta-adrenergic blockers, or calcium channel blocking agents.*

SPECIAL CASE:

AF WITH WIDE QRS COMPLEXES

The QRS complexes in atrial fibrillation are narrow except when there is a preexisting ventricular conduction problem, such as a bundle branch block. Despite the wide QRS complexes, the irregularly irregular ventricular rhythm still makes AF easy to detect (Figure 12–18).

ASHMAN'S PHENOMENON (ABERRANT CONDUCTION)

Short episodes of abnormal ventricular conduction of supraventricular impulses commonly occurs in AF and result in wide QRS complexes (Figure 12–19). Aberrant conduction typically follows a sequence of long-short R-R intervals, which produces delayed AV conduction. There are three useful rules concerning AF with distorted QRS complexes:

1. *When the short R-R interval that includes a distorted beat follows a long R-R interval, aberration is common.* This is termed **Ashman's phenomenon** and happens when the ventricles are not fully repolarized from the previous beat before the next impulse arrives.

2. *When consecutive wide QRS complexes occur during fibrillation, aberration is more likely than ventricular tachycardia.*

3. *QRS patterns that show an rsR' in MCL$_1$ heavily favors abnormal conduction rather than ventricular beats.*

These three rules help differentiate aberrant conduction from ectopic pacemakers, which will avoid unnecessary antidysrhythmic medication.

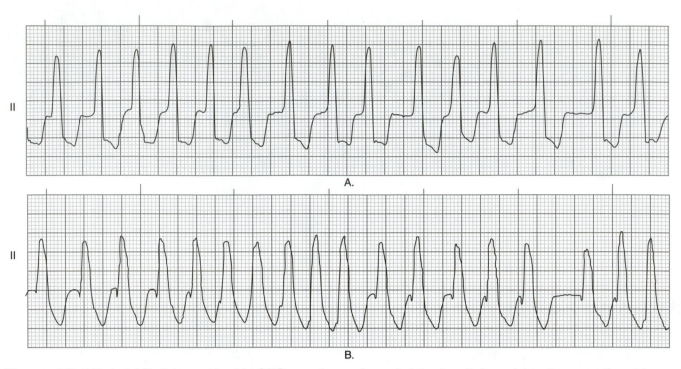

Figure 12-18 Atrial fibrillation with wide QRS complexes. An underlying bundle branch block causes the wide QRS complexes. The major clue pointing to atrial fibrillation is the variable ventricular rhythm. It is not easy to see the wavy baseline.

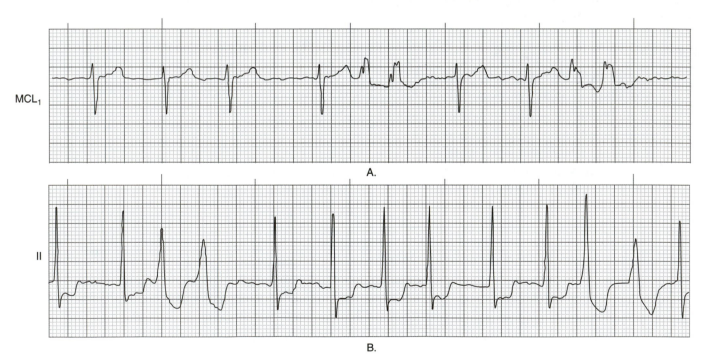

Figure 12-19 Atrial fibrillation with aberrant ventricular conduction (Ashman's Phenomenon). In strip A the 3rd and 10th beats are aberrantly conducted. In strip B, the two sets of two distorted QRS complexes (beats number 5 to 6 and 9 to 10) follow long-short R-R intervals. The QRS complexes have a rsR' configuration, which is a helpful clue to the presence of aberrancy. In strip C the 3rd and 4th beats, along with the 11th and 12th beats, are aberrantly conducted complexes

Table 12-5 Key ECG Features of Junctional Rhythms

■ **Atrial activity:**	Usually absent, or retrograde P′ waves following the QRS, or occasionally seen prior to the QRS complex with a shorter than normal PR interval
■ **AV conduction:**	Usually absent, sometimes retrograde atrial conduction
■ **Ventricular activity:**	Normal QRS-T complexes
■ **Ventricular rate:**	Three common ranges depending on mechanism:
■ **Basic (escape) rhythm:**	40 to 60/minute
■ **Accelerated junctional rhythm:**	60 to 100/minute
■ **Junctional tachycardia:**	above 100/minute
■ **Ventricular rhythm:**	Regular
■ **AV relationship:**	Usually absent; otherwise 1:1 if a P wave exists

ECG Interpretation Tip: The common causes of a regular, narrow QRS complex tachy-dysrhythmia include sinus tachycardia, paroxysmal supraventricular tachycardia, and atrial flutter.

ECG Interpretation Tip: Since escape junctional rhythms emerge when the sinus node function is depressed, escape junction rhythms are secondary to another pacemaker disorder. Therefore, accurate ECG interpretation should also include the primary problem such as "sinus arrest with an AV junctional escape rhythm at 50/minute."

AV JUNCTIONAL RHYTHMS

AV junctional rhythms are regular supraventricular rhythms arising, as the name indicates, in the AV junction. The rate of AV junctional depolarization can vary considerably, ranging from bradycardic to tachycardic. AV junctional pacemakers can be accelerated or depressed depending on the cause (Figure 12–20 and Table 12–5). When the sinus node fails as pacemaker, the next escape pacemaker to emerge is the AV junction, discharging between 40 and 60 per minute. In contrast, accelerated discharge of the AV junction occurs when the rate is faster than 60/minute but less than 100/minute. Should the rate be faster than 100/minute it would be a junctional tachycardia, which is included in the group of supraventricular tachycardias (SVTs). Accelerated junctional rhythms compete with the sinus node for pacemaker control in contrast to escape junctional pacemakers, which emerge when the sinus node fails.

Escape Junctional Rhythms

AV junctional escape rhythms are not primary ECG disorders, meaning that they arise secondary to sinus node depression or AV heart block (Figure 12–21). An AV junctional escape rhythm paces the heart at a slower rate than the lower rate of sinus node (60/minute). Escape junctional pacemakers have a regular rhythm, narrow QRS complexes, and depolarize between 40 and 60/minute. The characteristics of the various junctional rhythms are described in Table 12–5.

Junctional complexes are characterized by normal QRS-T complexes that usually lack P waves. P′ waves sometime appear when retrograde conduction spreads to the atria, in which case the P′ wave is seen *following*, or as a part of the end of the QRS complex. Occasionally, a retrograde P′ wave may appear prior to the QRS but it will have a shorter than normal PR interval (less than 0.12 second).

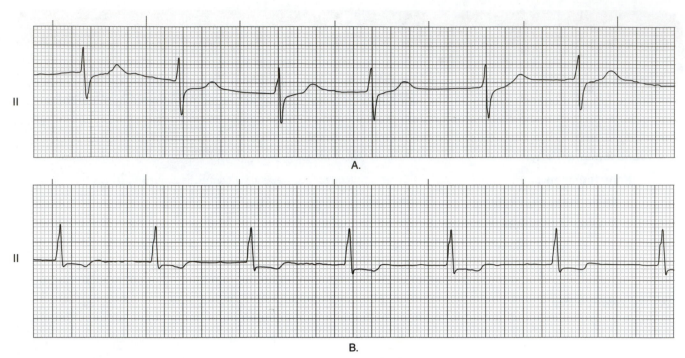

Figure 12-20 AV junctional escape rhythm. Regular narrow QRS complexes occur at a rate of 55/minute. Junctional rhythms pace the heart in the event of sinus node failure.

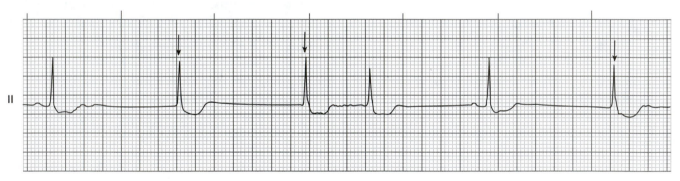

Figure 12-21 AV junctional escape rhythm. Strip A shows a very slow sinus rhythm with frequent escape junctional beats (number 2, 3, and 6). The escape beats are indicated by arrows.

Accelerated Junctional Rhythms

An accelerated junctional rhythm occurs when the rate is faster than expected based on the usual junctional escape rate of 40 to 60/minute. Accelerated junctional rhythms occur between 60 and 100/minute and look otherwise identical to junctional escape complexes with narrow QRS complexes and missing or retrograde P′ waves buried in the QRS or ST segments (Figure 12–22). The main difference from escape junctional rhythms is that the accelerated form challenges the underlying sinus rhythm due to increased AV junction automaticity. Accelerated junctional rhythms are benign because the ventricular rate is in the same range as

expected for a normal sinus rate (60 to 100/minute). Accelerated junctional rhythms subside spontaneously and do not require treatment.

Junctional Tachycardia

Junctional rhythms at rates over 100/minute are due to a reentry circuit involving the AV node. Junctional tachycardias are precipitated when a PJC occurs during the relative refractory period of a T wave. In Figure 12–23 retrograde P′ waves can be seen clearly immediately after the QRS complexes. Like other SVTs, junctional tachycardias have narrow QRS complexes,

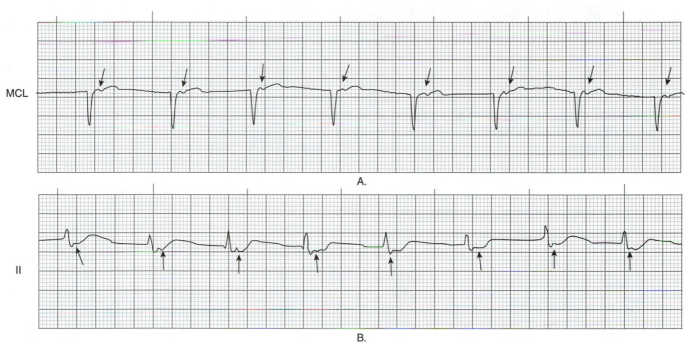

Figure 12–22 Accelerated junctional rhythms. Both examples show AV junctional rhythms at rates in the mid 70s, which is faster than expected for junctional escape rhythms (40–60/minute). Retrograde P′ waves occur immediately following the QRS complexes (arrows).

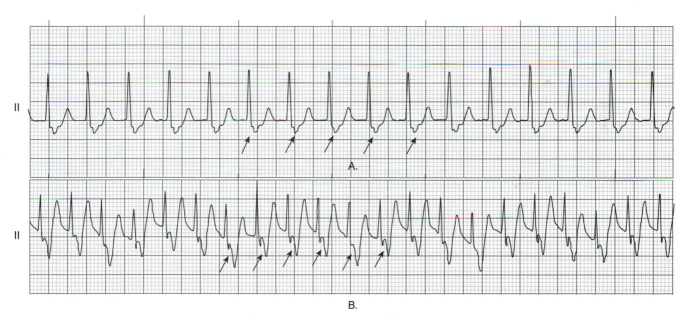

Figure 12–23 Junctional tachycardia. Strip A has a rate of 150/minute while strip B has a rate of 200/minute. Retrograde P′ waves can be seen immediately following the QRS complexes (arrows).

altered or missing P′ waves, and rates faster than 100/minute. Junctional tachycardia has the same significance and treatment as SVT. See the discussion of supraventricular tachycardia for more details.

Causes of Junctional Rhythms

Junctional *escape* rhythms occur when the sinus node fails to discharge and the AV junctional pacemaker passively discharges at 40 to 60/minute (Table 12–6). *Accelerated* junctional rhythms and junctional *tachycardias* compete with the SA node for pacemaker

Table 12–6 Conditions Associated with Junctional Rhythms

Escape Rhythms

- **Sick Sinus Syndrome (also known as "Brady-Tachy Syndrome).**

- **Sinus Bradycardia**

- **Inferior Wall Myocardial Infarction**

- **Digoxin, Calcium Channel Blocker, and Beta-Adrenergic Blocker Toxicity**

- **Hyperkalemia (high serum potassium)**

Accelerated Junctional Rhythms

- **Congestive Heart Failure**

- **Digoxin Toxicity**

- **Myocarditis (Inflammation of heart muscle)**

control because they occur at rates above the intrinsic junctional rate of 60/minute. The increased AV junctional discharge is due to a reentry rhythm or a rapid ectopic focus.

Clinical Significance of Junctional Rhythms

Junctional escape rhythms occur when sinus node functioning has become depressed. Like any escape rhythm, this backup pacemaker helps out in a time of need in order to stimulate the heart. Escape junctional pacemakers subside when a more rapidly discharging sinus node resumes control. Accelerated junctional pacemakers and junctional tachycardias discharge at a more rapid rate than escape pacemakers and challenge the sinus node for heart rate control. Accelerated junctional rhythms occur faster than 50/minute but less than 100/minute so they usually result in an adequate cardiac output and lack clinical complications. Junctional tachycardias occur around 120/minute so they cause an increased myocardial oxygen demand but do not result in major clinical complications.

Emergency Treatment for Junctional Disorders

- *Escape junctional rhythms* help provide a cardiac output. Therapy should be directed at accelerating sinus activity as the escape rhythm will subside spontaneously. Therapy should never be aimed

at suppressing junctional escape rhythms as they provide pacemaker activity in the face of higher pacemaker failure.

- *Accelerated junctional rhythms* have no clinical consequences since the rate is between 60 and 100/minute so they merely need observation to ensure adequate cardiac output.

- *Junctional tachycardias* are indistinguishable from other SVTs and the therpay is similar.

- *Junctional tachycardia* are indistinguishable from other SVTs and the therapy is similar. Junctional tachycardia is included in the 2000 ACLS guidelines for rapid narrow-complex dysrhythmias but it is a rare dysrhythmia in adults. As opposed to the vast majority of SVTs, which are due to a reentry mechanism, junctional tachycardia is due to an accelerated automatic pacemaker which suppresses the sinus node. Since the ventricular rate in junctional tachycardia ranges from 120 to 130 per minute, it is not rapid enough to compromise cardiac output and therefore, does not lead to an unstable condition. Electrical cardioversion is unlikely to be effective against an automatic ectopic pacemaker. Junctional tachycardia is commonly misinterpreted as paroxysmal supraventricular tachycardia and treated with adenosine, which is unsuccessful since it does not involve a reentry circuit.

The following agents are indicated for treatment:

- *Beta-adrenergic blocking agents*, such as metoprolol or atenolol, each are given in 5 mg slow IV doses that can be repeated in 5-10 minutes, or

- *Calcium channel blockers*, such as diltiazem, initially given in a 15 to 20 mg dose (0.25 mg/kg) over 2-5 minutes, which may be repeated if needed in 15 minutes at a dose of 20 to 25 mg (0.35 mg/kg) over two minutes. A maintenance infusion of 5 to 15 mg/hour can be titrated heart rate, or

- *Amiodarone* in an IV infusion of 360 mg over 6 hours at a rate of 1 mg/min.

Clinical Note: Junctional tachycardia in adults is rare and typically due to medication toxicity: digoxin, theophylline, and epinephrine. Withdrawal of the offending drug is necessary. Electrical cardioversion will not be successful.

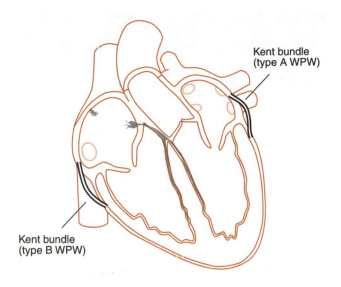

Figure 12–24 Diagram of the accessory pathways which lead to preexcitation.

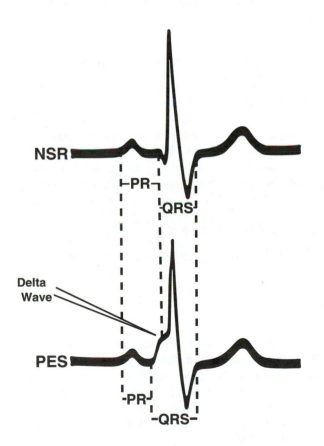

Figure 12–25 Preexcitation characteristics. The characteristics of preexcitation syndrome rhythms (PES) are contrasted to NSR. There are delta waves, shortened PR intervals, and distorted QRS complexes.

VENTRICULAR PREEXCITATION

Preexcitation (also termed **Short PR Interval Disorders**) is included with supraventricular disorders because preexcitation predisposes patients who develop atrial tachycardias, including PSVT, atrial fibrillation, and atrial flutter, to extremely fast ventricular rates. Preexcitation is caused by the presence of extra conduction tissue which connects the atria and ventricles (Figure 12–24). This additional conduction path bypasses the AV node and eliminates its "gatekeeper" function, which protects the ventricles from being overstimulated. The bypass tract is present at birth and is termed a "Kent Bundle," which makes the heart vulnerable should a rapid atrial dysrhythmia occur.

When an accessory path exists, a supraventricular impulse has two possible routes by which to enter the ventricles: (a) the usual route along the AV node or, (b) by bypassing the AV node and travelling via the accessory route. Since the Kent Bundle accessory path avoids the brief conduction delay afforded by the AV node, an impulse will arrive ahead of normal conducted impulses. This short-cut results in a less than normal PR interval—the hallmark ECG finding of preexcitation. There are two forms of preexcitation: W-P-W syndrome, which is the most common type, and L-G-L, which is uncommon.

Wolff-Parkinson-White (W-P-W) Syndrome and Lown-Ganong-Levine (L-G-L) Syndrome

Activation of the ventricles earlier than normal is characterized by:

■ a shortened PR interval

Two conditions cause short PR intervals: **Wolff-Parkinson-White (W-P-W) syndrome,** which has a slurred upstroke of the initial QRS component termed a "delta" wave (Figures 12–25 and 12–26), and **Lown-Ganong-Levine (L-G-L) syndrome,** which has a normal QRS complex that lacks a delta wave (Figures 12–27 and 12–28). W-P-W is far more common than Lown-Ganong-Levine (Table 12–7). The T wave has an opposite direction to that of the QRS complex deflection in W-P-W.

> **ECG Interpretation Tip:** *W-P-W Syndrome has a delta wave and a distorted QRS complex, whereas L-G-L Syndrome has a normal QRS complex and lacks a delta wave.*

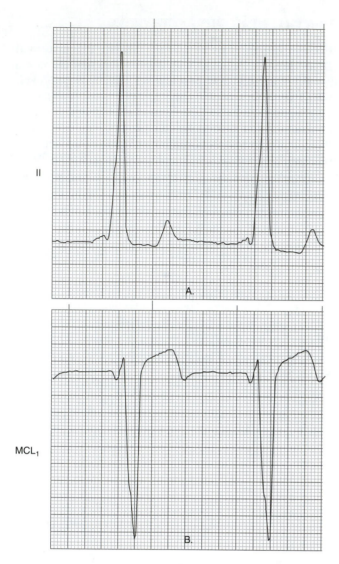

Figure 12-26 Preexcitation characteristics. The wide QRS, slurred delta wave, and shortened PR intervals are well illustrated in this case of Wolff-Parkinson-White Syndrome.

TABLE 12-7 ECG Findings of Preexcitation\

Wolff-Parkinson-White Syndrome

- **Short PR interval**
- **Slurred initial QRS component (delta wave)**
- **Wide QRS duration**
- **T wave direction is often opposite that of QRS complex**

Lown-Ganong-Levine Syndrome

- **Short PR interval**
- **Normal QRS shape and duration**

reaching the ventricles and result in a more tolerable rate of 150/minute. In W-P-W syndrome, however, the accessory pathway allows conduction of every atrial impulse.

Clinical Significance of Preexcitation Tachycardias

Preexcitation tachydysrhythmias are caused by an accessory pathway-mediated wide-complex tachycardia. Accessory pathways are present at birth but typically remain undetected until the first routine ECG is done or when the first bout of tachycardia occurs. Preexcitation can lead to a dramatic drop in cardiac output and have significant clinical consequences.

Causes of Preexcitation

Congenital presence of accessory conduction tissue.

Preexcitation and Tachydysrhythmias

Patients with accessory AV pathways are prone to developing extremely fast ventricular rates whenever a tachycardic rhythm develops because the AV node can not protect the ventricles from being overstimulated. Whether the tachydysrhythmia is a PSVT, atrial fibrillation or flutter, the bypass tract found in preexcitation allows the ventricles to be stimulated very rapidly because a circular reentry cycle can be established. Figure 12–22 illustrates the problem of preexcitation: the patient suddenly developed atrial flutter and the ventricles were paced 300/minute! Normally, the AV node would block at least half of the flutter waves from

Emergency Treatment for Preexcitation Tachycardias

If the patient's condition is unstable, immediate electrical cardioversion at an initial energy level of 100 to 200 Joules for atrial fibrillation and 50 to 100 Joules for atrial flutter is indicated. For patients with a stable hemodynamic status, drug therapy can be used but electrical cardioversion remains an option if hypotension results or the drugs fail.

Certain drugs are preferred for treating tachydysrhythmias associated with W-P-W syndrome due to their effects on the accessory pathway involved in preexcitation:

■ *amiodarone* is given in a IV infusion of 150 mg diluted in 100 cc of D_5W over 10 minutes and may be repeated in ten minutes as needed. An amiodarone infusion can be given as 360 mg over 6 hours, which equals 1mg per minute.

■ *procainamide* may be given up to a 20 mg/minute IV infusion until sinus rhythm results, significant hypotension occurs, the QRS duration widens by greater than 50% of baseline, or a total of 17mg/kg is given. The procainamide infusion may be slowed to minimize the hypotensive effects.

Impaired cardiac function. In patients with significantly impaired cardiac function and W-P-W—associated atrial fibrillation and flutter, amiodarone is the preferred agent since it depresses myocardial contractility less than procainamide. Electrical cardioversion is also acceptable and often preferred means to restore NSR. Amiodarone and procainamide must be used with caution when controlling the ventricular rate as they may chemically convert the dysrhythmias to sinus rhythm. When the atrial dysrhythmia has lasted for more than 48 hours, these agents need to be reserved until after the patient has been adequately anticoagulated of embolic events may occur.

Drugs to avoid. Some commonly employed drugs used to treat tachycardias which are not associated with

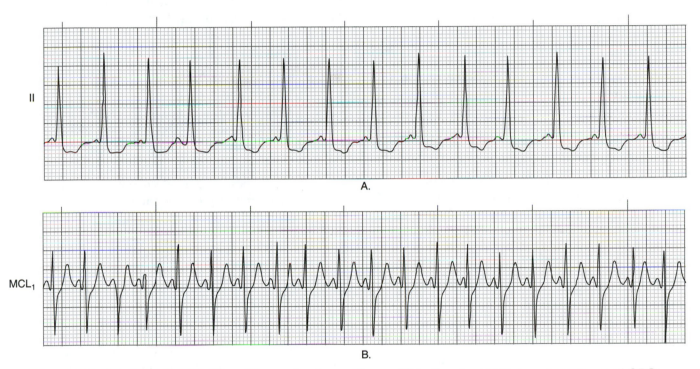

Figure 12-27 Preexcitation: Lown-Ganong-Levine syndrome. Note the short PR intervals and normal QRS complexes (no delta waves).

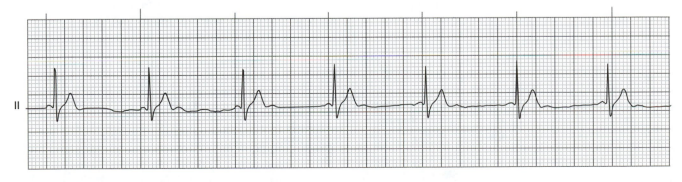

Figure 12-28 Lown-Ganong-Levine Syndrome. Note that the PR intervals are less than 0.10 second and the QRS complexes are normal.

W-P-W *must be avoided:* beta-adrenergic blockers, calcium channel blockers, adenosine, and digoxin. These agents can further accelerate the rapid heart rate because they selectively block the AV node while leaving the accessory pathway unaffected. The rapid atrial impulses will follow the path that offers the least resistance: the accessory bypass tract.

Alternative antidysrhythmics. The 2000 ACLS guidelines lists the following primary antidysrhythmic agents for possible use but they are not the agents of choice and are rarely used in emergency cardiac care:

■ *sotalol* in an IV dose of 1 to 15 mg/kg at a rate of 10 mg/min. Hypotension, bradycardia, and proarrhythmia are common side-effects. Ventricular tachycardia (Torsades de pointes) may result.

■ *flecanide* is approved in the US only in an oral form so it is almost never used in emergency cardiac care.

■ *propafenone* is also approved in the US only in an oral preparation so it rarely used.

> ***Clinical Note:*** *Most cases of W-P-W are identified during routine ECGs done in non-tachycardia states. W-P-W syndrome only becomes a concern when it is associated with tachydysrhythmias because the ventricular responses can be very, very fast, such as greater than 300 per minute.*
>
> ***Clinical Tip:*** *Amiodarone and procainamide are useful in treating W-P-W –associated tachycardias because they depress conduction in both the AV node as well as in the bypass tract, thereby slowing the ventricular response in atrial fibrillation and flutter. In cases of impaired cardiac functioning, amiodarone or electrical cardioversion is preferred.*

Drugs that preferentially slow AV nodal conduction, such as calcium channel blockers or digoxin, should be *avoided* as they can further speed the ventricular rate by favoring the accessory path.

> ***Clinical Note:*** *Drugs that preferentially depress AV nodal conduction favor transmission via the bypass tract and may paradoxically increase the rapid ventricular rate. Digitalis and calcium channel blocking agents are two such drugs that should be avoided. Verapamil (Isoptin®, Calan®) should be avoided in cases of W-P-W associated with atrial flutter or fibrillation.*

Chapter 13 presents twenty-five ECG tracings containing supraventricular dysrhythmias for interpretation practice.

Let's Review

1. Atrial flutter is a rapid, narrow QRS-complex dysrhythmia originating via a reentry mechanism.

2. Atrial flutter has distinct flutter waves usually occurring at 300/minute but may range from 250 to 350/minute.

3. The term *controlled* atrial flutter is applied to ventricular responses that are less than 100/minute and is encountered after treatment.

4. The term *uncontrolled* atrial flutter applies when the ventricular rate is over 100/minute.

5. The AV conduction ratio primarily determines the clinical consequences of tachycardic dysrhythmias, including atrial flutter. A 3:1 conduction ratio resulting in a ventricular rate of 100/minute is better tolerated than a 2:1 ratio yielding a heart rate of 150/minute.

6. Atrial fibrillation is a narrow complex tachycardia having an irregularly irregular rhythm.

7. Atrial fibrillation is the most common chronic dysrhythmia. AF is more common in patients over the age of 65 years and the incidence increases with age.

8. There is between a 20-25 percent decrease in ventricular filling caused by atrial fibrilla-

tion. As a result, stroke volume and cardiac output fall by the same amount.

9. A regular ventricular rhythm only occurs in atrial fibrillation when complete AV heart block also exists. AV heart block during AF is caused by medication such as adrenergic blocking agents, calcium channel antagonists, and less commonly, digoxin.

10. When the QRS complexes are wide (0.12 second or greater) in atrial fibrillation, a bundle branch block is present.

11. When one or several wide and distorted QRS complexes occur following long-short R-R intervals, they are due to aberrant conduction. The term "Ashman's Phenomenon" describes these distorted QRS complexes.

12. Emergency cardiac care of atrial fibrillation is directed toward slowing the ventricular response. Once this is accomplished, conversion to NSR can be done later.

13. A junctional rhythm arises in the AV junction, which is the tissue surrounding the AV node. Junctional rhythms are characterized by narrow QRS complexes and absent or distorted P waves along with shortened PR intervals.

14. Escape junctional rhythms occur in the range of 40 to 60/minute and averages 50/minute. Escape rhythms occur when the sinus node's automaticity is depressed.

15. Accelerated junctional rhythms occur at rates ranging between 60 and 100/minute. Accelerated junctional rhythms are due to increased automaticity or a reentry mechanism.

16. Preexcitation is a congenital disorder in which extra conduction tissue, termed an accessory pathway, connect the atria and ventricles.

17. When a supraventricular impulse bypasses the AV node, the ECG complex has a shortened PR interval and a distorted QRS complex with a slurred upstroke termed a delta wave.

18. Wolff-Parkinson-White (W-P-W) syndrome and Lown-Ganong-Levine (L-G-L) syndrome are two forms of preexcitation. Both have shortened PR intervals; W-P-W has a delta wave and L-G-L lacks a delta wave.

Glossary

Accessory pathway Congenital abnormality involving extra conduction tissue linking the atria and ventricles thereby allowing atrial impulses to bypass the AV node.

Ashman's phenomenon Aberrant ventricular conduction occuring in atrial fibrillation, characterized by long-short R-R intervals.

Atrial fibrillation Narrow QRS complex tachycardia that arises from multiple atrial foci and characterized by an irregularly irregular ventricular rhythm.

Atrial flutter Rapid regular, narrow QRS complex tachycardia caused by a reentry mechanism and characterized by an atrial rate of 250 to 350 bpm.

Bundle branch block (BBB) Conduction delay occurring in one or more bundle branches and resulting in a widened and distorted QRS complex.

Controlled ventricular response In atrial fibrillation the AV node forms a physiologic block resulting in a ventricular rate below 100/minute and preventing the ventricles from overstimulation.

Delta wave Slurred upstroke of the QRS complex due to preexcitation seen in W-P-W syndrome.

Fib (fibrillatory) waves P′ waves occurring in atrial fibrillation that may appear as fine or coarse ECG baseline fluctuations at a very rapid rate.

Fib-flutter Composite atrial dysrhythmia in which the ECG tracing has portions where it resembles atrial fibrillation and other areas where flutter waves predominate.

Flutter waves P′ waves typical of atrial flutter are regular and generally occur at 300/min. Flutter waves are more organized than fibrillatory waves.

FR interval Distance from the start of the flutter wave to the start of the QRS complex; analogous to the PR interval for sinus beats.

Kent bundle AV node bypass tract that is associated with ventricular preexcitation.

Lown-Ganong-Levine (L-G-L) syndrome
Form of preexcitation involving an accessory pathway and characterized by a short PR interval but lacking a delta wave.

Preexcitation   Condition that predispose patients to extremely fast ventricular rates that is caused by a congenital connection between the atria and ventricles that bypasses the AV node.

Short PR interval disorders   Another term for cases of ventricular preexcitation.

Thrombus   Blood clot forming in blood vessel of heart chanber.

Uncontrolled ventricular response   The ventricles respond to a rapid atrial dysrhytmia with a tachycardic heart rate in the range of 120 to 150/minute.

Wolff-Parkinson-White (W-P-W) syndrome
Form of preexcitation involving an accessory conduction pathway and characterized by a short PR interval and a delta wave.

Supraventricular Dysrhythmias— Self-Assessment ECG Tracings

LEARNING OBJECTIVES

Upon completion of this chapter, the reader should be able to:

- *Correctly identify the ECG disorder, given a series of sample ECG tracings displaying various supraventricular abnormalities.*
- *Accurately assess the rhythm, PR intervals, QRS durations, AV conduction ratios, and ST segments, given a sample of ECG tracings displaying various supraventricular dysrhythmias.*

CHAPTER OVERVIEW

The following ECG tracings contain supraventricular dysrhythmias that were presented in Chapters 11 and 12. Each tracing should be analyzed according to the systematic approach outlined earlier. Your interpretations should be compared with the answers provided in Appendix A. If further explanation is needed, the appropriate sections in the previous chapter should be reviewed.

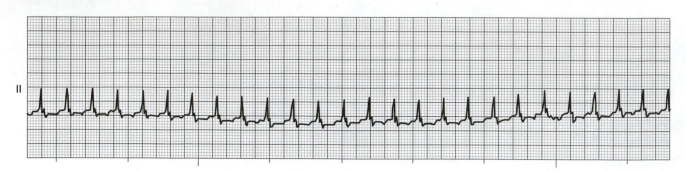

Figure 13–1
Rate _____
Rhythm _____
QRS Duration _____
PR Interval _____
AV Conduction Ratio _____
ST Segment _____
Interpretation _____
Reasoning _____

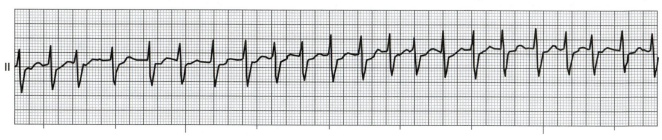

Figure 13–2
Rate _____
Rhythm _____
QRS Duration _____
PR Interval _____
AV Conduction Ratio _____
ST Segment _____
Interpretation _____
Reasoning _____

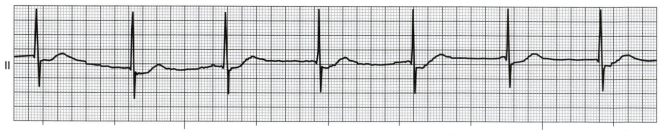

Figure 13–3
Rate _____
Rhythm _____
QRS Duration _____
PR Interval _____
AV Conduction Ratio _____
ST Segment _____
Interpretation _____
Reasoning _____

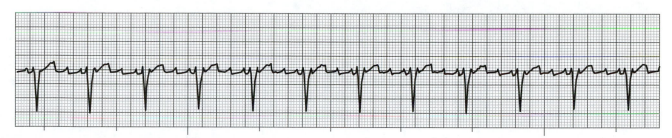

Figure 13-4   Rate _____
Rhythm _____
QRS Duration _____
PR Interval _____
AV Conduction Ratio _____
ST Segment _____
Interpretation _____
Reasoning _____

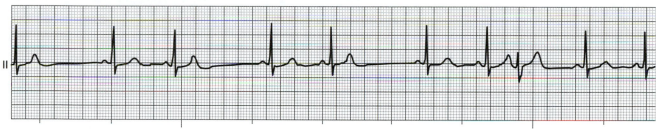

Figure 13-5   Rate _____
Rhythm _____
QRS Duration _____
PR Interval _____
AV Conduction Ratio _____
ST Segment _____
Interpretation _____
Reasoning _____

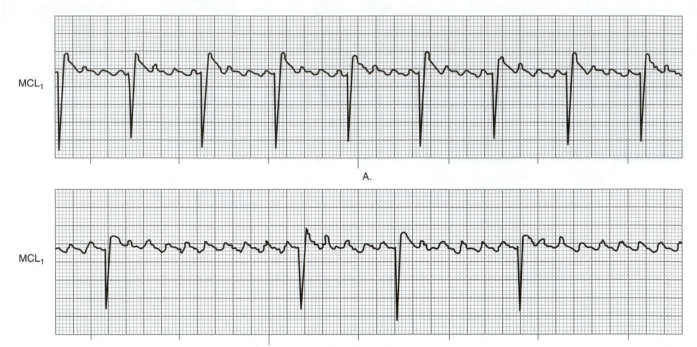

A.

B. 5 minutes later

Figure 13-6

Rate _____

Rhythm _____

QRS Duration _____

PR Interval _____

AV Conduction Ratio _____

ST Segment _____

Interpretation _____

Reasoning _____

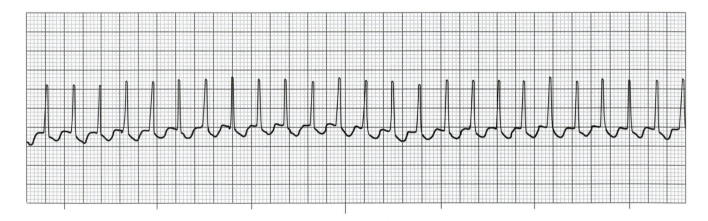

Figure 13-7

Rate _____

Rhythm _____

QRS Duration _____

PR Interval _____

AV Conduction Ratio _____

ST Segment _____

Interpretation _____

Reasoning _____

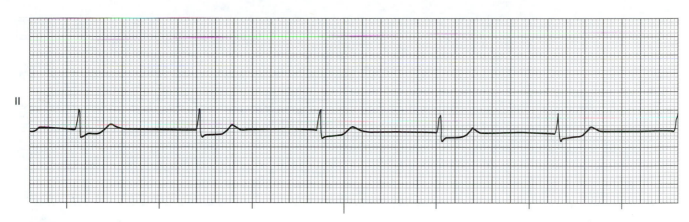

Figure 13-8   Rate _____
Rhythm _____
QRS Duration _____
PR Interval _____
AV Conduction Ratio _____
ST Segment _____
Interpretation _____
Reasoning _____

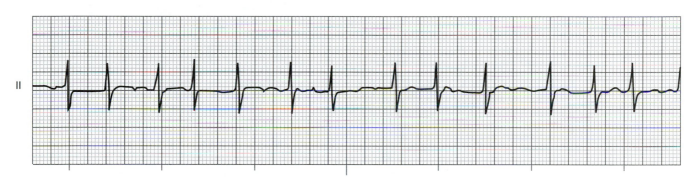

Figure 13-9   Rate _____
Rhythm _____
QRS Duration _____
PR Interval _____
AV Conduction Ratio _____
ST Segment _____
Interpretation _____
Reasoning _____

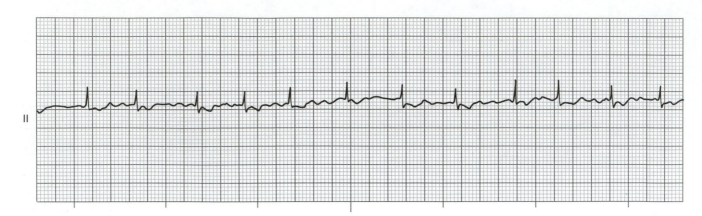

Figure 13–10 Rate _____
Rhythm _____
QRS Duration _____
PR Interval _____
AV Conduction Ratio _____
ST Segment _____
Interpretation _____
Reasoning _____

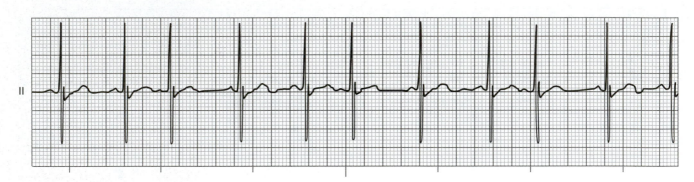

Figure 13–11 Rate _____
Rhythm _____
QRS Duration _____
PR Interval _____
AV Conduction Ratio _____
ST Segment _____
Interpretation _____
Reasoning _____

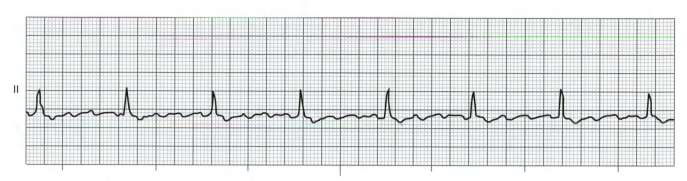

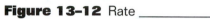

Figure 13–12 Rate _____
Rhythm _____
QRS Duration _____
PR Interval _____
AV Conduction Ratio _____
ST Segment _____
Interpretation _____
Reasoning _____

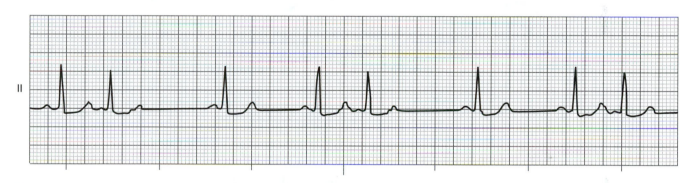

Figure 13–13 Rate _____
Rhythm _____
QRS Duration _____
PR Interval _____
AV Conduction Ratio _____
ST Segment _____
Interpretation _____
Reasoning _____

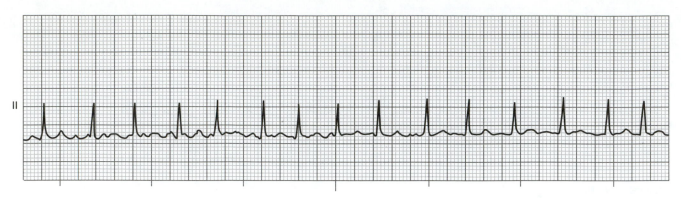

Figure 13-14 Rate _____
Rhythm _____
QRS Duration _____
PR Interval _____
AV Conduction Ratio _____
ST Segment _____
Interpretation _____
Reasoning _____

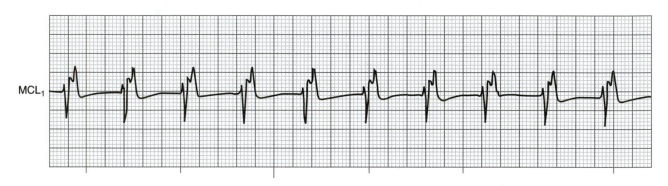

Figure 13-15 Rate _____
Rhythm _____
QRS Duration _____
PR Interval _____
AV Conduction Ratio _____
ST Segment _____
Interpretation _____
Reasoning _____

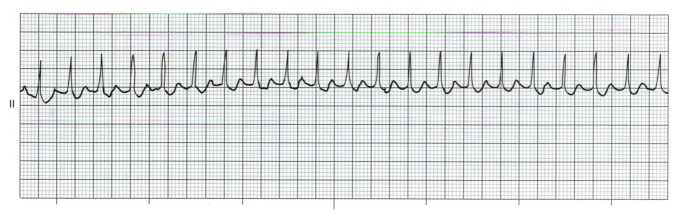

Figure 13-16 Rate _____
Rhythm _____
QRS Duration _____
PR Interval _____
AV Conduction Ratio _____
ST Segment _____
Interpretation _____
Reasoning _____

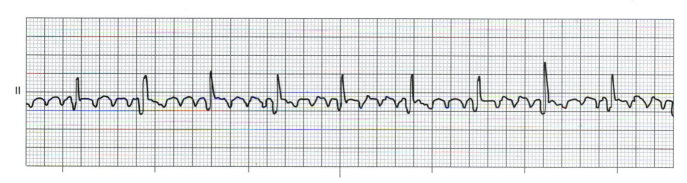

Figure 13-17 Rate _____
Rhythm _____
QRS Duration _____
PR Interval _____
AV Conduction Ratio _____
ST Segment _____
Interpretation _____
Reasoning _____

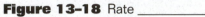

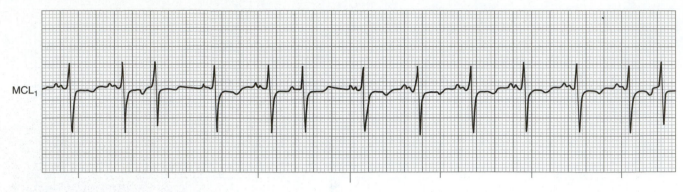

Figure 13–18 Rate _____
Rhythm _____
QRS Duration _____
PR Interval _____
AV Conduction Ratio _____
ST Segment _____
Interpretation _____
Reasoning _____

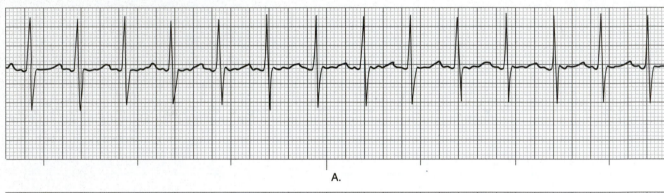

A.

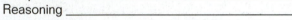

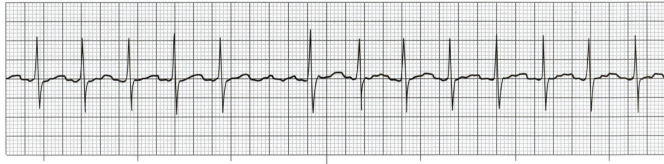

B. Continuous recording

Figure 13–19 Rate _____
Rhythm _____
QRS Duration _____
PR Interval _____
AV Conduction Ratio _____
ST Segment _____
Interpretation _____
Reasoning _____

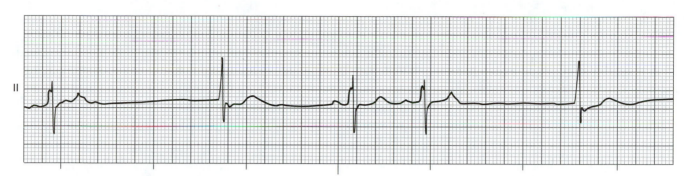

Figure 13–20 Rate _____

Rhythm _____

QRS Duration _____

PR Interval _____

AV Conduction Ratio _____

ST Segment _____

Interpretation _____

Reasoning _____

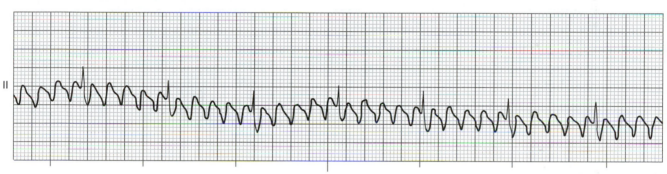

Figure 13–21 Rate _____

Rhythm _____

QRS Duration _____

PR Interval _____

AV Conduction Ratio _____

ST Segment _____

Interpretation _____

Reasoning _____

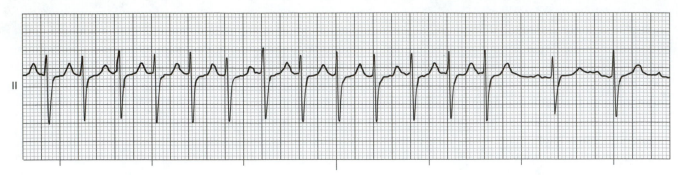

Figure 13–22 Rate _____
Rhythm _____
QRS Duration _____
PR Interval _____
AV Conduction Ratio _____
ST Segment _____
Interpretation _____
Reasoning _____

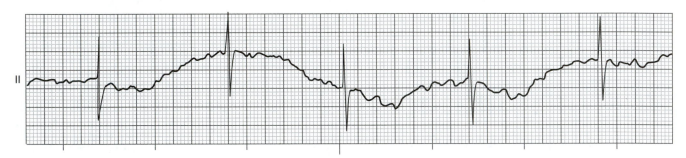

Figure 13–23 Rate _____
Rhythm _____
QRS Duration _____
PR Interval _____
AV Conduction Ratio _____
ST Segment _____
Interpretation _____
Reasoning _____

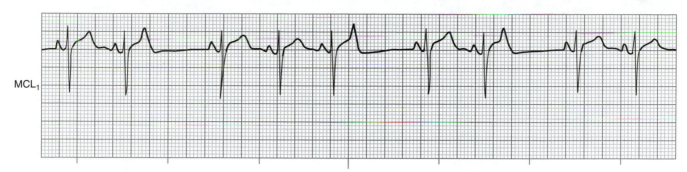

MCL₁

Figure 13–24 Rate _____
Rhythm _____
QRS Duration _____
PR Interval _____
AV Conduction Ratio _____
ST Segment _____
Interpretation _____
Reasoning _____

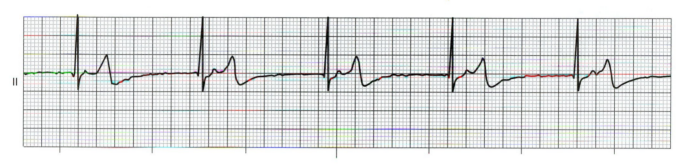

II

Figure 13–25 Rate _____
Rhythm _____
QRS Duration _____
PR Interval _____
AV Conduction Ratio _____
ST Segment _____
Interpretation _____
Reasoning _____

Atrioventricular Heart Blocks

LEARNING OBJECTIVES

Upon completion of this chapter, the reader should be able to:

- *List the components and functions of the atrioventricular (AV) conduction system.*

- *Name three parts of the conduction pathway at which an AV block can occur.*

- *Identify the area of the AV conduction pathway that has the slowest conduction velocity.*

- *Describe the ECG features that distinguish a sinus block from an AV block.*

- *Name the site of blockage causing a first-degree AV block.*

- *List the major ECG features that characterize a first-degree AV block.*

- *Discuss the clinical significance and treatment of a first-degree AV block.*

- *List the ECG characteristics of a Mobitz Type I form of second-degree AV block.*

- *Discuss the clinical significance of a Mobitz Type I form of second-degree AV block.*

- *List the ECG characteristics of a Mobitz Type II form of second-degree AV block.*

- *Name the possible sites at which conduction can be blocked in: (a) Mobitz Type I; and (b) Mobitz Type II forms of second-degree AV heart block.*

- *Describe the clinical significance of a Mobitz Type II form of second-degree AV block .*

- *List the ECG characteristics of a second-degree AV heart block with 2:1 conduction that distinguish Mobitz Type I from Type II.*

- *Name the ECG characteristics of a "high-grade" AV heart block.*

- *Describe the clinical importance of detecting a high-grade AV heart block.*

- *List the ECG features of an atrioventricular (AV) dissociation rhythm.*

- *Describe how AV dissociation differs from third-degree AV heart block.*

- *Name two forms of AV dissociation that are not caused by third-degree heart block.*

- *Explain the clinical significance of fixed PR intervals that are longer than 0.20 second.*

CHAPTER OVERVIEW

Atrioventricular conduction problems involve a disturbance in the transmission of sinus impulses to the ventricles. AV heart blocks share the following characteristics: nonconducted P waves, dropped QRS complexes, or prolonged PR intervals. The QRS complexes may be normal or wide and distorted. AV heart blocks are divided into partial and complete forms, depending on the adequacy of conduction. Some are benign while others can cause serious signs and symptoms. AV dissociation involves a lack of coordination between atrial activity and ventricular activity that can be caused by conditions other than heart block. AV dissociation is a benign disorder compared to third-degree AV heart block with a very different clinical significance. AV dissociation typically occurs in the absence of AV heart block.

INTRODUCTION TO AV HEART BLOCKS

Atrioventricular block involves a delay or interruption in the conduction of sinus impulses between the atria and ventricles. Impaired AV conduction is encountered fairly often in emergency care since advanced heart block types complicate 5 to 10 percent of myocardial infarctions. Being able to correctly identify particular forms of AV heart block is crucial because, while some AV heart block types are relatively benign, others cause a dramatic fall in cardiac output.

Many of those who are new to ECG interpretation become confused and unsure of how to proceed when faced with a tracing displaying more P waves than QRS complexes. Some form of conduction disturbance is suspected, but there is trouble organizing the assessment and identifying the particular heart block form. Such uncertainty will be replaced by confidence as the reader learns a simple and straightforward—yet comprehensive—approach to interpretation and by examining numerous examples.

ECG clues that point to the presence of a heart block include: more P waves than QRS complexes, changing PR intervals, prolonged PR intervals, grouped beats, QRS complexes lacking P waves, and P waves that appear to "march through" ventricular complexes. In some cases, the P waves occur in a random relationship to, or merge with, QRS complexes (Figure 14–1). While some of these findings are shared with dysrhythmias other then AV disorders, heart block should be a strong consideration when they are encountered.

Despite what is implied by the terminology, AV blocks do *not* occur only within the AV node since conduction can be interrupted at several locations in other areas of the conduction system as well (Figure 14–2).

P Wave and QRS Complex Relationship

Assessing the relationship between the atrial and ventricular activity is key to identifying the type of AV heart block. The various atrioventricular relationships that occur during heart block include: (1) a constant AV relationship having a 1:1 ratio and a prolonged PR interval; (2) fixed PR intervals having more than one P wave for each QRS; (3) changing PR intervals that have more than a single P wave for some QRS complexes; or (4) a changing PR interval without a fixed association between atrial and ventricular activity. These will be described further later in this chapter.

> *ECG Interpretation Tip:* Some dysrhythmias can easily be identified by viewing the ECG monitor, but heart blocks are an exception: it is best to analyze a printed ("hard") copy to confirm which conduction problem exists. Distinguishing second- from third-degree AV blocks, as well as sorting first-degree blocks from NSR, is easiest with a recorded ECG tracing because this makes measuring the intervals and assessing the atrioventricular relationship easier.

To aid in assessing whether a heart block exists, the following questions should be answered:

■ Is there a 1:1 AV relationship?

■ Is the PR interval fixed or does it change?

■ Is the PR interval normal or prolonged, that is, greater than 0.20 seconds?

■ Is there a single P wave before each QRS?

■ Is each P wave followed by a QRS complex?

■ Are there grouped beats? (Note: Not all grouped beats or nonconducted P waves signify a heart block.)

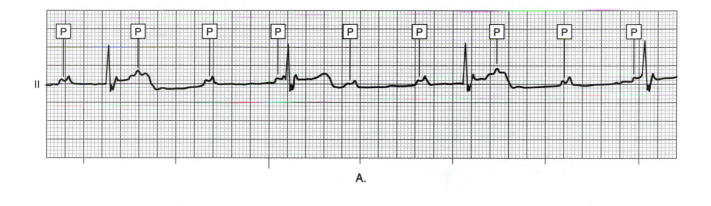

A.

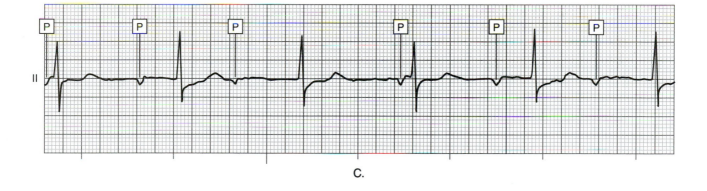

B.

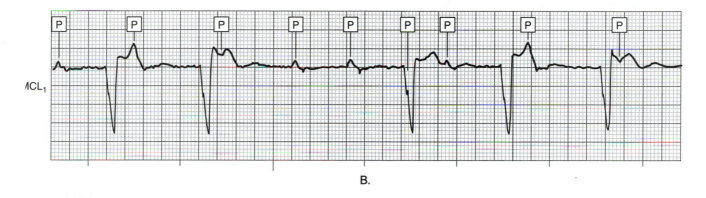

C.

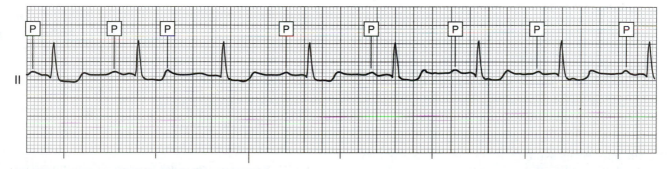

Figure 14–1 Some of the ECG clues that can point to the presence of an AV heart block include: more P waves than QRS-T complexes (A); consecutive P waves without intervening QRS-T complexes (B); changing PR intervals (C); and prolonged PR intervals (D). (The P waves in A are notched and in C are inverted.)

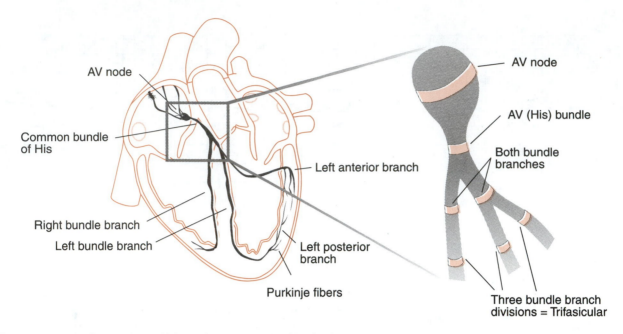

Figure 14–2 Sites where AV conduction can be blocked.

■ Is the ventricular rhythm regular or irregular?

■ If the rhythm is irregular, do the PR intervals change or are they constant?

Classification of AV Blocks

The traditional method for classifying heart blocks separates them into three types or "degrees." AV blocks are sometimes divided into two general groups ("complete" versus "incomplete" blocks). Such an approach could be criticized as being too simple but it is useful in assessing the need for emergency treatment (Table 14–1).
AV heart blocks involve a delay or conduction failure of one, some, or all sinus impulses being transmitted from the atria into the ventricles. The AV impulse transmission can be blocked at several points, involving: lower atrial tissue, AV node, His (AV) bundle, the bundle branches, or the smaller divisions of the bundle branches termed the fascicles (Table 14–2). Depending on the type of conduction disorder, the PR interval will be prolonged and/or the QRS-T complex(es) will not be conducted.

AV CONDUCTION

The PR interval measures the lag time between stimulation of the atria until activation of the ventricles. Normal AV conduction ensures a coordinated and effi-

Table 14-1 AV Heart Block Type

■ **Partial Block**
  ■ **First-degree**
  ■ **Second-degree**
    ■ **Type I**
    ■ **Type II**
■ **Complete Block**
  ■ **Third-degree**

Table 14–2 Sites of AV Heart Block

■ **Intra ("within") nodal**
■ **Infra ("below") nodal**
  ■ **His (AV) bundle**
  ■ **Bundle branches**
  ■ **Fascicles (bundle branch subdivisions)**

cient cardiac function. The QRS complex corresponds to the depolarization of the myocardium while the PR interval corresponds to conduction through the AV pathway and the ventricular system (Figure 14–3). The anatomic and functional properties of the AV node make it useful in slowing AV conduction velocity; however, the same properties lead to problems when disease develops. The AV node consists of specialized cardiac tissue whose fibers are arranged in a scattered fashion (Figure 14–4) which serve to delay the sinus impulse from stimulating the ventricles. The reduced conduction velocity permits the atria to finish contracting and the ventricles to completely fill before contraction. Impaired AV nodal conduction exaggerates the slowed conduction velocity. The mildest form of heart block, first-degree, involves a simple conduction delay, which causes PR interval prolongation.

Depressed Conduction

Conditions that increase the refractoriness in the AV pathway slow the impulse's conduction speed. Ischemia, fibrosis (scar tissue), increased parasympathetic/ vagal tone, drugs (including calcium channel blockers and beta-adrenergic blocking agents), inflammation of conduction tissue (as in myocarditis) increase the conduction pathway's refractoriness and leads to delayed or blocked conduction. Another relatively rare but increasing cause of AV block occurs in advanced Lyme disease (a tickborne illness), due to inflammation of the AV node.

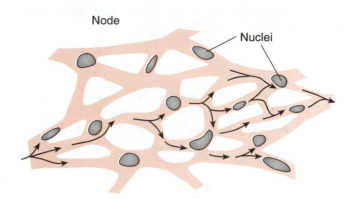

Figure 14–4 Illustration of AV nodal cellular fiber arrangement. There is a random arrangement of nodal fibers, which differs from the rest of the conduction system because it prolongs conduction. The arrow indicates the path taken by a sinus impulse.

In most people the blood supply to the AV node and the His bundle is provided by the right coronary artery. Developing an acute heart block may complicate myocardial infarctions. Inferior wall MIs commonly result in transient forms of second- and third-degree blocks. Anterior wall MIs are less frequently complicated by heart blocks, but when they occur, they tend to be permanent .

Clinical Considerations

The primary management consideration for patients with an AV block depends on the ventricular rate because it is the main determinant cardiac output. The ventricular rate depends on the sinus rate and the conduction ratio. For instance, a 3:2 AV conduction ratio for sinus rates of 100/minute, provides an adequate rate of 66/minute. However, the same conduction ratio for a sinus rate of 60/minute results in a bradycardic ventricular rate of only 40/minute.

> **ECG Interpretation Tip** *Complete ECG interpretations of AV heart blocks should include the conduction ratio, along with the ventricular rate, as they both affect cardiac output.*

Heart blocks, except for first-degree, cause a pause in ventricular activity. The prolonged pauses sometimes result in a patient's losing consciousness due to an abrupt fall in cerebral blood flow. Syncope caused by an AV heart block is termed **"Stokes-Adams Syndrome."** Syncopal episodes due to heart block are usually transient because the rhythm spontaneously

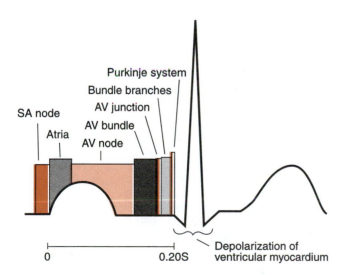

Figure 14–3 An illustration of the time components of a typical PR interval. Note that conduction through the AV node consumes the largest portion of the PR interval, and that the depolarization of the sinus node takes place before the P wave is formed.

reverts to normal or an escape pacemaker begins pacing the ventricles.

Escape Pacemakers

Escape complexes commonly follow ECG pauses. "Dropped" QRS complexes cause **asystolic pauses** that allow backup pacemakers to "escape" the normal inhibition by the sinus node. Figure 14–5 illustrates sites and rates of escape pacemakers.

FIRST-DEGREE AV BLOCK

The mildest form of AV heart block involves prolongation of the PR interval beyond 0.20 second yet all P waves are eventually conducted (Figure 14–6; Table 14-3). **First-degree AV block** involves delayed AV conduction after atrial depolarization, which leads to delayed ventricular depolarization (Figure 14–7). *A PR interval longer than 0.20 second is the hallmark ECG finding of first-degree block.* Asymptomatic cases of prolonged PR intervals have been found during routine examinations in approximately 2 percent of young healthy individuals. Again, every P wave is conducted and QRS complexes are not dropped (Figure 14–8). First-degree block is a benign dysrhythmia unless it occurs acutely in the setting of an acute myocardial injury, in which case it may lead to more significant forms of heart block.

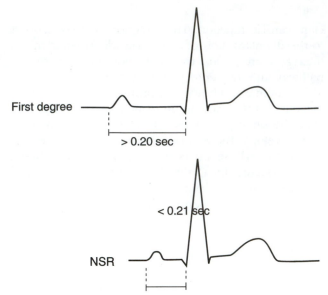

Figure 14–6 PR interval prolongation. A normal PR interval is compared with a prolonged PR interval.

> ***Clinical Note*** *While PR intervals that exceed 0.20 second are considered "abnormal," many healthy individuals have longer than normal PR intervals. In the absence of cardiac disease or medication toxicity, prolonged PR intervals are considered normal variants.*

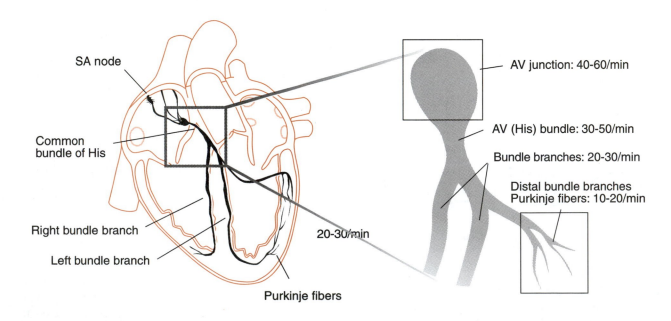

Figure 14–5 Escape pacemaker sites and relative depolarization rates. This illustration shows that higher pacemaker sites have faster discharge rates and emerge before slower back-up pacemakers.

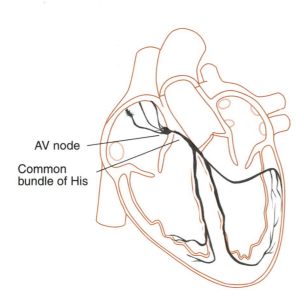

ECG Interpretation Tip *A PR interval greater than 0.20 second in the setting of a brady-cardic rate is usually due to increased vagal tone. As the heart rate rises above 60/minute, the prolonged PR interval usually shortens to normal.*

Figure 14–7 Site of first-degree AV block disturbance. The blockage site is in the proximal portion of the conduction pathway, either in the AV node or in the common AV bundle.

AV node

Common bundle of His

Table 14–3 Key ECG Features of First-Degree AV Block	
■ **P Waves:**	Normal
■ **Ventricular Activity:**	Normal
■ **AV Relationship:**	Prolonged, beyond 0.20 second
■ **Site of block:**	Within the AV node (intranodal)

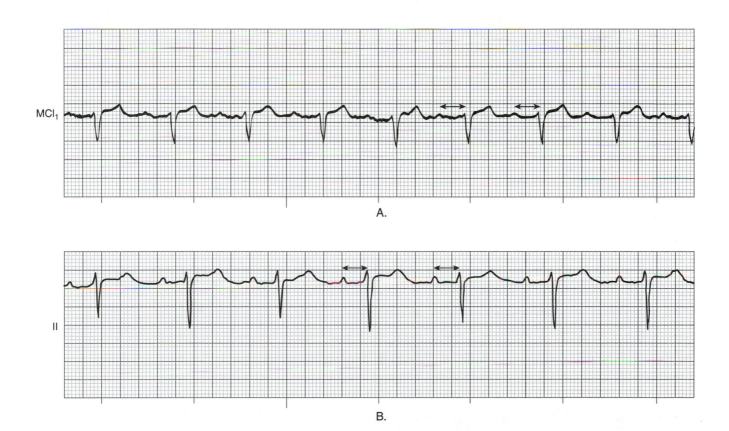

MCI₁

A.

II

B.

Figure 14–8 First-degree AV block. The PR intervals in both tracings exceed 0.20 second.

Causes of First-degree AV Block

First-degree block occurs when conduction through the AV node is depressed and can occur in several conditions as listed in Table 14–4. Increased vagal tone usually results in a slowed heart rate and a prolonged PR interval.

Clinical Significance of First-degree AV Block

Since every delayed sinus impulse is eventually conducted, first-degree AV block is not dangerous and therapy is not needed. However, PR prolongation that suddenly develops during a myocardial infarction, is caused by inflammation and swelling of AV nodal tissue and can be the earliest warning of progression to a more advanced block.

Around 10 percent of patients with myocardial infarc-

Table 14-4 Causes of First-Degree AV Block

■ **Degenerative Fibrosis**
(This is the most common cause and is due to aging)

■ **Idiopathic** (Unknown Cause); may be a normal variant

■ **Increased Vagal Tone**

■ **Drug Induced** (especially with digoxin, beta-adrenergic and calcium channel-blocking agents, quinidine, procainamide, and tricyclic antidepressant/phenothiazine toxicity)

■ **Myocardial Inflammation** (myocarditis, endocarditis, rheumatic heart disease, Lyme disease [tickborne infection], Lupus [autoimmune disease])

■ **Myocardial Ischemia/Infarction**

■ **Hyperkalemia** (high serum potassium level)

---

tions develop first-degree blocks but the majority spontaneously revert to NSR within two weeks. In the setting of drug toxicity, the development of a first-degree block should raise the possibility of progression to a more advanced block.

Emergency Treatment of First-degree AV Block

No therapy is indicated.

SPECIAL CASE: Prolonged PR Interval Associated with Bradycardia

The criteria for first-degree block apply only when the sinus rhythm has a *rate of at least 60/minute* because the PR interval is a function of the rate. A PR interval greater than 0.20 second in the setting of bradycardia is most commonly due to a high degree of vagal tone. Most prolonged PR intervals that are associated with bradycardia revert to normal when the heart rate accelerates above 60/minute. For example, Figure 14–9 A and C show two cases of prolonged PR intervals that occured during sinus bradycardia, but these should *not* be classified as a first-degree block *because the sinus rate is below 60/minute.*

SECOND-DEGREE AV BLOCK

In **second-degree AV block** some—but not all—atrial impulses fail to be conducted to the ventricles. The conduction problem may happen occasionally, occur regularly, or be permanent. The conduction disturbance can occur at any site along the conduction pathway. Second-degree heart block is divided into two types based on whether the PR interval changes before the QRS -T complexes are dropped.

ECG Interpretation Tip *When an ECG shows clustering of QRS complexes that are separated by pauses, heart block and premature beats are strong possibilities. Both ECG disorders can cause regularly irregular heart rhythm patterns*

Mobitz Type I (Wenckebach Type)

Mobitz Type I, the **Wenckebach form** of second-degree AV block, involves a partial blockage of sinus impulses and occurs within the AV node. Wenckebach AV block is characterized by grouped beating, PR intervals that progressively increase until a dropped beat occurs, coupled with shortening of the R-R intervals (Figure 14–10). The shortening of the R-R intervals is not as appreciated a finding as the increasing PR intervals but it develops as the QRS complex falls further behind the P wave. Table 14–5 highlights the ECG features found in this type of AV block.

Wenckebach is due to increased AV node refractoriness that is usually caused by increased parasympathetic tone or medication that slows AV conduction velocity. As a result, the conduction velocity through the AV

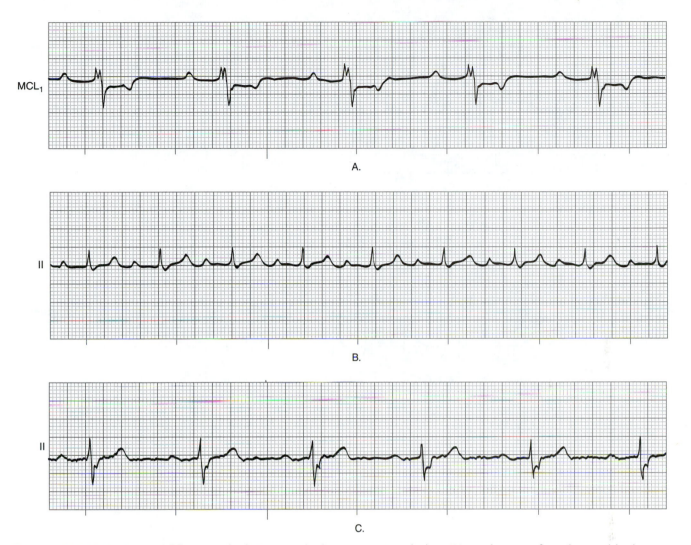

MCL₁

II

II

A.

B.

C.

Figure 14–9 Prolonged PR intervals. In tracing A, the sinus rate is below 50 so the term first-degree block cannot be applied because the rate must be at least 60/minute. In tracing B a first-degree AV block does exist because the sinus rate is at least 60/minute. Tracing C shows a sinus bradycardia with a prolonged PR interval. This is not considered a first-degree block because the heart rate is below 60/minute.

node decreases, eventually causing the last P wave of each group of beats not to be conducted. Nonconducted P waves are reflected by pauses in ECG activity at the point that QRS complexes are dropped. The first P wave arriving at the AV node following the dropped QRS has the *least difficulty* being transmitted. The first PR interval of each cycle also has the shortest interval of the group, because the nodal tissue has recovered during the preceding pause and is less refractory.

Causes of Wenckebach Block

Wenckebach is due to increased AV nodal refractoriness, which is caused by an abnormally long relative refractory period. High vagal tone and drugs, such as digox-

Table 14–5 ECG Features of Wenckebach Second-degree AV Block	
■ **Ventricular:**	Irregular R-R intervals due to grouped beating
■ **Atrial:**	Regular P-P intervals
■ **AV Conduction:**	Progressive PR interval prolongation
■ **R-R intervals:**	Become shorter as the PR intervals increase
■ **QRS-T complexes:**	Normal

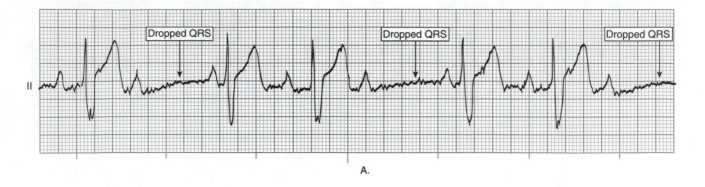

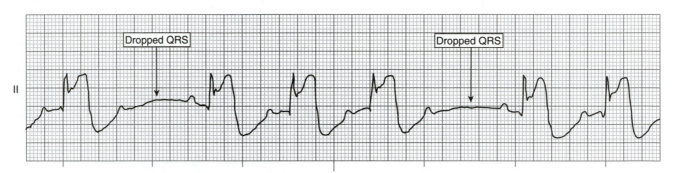

Figure 14–10 Second-degree AV block, Mobitz Type II (Wenckebach type). Tracing A shows one cycle of 2:1 and two cycles of 3:2 AV conduction, which is the most common ratio. Another common conduction ratio involves four P waves for each three QRS-T complex (4:3 conduction) as illustrated in tracing B.

in, beta-adrenergic blocking agents, or calcium channel blockers decrease conduction velocity and blocks some impulses travelling through the node (Table 14–6).

Clinical Significance of Wenckebach Block

The Wenckebach block is a relatively benign condition that typically subsides without treatment and does not cause a fall in cardiac output. Wenckebach dysrhythmias sometimes may, but not usually, progress to more serious forms of heart block, such as Mobitz Type II or complete AV block. Wenckebach block is a relatively common finding in athletes without symptoms. It often accompanies a resting bradycardia in patients with high vagal tone. As Table 14–6 notes, Wenckebach is usually associated with reversible problems and is therefore a temporary problem. Continuous ECG monitoring is prudent during an acute myocardial infarction until the condition has stabilized. In the vast majority of cases, Wenckebach is detected incidentally, during a routine screening examination and therapy is not needed.

Clinical Note Patients with the Wenckebach form of AV heart block are usually asymptomatic unless the ventricular rate is less than

45/minute. Most of the time, Wenckebach is found in healthy individuals with increased vagal tone.

Emergency Treatment of Wenckebach Block

Acute therapy is not needed unless the ventricular rate is so slow as to cause inadequate perfusion. In such cases, the approach to the treatment of adult symptomatic bradycardias is followed. It is included at the end of the chapter. The basic principle is to accelerate the ventricular rate only to the point needed to stabilize the patient's condition because a rapid rate will exacerbate ischemia. The following drugs are helpful:

- Atropine 0.5 mg rapidly administered via an intravenous bolus decreases the vagal tone; can be repeated up to a total 2 mg (at which point its full antivagal effect has occurred)

- An epinephrine infusion increases adrenergic tone

- Transcutaneous artificial pacing

Atropine is usually successful only when the block is located proximally in the AV conduction pathway, that

Table 14–6 Causes of Wenckebach AV Block

- **Increased Parasympathetic (Vagal) Tone**
- **Healthy Individuals (Especially Athletes)**
- **Drug Effect (Calcium Channel Blocker, Beta-Adrenergic Blocker, Digoxin)**
- **Rheumatic Fever**
- **Aortic Valve Disease**
- **Mitral Valve Prolapse**
- **Atrial Septal Defect (Congenital Opening Between Atria)**
- **Acute (Inferior Wall) Myocardial Infarction**

is, in the AV node, which is typical of Wenkebach. Atropine must be administered rapidly and in a minimum dose of 0.5 mg as paradoxical slowing has been reported. The two therapies besides atropine afford greater control over how fast the rate will increase.

Mobitz Type II (Second-degree AV Heart Block)

Just as with Mobitz I block, Mobitz Type II is a partial block during which some sinus beats are blocked (Figures 14–11 and 14–12, and Table 14–7) Mobitz Type II occurs *much less frequently than Mobitz Type I* but is a *significantly more serious* disorder. The block occurs below, or distally, to the AV node, typically develops *within the bundle branches* (Figure 14–13). Blockages at different sites will lead to a key ECG difference between types I and II: *the QRS complexes are wide and distorted in Mobitz II while they are normal in type I.* Identifying Mobitz Type II dysrhythmias are crucial

because they frequently and suddenly progress to complete heart block as shown in Figure 14–12.

> ***Clinical Note*** *Organic disease, such as myocardial injury or fibrosis involving the conduction pathway, is the major cause of failed AV conduction in Mobitz Type II AV block. Mobitz type I, in contrast, is a more benign disorder that usually occurs in the absence of organic heart disease.*

PR and R-R Intervals in Mobitz II Block

The key ECG feature of Mobitz Type II is that the PR intervals before the dropped beats do *not* change. The R-R interval that includes the nonconducted QRS complex is equal to two cardiac cycles (R-R intervals).

AV Conduction Ratio Patterns

In Mobitz Type II the blocked beats usually occur in fixed AV conduction ratios such as 4:3, 3:2, 4:1. The AV junction fails to respond to every third or fourth atrial impulse (3:2 or 4:3, respectively). A summary of Mobitz Type II ECG findings is presented in Table 14–7.

> ***ECG Interpretation Tip*** *Nonconducted PACs are frequently confused with second-degree AV blocks because both dysrhythmias display pauses in cardiac activity. It is helpful to remember that nonconducted PACs occur much more frequently than Mobitz Type II block and patients who have Mobitz Type II block tend to be much sicker.*

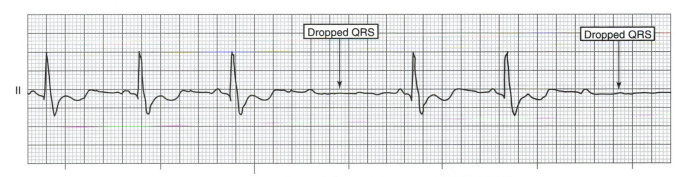

Figure 14–11 Second-degree AV block, Mobitz Type II. The 4th and 7th P waves are not conducted. In contrast to the Wenckebach block form, the PR intervals before the dropped QRS complexes are constant. Shortly after this tracing was recorded, the rhythm changed to a complete AV heart block, illustrating the seriousness of Mobitz Type II.

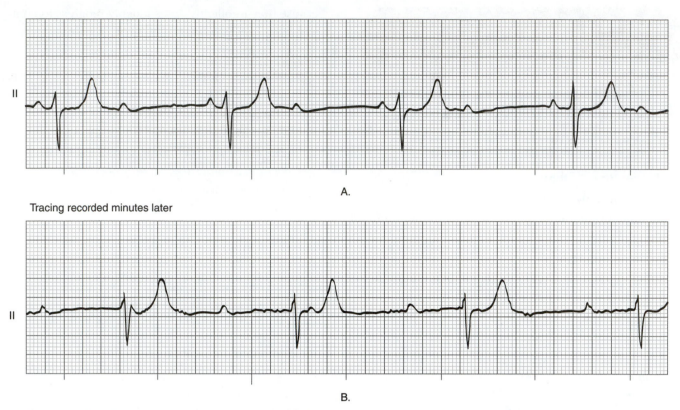

A.

Tracing recorded minutes later

B.

Figure 14–12 Second-degree AV block, Mobitz Type II changing to third-degree AV block. Strip A shows second degree block with 2:1 conduction, which was present for ten minutes before the block advanced to complete AV disruption in strip B. There is no relationship between the Ps or the QRS-T complexes in Strip B.

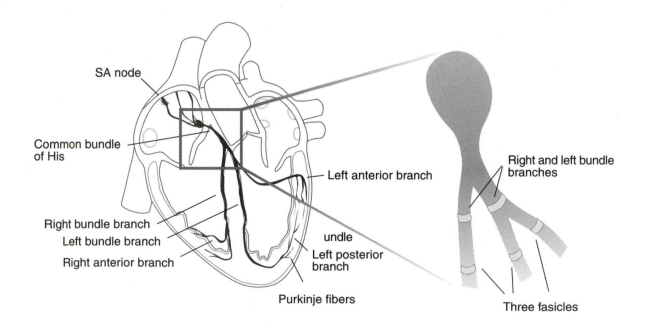

Figure 14–13 Sites of AV conduction disturbance in Mobitz Type II. The sinus impulse is blocked below the AV node, usually occuring simultaneously in both bundles or all these fasicles.

Causes of Mobitz Type II Block

Mobitz Type II heart block occurs with organic heart disease involving both bundle branches of the conduction system. Less commonly, the AV bundle is involved, leading to intermittent interruption of AV conduction. Common causes are listed in Table 14–8.

Clinical Significance of Mobitz Type II Block

Of the two types of second-degree block, type II is *much less common but is a more serious problem.* Type I block does not usually require treatment and subsides spontaneously in contrast to Mobitz type II which typically progresses to complete heart block and requires artificial pacing. Mobitz type II block commonly complicates anterior wall MIs, and occurs as the result of degeneration (fibrosis) of conduction's system. Patients experience near-syncope, fainting, light headedness and palpitations. The differences between Mobitz Type II and Mobitz Type I are summarized in Table 14–9.

Wenckebach Variations

It is not unusual to have the following variations from the classical Wenckebach pattern occur: (1) *every* PR interval does not necessarily increase; (2) the *last* PR interval usually shows the greatest PR increase; and (3) even the *first* PR interval of each group is often prolonged beyond 0.20 second (Figure 14–15).

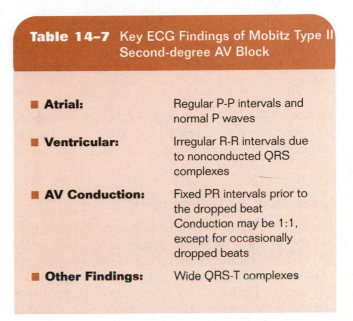

Table 14–7 Key ECG Findings of Mobitz Type II Second-degree AV Block

■ **Atrial:**	Regular P-P intervals and normal P waves
■ **Ventricular:**	Irregular R-R intervals due to nonconducted QRS complexes
■ **AV Conduction:**	Fixed PR intervals prior to the dropped beat Conduction may be 1:1, except for occasionally dropped beats
■ **Other Findings:**	Wide QRS-T complexes

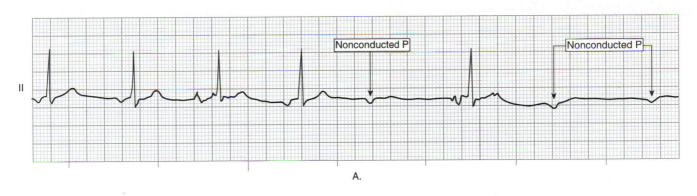

A.

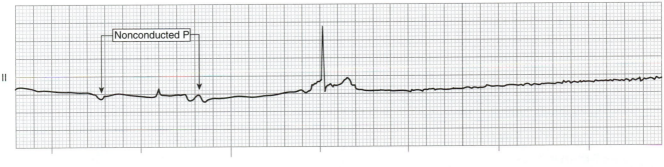

Continuous recording

B.

Figure 14–14 Second-degree AV block abruptly changing to a third-degree AV block with failure of an adequate escape pacemaker to develop. The 5th, 7th, and remaining P waves are not conducted. A single narrow QRS complex escape beat occurs in the middle of strip B. The patient sustained a cardiac arrest and required external and permanent artificial pacing.

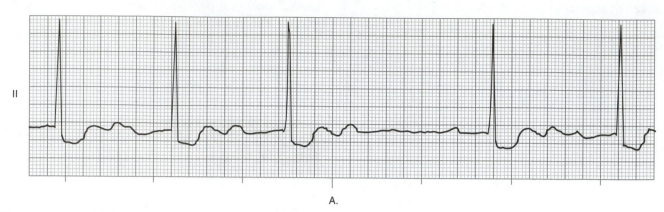

A.

Figure 14–15 Second-degree AV block with a first-degree block. Even the initial PR intervals of each set of grouped beats start out longer than 0.20 second and progressively increase. It is not uncommon to have both a first- and second-degree AV block.

Special Case: 2:1 AV Heart Block

Cases of 2:1 AV block are often incorrectly labeled as Mobitz Type II because the gradual prolongation of the PR interval typical of Wenckeback is not seen (Figures 14–16 and 14–17; Table 14–10). Both characterizations are wrong! During 2:1 AV conduction, it is often *not possible to determine with certainty whether Mobitz Types I or II exists* because conduction of two consecutive beats is needed to correctly determine the conduction pattern but it is absent.

> **ECG Interpretation Tip** *In order to classify a dysrhythmia as a Wenckebach form of second-degree block, at least two consecutively conducted P waves are needed.*

The term *Mobitz type: "nonspecific"* is more appropriate for 2:1 AV blocks than either Mobitz Type I or II. Helpful clues in determining whether a 2:1 block is a Mobitz Type I (Wenckebach) or Mobitz Type II include:

- Since Mobitz Type I reflects a nodal problem, it is associated with prolonged PR intervals and normal QRS complexes

- Since Mobitz II indicates a more distal (infranodal) blockage site, it has wide, distorted QRS complexes and a normal PR interval.

These rules help to classify most cases of 2:1 block, but if that is not possible, the term Mobitz type: "nonspecific" can be applied.

Table 14–8 Causes of Mobitz Type II Second-degree AV Block
■ **Drug Effect (Calcium Channel Blocker, Beta-Adrenergic Blocker, Digoxin)**
■ **Acute Myocardial Infarction**
■ **Lyme Disease (Rare)**
■ **Aortic Valve Disease**
■ **Degenerative Fibrosis**

Table 14-9 Second-degree AV Block Comparison

	Mobitz Type I	**Mobitz Type II**
Clinical Significance	Mostly benign and self- limited	Occurs with organic disease
ECG Differences	Progressive PR increase	Fixed PR interval
	Narrow QRS	Wide and distorted QRS
Defect Location	AV node	Bundle branches
Duration	Transient	Permanent
Progression to Complete Block	Rare	Common
Treatment	Atropine if symptomatic but usually no treatment is needed	Artificial pacemaker

High Grade Second-Degree AV Block

A second-degree AV block is classified as **high grade** when two or more consecutive P waves fail to be conducted (Figures 14–18 and 14–19). High degree AV block is very serious because it represents particularly

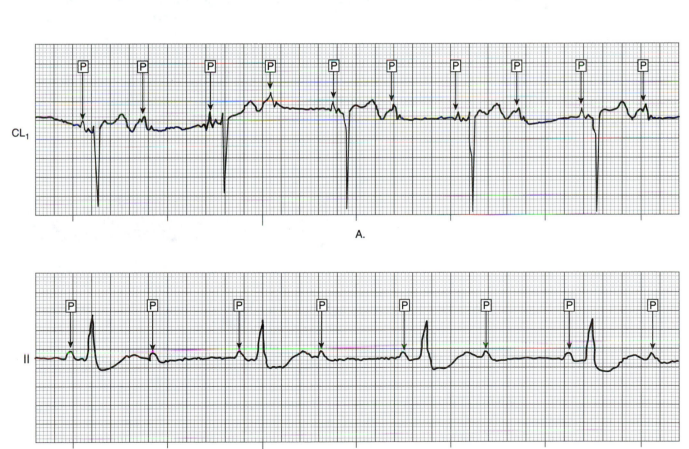

A.

B.

Figure 14–16 Second-degree AV block with 2:1 AV conduction. Each tracing has two P waves occurring for every QRS-T complex. While it is tempting to label these tracings as a Mobitz Type II form of second-degree because increasing PR intervals are not visible. However, at least two consecutively conducted P waves must be observed before the dropped QRS-T complex in order to identify the Mobitz type.

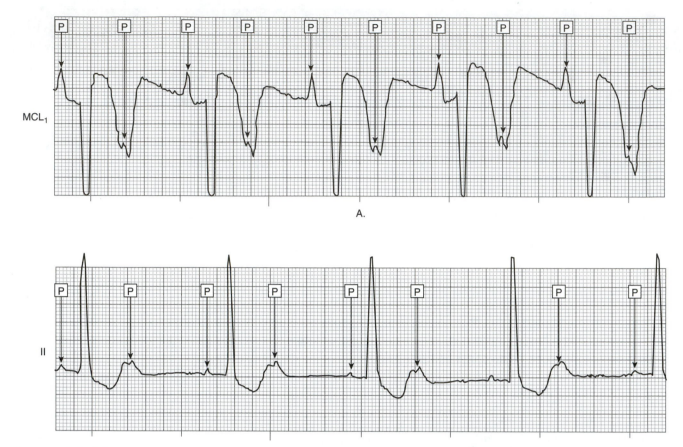

Figure 14–17 "Easy-to-miss" second-degree AV heart blocks with 2:1 conduction. This case of second-degree AV block with 2:1 AV conduction was misidentified as a sinus bradycardia in a patient experiencing a myocardial infarction. Lead MCL₁ (tracing A) was used for continuous monitoring and the second P wave landed in the middle of the T wave. Lead II (tracing B) clearly shows the nonconducted P waves. Using more than one lead to evaluate dysrhythmias is useful.

unstable AV transmission. Complete AV block quickly follows after the onset of high-grade heart block. Two ECG characteristics of a high-grade block include: (1) the atrial rate must *not* be abnormally fast, as happens in atrial flutter where nonconduction is actually a safety mechanism; and (2) an accelerated ectopic rhythm must be absent as it would interfere with P wave conduction even in the absence of a block.

Emergency Treatment for Mobitz Type II, Second-Degree Heart Block

Since the Mobitz Type II form of second-degree AV heart block only occurs with advanced organic heart disease and is likely to suddenly progress to complete block, immediate stabilization measures are indicated. Insertion of an intravenous artificial pacemaker will provide the most dependable rhythm. However, in an emergency, an external pacemaker will usually provide

Table 14–10 2:1 AV Block Classification		
	QRS Complexes	**PR Intervals**
■ **Mobitz Type I: (Wenckebach)**	Narrow	Prolonged
■ **Mobitz Type II:**	Wide, distorted	Normal

adequate myocardial capture until a transvenous pacemaker is inserted. Application of an external pacemaker does not require waiting for intravenous access and use of intravenous medication.

The adult emergency cardiac care treatment approach for bradycardia, included at the end of this chapter, includes the following therapy:

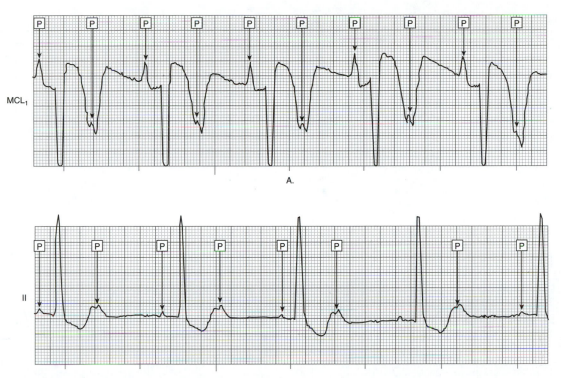

Figure 14-18 High-grade second-degree AV block. In strip A the P waves (numbers 1, 4, 6, 9, and 10 are not conducted leading to a 3:1 AV conduction ratio. Two consecutive P waves are blocked. The ventricular rate is extremely slow due to the bradycardic sinus rate. Since only 1 of every 3 P waves is conducted, the resulting ventricular rate is only 25/minute. In tracing B, P waves numbered 2, 3, 5, 6, 8, 9, and 11 are not conducted, leading to 3:1 AV conduction.

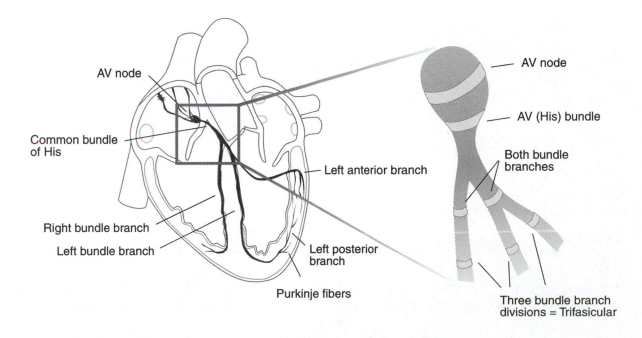

Figure 14-19 Sites of high-grade second degree and complete AV block conduction disturbances. The typical locations for a high-grade second degree and a third-degree block occur distally within the conduction system, such as in the bundle branches or simultaneously in the three fasicles. Third-degree block can occur more proximally in the AV node or AV bundle but it is much less likely.

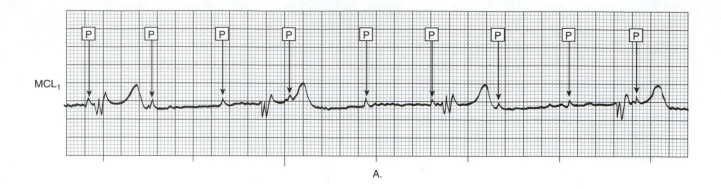

A.

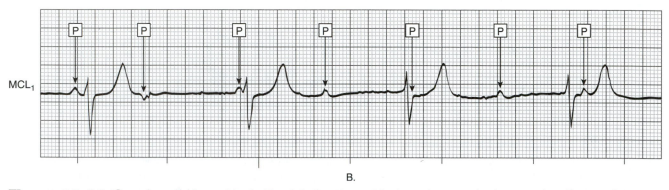

B.

Figure 14-20 Complete AV heart block. Third-degree heart block is shown in both examples. Some of the characteristics to note include atrial rates faster than ventricular rates, P waves having no relationship to the QRS-T complexes, bradycardic rates of 50/minute or less, and a regular ventricular and atrial rhythm—but without a relationship between each other.

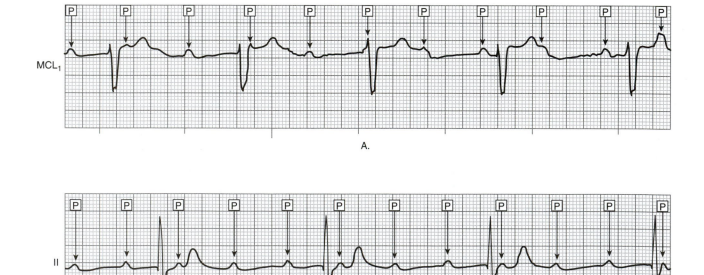

A.

II

Figure 14-21 Third degree (complete) AV heart block. The P waves and QRS-T complexes are completely independent of one another.

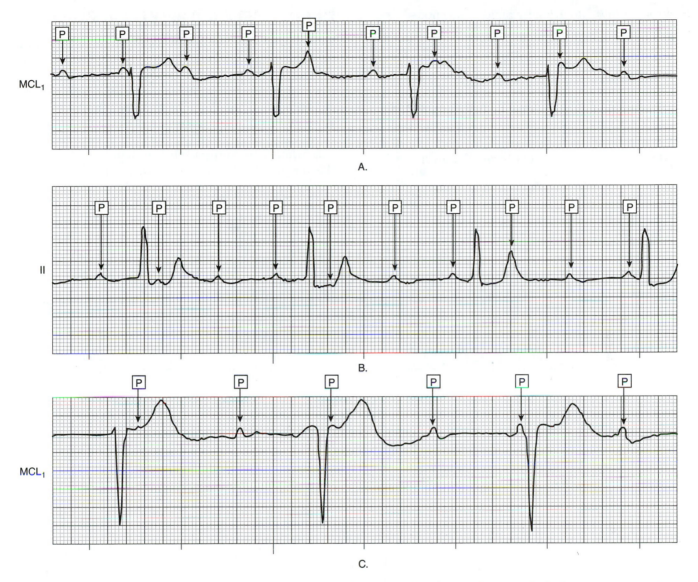

Figure 14–22 Complete AV heart block with bradycardic ventricular escape rhythms. In A, the ventricular rate is 40/minute, in B it is 35/minute, and in C it is just under 30/minute.

Table 14–11 Key ECG Features of Third-Degree Block	
■ **Atrial:**	Regular P-P intervals; P waves occur at a rate faster than the QRS complexes
■ **Ventricular:**	Regular R-R intervals; shape, width, and rate of QRS complexes depend on pacemaker site:
	■ AV junctional pacemakers: rate around 50 /minute with narrow, normal QRS-T complexes
	■ His bundle pacemakers: rate around 40/minute with narrow, normal QRS-T complexes
	■ Bundle branch pacemakers: rate 30–40/minute with wide, distorted QRS-T complexes
■ **AV Conduction:**	Absent
■ **Other Findings:**	Independent atrial and ventricular activity (AV dissociation)

- atropine in 0.5 to 1 mg by rapid intravenous administration up to 2 mg

- dopamine infusion at 5 to 20 µcg/kg/minute

- epinephrine infusion at 2 to 10 µcg/minute, and

- an infusion of isoprotenerol is mentioned out of historical reasons and because it is still included in the American Heart Association Advanced Cardiac Life Support protocols, but is rarely, if ever, used

THIRD-DEGREE (COMPLETE) AV BLOCK

The most serious form of AV heart block is **complete or third-degree block**. Conduction is so severely depressed that *no* sinus beats are conducted. The blockage occurs below the AV node, often in both bundle branches (Figures 14–20 and 14–21). Independent atrial and ventricular activity develops because two pacemakers are present: a sinus impulse controls the atria while a backup pacemaker stimulates the ventricles (Figures 14–21 and 14–22; Table 14–11).

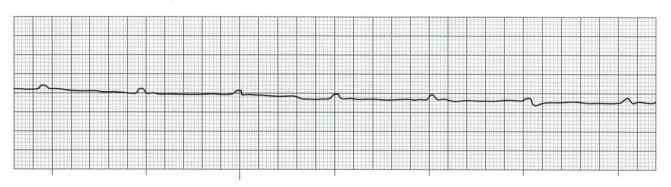

Figure 14–23 Ventricular standstill (asystole) in the setting of third-degree AV block. Only P waves without an escape ventricular pacemaker emerged in this case of third-degree AV block

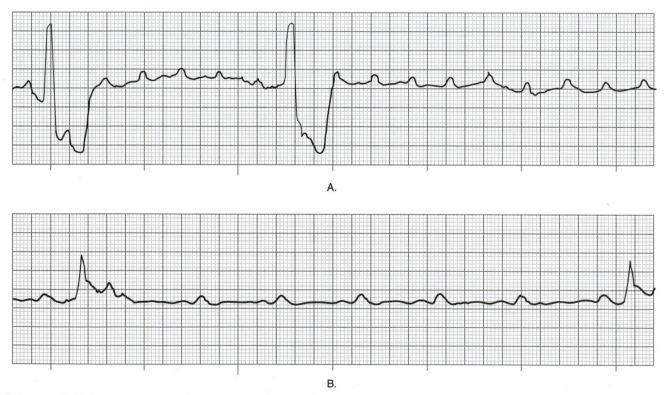

A.

B.

Figure 14–24 Failure of an effective escape rhythm to develop in complete AV heart block. In most cases of third-degree AV block, an escape pacemaker develops below the site of blockage to pace the ventricles. In these cases, a subsidiary paced rhythm did not develop, leading to cardiac arrest.

Fortunately, in most cases of third-degree block a "backup" pacemaker arises below the blockage site to keep the ventricles beating . Atrioventricular dissociation is present, meaning that atrial activity is not coordinated with ventricular activity. P waves are not associated with the QRS complexes. The atria are independently paced by the sinus node at a rate that is faster than the escape ventricular rate, resulting in two to three times as many P waves as QRS-T complexes. An ECG feature that is unique to complete block is that the *PR intervals are constantly changing*.

> **Clinical Note** *In third-degree AV block, the loss of coordinated cardiac activity, coupled with the bradycardic ventricular rate, causes a significant fall in cardiac output that leads to inadequate perfusion.*

Causes of Third-Degree Block

Third-degree block occurs as a result of advanced heart disease as listed in Table 14–12. Fibrosis of the conduction system that occurs with aging is a frequent cause. Third-degree block complicates 5 to 15 percent of

Table 14–12 Causes of Complete AV Heart Block

- **Myocardial Infarction**
- **Fibrotic Degenerative Changes Associated with Aging**
- **Congenital Cause**
- **Drug Toxicity: calcium channel blockers, digoxin, beta-adrenergic blockers**
- **Myocarditis (inflammation of the myocardium)**

myocardial infarctions. The location of the infarction generally determines whether the block is transient or permanent: anterior wall MIs usually cause a permanent block, while the block associated with inferior wall MIs typically subsides within a week or two as the swelling and inflammation diminishes. Advanced AV block in children is rare and pediatric cases are due to congenital conditions that are detected during infancy. Drug

toxicity, such as due to a calcium channel blocker or beta-adregenic blocker overdosage, commonly causes a block within the AV node that gradually resolves as the drug is metabolized.

Clinical Significance of Third-Degree Block

Third-degree AV block is a serious disorder that causes rate-related symptoms such as lightheadedness, dizziness, syncope, shortness of breath, and generalized weakness. How a patient tolerates third-degree block largely depends on the rate of the escape pacemaker. Escape pacemaker sites that are located relatively high in the ventricles have pacemaker rates around 50/minute and are well tolerated. High escape pacemakers located close to the AV node are also more dependable. Rates below 40/minute are generated by low escape pacemakers and are not as well tolerated. Low escape pacemakers, located further away from the AV node, are also less dependable and more likely to suddenly fail. Patients with third-degree AV block require an artificial pacemaker to stabilize the cardiac rhythm.

Escape Pacemakers in Third-Degree Block

An escape pacemaker discharges in either the AV bundle, bundle branches, or His-Purkinje system. The shape, rate, and duration of the QRS complexes provide useful clues in identifying the pacemaker site: (a) wide, slow (less than 40/minute) complexes arise low in the conduction pathway, while (b) narrow, rapid (50/minute) complexes arise high within the conduction pathway. Should an escape pacemaker fail to develop, ventricular standstill results and the ECG only shows P waves as shown in Figures 14–23 and 14–24.

> **Clinical Notes** *In third-degree AV block, the conduction disorder usually involves a problem in both bundle branches, rather than the AV node or His bundle. The lower within the ventricles that an escape pacemaker develops, the slower and the more unreliable the pacemaker's function. In contrast, the higher the escape pacemaker site, the more normal appearing the QRS complexes will be and the more dependable its function.*

Emergency Treatment of Third-Degree Block

Emergent treatment is indicated when severe bradycardia (usually below 45/minute) is associated with unsta-

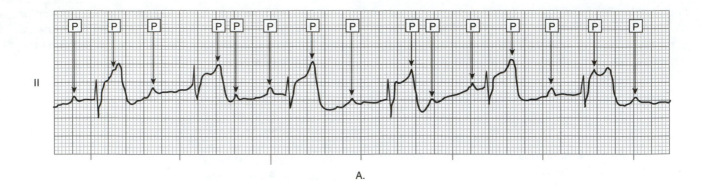

A.

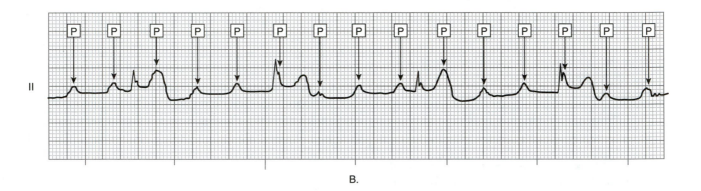

B.

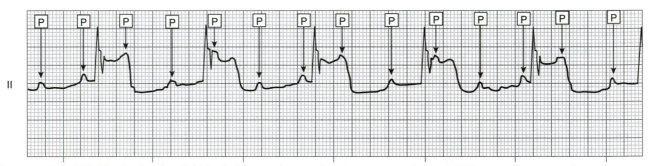

Figure 14-25 Third -degree AV block. The atrial rate for these examples is 150/minute because there are two large boxes between the Ps. The ventricular rates vary considerably: in A it is 60/minute, while in B the rate is 40/minute and in C it is 50/minute. Some P waves can be seen within the T waves and ST segments, while others are hidden by the QRS complexes.

ble vital signs or if inadequate perfusion is present. The approach to symptomatic bradycardias is included at the end of the chapter. Unlike second-degree block, atropine administration is *not* effective except for the few cases where the AV block is at or above the AV (His) bundle. Therapy for a complete AV block includes:

■ External and transvenous pacemaker

■ Dopamine infusion at 5 to 20 µg/kg/minute titrated to effect

■ Epinephrine infusion at 2 to 10 µg/minute titrated to desired heart rate

■ Permanent pacemaker insertion

Epinephrine may accelerate the ventricular heart rate but may not correct the heart block as shown in Figure 14–25.

AV DISSOCIATION

A frequent source of confusion concerns the difference

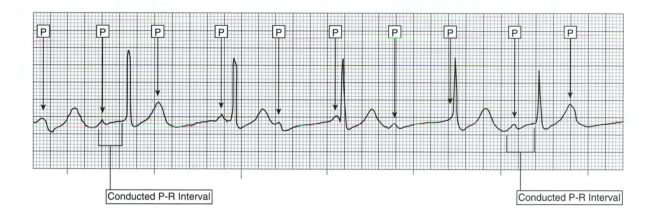

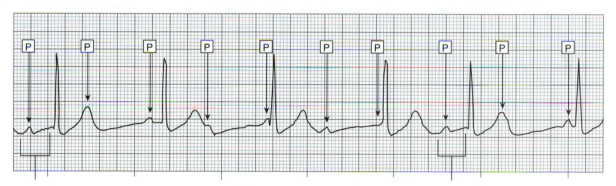

Figure 14–26 Atrioventricular dissociation. Four conducted beats (labelled) are found among the AV dissociated rhythm confirming that a high-grade second-degree AV block is present. The majority of atrial and ventricular complexes are dissociated from each other.

between AV dissociation and third-degree heart block. Every case of third-degree block involves AV dissociation. However, some cases of AV conduction is dissociated are due to transmission interference but a pathologic blockage. is not present AV dissociation exists when independent atrial and ventricular activity *interfere with one another*. AV dissociation develops secondary to another rhythm disorder when impulse formation or a conduction disturbance interferes with coordinated atrial and ventricular activity.

AV dissociation can result in the case of a sinus bradycardia or a Wenckebach AV block when the long R-R intervals allow escape pacemakers to develop (Figures 14–26 and 14–27). For a brief period, the escape rhythm interferes with sinus activity. This is a case of AV dissociation *without* AV heart block. In Figure 14–27 some conducted beats are clearly seen. The P waves and QRS-T complexes are unrelated and the dissociated state lasts until the sinus node regains control. When even a single "captured beat" is noted during a period of AV dissociation, it means that conduction is occurring and therefore, third-degree block cannot exist.

Another cause of AV dissociation occurs when an accelerated ventricular or junctional rhythm results in independent atrial and ventricular activity (Figure 14–28). For example, AV dissociation results when a rapid ventricular rate overtakes the sinus node rate and disrupts the coordinated atrioventricular rhythm. Some P waves are conducted while others are not associated with a QRS complex.

SPECIAL CASE: Isorhythmic AV dissociation

In some sinus bradycardias, the junctional escape and the sinus node discharge rate scan be so similar that they overlap, leading to pacemaker interference. For instance, a sinus bradycardia at a rate of 50/min. and an AV junctional rate at 50/min. overlap and will lead to sinus and junctional beats. That was the case in Figure 14–27. This form of AV dissociation is termed **isorhythmic dissociation**, which means the "same rate." This dissociated state is temporary, lasting for several seconds and ends as soon as the sinus node accelerates.

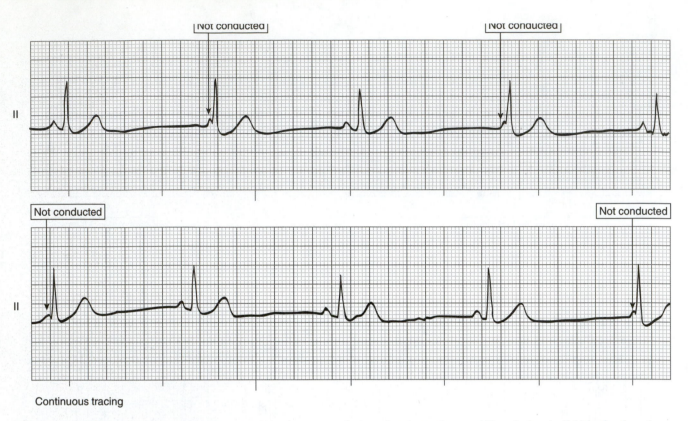

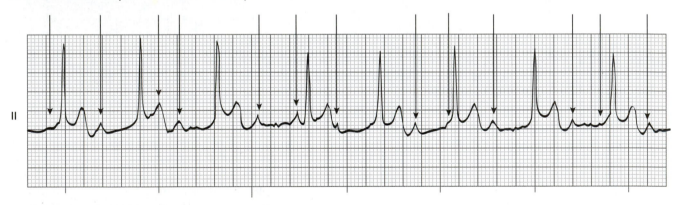

Figure 14-27 AV dissociation can result in the case of sinus bradycardia or a Wenckebach AV block when long R-R intervals allow pacemakers to develop.

Figure 14-28 AV dissociation can also result when an accelerated ventricular or junctional rhythm results in independent atrial and ventricualr activity.

Clinical Note *Every case AV dissociation is not due to complete heart block. There are three causes of AV dissociation: third-degree AV heart block is the most common cause. Less common causes include: accelerated ventricular or AV junctional pacemakers; and sinus node depression, which leads to interference by an escape junctional pacemaker.*

Table 14–13 correlates ECG findings common in AV heart blocks with the interpretation of those findings.

Table 14–14 summarizes the key findings of AV heart blocks. Chapter 15 contains twenty-five ECG tracings showing all types of AV conduction abnormalities for practice.

Treatment Approach of Adult Symptomatic Bradycardias

The following information will help explain the 2001 ACLS treatment guidelines for bradydysrhythmias:

■ **Correctly interpret the type of bradycardia.**
Correctly interpreting the type of heart block will

help determine the clinical significance and the likely need for treatment. Distinguishing a second degree AV block Mobitz Type I from a Mobitz Type II is important because the former almost never needs treatment while the latter almost always does. Sinus bradycardia rarely requires treatment and if such a patient is symptomatic, other causes should be evaluated before attributing the reason to the slow sinus rate. Most individuals do not become symptomatic until the heart rate drops below 40/minute.

- **Only symptomatic bradycardias require treatment.** The American marathon bicycle champion Lance Armstrong has a resting heart beat in the 30's and he clearly does not require treatment. Likewise, not all patients with slow heart rates need therapy. When the slow rate is the reason for the patient's symptoms, such as dizziness, fatigue, altered mental status, or syncope, treatment is indicated.

- **Slow dysrhythmias that are always pathologic.** Second degree AV block Mobitz Type II and third

likely not be effective because the ventricles have little vagal fibers and these blocks occur in the ventricular conduction system. Infusion of various beta-adrenergic drugs or vasopressor medication is reserved for cases where pacing does not work. The intervention order is:

- *atropine* in 0.5 mg IV boluses every 3 to 5 minutes up to a total of 0.03 mg/kg (a 2 mg dose for a 70 kg patient).

- *transcutaneous pacemaker*

- *dopamine* IV infusion at 5 to 20 µ/kg per minute

- *epinephrine* IV infusion at 2 to 10 µ/minute

- *isoproterenol* IV infusion at 2 to 10 µ/minute is the last choice drug for symptomatic bradycardias and is rarely used.

The infusion of medication are temporizing measures until a pacemaker becomes available. Infusing adrenergic and anticholinergic medications have the disadvantage of being unable to precisely control the desired rate in the way that using a pacemaker allows.

Table 14–13 Significance of ECG Findings Regarding the Relationship of P waves to QRS Complexes

ECG finding	Conclusion
More P waves than QRS complexes	A second- or third-degree AV block (or dissociation) is present
Some P waves—but not all—are not conducted	A second-degree (partial) block is present
P waves have no relationship to QRS-T complexes	Complete AV dissociation exists
Fixed PR intervals occur before dropped QRS-T complexes	Second-degree block; Mobitz Type I (Wenckebach) is present
Progressive increases in the PR intervals occur before dropped QRS-T complexes	Second-degree AV block; Mobitz Type II exists

degree (complete) AV heart block are likely to cause significant symptoms and are prone to sudden deterioration in the patient's condition. Aside from these two rhythm disorders, most others do not require emergent therapy.

Order of Treatment. Unless atropine is contraindicated, the approach to symptomatic bradycardia begins with atropine and quickly moves to transcutaneous pacing. In advanced forms of heart block, such as Mobitz type II and third degree AV block, atropine will

Clinical Tip: Atropine is not indicated for third degree heart block, wide complex escape ventricular pacemaker rhythms, or for Mobitz type II. Atropine works by blocking the effects of the vagus nerve but there are few such fibers in the ventricles. Atropine might increase the atrial rate but it is unlikely to reverse third degree block; it is better to go directly to transcutaneous pacing.

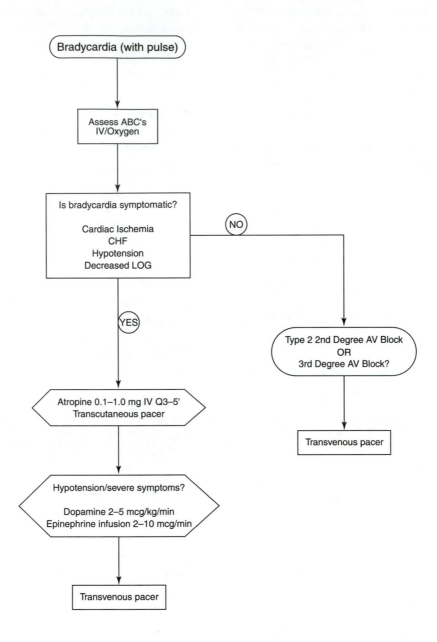

Figure 14-29 ACLS treatment algorithm for adult bradycardic rhythms. (Reprinted with permission EmedHome.com website (http://www.emedhome.com)

Let's Review

1. The mildest form of AV block, first degree, involves a PR interval greater than 0.20 second. There are no adverse effects as long as the sinus rate is adequate.

2. First-degree AV block differs from NSR only in that the PR interval is prolonged. Unlike other heart block, no QRS-T complexes are "dropped." Aside from the long PR interval, the pacemaker is sinus, the order of cardiac activation is normal, and the QRS-T complex is the same as in NSR.

3. When sinus bradycardia and a prolonged PR interval occur together, evaluation of the slow heart rate takes precedence over the prolonged PR interval because long PR intervals are harmless, whereas a slow rate can cause cardiac output to fall.

4. In the majority of cases of first-degree block, PR interval prolongation represents a benign and incidental finding.

5. When sinus bradycardia results from increased parasympathetic tone the PR interval commonly increasea as well. A prolonged PR interval should not be termed first-degree block unless the heart rate is at least 60/minute.

6. The conduction delay in first-degree block is located within the AV node.

7. There are two types of second-degree AV heart block: Mobitz Type I and Mobitz Type II. Mobitz Type I block is less serious as it is usually transient and self limited. Mobitz Type II represents a serious conduction problem and occurs in patients with heart disease.

8. Wenckebach (Mobitz Type II) usually develops within the AV node and is benign, while Mobitz Type II develops below the AV node and is pathological. Mobitz Type II is a clear indication for insertion of an artificial pacemaker, while Mobitz Type I usually requires only observation.

9. The first conducted PR interval of each grouped beat cycle in Wenckebach AV block is often prolonged beyond 0.20 second. A first-degree and a second-degree block is simultaneously present.

10. A Wenckebach heart block is much more common than Mobitz Type II, and is usually transient and benign compared to Mobitz Type II.

11. In Wenckebach, QRS complexes are usually narrow and have a normal shape in contrast to Mobitz Type II, which have wide and distorted QRS complexes. In Mobitz Type I the problem occurs intranodally, while in Mobitz Type II it is an infranodal problem, usually in the bundle branches.

12. The pauses in cardiac activity that result when beats are dropped in Wenckebach (Mobitx Type II) are less than twice the shortest R-R cycle. This is helpful because the PR intervals sometimes cannot be measured, yet the grouped beating and pauses are still readily apparent.

13. As the PR intervals lengthen in Wenckebach, the R-R intervals progressively shorten. As the PR intervals increase, the QRS complexes fall further behind the P waves, appearing closer to the QRS complexes that follow.

14. Mobitz Type II block occurs only with serious cardiac disease, in contrast to Wenckebach, which can be seen in normal individuals. Mobitz Type II block is likely to suddenly progress to complete heart block.

15. The PR intervals in Mobitz Type II are constant. The R-R interval that includes the dropped P wave is equal to two R-R intervals.

16. The main management concern for patients with Mobitz Type II, second-degree heart block depends on the ventricular rate.

17. "High grade" second-degree AV block involves failure of two or more consecutive P waves to be conducted. This is a very serious form of second-degree heart block. It will quickly progress to complete heart block.

18. Cases involving 2:1 AV conduction may be misinterpreted as a case of "marked sinus bradycardia" if the second P wave is hidden within the ST segment-T waves.

19. In 2:1 AV block, clues that help distinguish Type I from Type II include: a normal QRS complex with a prolonged PR interval is found because Wenckebach is usually due to an intranodal block. In contrast, Mobitz Type II shows a wide QRS complex but has

a normal PR interval.

20. Third-degree block occurring during inferior wall MIs often resolve over several days, whereas similar blocks found during anterior MIs are typically permanent.

21. High escape pacemakers pace the heart at 50/minute, are typically transient, and tend to be well tolerated. Low escape pacemakers discharge at rates below 40/minute, have a distorted QRS-T complexes, and are undependable.

22. Third-degree AV block is the most common type of AV dissociation, but there are conditions besides heart block that cause atrial and ventricular activity dissociation.

23. While all cases of third-degree AV block involve AV dissociation, the converse is not true. Every case of AV dissociation does not involve third-degree heart block. Atrial and ventricular dissociation activity can occur despite normal AV conduction if there is competition between a slow sinus pacemaker and a rapid junctionalk pacemaker, for instance.

Glossary

Asystolic pauses ECG pauses caused by nonconducted P waves missing QRS complexes.

Atrioventricular block Delay or interruption in impulse conduction between the atria and ventricles.

Atrioventricular (AV) dissociation Lack of coordination between atrial and ventricular activity that is due to heart block or disruption of pacemaker timing.

Complete AV block Same as third-degree AV block.

Dropped QRS complex Nonconducted P wave results in a missing QRS complex.

Fasciles Smaller divisions of the bundle branches.

Fibrosis Scar tissue.

First-degree AV block Delay in conduction that occurs after atrial depolarization, thus delaying ventricular depolarization.

High grade second-degree AV block Two or more consecutive P waves fail to be conducted.

Infranodal Location below the AV node; for example, in the bundle branches.

Intranodal Location within the AV node.

Isorhythmic dissociation The junctional escape rate and the sinus rate are similar and often leads to pacemaker interference.

Mobitz Type: nonspecific Term applied to cases of 2:1 AV conduction when there is uncertainty whether the block is Mobitz Type I or Mobitz Type II.

Mobitz Type I (Wenckebach type) block Fform of second-degree AV block involving partial blockage of sinus impulses and characterized by progressively increasing PR intervals.

Mobitz Type II block Form of second-degree AV block involving partial blockage of sinus impulses and characterized by fixed PR intervals and blocked QRS complexes.

Myocarditis Inflammation of the myocardium.

Second-degree AV block Interruption in conduction that allows some but not all atrial impulses to be conducted to the ventricles.

Stokes-Adams syndrome Syncope caused by complete AV heart block.

Syncope Loss of consciousness.

Third-degree complete AV block Complete interruption in conduction such that no sinus beats are conducted; characterized by independent atrial and ventricular pacemakers.

chapter 15

Atrioventricular Heart Blocks—Self-Assessment ECG Tracings

LEARNING OBJECTIVES

Upon completion of this chapter, the reader should be able to:

- *Correctly identify various types of AV blocks when presented with sample ECG tracings.*
- *Accurately assess the rhythm, PR intervals, QRS duration, AV conduction ratios, and ST segments, when given a sample of ECG tracings displaying various types of atrioventricular heart blocks.*

SELF-ASSESSMENT ECG TRACINGS

The following ECG tracings show a variety of atrioventricular block dysrhythmias. Each tracing should be analyzed according to the systematic approach outlined earlier and an interpretation made based on the dysrhythmia descriptions explained in Chapter 14. Answers can be checked with the interpretations provided in Appendix A. If any difficulties are encountered, the relevant sections in Chapter 14 should be reviewed.

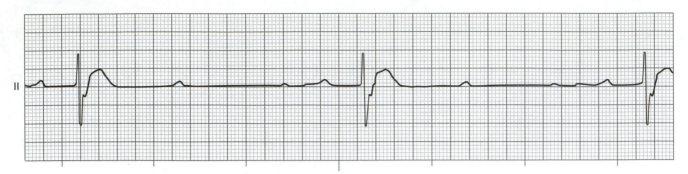

Figure 15-1   Rate _____
Rhythm _____
QRS Duration _____
PR Interval _____
AV Conduction Ratio _____
ST Segment _____ _____
Interpretation _____
Reasoning _____

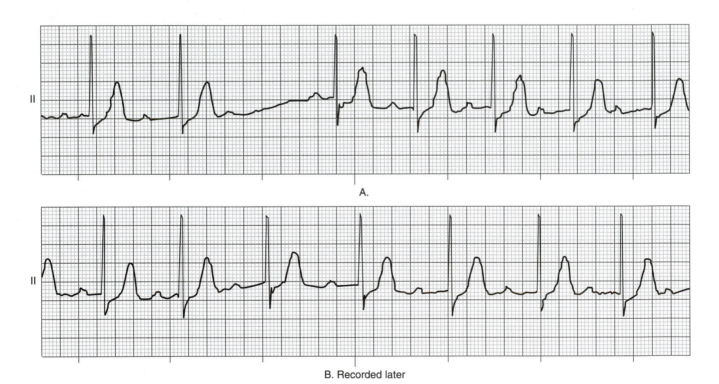

A.

B. Recorded later

Figure 15-2   Rate _____
Rhythm _____
QRS Duration _____
PR Interval _____
AV Conduction Ratio _____
ST Segment _____
Interpretation _____
Reasoning _____

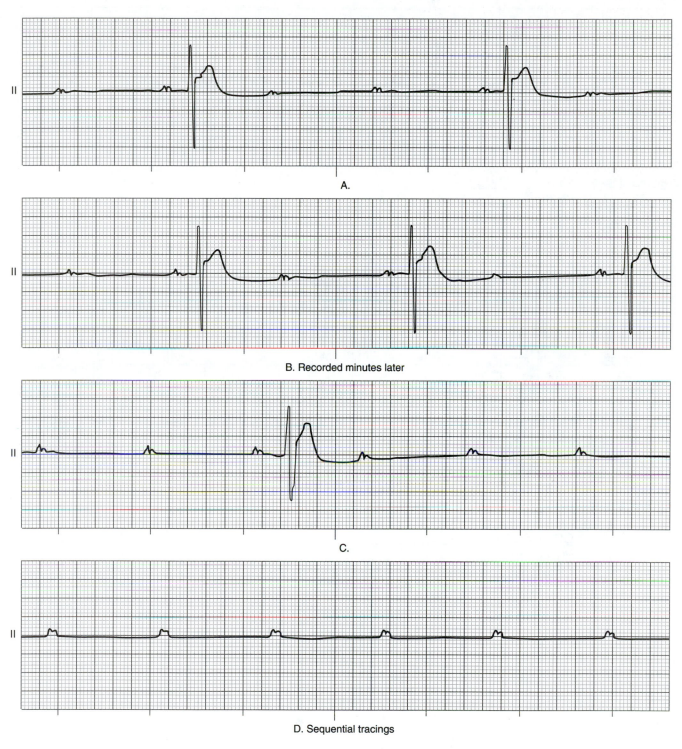

A.

B. Recorded minutes later

C.

D. Sequential tracings

Figure 15–3
Rate _____
Rhythm _____
QRS Duration _____
PR Interval _____
AV Conduction Ratio _____
ST Segment _____
Interpretation _____
Reasoning _____

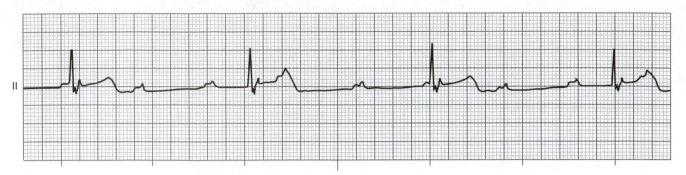

Figure 15–4   Rate _____

Rhythm _____

QRS Duration _____

PR Interval _____

AV Conduction Ratio _____

ST Segment _____

Interpretation _____

Reasoning _____

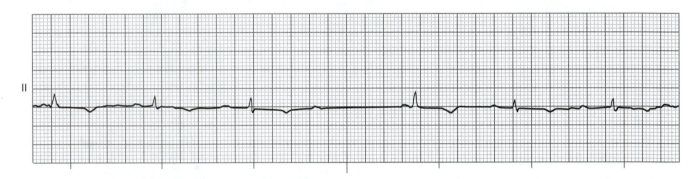

Figure 15–5   Rate _____

Rhythm _____

QRS Duration _____

PR Interval _____

AV Conduction Ratio _____

ST Segment _____

Interpretation _____

Reasoning _____

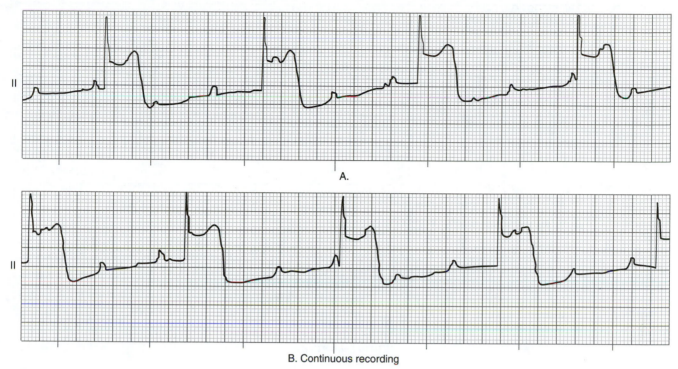

A.

B. Continuous recording

Figure 15–6   Rate _____
Rhythm _____
QRS Duration _____
PR Interval _____
AV Conduction Ratio _____
ST Segment _____
Interpretation _____
Reasoning _____

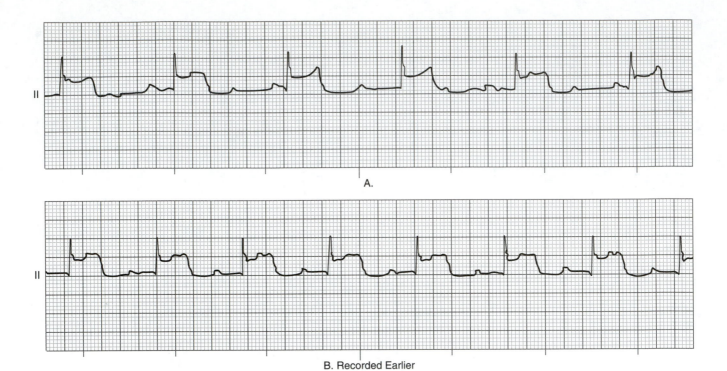

A.

B. Recorded Earlier

Figure 15–7   Rate _____
Rhythm _____
QRS Duration _____
PR Interval _____
AV Conduction Ratio _____
ST Segment _____
Interpretation _____
Reasoning _____

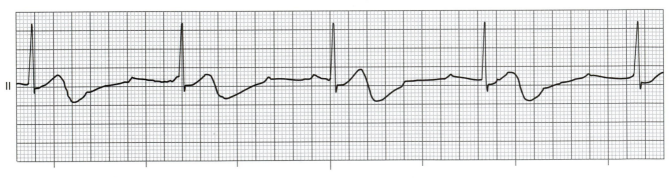

Figure 15–8   Rate _____
Rhythm _____
QRS Duration _____
PR Interval _____
AV Conduction Ratio _____
ST Segment _____
Interpretation _____
Reasoning _____

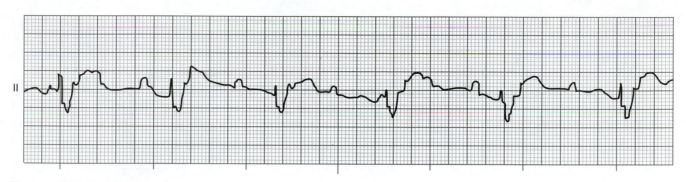

Figure 15–9   Rate _____
Rhythm _____
QRS Duration _____
PR Interval _____
AV Conduction Ratio _____
ST Segment _____
Interpretation _____
Reasoning _____

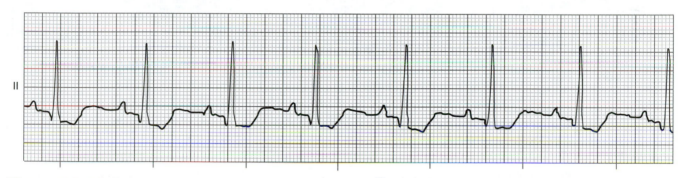

Figure 15–10   Rate _____
Rhythm _____
QRS Duration _____
PR Interval _____
AV Conduction Ratio _____
ST Segment _____
Interpretation _____
Reasoning _____

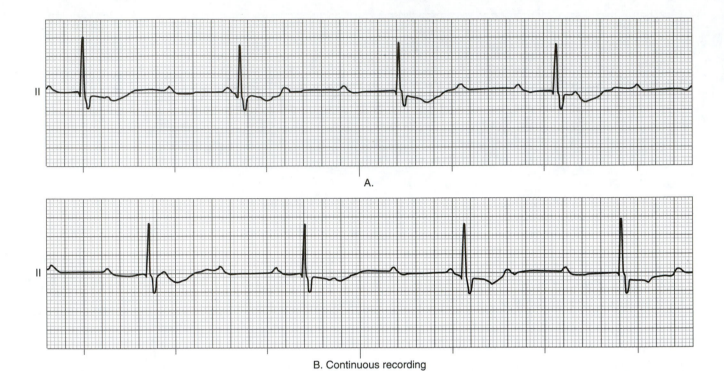

A.

B. Continuous recording

Figure 15-11 Rate _____
Rhythm _____
QRS Duration _____
PR Interval _____
AV Conduction Ratio _____
ST Segment _____
Interpretation _____
Reasoning _____

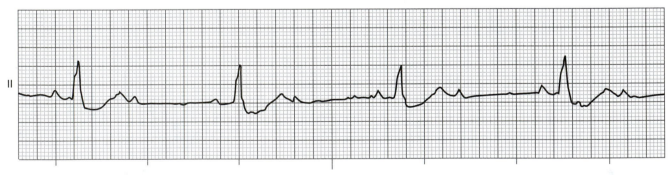

Figure 15-12 Rate _____
Rhythm _____
QRS Duration _____
PR Interval _____
AV Conduction Ratio _____
ST Segment _____
Interpretation _____
Reasoning _____

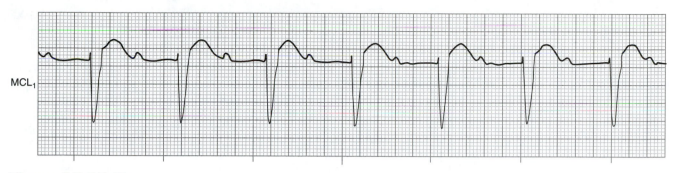

Figure 15-13 Rate _____
Rhythm _____
QRS Duration _____
PR Interval _____
AV Conduction Ratio _____
ST Segment _____
Interpretation _____
Reasoning _____

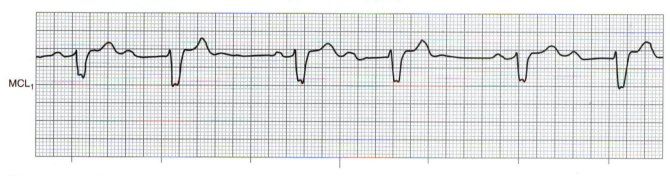

Figure 15-14 Rate _____
Rhythm _____
QRS Duration _____
PR Interval _____
AV Conduction Ratio _____
ST Segment _____
Interpretation _____
Reasoning _____

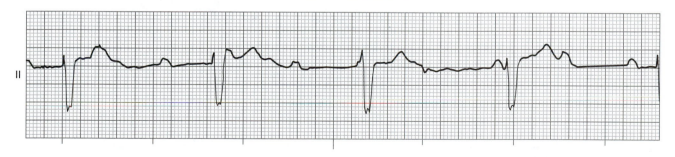

Figure 15-15 Rate _____
Rhythm _____
QRS Duration _____
PR Interval _____
AV Conduction Ratio _____
ST Segment _____
Interpretation _____
Reasoning _____

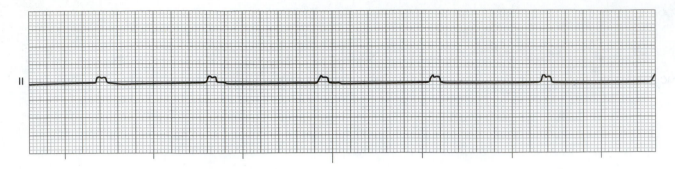

Figure 15-16 Rate _____
Rhythm _____
QRS Duration _____
PR Interval _____
AV Conduction Ratio _____
ST Segment _____
Interpretation _____
Reasoning _____

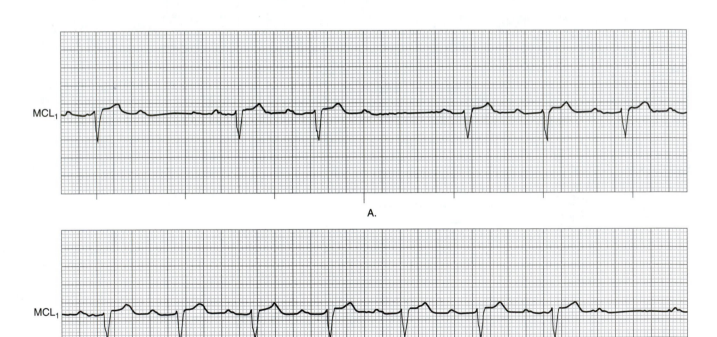

A.

B. Continuous tracing

Figure 15-17 Rate _____
Rhythm _____
QRS Duration _____
PR Interval _____
AV Conduction Ratio _____
ST Segment _____
Interpretation _____
Reasoning _____

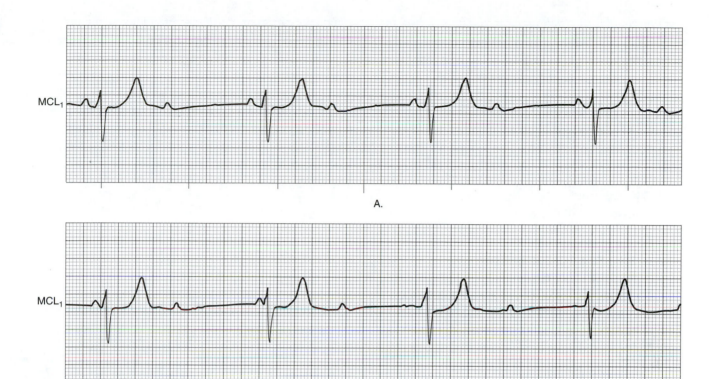

A.

B. Continuous tracing

Figure 15–18   Rate _____
Rhythm _____
QRS Duration _____
PR Interval _____
AV Conduction Ratio _____
ST Segment _____
Interpretation _____
Reasoning _____

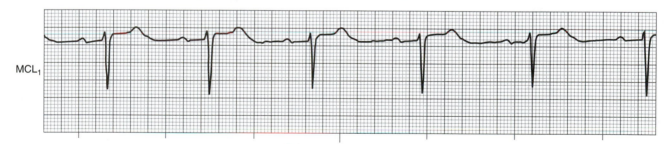

Figure 15–19   Rate _____
Rhythm _____
QRS Duration _____
PR Interval _____
AV Conduction Ratio _____
ST Segment _____
Interpretation _____
Reasoning _____

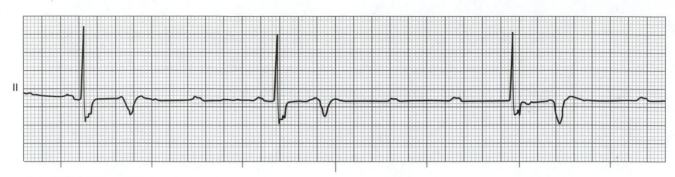

II

Figure 15–20 Rate _____
Rhythm _____
QRS Duration _____
PR Interval _____
AV Conduction Ratio _____
ST Segment _____
Interpretation _____
Reasoning _____

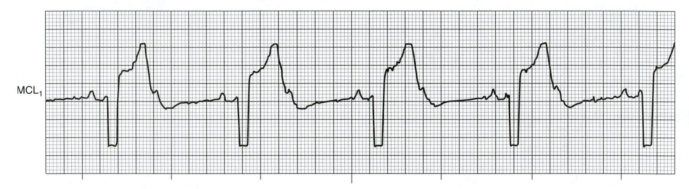

MCL₁

Figure 15–21 Rate _____
Rhythm _____
QRS Duration _____
PR Interval _____
AV Conduction Ratio _____
ST Segment _____
Interpretation _____
Reasoning _____

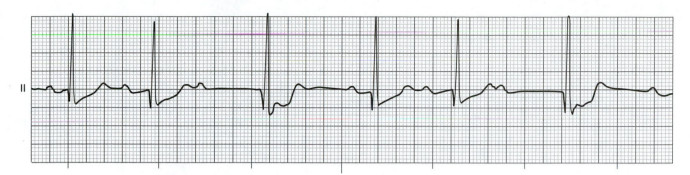

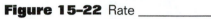

Figure 15–22 Rate _____
Rhythm _____
QRS Duration _____
PR Interval _____
AV Conduction Ratio _____
ST Segment _____
Interpretation _____
Reasoning _____

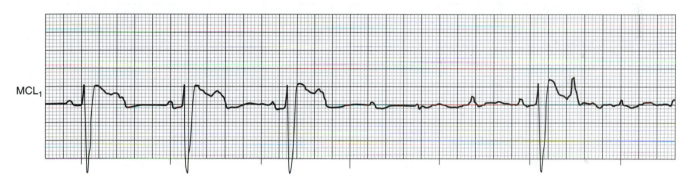

Figure 15–23 Rate _____
Rhythm _____
QRS Duration _____
PR Interval _____
AV Conduction Ratio _____
ST Segment _____
Interpretation _____
Reasoning _____

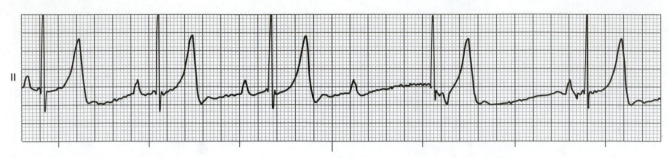

Figure 15–24 Rate _____

Rhythm _____

QRS Duration _____

PR Interval _____

AV Conduction Ratio _____

ST Segment _____

Interpretation _____

Reasoning _____

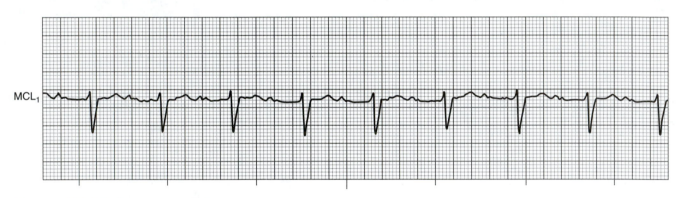

Figure 15–25 Rate _____

Rhythm _____

QRS Duration _____

PR Interval _____

AV Conduction Ratio _____

ST Segment _____

Interpretation _____

Reasoning _____

Ventricular Dysrhythmias—Part One

LEARNING OBJECTIVES

Upon completion of this chapter, the reader should be able to:

- *Define Key terms.*
- *List the ECG characteristics of ventricular complexes that distinguish them from supraventricular complexes.*
- *Define the passive and active mechanisms of dysrhythmia formation.*
- *List the ECG characteristics of premature ventricular complexes (PVCs).*
- *Describe the clinical significance of PVCs.*
- *List one indication for treating PVCs.*
- *List the ECG characteristics of monomorphic ventricular tachycardia (VT).*
- *Describe the reason that ventricular tachycardia must be promptly treated.*
- *List three drugs that can be used for treating monomorphic VT.*
- *State the therapy of choice for monomorphic VT that is associated with an unstable patient condition.*
- *Describe the clinical significance of monomorphic ventricular tachycardia.*
- *Describe the "proarrhythmia" complications of anti-dysrhythmic medication.*

CHAPTER OVERVIEW

Ventricular dysrhythmias "stick out like a sore thumb" because of their wide and bizarre appearance. Ventricular dysrhythmias are easy to distinguish from supraventricular disorders because they lack the sleek, narrow QRS complexes typical of sinus and AV junctional rhythms.

Abnormal ventricular rhythms are significant because they are usually associated with heart disease. Life-threatening ventricular dysrhythmias are common during an MI—in fact, they are the leading cause of early sudden cardiac death.

Ventricular dysrhythmias include a wide range of rhythm disorders. Premature ventricular complexes and short episodes of ventricular tachycardia usually do not require therapy, but sustained ventricular tachycardia can cause shock, ventricular fibrillation, and sudden death if not corrected.

INTRODUCTION TO VENTRICULAR DYSRHYTHMIAS

Ventricular dysrhythmias as a group are generally more serious than supraventricular rhythm disorders because they have the potential to cause impaired cardiac output and cardiac arrest. Ventricular tachycardia, for instance, is more likely to cause clinical deterioration than a supraventricular tachydysrhythmia.

The clinical setting during which a ventricular disorder occurs yields an important clue about how serious a dysrhythmia is and how rapidly therapy must be started. In contrast to supraventricular dysrhythmias, organic heart disease is commonly associated with ventricular disorders. Paroxysmal supraventricular tachycardia (PSVT), for example, usually occurs in the *absence of organic disease*, but ventricular tachycardia seldom, if ever, does. Similarly, certain types of premature ventricular complexes can lead to ventricular tachycardia or even ventricular fibrillation—a potentially lethal dysrhythmia—yet premature supraventricular complexes are only a minor nuisance.

Ventricular dysrhythmias are frequently encountered during the early stages of a myocardial infarction and this electrical instability accounts for the vast majority of early sudden cardiac deaths. Paradoxically, ventricular disorders that develop during thrombolytic therapy are actually a welcome sign, heralding myocardial reperfusion and indicates that coronary blood flow has been reestablished.

Passive Versus Active Dysrhythmia Mechanisms

Ventricular dysrhythmias can occur through either a "passive" and "active" mechanisms. Active impulse formation is due to ventricular irritability, which causes increased pacemaker discharge (automaticity) and disrupts sinus rhythm. Passive impulse formation, in contrast, results from a default situation when higher pacemakers fail. Escape pacemaker formation is an example of a passive pacemaker mechanism while the rapid discharge of an irritable ventricular site represents active development. Passive pacemakers do *not* compete with the sinus node for heart rate control and subside as soon as higher pacemaker function resumes.

Recognizing Ventricular Complexes and Rhythms

Previous chapters have concentrated on supraventricular dysrhythmias, including disorders originating in the sinus node, atria, AV node or early portion of the AV bundle. Supraventricular dysrhythmias share narrow QRS complexes and distorted P waves. Ventricular dysrhythmias, in contrast, share other characteristics: missing or retrograde P waves and an altered ventricular

depolarization, resulting in widened and distorted QRS complexes (Figure 16–1). The ST segments and T waves of ventricular dysrhythmias are also distorted because the repolarization phase is abnormal (Figure 16–2). The wide and distorted QRS-T complexes of ventricular dysrhythmias makes distinguishing them from the narrow QRS-T complexes of supraventricular rhythms easy.

PREMATURE VENTRICULAR COMPLEXES

A **premature ventricle complex (PVC)** is an early, extra depolarization that arises below the AV (His) bundle. A PVC is described as premature because it occurs before the next expected sinus beat (Figure 16–3). PVCs disrupt regular sinus rhythm and result in shortened R-R intervals (Table 16–1). PVCs generate less stroke volume than sinus beats because they occur before the ventricles have had a chance to maximally fill. The ventricles also contract sequentially rather than simultaneously as in sinus beats. The normal activation process is reversed because the impulse arises within the ventricle, depolarization is prolonged, and an abnormal conduction pathway is followed. This accounts for why the QRS complex is distorted and the QRS duration prolonged. Altered repolarization follows the abnormal depolarization process and results in a distorted ST-T complex shape.

PVC Appearance

The unusual appearance of the distorted QRS-T complexes allows these beats to easily be distinguished from supraventricular beats. The PVC QRS complex is distorted and widened to 0.12 second and beyond (Figure 16–4). P waves can often be seen distorting the ST-T wave segments (Figure 16–5). The ST-T waves occur in an opposite direction to that of the main deflection of the PVCs QRS complex. For instance,

---

Table 16-1 Key ECG Features of PVCs

- ■ **Atrial:**   Usually not visible

- ■ **Ventricular:**   Wide, distorted QRS-ST
                        complexes

- ■ **Other Findings:**

  - ■ Occurs early and are taller than sinus beats

  - ■ Compensatory pauses follow PVCs

  - ■ T wave of the ectopic complex occurs in direction opposite to the distorted QRS deflection

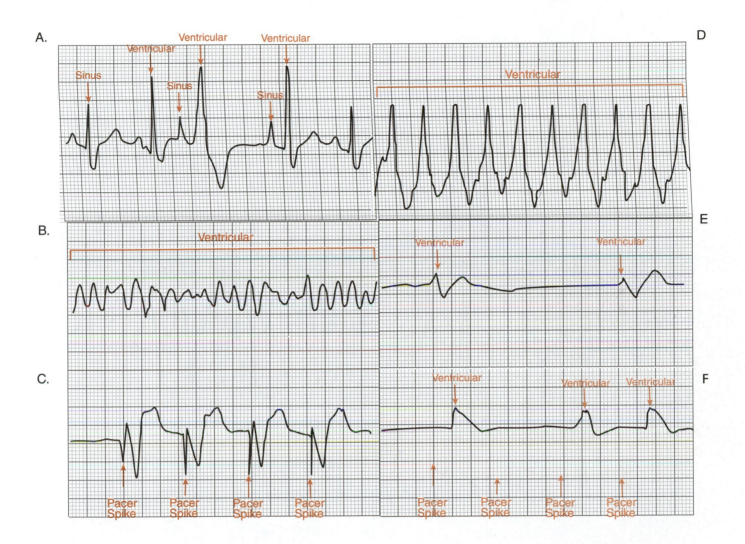

Figure 16–1 Ventricular complexes have wide and bizarre-appearing QRS-T complexes with absent P waves. Ventricular beats are easy to differentiate from sinus and junctional complexes because of their distorted shapes and delayed conduction. In tracing A the 1st, 3rd, and 5th beats are sinus while the remainder are ventricular. Tracing B shows irregular ventricular complexes. Tracing C shows artificial pacemaker beats that resemble ventricular beats because the electrical stimulus is discharged within the right ventricle, leading to an abnormal depolarization. Tracing D shows a rapid ventricular rhythm, while tracing E and F show very slow wide QRS complex rhythms.

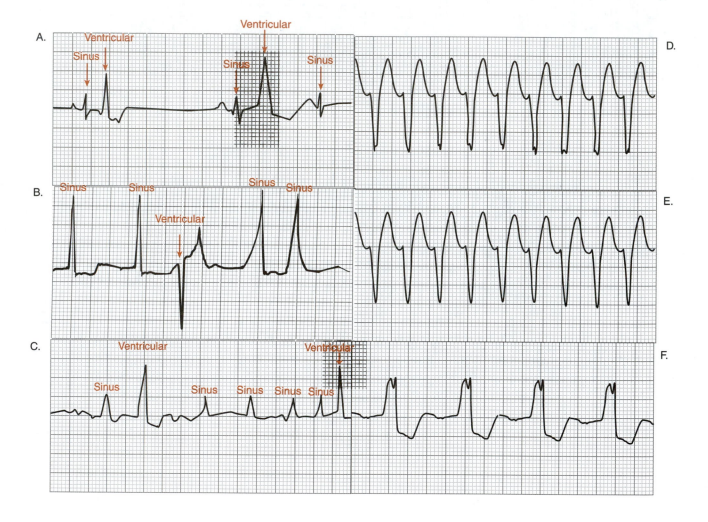

Figure 16–2 Wide and distorted ventricular complexes. In tracing A beats number 1, 3, and 5 are sinus while beats number 2 and 4 are ventricular. In tracing B the third beat is ventricular while in tracing C beats number 2 and 7 are ventricular. The remainder of the beats are ventricular. Tracings D and E show only rapid ventricular rhythms—every beat is ventricular. Tracing F shows a slower ventricular rhythm.

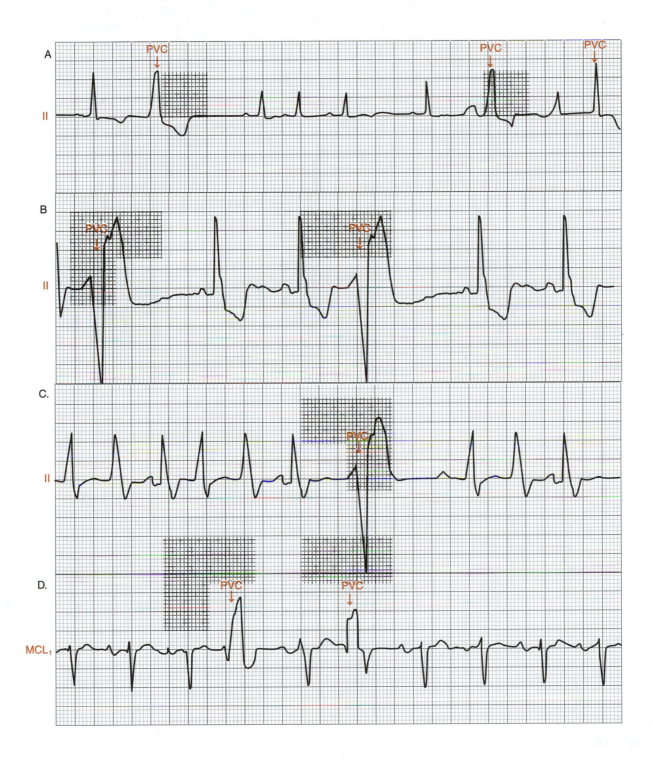

Figure 16–3 Premature ventricular complexes have been labeled with arrows. They occur early, have wide and distorted QRS-T complexes, lack P waves, and have T waves that point in a direction opposite to the QRS complexes.

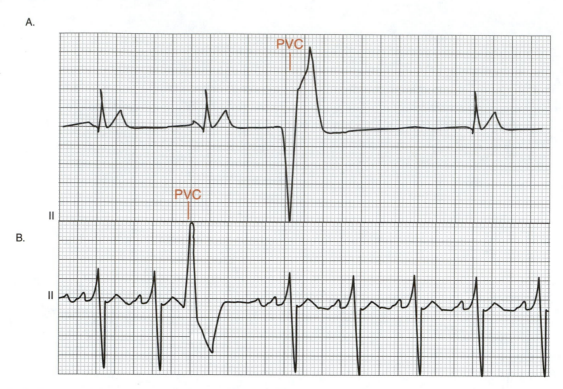

Figure 16–4 The third beat in each tracing is a PVC, that has wide and distorted QRS complexes. PVCs are premature, usually taller than surrounding sinus beats, and the ST-T waves face a direction opposite to the QRS complexes of the PVCs.

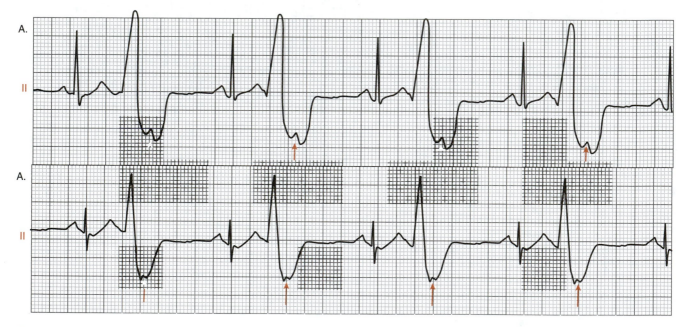

Figure 16–5 P waves in the ST segments of PVCs. The P waves occur during the PVCs following ventricular depolarization.

when the PVC QRS complex deflection is negative, the ST-T wave will be upright. Likewise, should the PVC QRS be positive, the ST-T wave portion will be negative.

Compensatory pauses follow PVCs and are equal to two normal R-R intervals (Figure 16–6). A compensatory pause consists of: (a) a shortened R-R interval of the PVC that is coupled to the prior sinus beat; and (b) the longer R-R interval that follows the PVC.

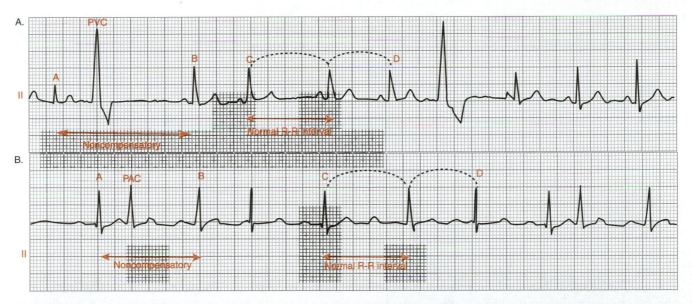

Figure 16–6 Compensatory pause. Strip A shows a PVC with full compensatory pause. The interval from the sinus beat before the PVC to the sinus beat after the PVC equals two R-R intervals. Thus, the distance from A to B is equal to the distance from C to D. Strip B shows a PAC with noncompensatory pause. The interval from the sinus beat preceding the PAC to the one following is less than two R-R intervals. Thus, the distance from A to B is less than the distance from C to D.

Mechanisms of PVC Development

Two mechanisms account for PVC formation: re-entry and automaticity.

Reentry

During re-entry a depolarization impulse encounters tissue which has devloped a unidirectional (one-way) conduction block, causing the impulse to circle around the blocked tissue. The impulse eventually arrives back at the original point but instead of ending, the depolarization cycle continues. When the PVC emerges, it encounters surrounding tissue that has had time to become repolarized and is ready to be re-stimulated. A rapid circular pathway can become established leading to an abnormal tachhycardia.

Automaticity

Enhanced automaticity is a less common way for PVCs to develop. Ischemia can change the local electrolyte composition and electrical condition of cardiac cells. Hypoxia and increased sympathetic tone lower the depolarization threshold, leading to ectopic pacemaker formation.

Unifocal (Uniformed) PVCs

PVCs tend to have the same shape within the same ECG lead because they arise from the same site and follow the same depolarization pathway (Figure 16–7). The term **"unifocal"** is applied to PVCs with the same shape. However, it is less accurate than **"uniformed"** because it implies that the development site determines the shape: Because of tradition, the less accurate term unifocal is more commonly used.

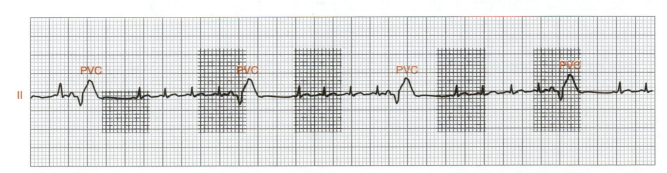

Figure 16–7 Unifocal or uniformed PVCs have identical shapes.

Multifocal (Multiformed) PVCs

Multifocal (Multiformed) PVCs, in contrast, have different configurations within the same ECG lead (Figure 16–8). Multiformed PVCs either arose from different sites or formed at the same place, but followed different depolarization paths. Again, a less accurate but more commonly used term "multifocal" is employed.

PVC Coupling Intervals

A **coupling interval** is the distance between a PVC and the sinus beat before it (Figure 16–9). Coupling intervals can be fixed or variable: In most cases there is a **fixed PVC coupling interval**, that is, the distance from the end of the sinus T wave until the PVC is constant. Fixed coupling intervals mean that the PVC is in

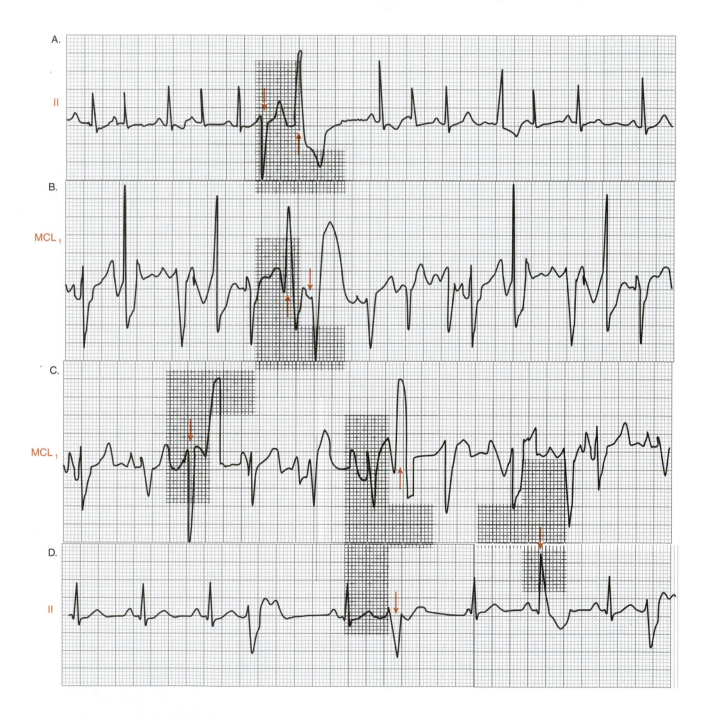

Figure 16–8 Multiformed PVCs have at least two different configurations (indicated by arrows).

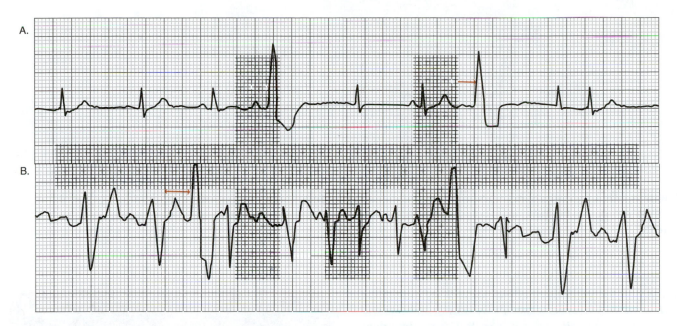

Figure 16–9 The coupling intervals that link the PVC to the preceding sinus beat are usually constant. In both examples the coupling intervals are variable. Variable coupling intervals are uncommon and occur when there is an automatic ventricular focus. There is a much greater chance of an R-on-T.

some way dependent on the sinus beat, and points toward a reentry mechanism. Fixed coupling intervals are by far the most common type.

Variable PVC coupling intervals involve changing distances between the PVC and the preceding sinus beat. When this happens, it strongly suggests that an independent automatic ectopic pacemaker is present. Variable coupling intervals occur only in a few cases of PVCs, but they have a greater chance of striking during the vulnerable T wave than does a PVC with fixed coupling intervals.

R-on-T Phenomenon

PVCs can trigger serious rhythm disturbances such as ventricular tachycardia and fibrillation, if they occur during a T wave. The **vulnerable period** corresponds to the downslope of the T wave. It is referred to as a vulnerable period because an ectopic beat occurring precisely during this point can result in an unstable tachydysrhythmia (Figure 16–10) and is referred to as a "R-on-T" phenomenon (Figure 16–11).

Very early PVCs or prolonged QT intervals increase the chance of developing ventricular fibrillation because they favor an R on T event. During the vulnerable period some cardiac fibers are repolarized, while others have only partially recovered. A PVC occurring at this point could destabilize the cardiac rhythm. During other parts of the cardiac cycle, PVCs can not lead to an R-on-T because the heart is refractory, or unresponsive, to further stimulation. This phase of ventricular unresponsiveness is termed the **refractory period**.

Causes of PVCs

PVCs are the most common cardiac dysrhythmias and are associated with many benign and pathologic conditions. While PVCs are uncommon in children, they fre-

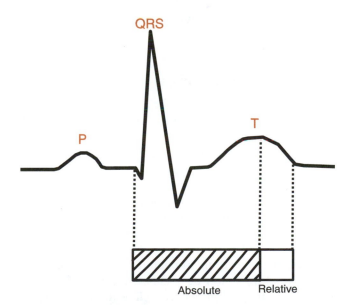

Figure 16–10 Refractory period. The ventricles are completely unresponsive during the absolute refractory phase. A stronger than normal impulse may cause another beat during the relative refractory period. The vulnerable period corresponds to the downslope of the T wave. PVCs that occur during the relative refractory period may cause a ventricular tachydysrhythmia.

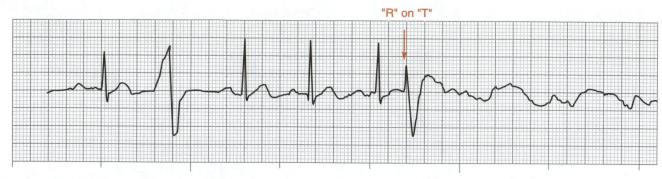

"R" on "T"

Figure 16–11 Vulnerable period. The second PVC strikes precisely during the downstroke of the T wave, causing ventricular fibrillation. The cardiac rhythm is vulnerable to electrical instability during the relative refractory period.

quently occur in healthy adults as well as in patients with structural heart disease. PVCs do not indicate the presence of organic disease, yet PVCs are found in greater frequency in patients with atherosclerotic heart disease and are more common during an MI.

An ischemic myocardium is sensitive to the effects of catecholamines, hypokalemia, hypomagnesemia, and acidosis. PVCs occur in a wide variety of settings: in congestive heart failure (CHF), stroke, myocardial ischemia, myocardial contusion, but also in non-cardiac conditions, such as drug toxicity, stimulant use including caffeine, nicotine, and cocaine, and hypoxia and acidosis (Table 16–2). Even antidysrhythmia medication can paradoxically cause dysrhythmias due to a **"proarrhythmia" effect**.

Clinical Significance of PVCs

The significance of PVCs varies greatly, depending on the patient's clinical condition and the frequency of PVCs. For instance, frequent PVCs occurring during an acute myocardial infarction—especially if they form couplets of successive ventricular beats—signify an irritable myocardium and can be a warning that more serious dysrhythmias may follow. However, sustained ventricular dysrhythmias can occur even in the absence of PVCs. PVCs occur in virtually all healthy adults and in such cases are of no clinical concern.

Frequent PVCs occurring in patients who have survived a myocardial infarction do increase the risk of sudden cardiac death. Unfortunately, clinical studies have shown that suppressing PVCs with chronic anti-arrhythmia medication does not produce improved survival. In fact, long-term anti-arrhythmic medication was associated with a significantly higher death rate that resulted from a paradoxical increase in dysrhythmia formation.

Table 16–2 Causes of PVCs

- **Congestive Heart Failure**

- **Myocardial Ischemia, Injury, Infarction and Occasionally Trauma (myocardial contusion)**

- **Drug Toxicity (theophylline, digoxin, and amphetamines)**

- **Valvular Heart Disease**

- **Hypoxia**

- **Acidosis**

- **Electrolyte Disorders (hypokalemia [low serum potassium], hypocalcemia [low serum calcium])**

- **Anti-dysrhythmic Drugs can paradoxically increase formation**

Clinical Note *A paradoxical side effect of anti-dysrhythmia treatment is the potential to worsen the dysrhythmias, known as a proarrhythmia effect. When a patient develops increased dysrhythmias while taking an anti-dysrhythmic agent, a proarrhythmia effect should be considered.*

Management of patients having recurrent ventricular tachycardia as well as survivors of ventricular fibrillation-associated cardiac arrest have had the best treatment results with automatic **implantable cardioverter-defibrillator (ICD) devices**, which deliver a series of shocks to terminate a sustained ventricular dysrhythmia. Despite the relatively high initial insertion cost, ICD devices have been remarkably effective without incurring a medication's side effects.

Emergency Treatment of PVCs

It is important to note that most PVCs do *not* require treatment, especially in the absence of cardiac disease. Initial treatment should be aimed at correcting any precipitating cause, such as hypoxia, ischemia, electrolyte disorders, or acidosis (Table 16–3). In cases of acute myocardial infarction, PVCs that occur with sinus tachycardia indicate increased autonomic sympathetic stimulation and intravenous beta-adrenergic blockers are usually successful.

The ACLS therapy guidelines concerning PVCs in the setting of an MI have changed dramatically during the last fifteen years as the understanding of the significance of ectopic beats has evolved. *Aggressive therapy is no longer used to suppress PVCs during an MI.* Our changing understanding and approach to PVCs is reflected in a more reasoned approach:

■ *Acute MI with frequent PVCs.* Initial treatment of PVCs involves correcting underlying conditions that may precipitate PVCs. Correcting electrolyte disorders, especially low potassium and magnesium serum levels, preventing ischemia by avoiding hypoxia or hypotension, and avoiding adrenergic stimulation by administering beta-adrenergic blocking agents are often effective (Table 16–3).

> *Clinical Note* PVCs that occur during an acute MI indicate the need to treat the ischemia/injury/infarction with oxygen, morphine, nitroglycerin and thrombolytic agents. Suppressing PVCs with lidocaine is simply treating the symptoms and not the underlying myocardial irritability. Routine suppression of PVCs has been abandoned because it did not work and was complicated by a high incidence of side effects, including asystole.

■ *"Malignant" PVCs.* Some PVC types cause more clinical concern, including those that strike during the T waves or occur in couplets of successive beats. In such cases, during the first hours after an MI, a short course of lidocaine therapy—less than

24 hours—may sometimes be indicated. Generally, the conditions that give rise to PVCs are remedied rather than suppressing the PVCs directly.

■ *Successive PVCs.* Successive PVCs that result in nonsustained—less than 30 second—episodes of ventricular tachycardia usually subside *without therapy.* During the early stages of an MI, especially during the prehospital phase, antidysrhythmic therapy may be implemented but it is unclear if this has positive survival benefits.

Table 16–3 Treatment for PVC's

■ **No antidysrhythmic agents for most cases**

■ **Correct underlying condition:**

  ■ **Ischemia**

  ■ **Acidosis**

  ■ **Electrolyte imbalance, especially low serum magnesium & potassium**

  ■ **Beta-adrenergic blockers if due to high sympathetic tone**

> *Clinical Note* Appropriate PVC treatment must be based on the likelihood that PVCs will cause deterioration in a patient's condition, along with the probability that they will lead to serious ventricular dysrhythmias. Aside from sustained ventricular tachycardia episodes and in patients who have been resuscitated from a ventricular fibrillation/tachycardic arrest, PVCs rarely require treatment.

CONSECUTIVELY OCCURRING PVCS ("MULTIPLES" OR "SALVOS")

Consecutively occurring PVCs increase the likelihood that a sustained ventricular tachycardia will develop. The following terms are applied to consecutively occurring ectopic ventricular complexes:

■ A **PVC couplet** is two PVCs occurring in a row. Consecutive PVCs predispose to further episodes of successive PVCs (Figure 16–12).

■ A **PVC triplet** refers to three consecutive ventricular beats. By definition, ventricular tachycardia exists when three or more consecutive PVCs occur at a rate greater than 100/minute (Figure 16–13).

■ **PVC "salvo"** is a term that describes a burst of nonsustained successive PVCs but it does not refer to a specific number of PVCs. Nonsustained dysrhythmias are episodes lasting less than 30 seconds.

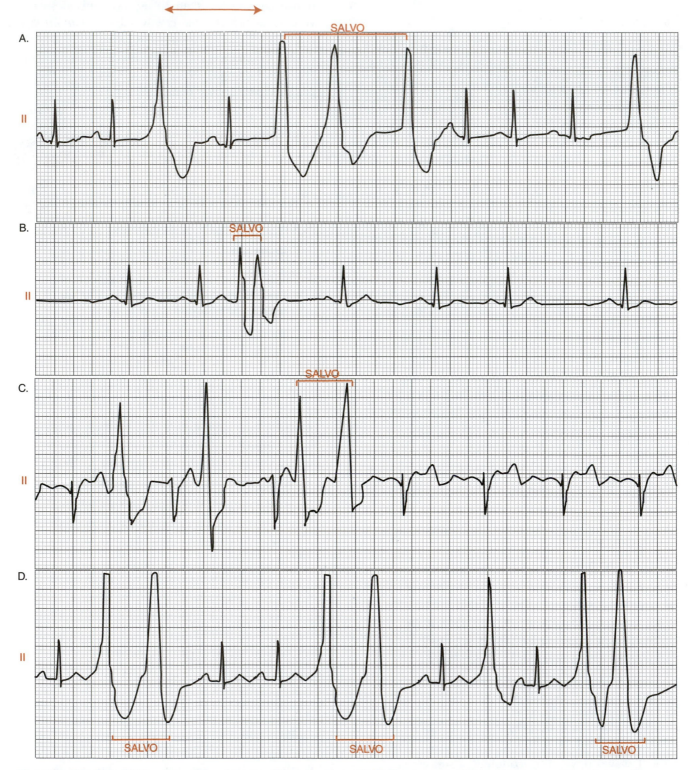

Figure 16-12 PVC salvos. Consecutive ("back-to-back") PVCs occur without intervening sinus beats. Tracing A shows three consecutive PVCs, which meet the minimum criteria for nonsustained episode of ventricular tachycardia. Tracings B, C, and D show two-beat salvos of consecutive PVCs. Tracing D shows three salvos.

INTERPOLATED PVCS

Some ectopic beats occur so early during the R-R interval that there is time for the heart to repolarize before the next expected sinus beat arises. As a result, interpolated PVCs do not have compensatory pauses.

Interpolated PVCs are "squeezed" between two regular R waves without disrupting the underlying sinus rhythm (Figure 16–14). Interpolated PVCs are uncommon and have no clinical significance apart from other PVC types.

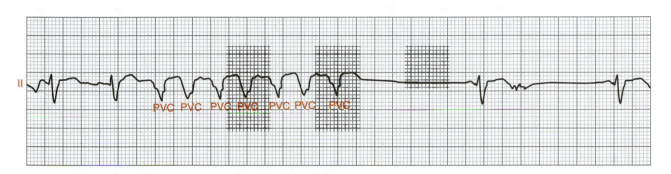

Figure 16-13 Nonsustained ventricular tachycardia. The 3rd through 9th beats are successive and rapid PVCs.

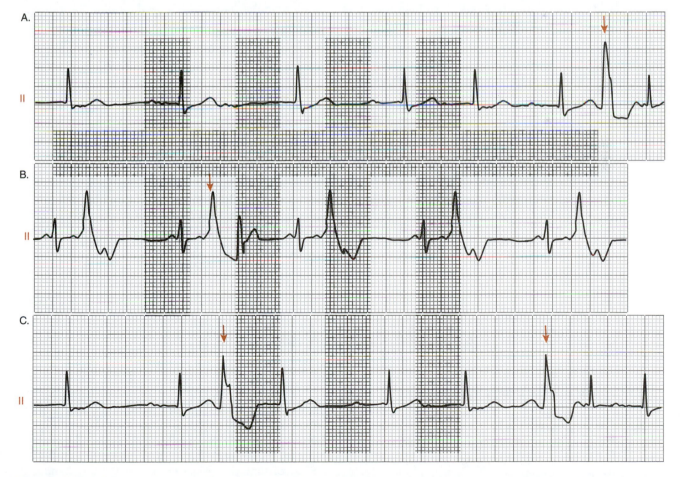

Figure 16-14 Interpolated PVCs, which are indicated by arrows, occur between sinus beats without causing a compensatory pause. Interpolated PVCs without compensatory pauses are much rarer than PVCs with compensatory pauses. Because these very early PVCs do not disrupt the sinus rhythm, they occur early enough to be squeezed between regularly occurring sinus beats. In strip B the second PVC is interpolated.

FUSION BEATS

Fusion beats share components of sinus beats, as well as, ectopic beats (Figure 16–15). Fusion beats are caused when two pacemakers simultaneously discharge. Figure 16–15 shows how a sinus impulse and a ventricular impulse can occur nearly at the same time and results in a "composite" beat that looks like a cross between a PVC and sinus beat. As a result, fusion beats do not look quite as normal as a sinus beat nor as bizarre as a PVC. Fusion beats are somewhat widened but still resemble a sinus beat.

REGULARLY OCCURRING PVC PATTERNS

When PVCs occur in a set pattern in relationship to normal beats, the following terms are applied based on the number of normal beats-to-PVCs.:

■ **Ventricular bigeminy**: every other beat is a PVC (Figure 16–16).

■ **Ventricular trigeminy:** a PVC occurs after two normal beats (Figure 16–17). Every third beat is a PVC.

Because the patterns have fixed PVC coupling intervals, there is no danger that they will cause an R-on-T episode. Bigeminy and trigeminy form interesting ECG patterns but have no clinical significance apart from other PVCs.

> *ECG Interpretation Tip* *PVCs can be mimicked by PACs that are aberrantly conducted. Figure 16–18 illustrates some examples. Distorted PACs are caused when atrial beats encounter a partially refractory ventricular conduction system. P′ waves are usually present.*

Table 16–4 Treatment for Escape Ventricular Complexes/Rhythms

■ **No therapy needed unless symptomatic**

■ **For symptomatic cases- accelerate the sinus rhythm with:**

  ■ **Atrophine IV bolus**

  ■ **External Pacing,or**

  ■ **Epinephrine infusion**

ESCAPE VENTRICULAR BEATS

PVCs and **escape ventricular beats** have a similar appearance because they both arise within the ventricles; however, they differ in major ways regarding their clinical significance and treatment (Table 16–4). When escape ventricular beats arise during bradycardic rhythms, they provide additional cardiac output and stimulate the slow heart. Escape pacemakers originating in the His-Purkinje fibers resemble PVCs because they both have wide, bizarre shapes, but unlike PVCs, they occur *during the later portion of the R-R cycle* (Figure 16–19). If the patient is symptomatic and having escape beats due to a slow rhythm, treatment should be directed at speeding the sinus rate. Escape ventricular beats spontaneously subside when they no longer are needed to stimulate the heart.

> *Clinical Note* *Escape ectopic beats should not be suppressed because the patient may be left with only a very slow rhythm. If the patient relies on a slow escape idioventricular rhythm because the sinus node and AV junctional failed to pace, lidocaine administration could cause asystole.*

VENTRICULAR TACHYCARDIA (VT)

Ventricular tachycardia is defined as three or more successive PVCs occurring at a rate greater than 100 /minute (Figures 16–20 & 16–21). The ventricular rate of this serious tachydysrhythmia usually occurs between 150 and 220/minute, although it can range from just over 100/minute to as fast as 250/minute. Ventricular tachycardia has a regular rhythm that resembles a series of rapidly occurring PVCs that have been strung together. Ventricular tachycardia can be episodic, lasting for several seconds or for several beats, to several hours. In its most common form, all the QRS complexes appear the same, and is termed **monomorphic** VT. (A much less common type is the **polymorphic** form in which the QRS complexes change shape and will be discussed in the next chapter.)

Ventricular tachycardia occurs when myocardial irritability causes increased automaticity of an ectopic focus, or when a reentry circuit develops. Ventricular tachycardia is a serious dysrhythmia that produces significant signs and symptoms, such as hypotension and altered mental states. While some patients are able to tolerate ventricular tachycardia reasonably well for a period of time, in others it can be life-threatening. VT is a highly unstable dysrhythmia that can precipitate acute heart failure and even deteriorate into ventricular fibrillation. For these reasons it is important to aggressively treat ventricular tachycardia.

Clinical Note *Ventricular tachycardia is much more serious than supraventricular tachycardias despite the faster ventricular rates seen with SVTs. Ventricular tachycardia causes an unstable patient condition more commonly than SVT because ventricular depolarization is abnormal in VT and preserved in SVT.*

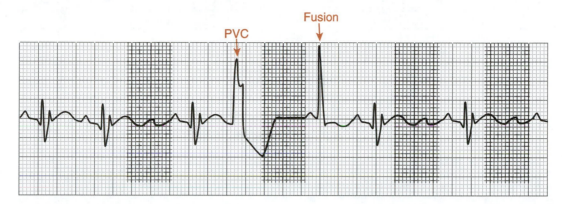

Figure 16–15 The fifth complex is a fusion beat that is narrower than a typical PVC, yet it also appears different from sinus beats: it is taller and also has a T wave that is oriented opposite to the QRS complex. Because the ectopic beat and the sinus beat develop almost simultaneously, the QRS complex will be a distorted ("fusion") composite of both impulses.

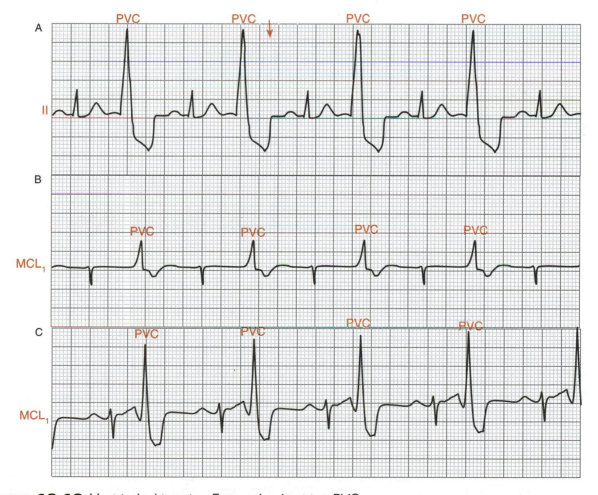

Figure 16-16 Ventricular bigeminy. Every other beat is a PVC.

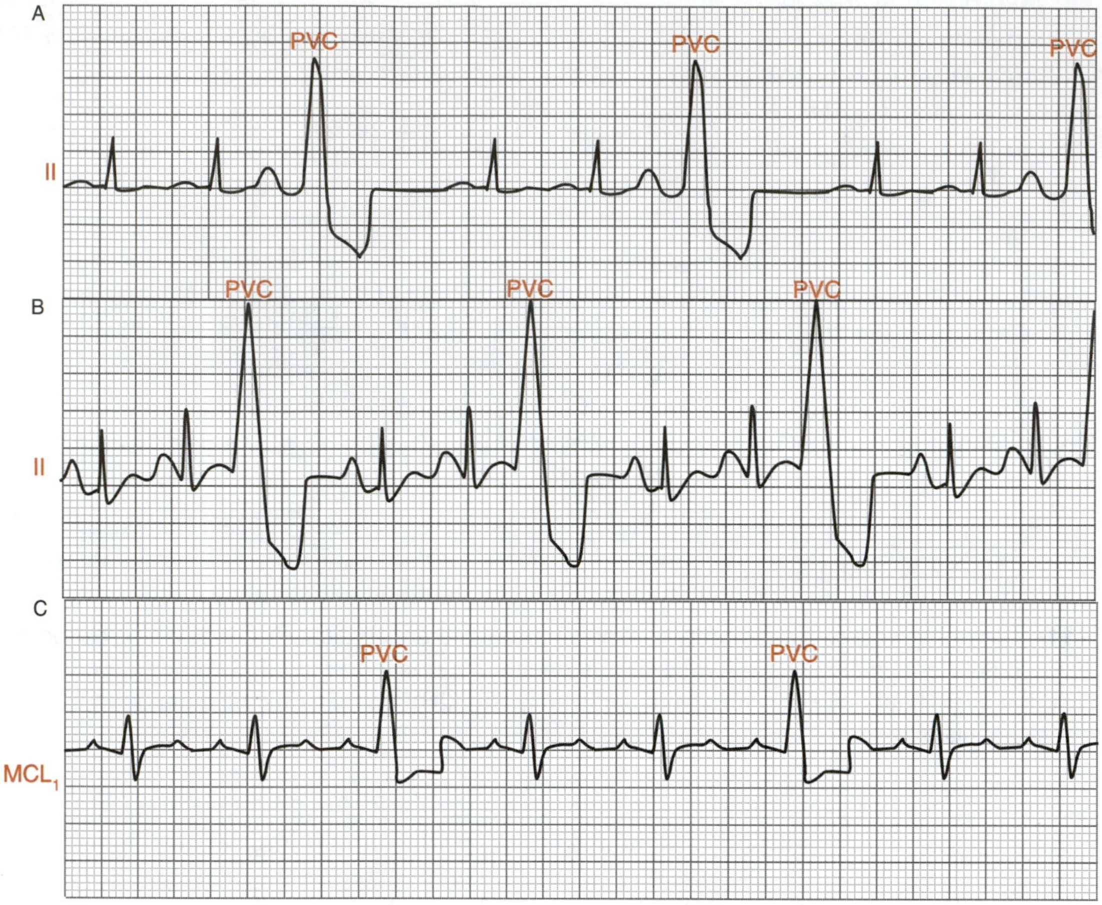

Figure 16–17 Ventricular trigeminy. Every third beat is a PVC. The pattern of two sinus beats followed by a PVC (beats number 3, 6, 9, and 12) repeats itself.

VT Characteristics

Ventricular tachycardia has the following ECG characteristics (Table 16–5):

- *AV dissociation.* AV dissociation is present because sinus node activity continues causing atrial depolarization. P waves are often hard to detect because they are scattered among the distorted QRS-T complexes.

- *AV conduction/"capture" beats.* Conduction from the atria and ventricles occasionally occurs during VT. The capture beat has a normal, or almost normal, QRS complex. The term "capture" signifies that the ventricles were stimulated by a sinus beat for one or a few beats while the rest of the QRS complexes are wide and distorted. **Capture beats** are seldom seen because the rapid ventricular rate causes long refractory periods.

Table 16–5 Key ECG Features of Monomorphic VT	
■ **Atrial:**	Occasional P waves are seen due to AV dissociation
■ **Ventricular:**	Wide and distorted QRS complexes
■ **AV Relationship:**	Dissociation
■ **Other Findings:**	
■ Resembles a series of rapidly occurring PVCs usually regular but may be slightly irregular	

- *VT occurring during thrombolytic therapy.* VT that occurs during coronary reperfusion from throm-

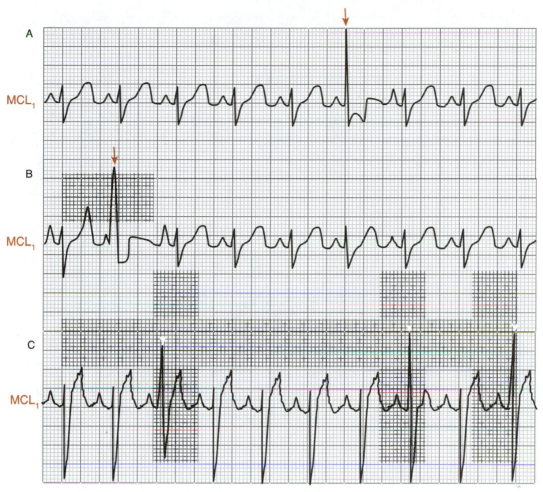

Figure 16-18 PACs with aberration. The PACs, which are indicated by arrows, occur early and encounter a conduction system that is relatively refractory from the previous sinus beat, causing the premature atrial beats to be abnormally conducted.

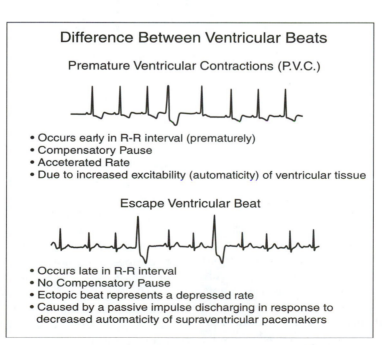

Difference Between Ventricular Beats

Premature Ventricular Contractions (P.V.C.)

- Occurs early in R-R interval (prematurely)
- Compensatory Pause
- Acceterated Rate
- Due to increased excitability (automaticity) of ventricular tissue

Escape Ventricular Beat

- Occurs late in R-R interval
- No Compensatory Pause
- Ectopic beat represents a depressed rate
- Caused by a passive impulse discharging in response to decreased automaticity of supraventricular pacemakers

Figure 16-19

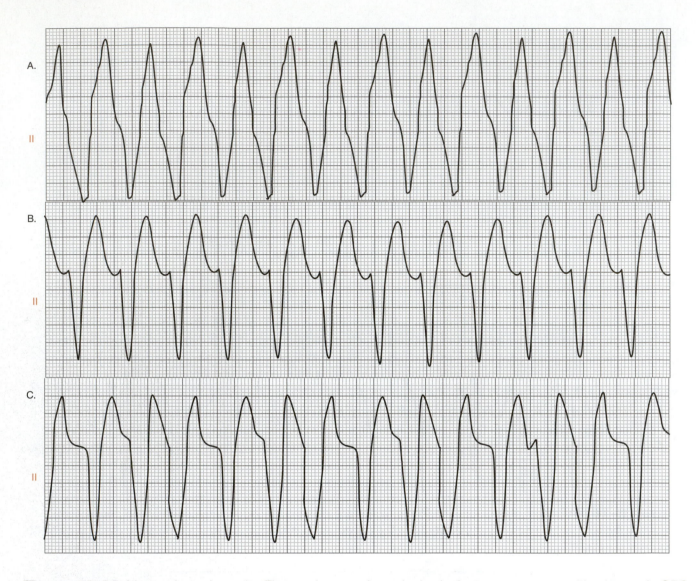

Figure 16–20 Ventricular tachycardia. The rapid ventricular tachydysrhythmias are recognized by their wide QRS complexes and generally regular rhythm. Every example has a rate in the range of 140/minute.

bolytic therapy is easily treated and is a favorable sign that injured myocardium is being salvaged. VT developing during treatment of an MI typically lasts for 10 to 20 seconds and subsides spontaneously.

Sustained Versus Nonsustained VT

Ventricular tachycardia can be divided into two types based on how long the dysrhythmia persists. **Sustained VT** exists for *at least 30 seconds*. Sustained VT usually occurs in the setting of coronary artery disease when a PVC and occurs during the relative refractory period establishes a reentry mechanism in ischemic tissue. Less commonly, a rapid firing ectopic pacemaker is the cause. Sustained VT often produces hypotension, ischemic chest pain, cardiovascular collapse, or ventricular fibrillation. Sustained VT in the setting of an MI requires aggressive antidysrhythmia medication and/or electrical countershock.

Non-sustained VT consists of short episodes of VT lasting for *less than 30 seconds*. Because the episodes are brief—most last for fewer than ten beats—they cause minimal hemodynamic effects and typically subside without therapy. However, during an MI, especially during the prehospital phase where the risk for sudden cardiac death is highest, antidysrhythmic therapy is usually instituted. Current evidence shows that stable patients who are in an intensive care monitored setting, and who experience short episodes of VT that spontaneously subside, do *not* require antidysrhythmia medication.

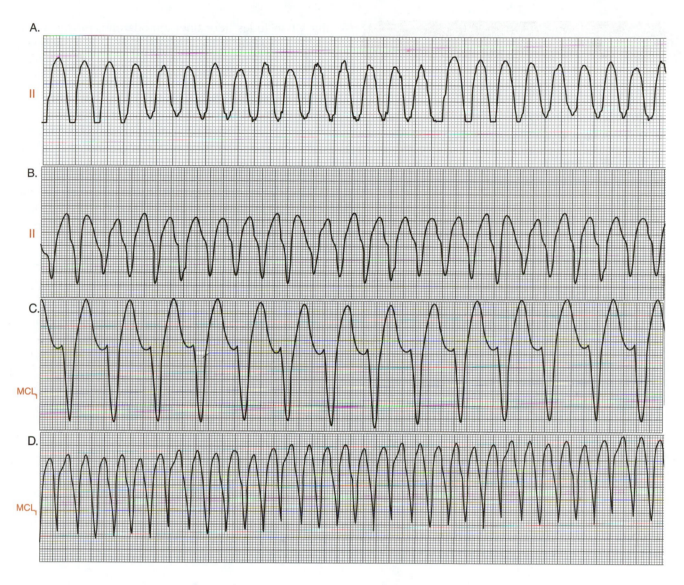

Figure 16–21 Ventricular tachycardia. These wide and bizarrely shaped QRS complexes resemble a series of rapid PVCs. VT is a serious dysrhythmia that has the potential to deteriorate into ventricular fibrillation.

Causes of VT

Cases of adult VT are usually due to ischemic or organic heart disease. In patients who are recovering from an MI, myocardial scar tissue may be the location for the VT development. Conditions that are associated with VT development are listed in Table 16–6. When ventricular tachycardia occurs in children, the usual cause is cardiomyopathy, congenital cardiac disease, myocarditis, or electrolyte disorder, such as, low serum potassium or magnesium levels.

Clinical Significance of VT

Some patients tolerate short episodes of VT reasonably well, while most are symptomatic and experience

hypotension, shock, dizziness, chest pain and shortness of breath, or are on the verge of cardiac arrest. How a patient tolerates VT primarily depends on whether underlying heart disease is present.

Emergency Treatment of VT

VT without associated pulses, that is, for patients in cardiac arrest, is treated the same as ventricular fibrillation and is discussed in Chapter 17. Treatment generally depends on whether the patient is stable or unstable. Sustained VT in patients with *unstable hemodynamics* such as those with hypotension, ischemic chest discomfort, alteration of mental status, or pulmonary edema, the goal is immediate stabilization by using-

Table 16–6 Causes of Monomorphic VT

- **Myocardial Ischemia/ Infarction**
- **Ventricular Aneurysm**
- **Reperfusion Dysrhythmia** During Thrombolysis
- **Cardiomyopathy**
- **Prodysrhythmic Effects** of Anti-disrhythmic Drugs
- **Electrolyte Disorders:** hypokalemia and hypomagnesemia
- **Mechanical Irritation** from Misplaced Central Venous and Pulmonary Artery Catheters
- **Pediatric Cases: cardiomyopathy, myocarditis, hypokalemia**

electrical cardioversion. Monomorphic VT is treated with synchronized cardioversion beginning at 100 joules (watt/seconds).

Sustained VT in patients with *stable hemodynamics*

Table 16–7 Treatment of Monomorphic VT

STABLE CONDITION

Normal Cardiac Function (No CHF)

- **Procainamide (or Sotolol)**
- **Others acceptable:**
  - Amiodarone or Lidocaine (does below)
  - Option: Proceed Directly to Synchronized Electrical Cardioversion
- **Impaired Cardiac Function (CHF Present)**
  - Amiodarone 150mg IV over 10min. or
  - Lidocaine 0.5 to 0.75 mg/kg IV push;thenMisplaced Central Venous and Pulmonary
  - Synchronized electrical cardioversion

UNSTABLE CONDITION

- **Electrical synchronized cardioversion starting at 100J**

undergo a trial of medication before resorting to electrical cardioversion (Table 16–7). Medication for treat-

ing VT includes lidocaine, amiodarone, procainamide, and magnesium. If these medications are unsuccessful or if the patient's condition deteriorates, synchronized cardioversion should be used. Treatment includes:

- Lidocaine with an initial dose of 1-1.5 mg/kg followed by doses of 0.5–0.75 mg/kg every 5 to 10 minutes as needed up to a maximum of 3 mg/kg. (Maintenance infusion of 1–4 mg/minute is started after conversion.)

- Amiodarone with an initial loading dose of 150 mg over 20 minutes followed by a continuous infusion of 1 mg/minute for the intial six hours and then decreased to 0.5 mg/minute thereafter.

- Procainamide at an initial loading dose of 12–17 mg/kg over 20 to 30 minutes followed by a maintenance infusion of 1–4 mg/ minute.

Clinical Note *Current ACLS recommendations discourage the use of multiple antidysrhythmic drugs. If one drug is unsuccessful, the next treatment should be electrical cardioversion.*

Most patients with short runs of nonsustained VT will be asymptomatic and not require therapy. However, patients who are likely to deteriorate, such as those patients during the very early phase of their MI—especially those encountered by EMS—will benefit from treatment. Correcting underlying electrolyte disorders or ischemia is important in preventing the recurrence of VT.

Clinical Note *Patients who are in cardiac arrest and whose ECG shows ventricular tachycardia ("pulseless VT") are treated the same as if they were in ventricular fibrillation.*

Cases of unstable VT are best treated with electrical cardioversion.

A CLINICAL CHALLENGE: VT OR SVT WITH ABERRANT CONDUCTION?

The wide, bizarre-looking ECG rhythm of VT is sometimes mimicked when a supraventricular tachydysrhythmia follows an abnormal ventricular conduction route. Most cases of SVT have normal appearing QRS complexes with a QRS duration of less than 0.12 second. However, when a bundle branch block exists, or the conduction system becomes fatigued owing to the rapid rate, the QRS complexes of an SVT will be wide and distorted. Because it is not practical to distinguish between these two dysrhythmias during an emergency, it is safer to treat patients who have hemodynamic compromise, or those with a past MI, or when the QRS complex is wider than 0.14 second as if the wide QRS tachycardia is VT and electrically cardiovert the dysrhythmia. See Table 16–8 for a summary of treatment of stable, wide complex tachycardias.

Table 16–8 Treatment for Stable, Wide-complex Tachycardia

Establish a specific dysrhythmia interpretation if possible using 12-lead and clinical informaiton to place into 1 of 3 groups:

- **Confirmed stable VT: use stable VT algorithm**
- **Confirmed SVT: use narrow complex tachycardia algorithm**
- **Wide Complex uncertain type**

• normal cardiac function (no CHF or low ejection fraction)

  • electrical cardioversion or

  • Procainimide or Amiodarone

• impaired cardiac function (CHF or low ejection <40%)

  • electrical cardioversion or Amiodarone

Clinical Note *Deciding whether a wide complex tachydysrhythmia is VT or PSVT with aberration based on how well the patient appears is often incorrect and can be dangerous. Some patients with SVT and aberrant conduction can be unstable, while some experiencing VT can tolerate the dysrhythmia and appear deceptively well for a period of time but can suddenly deteriorate.*

Clinical Note *Administering a calcium channel blocking agent, such as verapamil to a patient with VT in the mistaken belief that*

the dysrhythmia is SVT with aberration can cause profound hypotension, cardiovascular collapse, and even death.

Let's Review

1. Ventricular dysrhythmias are the leading types of unstable dysrhythmias and number one cause of sudden cardiac death.

2. Ventricular dysrhythmias can be caused by increased automaticity or a reentry mechanism.

3. Ventricular dysrhythmias have wide, distorted QRS complexes that lack P waves. The ST-T wave components occur in a direction opposite to the distorted QRS complexes.

4. A PVC is an early ectopic depolarization that happens before the next expected sinus beat.

5. PVCs are one of the most common dysrhythmias and are associated with cardiac as well as non-cardiac conditions.

6. Unifocal (uniformed) PVCs have identical QRS shapes. Multifocal (multiformed) PVCs have different QRS shapes.

7. PVCs occurring during the downstroke of the T wave of a sinus beat can precipitate ventricular fibrillation or ventricular tachycardia (R-on-T phenomenon).

8. A PVC couplet occurs when there are two consecutive PVCs. A PVC triplet occurs when three PVCs occur in a row. Three successive PVCs at a rate over 100/minute is defined as ventricular tachycardia.

9. In ventricular bigeminy a PVC follows every other sinus beat. In ventricular trigeminy a PVC follows every two sinus beats.

10. PVCs are best treated by correcting the underlying conditions that precipitate their development, such as electrolyte disorders, hypoxia, acidosis, and high adrenergic tone.

11. Escape ventricular complexes are *not* PVCs. Unlike PVCs, which are early ventricular beats that disrupt normal sinus activity, late occurring escape ventricular complexes develop when there is a pause in sinus activity or the ventricles are not activated.

12. Escape ventricular rhythms occur via a passive mechanism when pacemakers fail.

13. Lidocaine therapy should not be used to treat escape ventricular beats because back-up pacemakers are helpful in the event of a very slow rate or pauses in cardiac activity.

14. VT occurs during organic heart disease and typically produces serious symptoms or hypotension.

15. Nonsustained VT lasts for less than 30 seconds and usually spontaneously subsides. Nonsustained VT does not adversely affect the patient.

16. Sustained VT lasts for at least 30 seconds and requires aggressive therapy. Sustained VT can result in cardiovascular collapse and cardiac arrest.

Glossary

Capture beat Narrow, normal appearing QRS complex occuring during ventricular tachycardia.

Coupling interval Distance between an early beat (PVC) and the sinus beat that precedes it.

Escape ventricular beats Ventricular escape beats that occur when the sinus and AV junction fails to initiate a cardiac cycle.

Fixed PVC coupling intervals Constant distance from the PVC to the previous sinus T waves, indicating a reentry mechanism.

Fusion beat Complex that shares the components of a sinus beat as well an ectopic beat.

ICD devices Automatic implantable cardioverter defibrillator (ICD) that is surgically implanted and delivers an electrical shock to terminate a sustained serious ventricular dysrhythmia.

Interpolated PVC PVC occuring between two sinus beats without disrupting the sinus rhythm.

Monomorphic VT Common form of ventricular tachycardia in which all of the QRS complexes have the same appearance.

Multifocal/Multiformed PVCs PVCs with varying QRS shapes.

Nonsustained VT Ventricular tachycardia consisting of short episodes lasting less than 30 seconds.

Polymorphic VT Unusual form of ventricular tachycardia in which the QRS complexes change shape.

Premature ventricular complex (PVC) An early, extra ventricular depolarization that arises below the bundle of His and disrupts sinus activity.

Proarrhythmia effect Paradoxical effect whereby anti-arrhythmic medication results in increased disrhythmias.

PVC couplets Two consecutive PVCs.

PVC salvos Consecutively occuring PVCs.

R-on-T phenomenon Development of an unstable ventricular tachydysrhythmia when a PVC occurs during the vulnerable period.

Refractory peroid Ventricular tissue is unresponsive to electrical stimuli (PVC) during depolarization and repolarization.

Sustained VT Ventricular tachycardia lasting at least 30 seconds.

Unifocal/Uniformed PVC PVCs having the same QRS shape.

Variable PVC coupling interval Changing distances from the PVC to the previous sinus T waves, indicating an independent pacemaker mechanism.

Ventricular bigeminy Regularly occuring PVC rhythm; every other sinus beat is a PVC

Ventricular tachycardia (VT) Dysrhythmia characterized by three or more successive PVCs occurring at a rate greater than 100/minute.

Ventricular trigeminy Regularly occuring PVC rhythm; every two sinus beats are followed by a PVC.

Vulnerable period Portion of the cardiac cycle prone to developing unstable ventricular dysrhythmias should a premature beat occur during the downslope of the T wave.

Ventricular Dysrhythmias—Part Two

LEARNING OBJECTIVES

Upon completion of this chapter, the reader should be able to:

- *Define key terms*

- *List the ECG characteristics of polymorphic ventricular tachycardia, which is also known as Torsade de Pointes (TdP).*

- *Contrast polymorphic ventricular tachycardia to monomorphic VT in terms of causes and treatment.*

- *Describe the clinical significance of polymorphic ventricular tachycardia (Torsade de Pointes).*

- *List the ECG characteristics of an idioventricular escape rhythm.*

- *List two reasons why idioventricular escape rhythms should not be suppressed with antidysrhythmic medication.*

- *Describe the clinical significance of an idioventricular escape rhythm.*

- *Discuss their clinical significance of reperfusion-associated ventricular dysrhythmias.*

- *List the ECG characteristics of an accelerated idioventricular rhythm (AIVR).*

- *Define the clinical significance of an accelerated idioventricular rhythm.*

- *State the usual rates at which the pacemaker discharges in the following dysrhythmias: (a) escape idioventricular rhythms; (b) accelerated idioventricular rhythms; and (c) ventricular tachycardia.*

- *List the ECG characteristics of ventricular fibrillation (VF).*

- *Contrast the ECG findings between fine ventricular fibrillation and coarse VF.*

- *List two differences between primary ventricular fibrillation and secondary VF.*

- *Contrast the relative incidence of ventricular fibrillation in primary ventricular fibrillation for adults and children.*

- *List the ECG characteristics of asystole.*

- *Describe the clinical significance and treatment of asystole.*

- *Explain the terms pulseless electrical activity (PEA) and electro-mechanical dissociation (EMD).*

- *Describe the clinical significance and treatment of PEA.*

CHAPTER OVERVIEW

Polymorphic VT is the less common form of ventricular tachycardia that has different causes, ECG appearance, and treatment than monomorphic VT. QT interval prolongation is the major cause of polymorphic VT, which is also known as Torsade de Pointes. Ventricular escape rhythms develop due to failure of higher pacemakers and rescues the heart from asystole. Slow, agonal ventricular rhythms are difficult to treat. The most common ECG rhythm causing sudden cardiac death is ventricular fibrillation.

TORSADE DE POINTES (TDP)

Torsade de Pointes (also known as **polymorphic VT**) is distinctly different and much less common form of ventricular tachycardia than monomorphic VT. The size and shape of QRS complexes rhythmically change in Torsade de Pointes (Figures 17–1 and 17–2). The colorful name "Torsade de Pointes" derives from French meaning "twisting of points." In the monomorphic form of VT that was discussed in Chapter 16, each ventricular complex had the same shape and size. In contrast, during Torsade de Pointes the QRS complexes rhythmically alternate from a positive to negative deflection—as if swinging above and below the ECG baseline (Figures 17–3 and 17–4). TdP is a very serious dysrhythmia because if not treated appropriately, it can suddenly degenerate into ventricular fibrillation and lead to sudden cardiac death. Being able to distinguish Torsade de Pointes from monomorphic VT is crucial because they are caused by different conditions and have different treatments (Figures 17–3 17-5, and 17–6; Table 17–1).

> **ECG Interpretation Tip** *The hallmark appearance of Torsade de Pointes or polymorphic VT shows waxing and waning sizse of the ventricular complexes that resemble the shape of bow-ties as the QRS complexes alternate from a positive to negative deflection.*

Causes of Torsade de Pointes

Torsade de Pointes develops where ventricular repolarization is delayed and is manifest by QT interval prolongation. A prolonged QT interval corresponds to a prolonged refractory period, which involves a disordered repolarization phase and increases the chance of a reentry dysrhythmia forming. Two leading causes of Torsade de Pointes are electrolyte disorders and medications. Certain antidysrhythmic drugs, such as pro-

cainamide, disopyramide, quinidine, and tricyclic antidepressants, along with many other drug combinations can precipitate TdP by prologing the refractory period. Commonly associated conditions resulting in TdP are listed in Table 17–2.

Women may be more likely to develop polymorphic VT while taking antidysrhythmic medication due to unclear reasons. Less common causes of QT interval prolongation include significantly bradycardic rhythms, electrolyte disorders, congenital QT prolongation, and the interaction between drugs that delay repolarization. Most ECG machines automatically calculate corrected QT intervals and flag abnormal values. *A clinically useful rule is: For heart rates between 60 and 100/minute, a QT interval beyond 0.44 second is prolonged.*

Clinical Significance of Torsade de Pointes

TdP is a special form of VT that can be caused by diverse conditions, some major ones are due to an acquired non-cardiac form. TdP is a major ventricular dysrhythmia that produces severe signs and symptoms. Drug interactions, electrolyte disorders, and toxic ingestion are common causes. The diverse causes all the QT interval, which reflects a delayed ventricular repolariza-

Table 17-1 Key ECG Features of Torsade de Pointes	
■ **Atrial:**	Absent
■ **Ventricular:**	Waxing and waning pattern; QRS complexes appear to twist around the ECG baseline from a positive to negative direction.
■ **AV Relationship:**	Absent
■ **Other Findings:**	Direction of ventricular complexes varies in cycles
	Associated with prolonged QT intervals

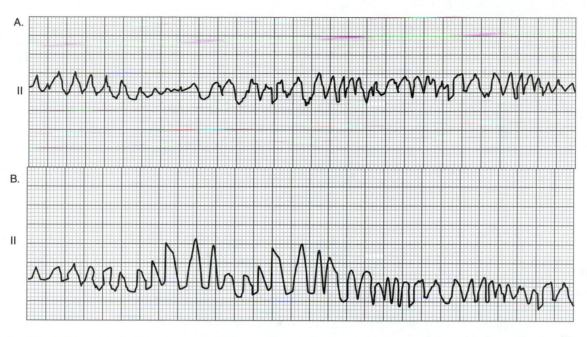

Figure 17-1 Torsade de Pointes. The QRS complexes vary rhythmically in shape, size, and direction.

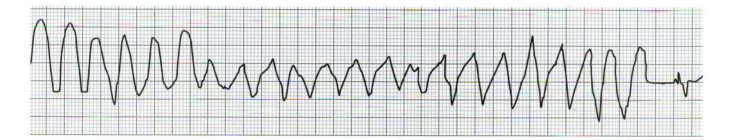

Figure 17-2 Torsade de Pointes variation of VT converting spontaneously to sinus rhythm.

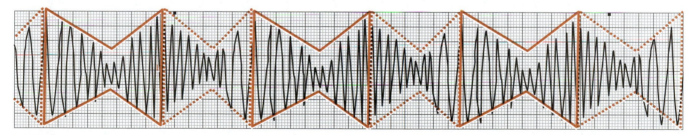

Figure 17-3 "Bow-tie" appearance of Torsade de Pointes analogy can be appreciated in this illustration.

tion phase. Patients with TdP are critically ill and at risk for sudden death owing to deterioration into ventricular fibrillation.

Emergency Treatment of Torsade de Pointes

The therapeutic goal for treating Torsade de Pointes is to shorten the QT interval, which reduces the refractory period. Because the causes of polymorphic VT are diverse, therapy needs to be tailored to the specific problem:

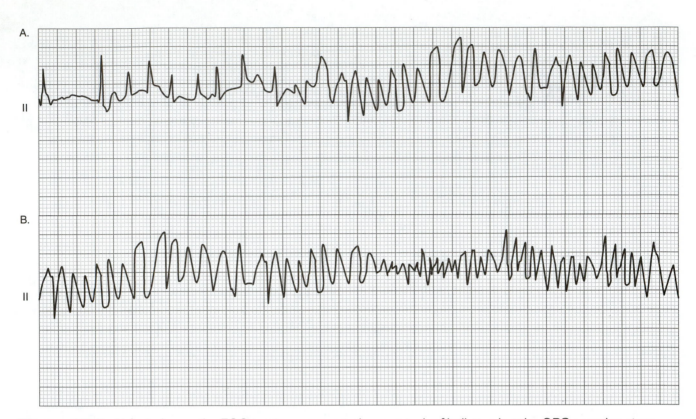

Figure 17-4 At first glance, the ECG tracing appears to be ventricular fibrillation but the QRS complex sizes rhythmically increase and decrease, revealing that this is Torsade de Pointes.

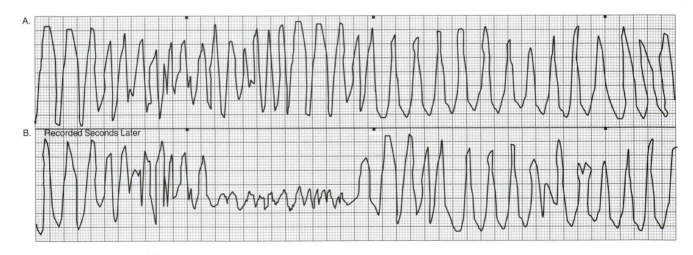

Figure 17-5 The size and direction of QRS complexes show a cyclic change between a positive to a negative direction and back again. Tracing A shows classical Torsade de Pointes which quickly deteriorates (tracing B) into ventricular fibrillation.

- Unstable cases should be electrically cardioverted using an unsyncronized mode

- Magnesium is the drug of choice, given 2 grams intravenously over 3 to 5 minutes.

- Overdrive pacing with an external pacemaker at a rate of 180 beats per minute suppresses TdP.

- Calcium chloride 500 mg to 1 gram given intravenously over 3 to 5 minutes.

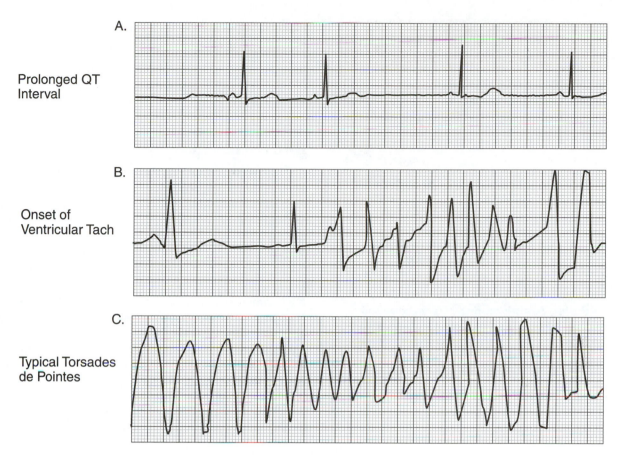

Figure 17-6 (A) A markedly prolonged QT interval developed due to quinidine therapy. (B) A PVC occurs during the T wave, and Torsade de Pointes VT results. (C) The typical alternating pattern of Torsade de Pointes is present. (Used with permission from Waugh RA, Ramo BW, Wagner GS. Cardiac Arrhythmias: A Practical Guide for the Clinician. Philadelphia: FA Davis Co; 1994: 278.)

Table 17-2 Treatment for Polymorphic VT (Torsade de Pointes)

UNSTABLE CASE: Unsynchronized electrical cardioversion

STABLE CASE: Normal baseline QTc interval
- Treat Ischemia
- Correct electrolyte abnormalities
- Beta blockers or Lidocaine or
- Amiodarone or Procainamide (or Sotalol)
- May proceed directly to synchronized cardioversion without medication

■ **Prolonged Baseline QTc interval**

Normal cardiac function (No CHF /low ejection fraction)
- Treat Ischemia
- Correct electrolyte abnormalities
- Magnesium or overdrive cardiac pacing
- Isopoterenol, or Phenytoin, or Lidocaine

Impaired cardiac function (CHF or low ejection fraction)
- Amiodarone 150 mg IV over 10 min or Lidocaine 0.5 mg/kg IV push, then
- Synchronized electrical cardioversion (100J, 200J, 300J, 360 J

■ Sodium bicarbonate 44 to 88 mEq given in a bolus administration to alkalinize the blood has been very effective in cases of tricyclic antidepressant medication overdosage. This dose can be followed by a constant infusion by adding 1 to 2 ampules of bicarbonate to a liter of normal saline. Fortunately, newer antidepressants have replaced tricyclics and do not cause TdD.

■ For hypokalemia, controlled replenishment using a potassium infusion is needed.

Table 17–3 summarizes the treatment of TdP.

Clinical Note Polymorphic VT is usually an acquired problem caused by drug and electrolyte abnormalities. Since electrolyte disorders are common in patients receiving hemodialysis, taking diuretics, or recovering from surgery, in emergency situations repleting magnesium, calcium, and potassium should be considered.

Table 17-3 Causes of Torsade de Pointes

- **Electrolyte Disorders** (hypomagnesemia, hypocalcemia, and hypokalemia)

- **Congenital QT Prolongation and Familial QT Prolongation**

- **Acute MI**

- **Tricyclic Antidepressant and Phenothiazine (Psychotropic) Toxicity**

- **Subarachnoid Hemorrhage**

- **Proarrhythmia Effect of Antidysrhythmics** (Class IA drugs: amiodarone, procainamide, disopyramide, quinidine; Class III drugs: amiodarone, bretylium, and sotolol)

- **Nonsedating Antihistamines** (Terfenadine and Astemizole); **When Used in Combination with Drugs That Inhibit Their Metabolism**, such as ketoconazole, itraconazole, fluconazole, erythromycin, clarithromycin, and toleandomycin

VENTRICULAR FLUTTER

Ventricular flutter is not actually a distinct dysrhythmia; rather, it is an accelerated form of ventricular tachycardia (Figure 17–6; Table 17–4). Ventricular flutter should be viewed as a transitional dysrhythmia, which is sometimes briefly observed before VT degenerates into ventricular fibrillation. Ventricular flutter is a life-threatening dysrhythmia that resembles a sine wave whose QRS complexes have a regular, smooth, rounded shape. Ventricular flutter occurs at a much faster rate than VT—between 250 and 300/minute. Monomorphic ventricular tachycardia is usually much slower—between 150 and 220/minute. Pulses are not present during ventricular flutter so an unsynchronized defibrillation countershock should immediately be performed.

Table 17-4 Key ECG Features of Ventricular Flutter

Ventricular:	Distinctive pattern: a rapid, wide, smooth, sine wave
Atrial:	Not observed
AV Relationship:	Absent
Other Findings:	Rate is more rapid than VT: 250+/minute

Causes, Significance, and Emergency Treatment of Ventricular Flutter

Same as for ventricular fibrillation/pulseless ventricular tachycardia and is discussed later in this chapter (see Table 17–15).

IDIOVENTRICULAR RHYTHMS

An **idioventricular rhythm** develops when a slow ventricular escape focus develops after failure of higher pacemakers. Idioventricular escape rhythms represent an unstable ventricular pacemaker discharging between 20 and 40/minute (Figures 17–8 and 17–9; Tables 17–5 and 17–6). Idioventricular impulses form spontaneously in Purkinje fibers or myocardial tissue. Becuase the rhythm originates within the ventricles, the QRS complexes have a wide and distorted appearance (Figure 17–10). P waves are not present because the atria are not stimulated.

Extremely slow idioventricular rates in the range of 5-15 complexes per minute are referred to as **"agonal" dysrhythmias** because they are seen just prior to death. Idioventricular rhythms are commonly encountered during resuscitation efforts as pulseless rhythms, especially following high dosages of epinephrine.

Causes of Idioventricular Escape Rhythms

Idioventricular escape rhythms develop when higher pacemakers, such as the sinus node and AV junction, fail. The bradycardic rate and lack of atrial depolariza-

Table 17-5 Ventricular Dysrhythmia Rates

- **Idioventricular escape rhythms:** 20–40/minute (averages 30/minute)

- **Accelerated idioventricular rhythms:** 50–100/minute (averages 75/minute)

- **Ventricular tachycardia:** 101 to 200/minute (averages 150/minute)

Table 17-6 Key ECG Features of Idioventricular Escape Rhythms

Atrial :	Absent
Ventricular:	Wide and distorted; regular, slow rhythm
AV Relationship:	Absent

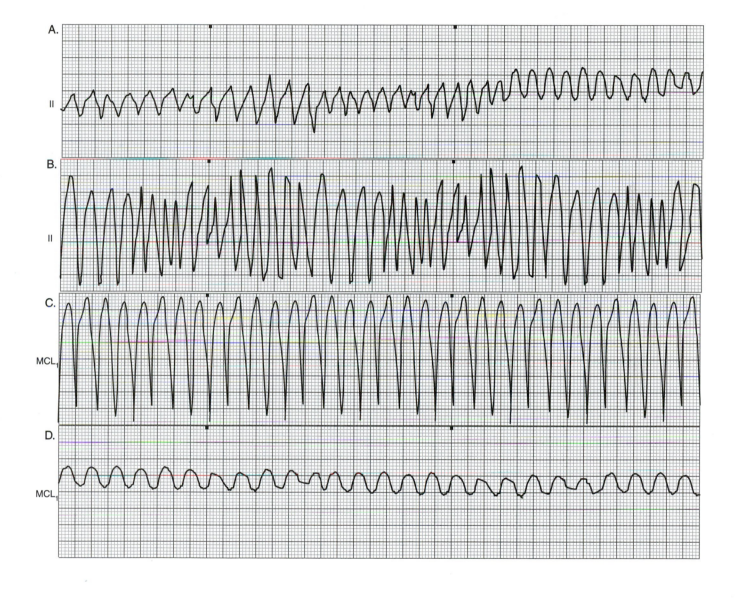

Figure 17-7 Ventricular flutter. The ECG tracings display the "sine wave" appearance that is typical of this very rapid regular form of ventricular tachycardia known as ventricular flutter.

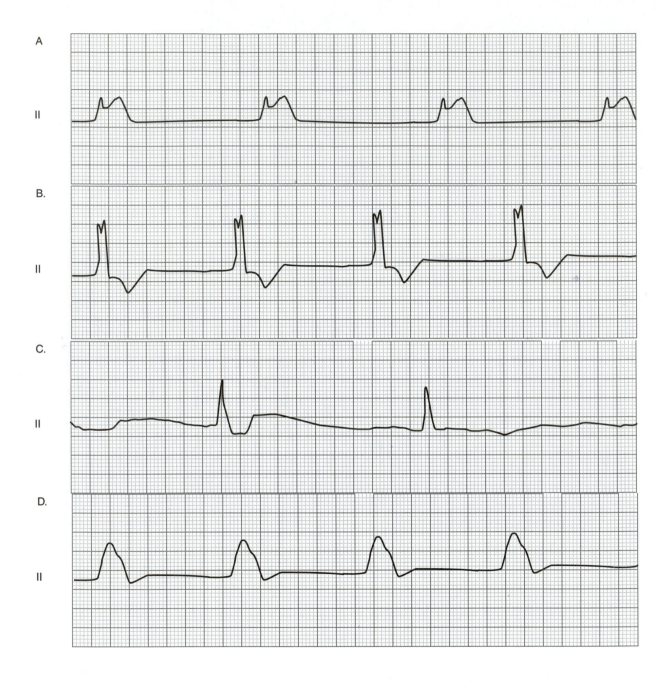

Figure 17-8 Idioventricular escape rhythms. Slow, wide QRS complexes are typical. Sinus and AV junctional pacemaker activity is not present. The rhythm in tracing C is too slow to support life and for that reason is sometimes termed "agonal."

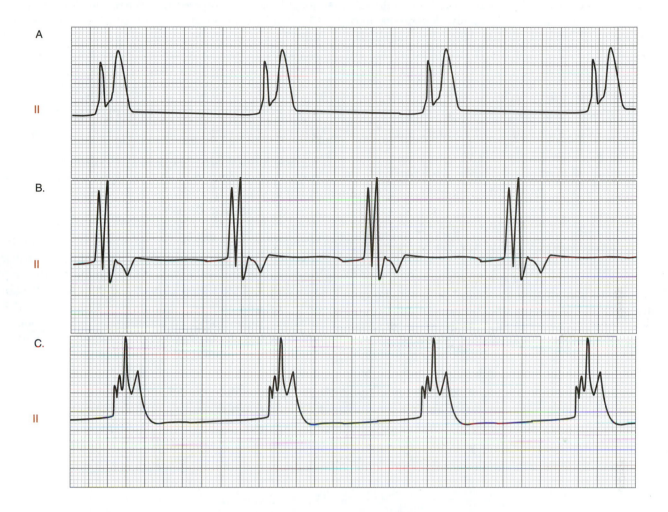

Figure 17–9 Idioventricular escape rhythms. The ECG tracings were recorded during episodes of cardiogenic shock and dying hearts. The QRS complexes are slow and very distorted.

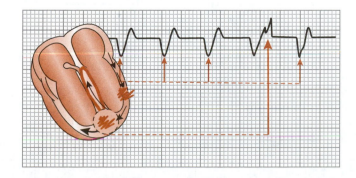

Figure 17–10 Etiology of an idioventricular rhythm. The illustration depicts two ventricular escape foci discharging.

tions result in a markedly reduced cardiac output. Idioventricular escape pacemakers are unstable and cannot reliably pace the heart for long periods. Idioventricular rhythms can suddenly degenerate into to ventricular fibrillation or asystole. The unreliable nature of this backup rhythm is illustrated in Figure 17–11).

> ***Clinical Note*** *Idioventricular escape rhythms only emerge after both sinus and AV junctional pacemakers have failed.*
>
> *Idioventricular escape rhythms preserve some cardiac output when the heart is faced with pacemaker failure. This rhythm should be viewed as a temporary solution until an artificial pacemaker can be used.*

Emergency Treatment Escape Rhythms

An idioventricular rhythm associated *with a pulse* can be treated with an epinephrine infusion or an isoproterenol infusion or artificial pacing. If a *pulseless* idioventricular rhythm exists, resuscitation measures for

pulseless electrical activity (PEA) should be implemented, including CPR, endotracheal intubation, and frequent boluses of intravenous epinephrine and atropine. The ACLS treatment algorithm for PEA is shown in figure 17–12. A search for correctable underlying precipitating causes should be done. The treatment is summarized in Table 17–18.

ACCELERATED IDIOVENTRICULAR RHYTHM (AIVR)

An **accelerated idioventricular rhythm** is an independent ventricular rhythm originating within the His-Purkinje system at a rate between 50 and 100/minute. Like all ventricular disorders, the QRS complexes are wide and distorted (Table 17–7). AV dissociation is present but the P waves are usually hidden within the distorted QRS complexes. Accelerated idioventricular rhythms, which are abbreviated AIVR, typically develop suddenly, last for a brief period, and then abruptly subside. Despite arising within the ventricles, AIVR rhythms usually produce an adequate cardiac output unlike ventricular tachycardia and slow *escape* idioven-

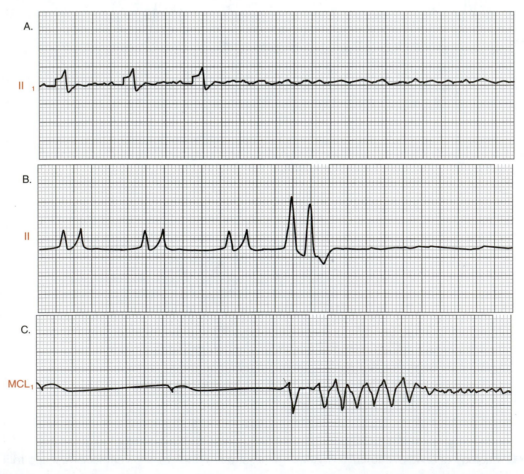

Figure 17–11 Degeneration of idioventricular escape rhythms into cardiac arrest. These tracings depict the unreliability of idioventricular rhythms.

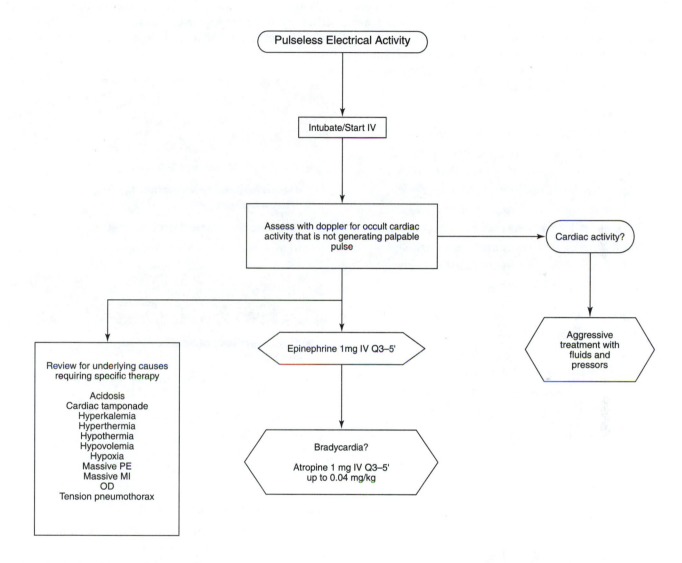

Figure 17-12 Pulseless Electrical Activity (PEA) Treatment Algorithm. (Reprinted with permission from EMedHome.com website (http://www.emedhome.com/).)

tricular rhythms (Figure 17–13; Table 17–7). AIVRs are commonly noted during recovery after an MI, as well as during thrombolytic therapy. AIVRs are generally harmless disorders that last for a short while without causing serious symptoms or compromising cardiac output. Accelerated idioventricular rhythms occur faster than escape rhythms—in the range of 50 to 100 per minute—and do not because of sinus pacemaker failure. Patients are usually unaware of the AIVRs because the rate is in the range that is expected for sinus rhythms. Unlike VT, accelerated idioventricular rhythms do not deteriorate into ventricular fibrillation.

ECG Interpretation Tip Artificial pacemaker rhythms resemble accelerated idioventricular rhythms because they both share the ECG characteristics of wide, distorted QRS T-wave complexes at rates of about 70 per minute. AIVR rhythms can be distinguished because they lack pacemaker spike artifacts which are typically tiny and can be overlooked (Figure 17–14).

ECG Interpretation Tip "Slow ventricular tachycardia" is a term that is sometimes incorrectly applied to accelerated idioventricular rhythms but there is no similarity to VT's malignant nature. AIVRs are benign dysrhythmias and occur at rates below 100/minute.

Clinical Significance of AIVR

AIVR does not have a detrimental effect on cardiac

Table 17–7 Key ECG Features of Accelerated idioventricular rhythms (AIVR)	
■ **Atrial:**	Independent P wave activity hidden among the QRS complexes
■ **Ventricular:**	Wide and distorted QRS complexes
■ **AV Relationship:**	AV dissociation
■ **Other Findings:**	Regular rate above 40/minute up to 100/minute
	AIVRs disrupt NSR for brief periods

functioning—possibly because it is short-lived and because AIVR rate is neither too fast nor too slow. AIVR does not lead to more serious dysrhythmias (Table 17–8). In fact, AIVR is viewed as a favorable marker of myocardial reperfusion after thrombolytic therapy (Figure 17–15). The ventricular pacemaker focus in AIVRs represents a mild form of ventricular excitation. Therapy is *not required* because the dysrhythmia quickly reverts to NSR and does not produce symptoms.

Table 17–8 Causes of Accelerated Idioventricular Rhythms (AIVR)
■ **Acute MI Recovery Phase**
■ **Reperfusion Dysrhythmia During Thrombolysis**
■ **Cardiac Resuscitation Dysrhythmia**

Table 17–9 Intrinsic Rates for Ventricular Rhythms
■ **Escape Idioventricular Rhythms:** 20–40/minute
■ **Accelerated Idioventricular Rhythms:** 40–100/minute
■ **Ventricular Tachycardia:** l00–250/minute

Emergency Treatment of AIVR

In the event that a patient's condition becomes unstable, therapy should be based on the rate of the AIVR. If the AIVR rate becomes slower than 40 /minute, therapy should be directed at accelerating the rate by using atropine or an external pacemaker. (Table 17–10) If an AIVR becomes faster than 100/minute, the therapy for ventricular tachycardia should be started, including lidocaine (1–1.5 mg/kg IV can be repeated at 1–1.5 mg/kg dose in 3–5 minutes) and/or electrical cardioversion. Table 17–9 lists the common rates for ventricular rhythms.

AIVR Occurring During Cardiac Resuscitations

The appearance of AIVR during cardiac resuscitations is a special case because an accelerated idioventricular rhythm in those circumstances is a highly unreliable

Table 17–10 Treatment for AIVR

■ **Rate:** 50-100/min.: no treatment as rhythm subsides spontaneously; consider Vasopressor infusion if hypotensive

■ **Rate:** >100/min.: treat as for monomorphic VT

- Amiodarone
- Lidocaine
- synchronized cardioversion

disorder and likely to degenerate into ventricular fibrillation or asystole (Figure 17–16). Short bursts of accelerated idioventricular rhythms during resuscitation efforts only produce a marginal cardiac output if any at all. In such cases, the AIVR gradually slows until it becomes agonal.

VENTRICULAR FIBRILLATION (VF)

Ventricular fibrillation is a life-threatening dysrhythmia characterized by chaotic electrical activity and completely disorganized myocardial activity in which cardiac output is absent (Figure 17–17; Table 17–11). Ventricular fibrillation is the leading cause of sudden cardiac arrest and is a lethal condition if not promptly corrected. The bizarre appearance of this dysrhythmia

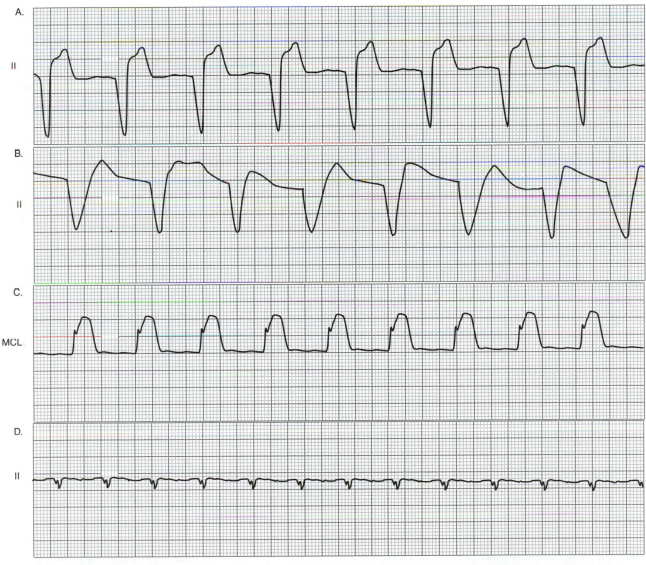

Figure 17–13 Accelerated idioventricular rhythms. Tracings A–D show ventricular rhythms at rates that are considerably faster than normal for ventricular escape rhythms (20–40/minute). They occur below 100/minute, however, or they would be termed VT.

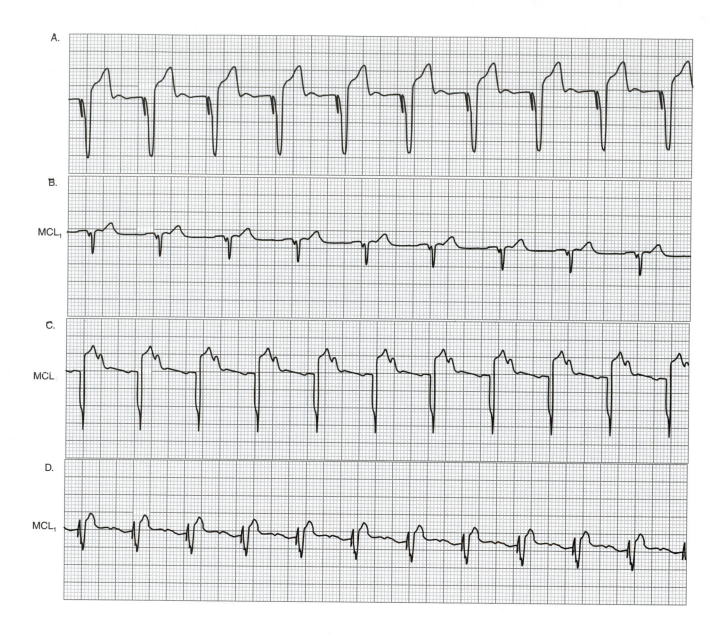

Figure 17-14 Similarity of artificially paced rhythms and accelerated idioventricular rhythms. Tracings A & D are artificial pacemaker rhythmsthat have pacer wires in the right ventricle and cause wide QRS complexes rhythms. Since artificial pacemakers stimulate the ventricle sequentially—rather than simultaneously as with sinus beats—they resemble accelerated idioventricular rhythms (tracings B and C).

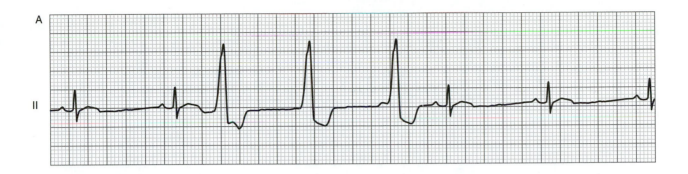

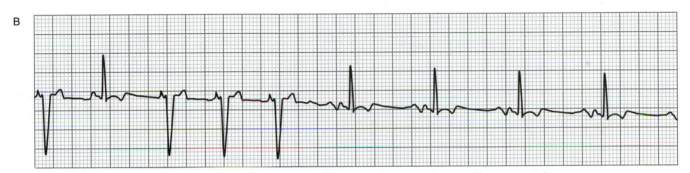

Figure 17-15 Short runs of accelerated idioventricular rhythms. The brief episodes subsided without treatment.

makes VF relatively easy to identify. This dysrhythmia can be mimicked by movement artifact or dislodged ECG electrodes but VF is obviously not present in an awake patient.

Coarse Versus Fine VF

The terms coarse and fine VF apply to the amplitude of the fibrillatory waves. Large waves are present in **coarse ventricular fibrillation** and there is a better chance of successfully converting the dysrhythmia to NSR. The briefer the VF episode, the coarser the waves will be. The longer that VF lasts, the finer and flatter the waves will appear.

- In **coarse amplitude ventricular fibrillation**, the VF waves are at least 3 mm high (Figure 17–18A). As the fibrillation episode continues, the degree of acidosis and hypoxia worsen, resulting in fibrillatory waves that become progressively smaller until asystole occurs.

- In **fine amplitude ventricular fibrillation**, VF wave height is 2 mm or less (Figures 17–18B and 17–19). The chances of successfully countershocking VF is less with fine waves than with coarse VF waves.

Primary Versus Secondary VF

Ventricular fibrillation is classified as either a primary problem or a secondary disorder based on the dysrhythmia's cause. **Primary VF** applies when the dysrhythmia is caused by an underlying *cardiac disorder*. **Secondary VF** develops from *non-cardiac*, non-ischemic disorders.

- *Primary VF cases*. Myocardial ischemia and injury, which occur during acute coronary syndromes, are the major causes of primary cardiac-related rhythm disorders.

- *Secondary VF cases*. Secondary ventricular fibrilla-

Table 17-11	Key ECG Findings of Ventricular Fibrillation
■ **Atrial:**	Absent
■ **Ventricular:**	Absent
■ **AV Relationship:**	Absent
■ **Other Findings:**	Chaotic complexes; no organized pattern
	Wavy undulating baseline

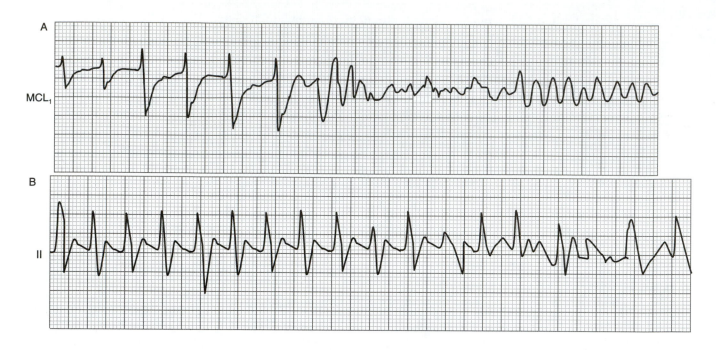

Figure 17–16 Accelerated idioventricular rhythms degenerating into ventricular fibrillation. Both tracings were obtained during cardiac resuscitation efforts.

tion occurs as a result of circulatory or respiratory failure or from extensive systemic disease. Ischemic coronary artery disease is *not* a cause. For instance, a teenager may sustain a cardiac arrest due to an obstructed airway, electrocution, poisoning, or drowning. VF occurs as a terminal ECG rhythm not caused by heart disease. VF is the final common pathway by which the heart's conduction system fails due to a variety of non-cardiac conditions such as from overwhelming sepsis, cancer, or trauma. Resuscitation of secondary ventricular fibrillation cases is more difficult because the underlying multiorgan system failure must be corrected.

Mechanism of VF Development

VF results from a chaotic ventricular reentry mechanism; which is sometimes caused when an ectopic premature ventricular complex strikes during the vulnerable T wave. The greatest risk for sudden cardiac death exists during the initial hours following an MI when the incidence of VF is greatest (Table 17–11). In cases of secondary ventricular fibrillation, which is caused by non-ischemic, non-cardiac disease, ventricular fibrillation is typically a "final common pathway" by which death occurs.

Clinical Significance of VF

VF is a life-threatening dysrhythmia that must be corrected with immediate defibrillation and resuscitative measures. The clinical significance of VF depends on whether the ventricular fibrillation is a primary or secondary disorder. Brief cases of VF that occur in a monitored setting have a successful conversion rate well over 90 percent. In contrast, ventricular fibrillation that exists for ten minutes without bystander CPR usually has a dismal resuscitation rate (less than 1 percent).

Emergency Treatment of VF

The most important therapy for primary ventricular fibrillation is rapid defibrillation. Widespread public access defibrillation, using automatic defibrillators that are available in locations where many people assemble at work, is an important measure in treating VF. The emergency cardiac care ACLS treatment algorithm for pulseless ventricular tachycardia and ventricular fibrillation are listed in Figure 17–20. Survivors of ventricular fibrillation need to considered for **implantable cardiodefibrillator (ICD)** placement due to the high recurrence rate, especially during the next twelve months. . ICDs are very effective in detecting and treating VF. Implanted cardioverter defibrillators (CID) detect unstable ventricular dysrhythmias and deliver a

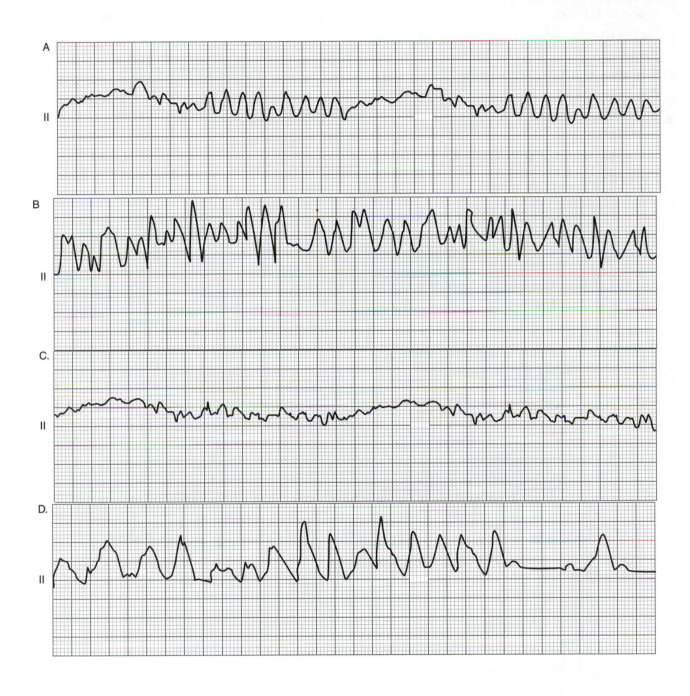

Figure 17-17 Coarse ventricular fibrillation.

Table 17–12 Causes of Ventricular Fibrillation

- **Myocardial Ischemia/ Infarction—major cause of primary VF**
- **Electrolyte Disorders (Hypokalemia and Hyperkalemia)**
- **Electrical Shock/ Electrocution**
- **Cardiomyopathy**
- **Drug Toxicity (cocaine use, tricyclic overdose)**
- **Untreated Ventricular Tachycardia**
- **Hypothermia**

Table 17–13 Treatment for V. Fibrillation and Pulseless VT

- **Defibrillation: 200J, 300J, 360J**
- **Epinephrine 1mg IV every 3-5 min. or Vasopressin 40 unit single IV dose**
- **Defibrillate at 360J**
- **Consider Amiodarone or Lidocaine or Magnesium or Procainamide**
- **Consider buffers**
- **Reattempt defibrillation**

series of shocks. Automatic ICDs have a much higher success rate and fewer side effects than long-term anti-dysrhythmic medication. Despite the higher initial cost and need for surgical insertion, ICDs are an effective treatment for recurrent VT/VF.

Therapy for VF can be summarized (Table 17–13) as initial defibrillation, frequent epinephrine doses, and repeat defibrillations after the following medications: lidocaine, amiodarone, procainamide, and magnesium. Only one antidysrhythmic drug should be used.

Useful medications include:

- Epinephrine as a 1mg IV push, repeated every 3 to 5 minutes.

- Lidocaine at an initial dose of 1–1.5 mg/kg IV bolus In refractory cases, repreat 1–1.5 mg/kg IV push in 3 to 5 minutes; maximum total dose, 3 mg/kg.

- Amiodarone 300 mg infusion over 10 minutes (15 mg/minute). This is followed by a slow infusion 1 mg/minute over the next 6 hours. A maintenance infusion of 0.5 mg/minute for the remaining 18

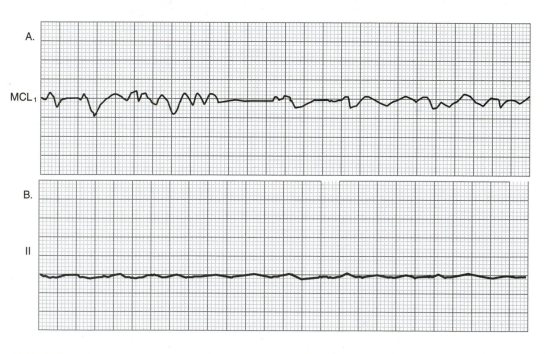

Figure 17-18 Coarse VF compared with fine amplitude VF. Tracing A shows large fibrillatory waves, while B has fine waves.

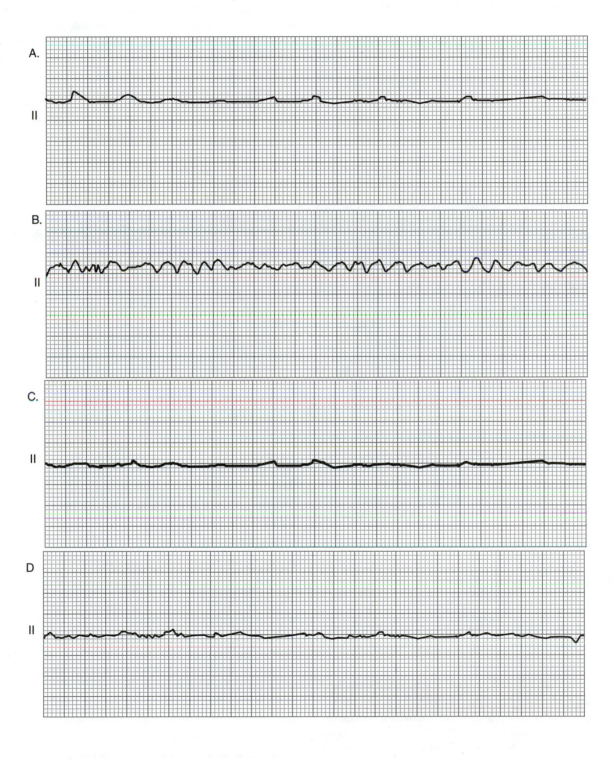

Figure 17-19 Fine amplitude VF.

hours.

■ Procainamide as a 30 mg/minute IV infusion up to a maximum dose of 17mg/kg. In refractory cases, can also be given as 100 mg IV push every 5 minutes.

■ Magnesium sulfate as a 1–2 gram dose diluted in 10 cc of 5% dextrose given as an IV push for Torsade de Pointes, suspected hypomagnesemia, or refractory VF

Normal Hearts and VF

VF may occur in normal hearts but only if there is an intense precipitating trigger such as illicit drug use (especially cocaine use), intense hypoxia (as seen with fatal asthma syndrome or foreign body airway obstruction), electrocution, or a severe electrolyte disorder.

Pediatric Cardiac Arrest Dysrhythmias

In infants and children, ischemic heart disease is almost unheard of and primary VF is rare. Most cases of cardiac arrest in young children are secondary to overwhelming sepsis, respiratory insufficiency, or congenital heart abnormalities. Sudden Infant Death Syndrome is a leading cause of death in infants less than two years of age, while accidents are the major cause of death in older children. Most pediatric cardiac arrests present with **brady-asystolic cardiac rhythms** which are characterized by slow, irregular cardiac rhythms with long periods of absent electrical activity. For example, the ECG shown in Figure 17–21 was recorded in a child with Down syndrome who had multiple congenital cardiac abnormalities.

ASYSTOLE

Asystole is the complete absence of electrical and mechanical activity (Figure 17–22; Table 17–14). The SA node and all other escape pacemakers fail. The ECG shows a flat line which indicates that there is extensive damage to the heart's electrical conduction system.

Table 17–14 Key ECG Features of Asystole

■ **Atrial:**	Absent
■ **Ventricular:**	Absent
■ **AV relationship:**	Absent

Asystole is usually a terminal cardiac activity since resuscitation measures are rarely successful.

Although asystole can be a primary cardiac arrest rhythm, it usually follows a period of ventricular fibrillation. In children, brady-asystolic arrests are much more common than VF. In a dying heart, isolated idioventricular beats typically punctuate long periods of asystole (Figure 17–23).

> ***ECG Interpretation Tip*** *Fine amplitude VF may masquerade as asystole so it is important to confirm asystole in at least two leads. Selecting a lead perpendicular to the initial lead will ensure that the maximal amplitude is obtained. A properly calibrated ECG monitor will prevent fine ventricular fibrillation from being mistaken for asystole.*

Causes of Asystole

Extensive atherosclerotic heart disease is the primary cause of this dysrhythmia. Asystole occurs when the cardiac impulse generation system completely fails. Asystole is a terminal rhythm and usually develops in adults following a period of ventricular fibrillation. In children, asystole is a common primary cardiac arrest dysrhythmia.

Clinical Significance of Asystole

Asystole represents the complete failure of myocardial electrical activity and is a terminal rhythm. Resuscitation is usually not successful.

Emergency Treatment of Asystole

Resuscitation efforts need to be directed at administering epinephrine and atropine, along with CPR and correcting underlying conditions such as acidosis, hypoxia, or electrolyte disturbance (Table 17–17). An emergency cardiac care treatment algorithm for asystole is contained in Figure 17–24. Artificial pacing should be tried early during resuscitation efforts but is usually ineffective. Prolonged resuscitation efforts and transportation by EMS units is not indicated.

PULSELESS ELECTRICAL ACTIVITY (PEA)

Pulseless electrical activity refers to the finding of electrical ECG activity without pulses (Figure 17–25; Table 17–18). PEA applies to a diverse group of dys-

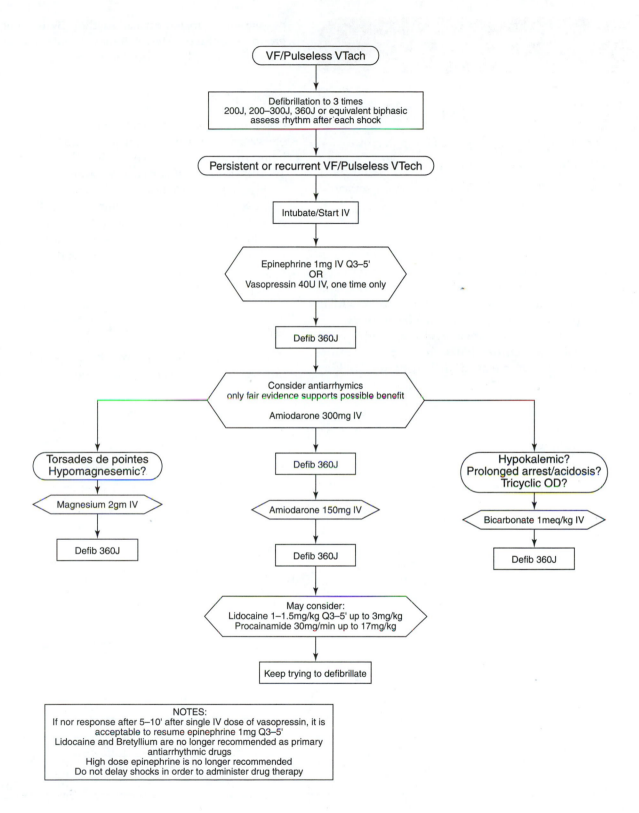

Figure 17–20 Adult Ventricular Fibrillation and Pulseless Ventricular Tachycardia Treatment Algorithm. (Reprinted with permission from EMedHome.com website (http://www.emedhome.com/).)

Table 17-15 Key ECG Features of Pulselss Electrical Activity

- ■ **Atrial:** Usually missing or else there are isolated P waves
- ■ **Ventricular:** Slow and wide complexes
- ■ **AV Relationship:** Absent
- ■ **Other Findings:** Organized electrical activity with absent pulses

rhythmias that have an organized ECG rhythm, including electromechanical dissociation, idioventricular rhythms, and bradyasystolic rhythms. Ultrasound examination during cardiac arrests have shown weak cardiac contraction that did not generate a palpable pulse. One form of PEA was previously termed **electrical mechanical dissociation (EMD)** because it was incorrectly assumed that mechanical activity was lacking despite an organized cardiac rhythm. By renaming this group of pulseless dysrhythmias as PEA the need to search for underlying treatable causes was stressed.

Causes of PEA

Common causes of PEA include massive MI, pulmonary embolism, cardiac tamponade, and exsanguinating hemorrhage, which have a dismal outcome (Table 17–19). However, if correctable causes are treated early during the resuscitation phase, chances for success improve. For instance, calcium administration is an effective therapy for calcium-channel overdosage, as is needle decompression in the case of a tension pneumothorax. Treating electrolyte disorders and correcting hypovolemia are useful in renal dialysis patients who have pulseless electrical activity.

Emergency Treatment of PEA

If a Doppler stethoscope or ultrasonographic evaluation reveals faint blood flow during PEA, aggressive

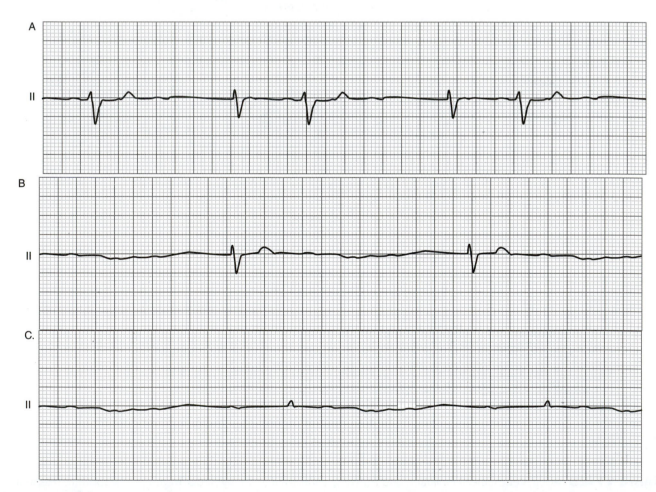

Figure 17-21 Brady-asystolic dysrhythmias. This rhythm disturbance is the most common type that occurs during pediatric cardiac arrests.

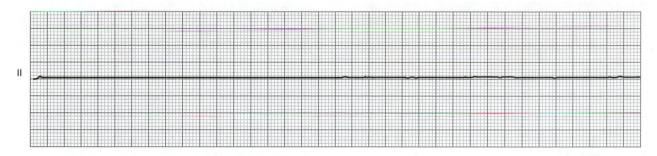

Figure 17-22 Asystole. Absence of electrical activity.

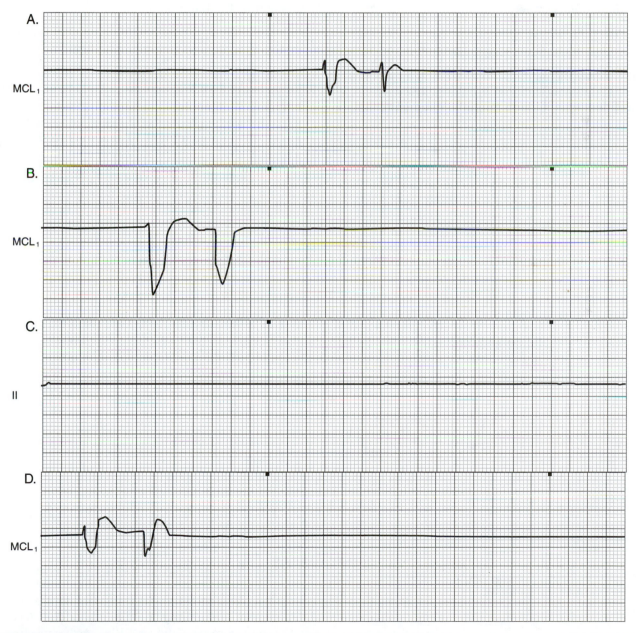

Figure 17-23 Asystole and isolated agonal beats. Slow, wide distorted beats are seen among a flat line tracing. Occasional agonal beats, which do not generate a cardiac output, are often seen for several minutes after resuscitation efforts have ceased.

Table 17-16 Causes of Pulseless Electrical Activity

- Massive Myocardial Damage
- Hypovolemia Due to Hemorrhage
- Hyperkalemia (High Blood Potassium Levels)
- Hypothermia
- Hypoxia
- Acidosis
- Cardiac Tamponade
- Tension Pneumothorax
- Massive Pulmonary Embolism
- Drug Overdoses (Especially Beta Antagonists, Calcium Channel Blockers, Tricyclic Antidepressants, and Digitalis Preparations)

Table 17-17 Treatment for Asystole

- Transcutaneous pacing
- Epinephrine 1 mg IV push every 3-5 min.
- Atropine 1 mg IV push every 3-5 min. to maximum of 0.04 mg/kg

Table 17-18 Treatment for PEA

- Epinephrine 1 mg IV push every 3-5 min.
- Atropine 1 mg IV push every 3-5 min. to maximum of 0.04 mg/kg (if ECG complex rate is slow)
- Other: norepinephrine infusion or dopamine infusion or dobutamine infusion; IV fluid volume challenge

therapy with vasopressors, including epinephrine, norepinephrine, dopamine, and dobutamine, along with volume expanders is reasonable (Table 17–20). Correction of electrolyte disorders, acidosis, and hypoxia should also be done. Although most resuscitation efforts for PEA fail, attention to underlying causes can lead to some success. The emergency cardiac care ACLS treatment algorithm for Pulseless Electrical Activity Algorithm is found in Figure 17–12 .

Tables 17–15 and 17–16 summarize characteristics of ventricular rhythms and ectopic complexes.

Let's Review:

1. Torsade de Pointes (TdP) is an uncommon polymorphic form of VT that has diverse causes.

2. Torsade de Pointes has QRS complexes that rhythmically increase and decrease in size as they rotate above and below the ECG baseline.

3. Torsade de Pointes occurs in conditions is associated with delayed ventricular repolarization and prolonged QT intervals.

4. Ventricular flutter is a rare transient dysrhythmia that is a very rapid form of ventricular tachycardia. The QRS complexes resemble a sine wave. The etiology, significance, and treatment of ventricular flutter are the same as for ventricular tachycardia.

5. Idioventricular escape rhythms occur when the sinus node and AV junctional pacemakers fail. Idioventricular escape rhythms have wide and distorted QRS complexes at a rate of 20 to 30 beats per minute.

6. Accelerated idioventricular rhythms (AVIR) arise from a reentry process or an automatic focus. The ventricular rate ranges from 50–100/minute.

7. Ventricular dysrhythmias, like supraventricular dysrhythmias, can result from both passive and active mechanisms. Passive mechanisms become active when higher pacemakers fail to pace the ventricles. Active mechanisms result from ventricular irritability and involve competition with the sinus node.

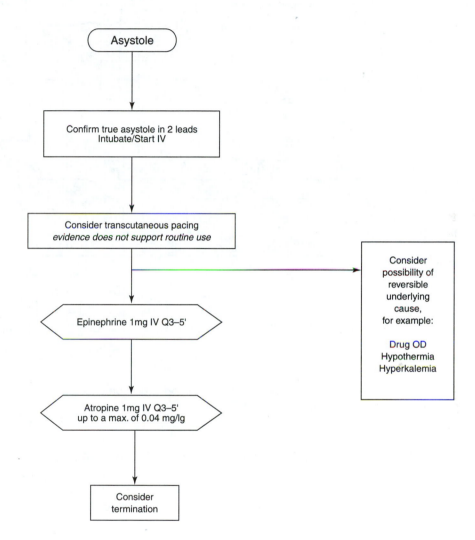

Figure 17-24 Adult Asystole Treatment Algorithm. (Reprinted with permission from EMedHome.com website (http://www.emedhome.com/).)

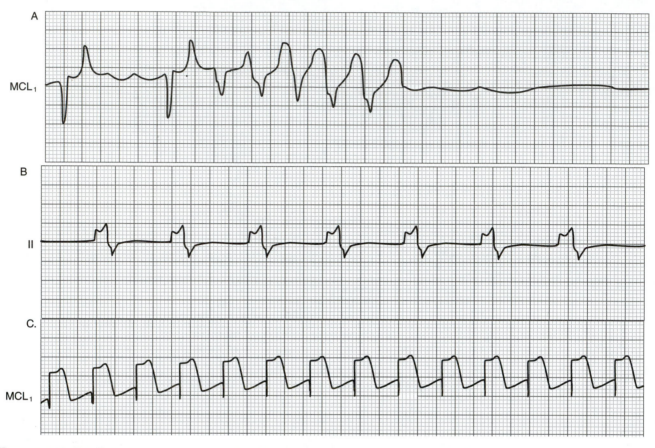

Figure 17–25 Pulseless electrical activity. The distorted and wide complex rhythms were recorded during cardiac resuscitations. Pulses were absent during each ECG tracing.

8. Ventricular fibrillation (VF) accounts for the vast majority of deaths from coronary artery disease, especially those occurring before the patient reaches the emergency department.

9. The coarser the waves in ventricular fibrillation (VF), the greater the chance of cardioversion success.

10. Primary VF is distinctly uncommon in pediatric cardiac arrests as ischemic heart disease is a disease of older patients.

11. Asystole has a flat ECG line because electrical activity is absent.

12. Pulseless electrical activity (PEA) is a cardiac arrest rhythm in which an organized electrical rhythm is present but pulses are absent.

13. To confirm asystole, the ECG monitor should be properly calibrated and the rhythm should be confirmed in a perpendicular lead.

Glossary

Accelerated idioventricular rhythms (AIVR) Independent rhythm originating within the His-Purkinje system at a rate between 50 and 100/minute.

Agonal dysrhythmias Extremely slow and unreliable idioventricular rhythms seen just prior to death.

Asystole Absence of electrical cardiac rhythm; resembling a flat ECG line.

Brady-asystolic cardiac rhythms Dysrhythmias observed during cardiac arrest consisting of slow complexes and asystolic periods.

Coarse amplitude VF Amplitude of fibrillatory waves is 3mm or more.

Electrical mechanical dissociation (EMD) Organized cardiac rhythm in the absence of heart contractions.

Fine amplitude VF Amplitude of fibrillatory waves is less than 3mm.

Idioventricular rhythm Bradycardic rhythm that develops from a ventricular escape focus due to the failure of higher pacemakers.

Implantable cardiodefibrillator (ICD) Device that is implanted on the chest wall and automatically delivers electrical shocks when VT or VF is detected.

Polymorphic VT Another term for Torsade de Pointes.

Primary VF Life threatening dysrhythmia resulting from an underlying cardiac disorder.

Pulseless electrical activity (PEA) Electrical ECG activity without pulses.

Secondary VF Life threatening dysrhythmia resulting from a non-cardiac disorder.

Torsade de Pointes (TdP) Uncommon form of ventricular tachycardia in which the size and shape of the QRS complexes vary rhythmically.

Ventricular fibrillation (VF) Life-threatening dysrhythmia characterized by chaotic electrical activity and completely disorganized myocardial activity; cardiac output ceases.

Ventricular flutter Accelerated form of ventricular tachycardia that exists briefly, resembles a sine wave, and deteriorates into ventricualr fibrillation.

Ventricular tachydysrhythmias Rapid, unstable ventricular dysrhythmias (VT and VF).

Ventricular Dysrhythmias— Self-Assessment ECG Tracings

LEARNING OBJECTIVE

Upon completion of this chapter, the reader should be able to:

- *Correctly interpret ventricular dysrhythmias, when given a series of sample ECG tracings displaying various ventricular abnormalities.*

- *Accurately assess the rhythm, PR intervals, QRS durations, AV conduction ratios, and ST segments, given a sample of ECG tracings displaying various ventricular dysrhythmias.*

VENTRICULAR DYSRHYTHMIAS—SELF ASSESSMENT ECG TRACINGS

The next twenty-five ECG tracings display a wide variety of ventricular dysrhythmias for practice. Suggested interpretations are provided in Appendix A. If any difficulties are encountered, refer back to related sections of Chapters 16 and 17.

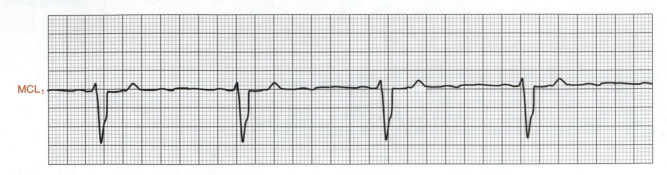

Figure 18–1   Rate _____
Rhythm _____
QRS Duration _____
PR Interval _____
AV Conduction Ratio _____
ST Segment _____
Interpretation _____
Reasoning _____

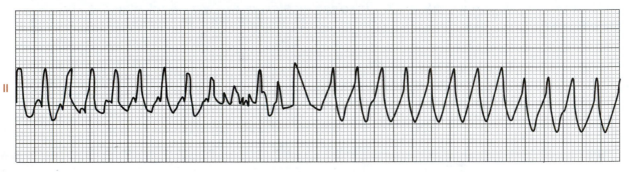

Figure 18–2   Rate _____
Rhythm _____
QRS Duration _____
PR Interval _____
AV Conduction Ratio _____
ST Segment _____
Interpretation _____
Reasoning _____

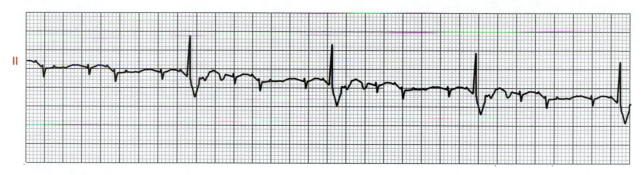

Figure 18-3   Rate _____
Rhythm _____
QRS Duration _____
PR Interval _____
AV Conduction Ratio _____
ST Segment _____
Interpretation _____
Reasoning _____

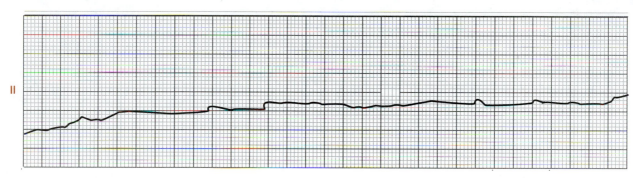

Figure 18-4   Rate _____
Rhythm _____
QRS Duration _____
PR Interval _____
AV Conduction Ratio _____
ST Segment _____
Interpretation _____
Reasoning _____

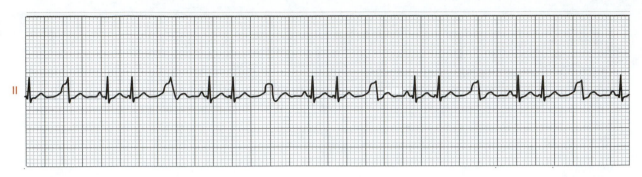

Figure 18–5   Rate _____
Rhythm _____
QRS Duration _____
PR Interval _____
AV Conduction Ratio _____
ST Segment _____
Interpretation _____
Reasoning _____

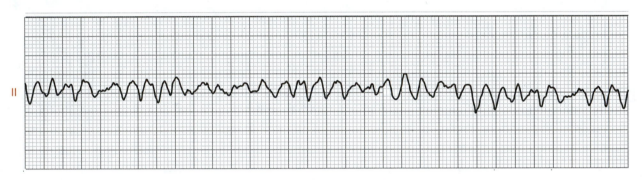

Figure 18–6   Rate _____
Rhythm _____
QRS Duration _____
PR Interval _____
AV Conduction Ratio _____
ST Segment _____
Interpretation _____
Reasoning _____

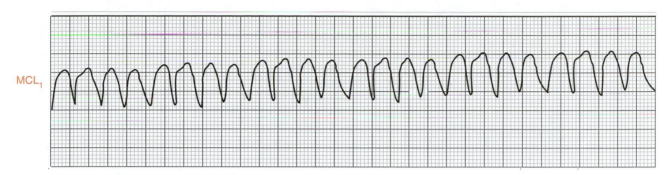

Figure 18–7   Rate _____
Rhythm _____
QRS Duration _____
PR Interval _____
AV Conduction Ratio _____
ST Segment _____
Interpretation _____
Reasoning _____

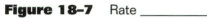

Figure 18–8   Rate _____
Rhythm _____
QRS Duration _____
PR Interval _____
AV Conduction Ratio _____
ST Segment _____
Interpretation _____
Reasoning _____

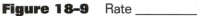

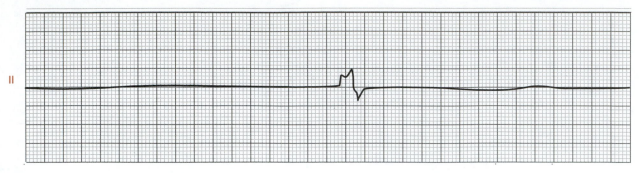

Figure 18-9   Rate _____
Rhythm _____
QRS Duration _____
PR Interval _____
AV Conduction Ratio _____
ST Segment _____
Interpretation _____
Reasoning _____

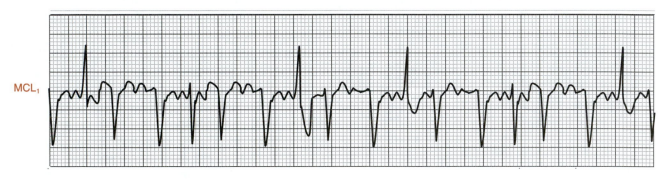

Figure 18-10   Rate _____
Rhythm _____
QRS Duration _____
PR Interval _____
AV Conduction Ratio _____
ST Segment _____
Interpretation _____
Reasoning _____

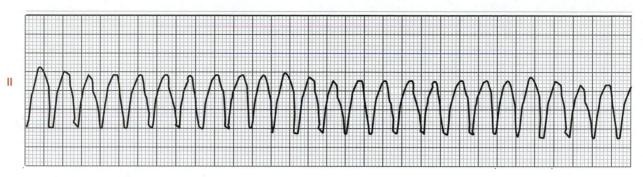

Figure 18–11 Rate _____
Rhythm _____
QRS Duration _____
PR Interval _____
AV Conduction Ratio _____
ST Segment _____
Interpretation _____
Reasoning _____

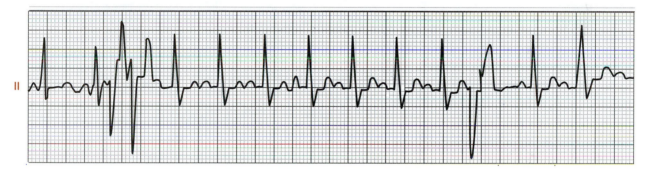

Figure 18–12 Rate _____
Rhythm _____
QRS Duration _____
PR Interval _____
AV Conduction Ratio _____
ST Segment _____
Interpretation _____
Reasoning _____

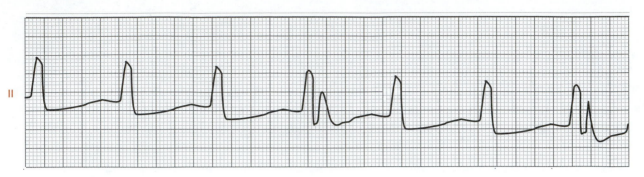

Figure 18–13 Rate _____

Rhythm _____

QRS Duration _____

PR Interval _____

AV Conduction Ratio _____

ST Segment _____

Interpretation _____

Reasoning _____

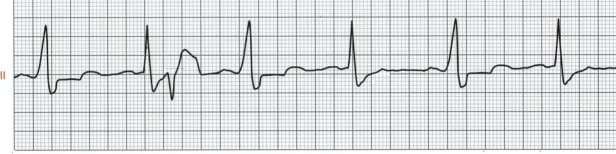

Figure 18–14 Rate _____

Rhythm _____

QRS Duration _____

PR Interval _____

AV Conduction Ratio _____

ST Segment _____

Interpretation _____

Reasoning _____

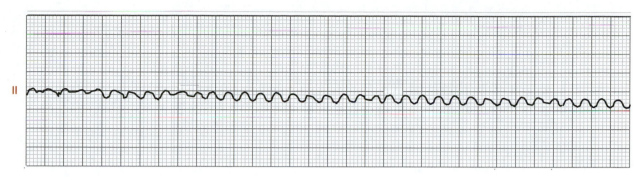

Figure 18–15 Rate _____
Rhythm _____
QRS Duration _____
PR Interval _____
AV Conduction Ratio _____
ST Segment _____
Interpretation _____
Reasoning _____

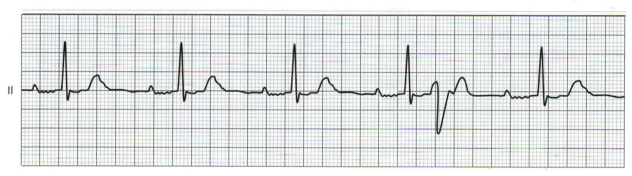

Figure 18–16 Rate _____
Rhythm _____
QRS Duration _____
PR Interval _____
AV Conduction Ratio _____
ST Segment _____
Interpretation _____
Reasoning _____

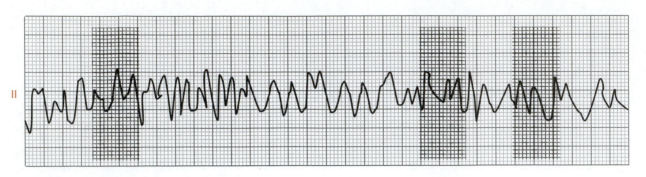

Figure 18–17 Rate _____
              Rhythm _____
              QRS Duration _____
              PR Interval _____
              AV Conduction Ratio _____
              ST Segment _____
              Interpretation _____
              Reasoning _____

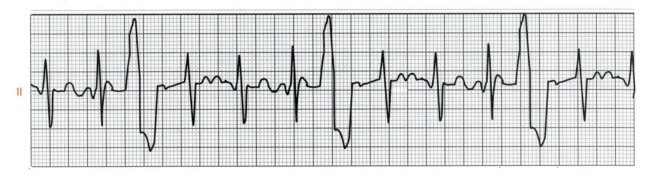

Figure 18–18 Rate _____
              Rhythm _____
              QRS Duration _____
              PR Interval _____
              AV Conduction Ratio _____
              ST Segment _____
              Interpretation _____
              Reasoning _____

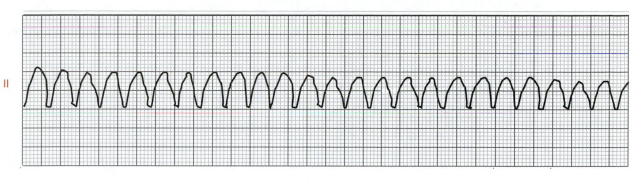

Figure 18–19 Rate _____
Rhythm _____
QRS Duration _____
PR Interval _____
AV Conduction Ratio _____
ST Segment _____
Interpretation _____
Reasoning _____

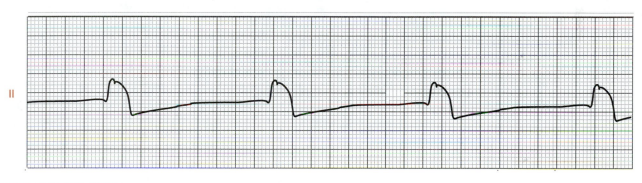

Figure 18–20 Rate _____
Rhythm _____
QRS Duration _____
PR Interval _____
AV Conduction Ratio _____
ST Segment _____
Interpretation _____
Reasoning _____

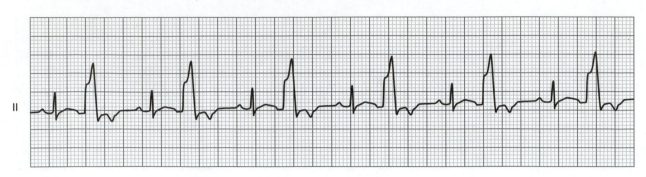

II

Figure 18–21 Rate _____
Rhythm _____
QRS Duration _____
PR Interval _____
AV Conduction Ratio _____
ST Segment _____
Interpretation _____
Reasoning _____

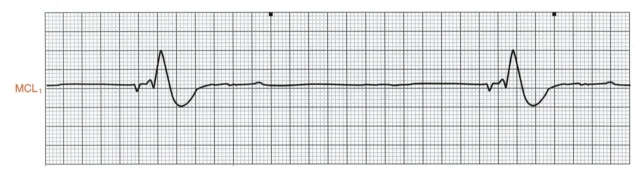

MCL₁

Figure 18–22 Rate _____
Rhythm _____
QRS Duration _____
PR Interval _____
AV Conduction Ratio _____
ST Segment _____
Interpretation _____
Reasoning _____

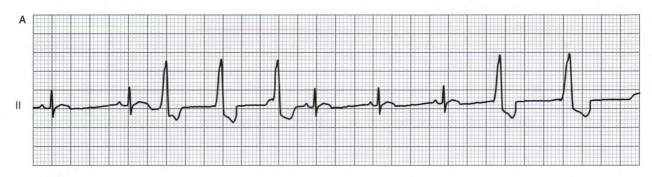

Figure 18-23 Rate _____
Rhythm _____
QRS Duration _____
PR Interval _____
AV Conduction Ratio _____
ST Segment _____
Interpretation _____
Reasoning _____

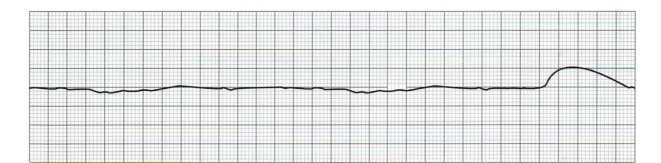

Figure 18-24 Rate _____
Rhythm _____
QRS Duration _____
PR Interval _____
AV Conduction Ratio _____
ST Segment _____
Interpretation _____
Reasoning _____

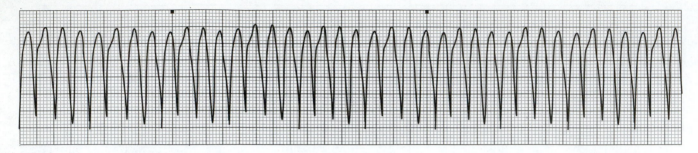

Figure 18–25 Rate _____
Rhythm _____
QRS Duration _____
PR Interval _____
AV Conduction Ratio _____
ST Segment _____
Interpretation _____
Reasoning _____

Artificial Pacemakers and Implantable Cardioverter-defibrillators (ICDs)

LEARNING OBJECTIVES

Upon completion of this chapter, the reader should be able to:

- *Identify the fundamental components of an artificial pacemaker system.*

- *List at least four primary indications for artificial pacemaker use.*

- *Describe the primary indications for use of the following common artificial pacemaker types: temporary, permanent, transthoracic (external), and transvenous.*

- *Describe the common lead placement(s) for most permanent single- and dual-chamber pacemakers.*

- *Given a sample ECG tracing, determine if the artificial pacemaker is properly functioning in terms of sensing and capturing operation.*

- *Describe the malfunction when a pacemaker fails to sense.*

- *Describe the malfunction when a pacemaker fails to capture.*

- *List two common causes for a pacemaker device's failure to capture.*

- *Explain what is meant when a pacemaker "oversenses" and describe the ECG appearance.*

- *Describe how the presence of an artificial pacemaker changes the evaluation and care of a patient with: a) ischemic chest pain; and b) a patient who is in cardiac arrest.*

- *Given sample ECG tracings, identify a failure of the artificial pacemaker to pace.*

- *Given sample ECG tracings, identify a failure of the artificial pacemaker to sense.*

- *Given sample ECG tracings, identify properly functioning artificial pacemaker with 1:1 capture.*

- *Describe a method for applying an external pacemaker device and ensuring proper capture by adjusting the discharge rate and pulse generator output level.*

- *Define the following pacemaker-related terms: escape interval, stimulation (capture) threshold, sensing threshold (sensitivity), pulse generator, refractory period, automatic interval, and output pulse.*

- *Explain what happens when a strong magnet is held over the chest of a patient with an implanted pacemaker.*

- *Identify the basic components and functions of an ICD.*

- *Explain the manner in which an implantable cardioverter-defibrillator (ICD) generates an electrical countershock.*

- *Describe the care of a patient who experiences ventricular tachycardia that is refractory to ICD cardioversion.*

- *Describe an emergent therapy that can be instituted in the emergency department or critical care unit for a malfunctioning ICD that is delivering inappropriate cardioversion shocks for sinus tachycardia.*

CHAPTER OVERVIEW

Patients with artificial pacemakers and implanted cardio-defibrillators (ICD) are frequently encountered in emergency care. The ECG provides important clues about the functioning of ICD and artificial pacemaker devices. Although extremely reliable, malfunction of ICDs and pacemakers is possible and the ability to do basic "troubleshooting' is a valuable clinical skill. The indications for pacemaker use and ICD insertion will be discussed and the basic components of artificial pacemakers and ICDs will be described.

INTRODUCTION TO ARTIFICIAL CARDIAC PACEMAKERS

Extreme bradycardia and prolonged asystolic pauses are types of cardiac electrical failure caused by atrioventricular conduction disturbances and impulse formation disorders. **Artificial pacemakers** are used to treat failure of the heart's electrical system by producing tiny electrical discharges that activate heart muscle and cause cardiac contraction when the body's natural system of escape pacemakers fail.

Artificial pacemakers were first implanted in the late 1950s and there are currently about 1 million people in the United States with implanted pacemakers so it is very likely that patients with these devices will be encountered frequently in EMS systems, emergency departments, and critical care units. Knowing how to assess whether a pacemaker is functioning properly is important.

Artificial cardiac pacemakers consist of a pulse generator, which contains the battery, and the electrodes which serve a dual purpose of sensing intrinsic cardiac activity as well as transmitting the electrical impulse to stimulate the heart (Figure 19–1). Figure 19–2 illustrates a typical device.

Pacemakers can be used either temporarily for transient conduction problems, or be permanently implanted for chronic disorders. Common indications for pacemaker implantation are listed in Table 19–1. Bradycardia and conduction disorders are commonly treated with pacemaker insertion if significant symptoms are present. Symptoms that are caused by slow heart rates include dizziness, lightheadedness, palpitations, syncope,

fatigue and generalized weakness, as well as shortness of breath, dyspnea on exertion, and chest pain. A frequent cause of permanent conduction system failure involves age-related degenerative fibrosis of the His bundle and bundle branches leading to impaired AV conduction.

Table 19-1 Common Indications for Permanent Pacemakers

Advanced Heart Block

- Third-degree AV block

- Third-degree AV block associated with an escape rate less than 40 bpm or asystolic periods lasting 3 seconds or longer.

- Symptomatic second-degree (Mobitz Type I or II) AV block

- Symptomatic atrial fibrillation with a ventricular rate less than 40 bpm

Dysrhythmias Associated with Myocardial Infarction

- Third-degree AV block

- Mobitz Type II second-degree AV block with bundle branch block

Symptomatic Sick Sinus Syndrome with Rates less than 40 bpm

Hypersensitive Carotid Sinus Syndrome Associated with Recurrent Syncope

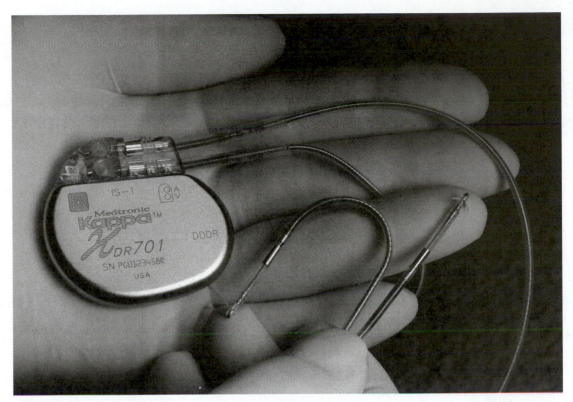

Figure 19–1 This dual-chambered pacemaker has an oblong shaped generator battery attached to two silicone insulated leads (wires). One end of the leads has barbs designed to be embedded into the ventricular heart muscle to prevent lead dislodgment. (Courtesy of Medtronic Inc.)

While most pacemakers are used to treat symptomatic bradycardias, some of the newer devices also have defibrillation and anti-tachycardia features. (Figure 19–3). The latest generation of pacemakers involve **dual–chamber devices** that are smaller and able to pace the atria as well as the ventricles. While older devices had limited commands that required the parameters to be determined *before* insertion, current devices have variable functions that can be reprogrammed as often as needed *after* insertion. For instance, newer pacemakers are capable of adjusting their discharge rate to meet the body's changing metabolic needs, such as, increasing when muscle activity is sensed during physical activity (Figure 19–4). Despite these advanced features, pacemakers remain relatively straight forward devices that are reliable and easy to troubleshoot.

Pacemaker Components

Pacemakers must be able to sense the patient's own natural beats in order to avoid competition between the device and the sinus node. Two terms that are used to describe the body's natural beats are **native beats** and **intrinsic cardiac activity** to distinguish them from an

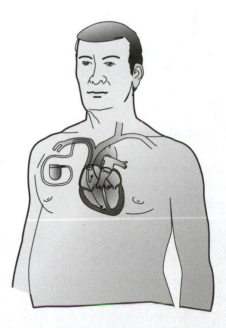

Figure 19–2 Dual-chamber pacemaker leads in place in the atrium and ventricle enable the pacemaker to simultaneously sense and pace both chambers.

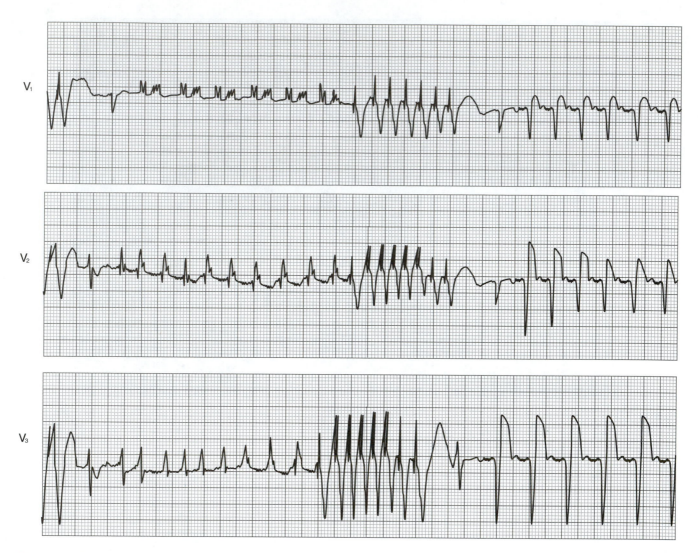

Figure 19–3 A seven-pulse pacing burst was delivered during an episode of VT. The rapid pacer pulses (indicated by the bracketed region) capture the ventricle and terminate the ventricular tachycardia. This is termed overdrive pacing

artificially paced beat. Pacemakers have three basic components:

■ The **pulse generator** contains the battery and produces the electrical discharge (Figure 19–5). The pulse generator is enclosed in a durable titanium shell and weighs only a few ounces, in contrast to earlier models that weighed nearly one quarter of a pound.

■ The **pacemaker battery** is contained within the pulse generator and modern lithium batteries last 8 to 10 years. As the battery becomes depleted, the voltage drops and the conduction resistance increases. Some models send a telemetry signal that a battery change is needed, while other pacers experience a gradual fall in pacing rate.

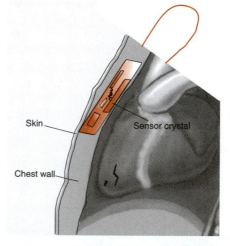

Skin

Sensor crystal

Chest wall

Figure 19–4 Motion-responsive pacemaker. A sensor inside the pulse generator responds to body motion by increasing the pacing rate. This adaptive pacing mode automatically adjusts to changing body needs.

■ The **pacing leads** transmit the generator-initiated electrical impulse to the myocardium. There are one or two pacing leads, which are thin wire electrodes made from platinum or metal alloys and covered by insulating silicone that attach to the heart. The electrode tip is attached to the heart from inside the chamber via a spiral screw-like ending or a flanged fin, anchor type (Figure 19–6). Pacing leads simultaneously sense intrinsic cardiac activity and relay the data to the pulse generator to coordinate pacemaker function.

Clinical Note Pacemaker battery status is usually evaluated by having the pulse generator "interogated" via telephone telemetry. Battery depletion causes a gradual decrease in paced pulse rate. Battery failure should be suspected when a patient's heart rate is 10 or more beats below the programmed paced rate. The programmed paced rate is listed on the pacemaker card carried by patients.

Bipolar Versus Unipolar Pacemaker Leads

Pacemaker electrodes are of two types:

■ A bipolar lead system is the most common design used in modern pacemakers and contains its leads within the same chamber it paces.

■ Unipolar leads were used in older models, as well as in external (transcutaneous) pacemakers. Some unipolar pacemakers are still in use and can be recognized by the large artifact pacer spike produced on the ECG.

Pacemaker Controls

The typical pulse generator (Figure 19–5) has the following controls:

■ *On-Off Switch:* Activates or deactivates the pacemaker.

■ *Output/Current (mA):* Changes the energy level generated that is needed to capture the heart. The output is measured in milliamperes (mA). This adjusts the strength of the generated impulse. Turning the dial higher increases the output.

■ *Basic Pacing Rate:* Sets the pacing rate as impulses per minute.

■ *Sensing Ability/Sensitivity:* Adjusts the pacemaker's sensitivity for detecting natural cardiac activity. The sensitivity selector sets the native beats's signal strength in millivolts (mV) that will inhibit the pacemaker. The sensitivity ranges between 1.0 mV (most sensitive) and 20 mV (least sensitive).

Clinical Note During emergency pacemaker application, a pacemaker's sensitivity dial should be set to the most sensitive level (1.0 mV), which will cause the pacemaker to register even a very weak signal. The sensitivity dial should be slowly decreased to avoid having the pacemaker respond to artifact. The highest setting, 20 mV, makes the device least sensitive, causing the pacemaker to respond to only the strongest cardiac signals .

Clinical Note During emergency pacemaker application, once the pacemaker rate is set, the output dial should set to the upper mA limit to ensure immediate cardiac capture. Then it should be gradually decreased until capture is lost. The milliamperage output should be increased until recapture occurs.

Pacemaker Functions

Every pacemaker shares the following basic functions of pacing and capture, pacing threshold, programmability, sensing and inhibition.

Pacing and Capture

A small electrical pulse stimulus is formed by the generator and sent via the pacing electrode to cause the myocardium to depolarize (Table 19–2). When a pacemaker impulse results in myocardial depolarization, the pulse stimulus is said to have "captured the ventricle." The ECG tracing shows a **capture beat** as a depolarization complex that immediately follows a pacemaker spike signal (Figure 19–7). A properly functioning pacemaker results in a cardiac depolarization for each pacemaker spike, and is referred to as 1:1 capture, indicating that one depolarization is present for each pacing stimulus (Figure 19–8). Normal 1:1 capture is shown in Figure 19–9. When the pacemaker has a single lead activating the right ventricle, the ECG shows a single spike per com-

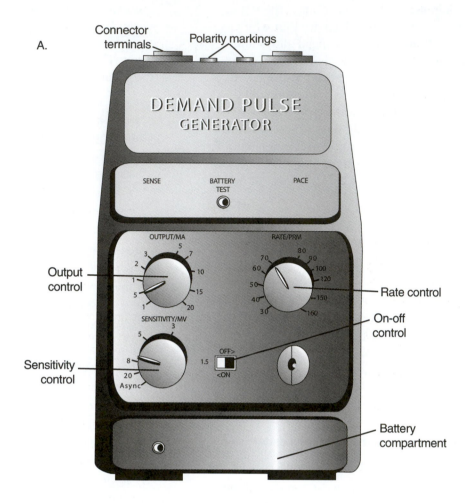

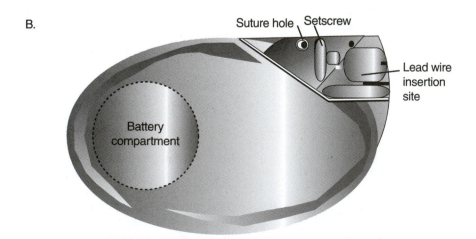

Figure 19–5 (A) A temporary pulse generator that is not implanted in the patient. The exrenal pulse generator is secured to the patient's body. Controls on the face allow the operator to adjust the settings. (B) Permanent generator that is implanted inside the patient's chest, and initial settings are programmed before insertion. The settings can be adjusted after implantation by using a programming device that is held over the patient.

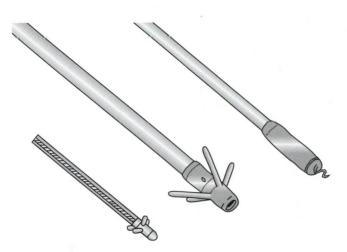

Figure 19–6 Transvenous electrode tips are designed to securely anchor the ends to the myocardium.

plex followed by a distorted QRS complex having a left bundle branch block shape (Figure 19–11). Since dual-chamber pacemakers stimulate both the atria and the ventricles, the ECG shows an atrial spike followed by a P wave, as well as, a ventricular spike associated with a wide QRS complex a short time later (Figure 19–11).

Pacing Threshold

The pacing threshold is the minimum amount of energy output needed to cause consistent cardiac capture.

Table 19–2 Pacemaker Properties

- **Discharging/ Firing:** Pulse generator discharges at a set rate per minute.

- **Output Pulse:** Electrical pulse intended to stimulate the myocardium and the energy level is expressed in voltage.

- **Sensing:** Pacemaker detects natural cardiac (electrical) activity.

- **Capturing/ Depolarization:** Pulse-generated impulse causes a cardiac depolarization or "captures" the heart.

- **Inhibition:** Pulse generator is inhibited when intrinsic cardiac activity is sensed.

- **Programmability:** Pacemaker functions can be adjusted noninvasively after insertion.

- **Sensing Threshold:** Minimal amount of energy needed to ensure consistent myocardial depolarization.

Programmability

In the past, pacemaker functions could only be set prior to insertion. Pacemakers are now fully programmable after implantation using noninvasive methods.

Sensing and Inhibition

Pacemakers must be able to sense intrinsic cardiac activity in order to prevent competition with native cardiac activity. When the pacemaker senses a native beat it will be inhibited. When a patient with a pacemaker has a natural heart rate that is faster than the programmed paced rate, any artificial pacemaker activity will not occur because the pacemaker has been inhibited (Figure 19–12).

ECG Interpretation Tip *The ECG tracing of an artificial pacemaker that fails to sense will show pacemaker spikes that are superimposed on the intrinsic P-QRS-T complexes. A pacemaker that fails to discharge due to oversensing will be inhibited by ECG artifact and pacemaker spikes will not occur where expected.*

Pacemaker Types

There are several basic types of pacemakers, some of which can be implanted internally, or applied externally on the chest wall, and can be used on an emergent, temporary, or permanent basis.

Internal Versus External Pacemakers

Internal and external pacing refers to the location of the pacing electrodes relative to the patient's chest wall. External pacemakers are the easiest and quickest way to pace during an emergency. For **transcutaneous pacing**, the pacing energy is applied to the chest wall using large adhesive electrodes, typically placed in an anterior-posterior position (Figure 19–13). This is also referred to as **transthoracic or external pacing**. Emergent external pacing is intended to temporarily stabilize the patient's rhythm until a more dependable device can be used. External pacing is the treatment of choice for symptomatic bradycardia.

Internal pacing electrodes are attached directly to the heart via wires that are advanced or "floated" into the right ventricle via large central veins, such as the subclavian. Internal electrodes can be permanently attached to an internally placed pulse generator or connected to a temporary external pacemaker that is securely attached to the patient.

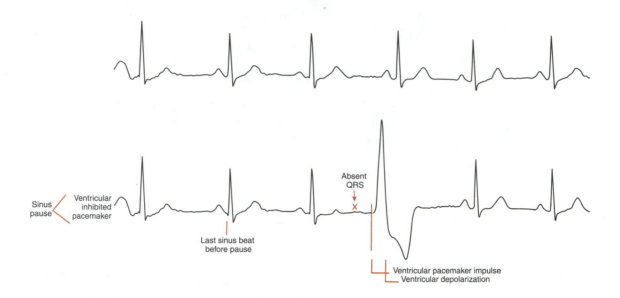

Figure 19-7 A normal functioning ventricular inhibited pacemaker is shown. (A) shows NSR; (B) shows a sinus pause.

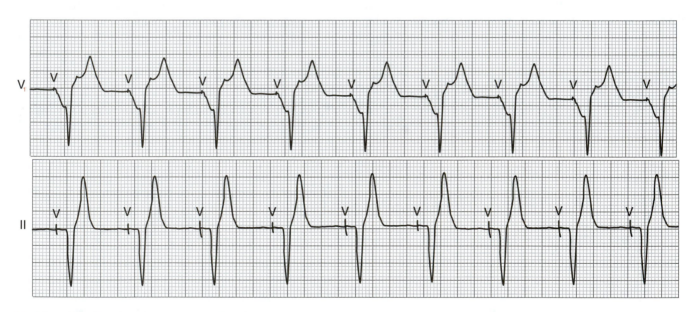

Figure 19-8 Normal ventricular capture. Ventricular spikes, which are labeled V, precede wide QRS complexes in the two ECG leads. No intrinsic rhythm is present and the pacemaker is set at a rate of 60 impulse/minute, which corresponds to a one second interval between beats. If an intrinsic complex is not sensed a pacing spike will occur after a one second escape interval.

Permanent Versus Temporary Devices

Pacemakers can be used permanently or for short-term emergent therapy, as in transient cases of advanced AV heart block. Temporary pacemakers may either be an external type, such as the transthoracic pacer, or transvenously inserted. Transthoracic external pacers are only employed for a few hours until a more stable pacing method can be accomplished. The transvenous route for emergent pacing can be used for several days

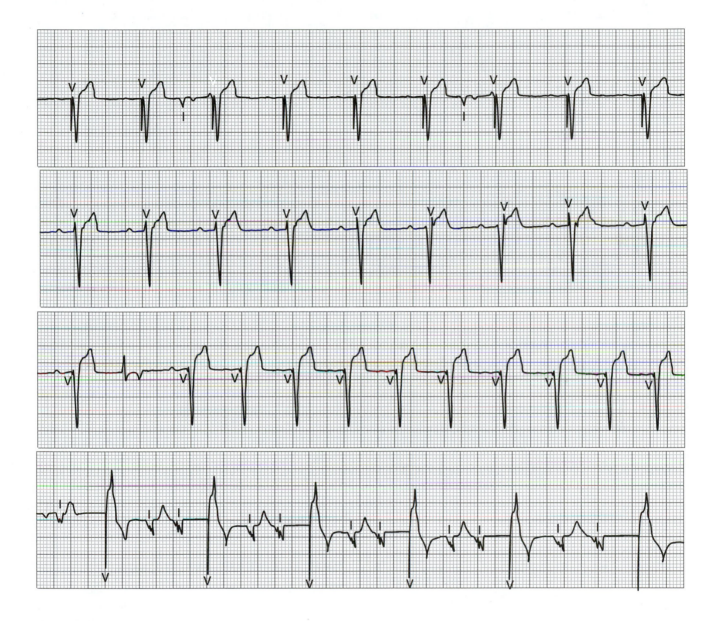

Figure 19-9 Ventricular capture examples. (A) The larger complexes (number 1, 2, 4–7, and 9) are paced impulses (labeled "V"), while the underlying rhythm is atrial fibrillation. Intrinsic beats are labeled as "I." (B) All of the beats are pacemaker complexes. The underlying rhythm is complete AV heart block. (C) All beats except for the second beat are pacemaker complexes. The underlying rhythm cannot be assessed because most of the tracing shows pacing function. (D) Beats number 2, 5, and 8 are pacer complexes. The underlying rhythm is a bundle branch block.

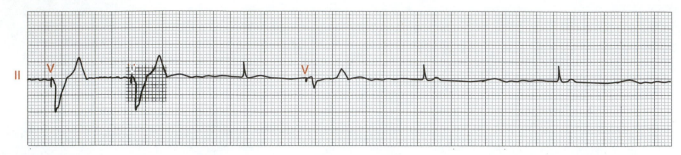

Figure 19–10 Normal ventricular sensing with pacemaker-related bundle branch block shapes. The underlying rhythm is atrial fibrillation. The artificial pacemaker rate is set at 50 bpm and has an escape interval of 1.2 seconds, which can be determined by evaluating the first two complexes labeled as V. The third complex is narrow and inhibits the artificial pacemaker. The 4th complex demonstrates a ventricular spike ("V") with a wide QRS complex. The last two beats occur following a period that is clearly less than the escape interval and inhibits the pacemaker.

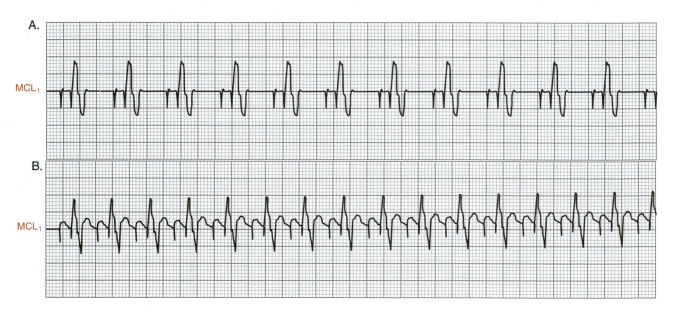

Figure 19–11 AV sequential pacing with a dual-chamber pacemaker. There are two pacemaker spikes for each cardiac complex. (A) The first impulse spike is followed by a P wave, while the second spike stimulates a QRS-T complex. (B) AV sequential pacemaker in which both atrial and ventricular pacer spikes are associated with P waves and QRS complexes, respectively.

until the need for permanent pacing is determined. In some patients, when the heart block or bradycardia subsides, the pacemaker can be discontinued.

Permanent pacemakers are used to treat chronic conditions, such as a slow heart rate caused by sick sinus syndrome. Permanent pacemaker insertion requires a brief surgical procedure, which is accomplished using local anesthesia, during which the pulse-generator is inserted into the subcutaneous tissue of the upper chest. The leads are transvenously threaded into place within the right ventricle (Figure 19–14).

Single Versus Dual Chamber Pacing

Pacemakers can stimulate either the ventricles, the atria, or the atria and ventricles, known as single- or dual-chamber devices, respectively. Most **single-chamber pacemakers** pace the right ventricle although if AV conduction is normal but the sinus node is defective, an atrial pacemaker can be used (Figure 19–15). Until recently, most pacemakers were single-chamber devices but because of clear advantages in certain groups of patients, more dual-chamber pacemakers are now being implanted.

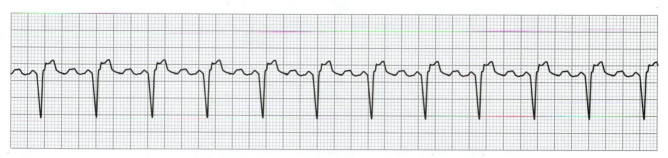

Figure 19–12 Sinus rhythm with a first degree AV block in a patient with an artificial pacemaker. The artificial pacemaker does not discharge when there is normal cardiac activity. In this case, the pacemaker was implanted for periods of sick sinus syndrome associated with symptomatic episodes of bradycardia.

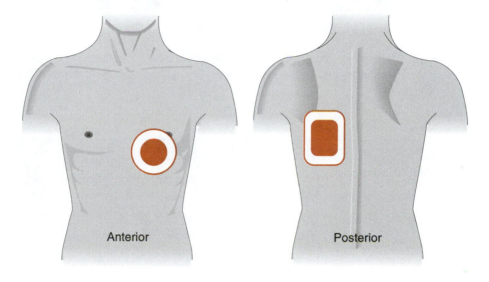

Anterior   Posterior

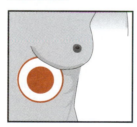

Female patients:
Position electrode
under breast

Figure 19–13 External pacing electrodes. Special pacing pads, which contain the electrodes surrounded by adhesive, are attached to the anterior and posterior chest wall. The relatively large size is needed in order to decrease the resistance from the chest wall.

Single-chamber pacemakers usually pace the right ventricle and the atria continue to beat without regard to ventricular activity. The resulting lack of AV coordination leads to a lower stroke volume than obtained with atrial or dual chamber pacing.

The major advantage of dual-chamber pacemakers over single-chamber devices is that their function more closely simulates natural cardiac activity because of coordinated atrial and ventricular function. Dual-chamber pacers produce a higher cardiac output than single-

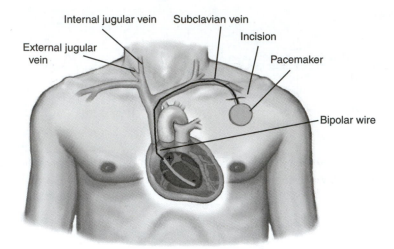

Figure 19-14 Permanently implanted pacemaker. The pulse generator is implanted in the subcutaneous tissue of the right or left anterior upper chest area just below the clavicle. The typical scar and pacemaker bulge can be easily detected.

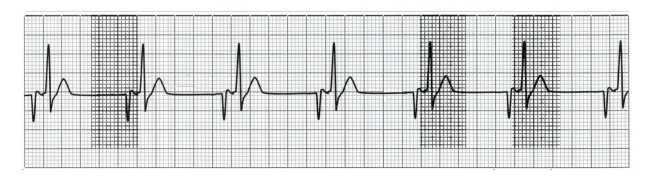

Figure 19-15 Atrial pacing with normal A-V conduction. An atrial pacemaker stimulates the atria if intrinsic P waves are not sensed within the programmed period (for example, one second when the rate is set at 60/minute).

chamber devices since atrial contraction precedes ventricular stimulation and the ventricles fill completely before contraction. The increased sophistication of dual-chamber pacemakers causes a greater battery drain and a shorter battery life.

Dual-chamber pacemakers have one lead in the atrium and another in the ventricle (Figure 19–2). In dual-chamber systems, when a P-wave is sensed a ventricular pulse is triggered if an associated QRS is not detected within a 0.2 second interval. This is an effective way of maintaining normal atrial-ventricular coordination, especially when the sinus node is functioning normally and can regulate the heart rate, such as during complete heart block. Dual-chamber pacemakers are especially suited for younger and active individuals who benefit from a higher cardiac output and the ability to quickly change cardiac output.

When stable sinus activity is present, a dual-chamber pacemaker is often used because the sensed P wave can

be used to trigger the ventricular impulse (Figure 19–16). Dual-chamber pacemakers allow the sinus node to continue to set the cardiac rate and be responsive to changing conditions requiring different heart rates. The patient still has the ability to increase the sinus discharge as more cardiac output is needed and the pacer will trigger the ventricles to "keep pace" with the atria.

PACEMAKER PACING RATES AND INTERVALS

The pacing rate is the number of times per minute the pacemaker is set to discharge if there is no sensed cardiac activity. The **pacing rate** is also referred to as the backup or demand rate and is analogous to how the body's own escape pacemakers function. For example, if the pacemaker is set to discharge at 60 impulses/minute, the ECG will show a pacemaker spike every

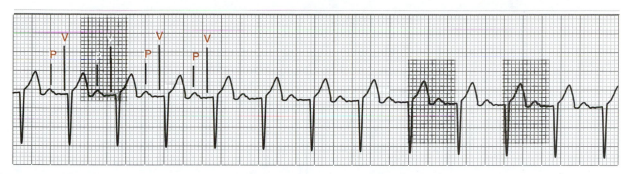

Figure 19-16 Normal pacing in dual-chamber pacemaker. The underlying rhythm is regular sinus with a dual-chamber pacemaker. The P waves, labeled P, are sensed and an atrial spike does not occur. After a programmed AV delay, because QRS complexes are not sensed, a ventricular pacing spike, labeled V, is triggered to maintain AV coordination. The major advantage of this system is that it allows a functioning sinus node to retain control of the rate.

second. As a safety function, a **ceiling pacer rate** is also set, above which the pacemaker will not discharge. A ceiling rate 150 impulses/minute, for instance, protects the heart from being overstimulated. The **automatic interval** is the time period between successively paced beats (Figure 19–17). A related concept is the **paced** or **escape interval**, which refers to the time period between when a pacer senses a spontaneous complex and when the succeeding paced beat occurs. The escape interval determines how long the pacemaker device waits before discharging after a cardiac pause. For instance, if the pacing rate was set at 60 per minute, the escape interval would be one second (Figure 19–18). Another example involves an artificial pacemaker that has been set to fire 50 times per minute; the pacer will discharge every 1.2 seconds until intrinsic cardiac activity is detected.

Pacemaker Discharge Modes

The earliest pacemakers discharged at regular intervals regardless of the underlying cardiac activity and this mode is termed an asynchronous device.

Asynchronous pacing, also termed fixed rate discharge, is mentioned mainly out of historical interest because this mode is no longer used except during emergency situations (Table 19–3). An asynchronous pacemaker does not utilize a sensing function. A major disadvantage of an asynchronous discharge mode is that the pacemaker stimulation interferes with intrinsic cardiac activity. An asynchronous pacemaker can not be coordinated with natural pacemaker function. There is a slight chance that an asynchronous pacing impulse can strike during the vulnerable phase and cause ventricular tachycardia (Figure 19–19).

Demand pacing is the mode used in permanent pacemakers. The demand mode functions in a standby role, during which the pacemaker's discharge is inhibited by sensed intrinsic cardiac activity and waits until a prolonged ECG pause is detected before discharging. The demand mode allows a pacemaker to work only when needed, thereby preserving battery life. Demand pacemaker function also prevents competition between the artificial pacemaker and natural cardiac activity. Figure 19–20 demonstrates how a pacemaker's demand function is applied to an isolated case of SA block as well as cases of combined SA and AV block.

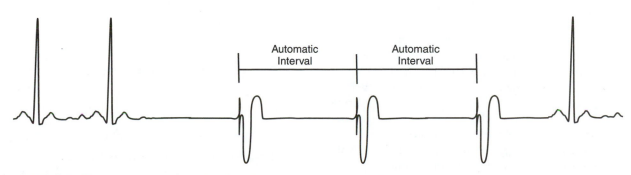

Figure 19-17 The automatic interval is the distance between paced beats.

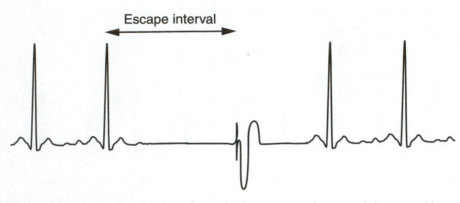

Figure 19–18 The escape interval is distance from the last intrinsic beat until the paced beat. It may be longer or equal to the automatic interval (Figure 19–17).

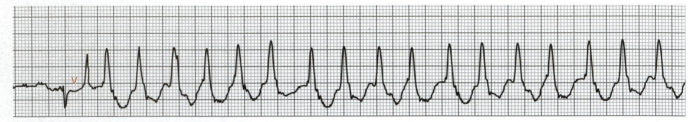

Figure 19–19 An asynchronous pacemaker stimulus occurred during the vulnerable period and caused ventricular tachycardia. The pacemaker spike occurs during the vulnerable phase of the T wave of the 2nd intrinsic beat. Ventricular tachycardia resulted.

Rate Responsive Pacemakers

A special feature employed in some pacemakers allows the device to respond to a patient's changing activity level. To increase the heart's cardiac output, the pacemaker automatically increases the discharge rate. This programmable rate function allows the pacemaker to match its discharge rate with the patient's activity level and is termed **rate responsive pacing**. Rate responsiveness allows a pacemaker to adapt to patients' changing activity levels, similar to how a natural sinus node functions. For instance, the pacer may be set to deliver a baseline rate of 70 pacing impulses per minute, but a rate responsive function would allow the pacer to gradually increase to 120/minute when the patient jogs or swims. An activity sensor monitors one of several bodily functions and then alters the pacemaker rate to match the cardiac needs. The most common rate adaptive sensor detects muscle activity or pressure-vibration (see Figure 19–4). When the sensor is activated, the pacemaker increases the pulse generator's discharge rate. Walking or running produces upper arm or chest vibrations that stimulates the sensor, which, in turn, increases the paced heart rate. Conversely, as muscle activity decreases or as the walking person slows down, the sensor is stimulated less frequently and the pulse generated rate decreases. Rate modulation allows a pacemaker to more closely mimic the sensing activity of the sinus node.

PACEMAKER PROGRAMMING

To adjust the pacemaker's function after insertion, each manufacturer produces a magnetic field programmer, which is able to send commands to the device.

Table 19–3 Comparison of Pacemaker Modes

Fixed Rate/ Asynchronous Discharge:

- Pacemaker discharges without regard to intrinsic cardiac activity.
- Lacks sensing mode.
- Interferes with intrinsic cardiac activity.
- Used only during emergencies

Demand/ Inhibited Discharge:

- Discharges in absence of intrinsic cardiac activity.
- Incorporates sensing function.
- Coordinates function with intrinsic cardiac activity
- Inhibited by intrinsic cardiac activity
- Used in all current pacemakers.

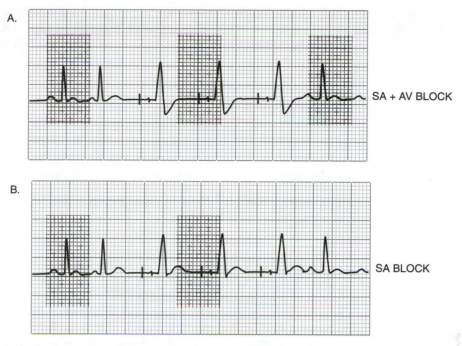

Figure 19-20 Diagram of QRS-inhibited sequential atrial and ventricular pacing. (A) In the presence of both SA and AV blocks, failure of a ventricular depolarization to occur after atrial capture will trigger ventricular pacing. Both chambers will be paced. (B) In an isolated SA block, when atrial impulses and ventricular depolarizations are not sensed within the set intervals, a paced atrial impulse occurs. Since AV conduction is normal, the atrial impulse is conducted into the ventricles resulting in a QRS complex.

Pacemakers are well insulated and there is little risk for inadvertent reprogramming from other magnetic sources, such as motors, microwave ovens, or small "refrigerator" magnets. But strong magnetic fields from power generators and MRI scanners *may interfere* with normal pacemaker function.

Pacemaker Identification Codes

The pacemaker device type or model can be identified by using a standard code that describes the lead location, as well as the pacing modes available for the pulse generator. The code has a three or four letter designation that refers to the chamber(s) paced, chamber(s) sensed, response mode, and indicates if the device is programmable (Table 19–4).

Common Program Modes

The most common program modes are designated with the following codes:

- **V-O-O:** the ventricle is paced in an asynchronous (fixed rate) mode that lacks sensing ability. This is the most commonly used temporary device in emergency cardiac care.

- **V-V-I:** the ventricle is both paced and sensed. When a QRS or R wave is detected, the pulse generator is inhibited (Figure 19–21A). This is the simplest type of permanently implanted demand device.

- **V-V-I-R:** the same pacemaker as the V-V-I type aside from the addition of a rate modulating sensor. This mode is commonly used in cases of atrial fibrillation to obtain a greater cardiac output.

- **D-V-I:** pacing occurs in the atrium as well as the ventricle. When R waves are sensed, atrial and ventricle pacing is inhibited (Figure 19–21B).

- **D-D-D:** pacing and sensing occur in both chambers, inhibiting either atrial or ventricular output when a P and/or R wave is detected. This type of pacemaker requires sinus rhythm to function optimally (Figure 19–22).

- **D-D-D-R:** same as a D-D-D mode but also has a rate modulating sensor.

The pacemaker code can be also used to describe all possible modes for any particular pacing generator, including indications such as cardioversion or anti-tachycardiac functions (Table 19–5).

Table 19–4 Pacemaker Code Letter Options

- **Chamber:** A = atrium, V = ventricle, D = dual (atrium and ventricle), O = neither atrial nor ventricle
- I = **inhibited pacing mode** after a sensed native P or R wave
- T = **triggered ventricular pacing** following a sensed P wave
- D = **dual mode** (I + T)
- R = **rate responsive**

First letter: chamber paced	Second letter: chamber sensed	Third letter: mode of response	Fourth Letter: programmable
A, V, D	A, V, D, O	I, T, D, O	R

The most widely used external pacing systems are the simple V-V-I or V-O-O devices, which indicate that the ventricles are paced while the ventricle may or may not be sensed. If intrinsic cardiac activity is present, the external pacemaker can be set in either a sensing or demand mode.

External transcutaneous pacing (TCP) is the major non-drug intervention for the treatment of life-threatening bradycardia and early asystolic arrest but is *not* effective in capturing the ventricle during ventricular fibrillation (Figure 19–23). TCP is now routinely done during out-of-hospital resuscitations because newer components and smaller size. Almost all currently available portable defibrillators now include a pacemaker option.

PACEMAKER MALFUNCTION

There are two basic types of pacemaker malfunction: problems with capturing the myocardium and problems with sensing intrinsic cardiac activity. In order for mechanical capture of either the atrium or ventricle to occur, an adequate amount of electrical energy must be delivered so that the chamber can depolarize. Sensing disorders interfere with a pacemaker's ability to detect the need for pacing as well as coordination betweeen artificial and intrinsic pacemaker activity (Table 19–6).

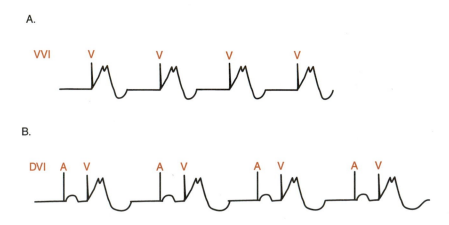

Figure 19–21 Pacing modes. (A) During V-V-I pacing, only the ventricle is sensed and paced. (B) During D-V-I or fixed rate AV sequential pacing, the atrium and ventricle are each paced at. Atrial and ventricular pacing stimuli are separated by the programmed AV interval. ("A" is atrial pacing stimulus; "V" is ventricular pacing stimulus.)

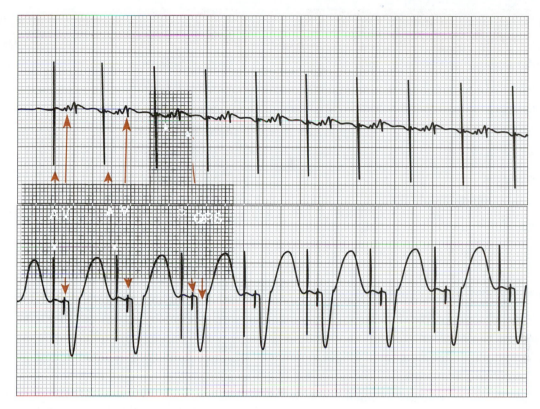

Figure 19–22 Normal AV pacing by a D-D-D pacemaker recorder on a simultaneous two-lead ECG tracing. This dual chamber pacemaker is pacing at f 85 bpm. Atrial pacing spikes ("A") occurs just ahead of associated P waves, demonstrating normal atrial capture. After a short predetermined AV delay, a ventricular pacing spike ("V") follows with normal ventricular capture. In two simultaneously recorded leads, the appearance of the pacing spikes, P waves, and QRS complexes appear different in each lead but record the same electrical activity. The ventricular pacing spike can be barely seen in V1 (strip A) whie the P waves are best seen in lead II in strip B.

Output Failure

The pacemaker generator can fail to deliver a sufficient because of several problems:

- *Battery depletion, a fractured or dislodged lead, or pacemaker oversensing are causes of failure to generate a pacemaker stimulus.* This type of malfunction usually presents dramatically as fatigue or lightheadedness, abrupt loss of consciousness, or even a sudden brady-asystolic arrest in pacemaker-dependent patients (Figure 19–24).

- *Failure to capture the chamber.* A weak pacemaker impulse will not have enough energy to stimulate the myocardium. The ECG will reflect failure to capture as a pacing (impulse) spike without an associated P wave or QRS-T complex (Figure 19–25).

> ***ECG Interpretation Tip*** *It is important to be aware that bipolar leads often produce tiny pacing artifacts in some ECG leads; sometimes pacing impulses can be identified only after evaluating multiple leads (Figure 19–26).*

- *Increased capture threshold* occurs when the heart requires a higher than normal stimulus to be activated. Increased capture threshold can occur due to infarction or ischemia, acidemia, hyperkalemia, new medications—especially antidysrhythmic and antiseizure drugs. A higher then expected depolarization threshold typically occurs during the first month following pacemaker insertion.

Sensing Failure

Failure to sense, or undersensing, occurs when a pacemaker is unable to detect intrinsic cardiac activity.

Table 19-5 Types of Pacing Modalities

Ventricular Pacing

- Continuous asynchronous (V-O-O)
- QRS-inhibited (V-V-I)
- QRS-triggered (V-V-T)
- P-triggered (V-A-T)

Atrial Pacing

- Continuous asynchronous (A-O-O)
- P-inhibited (A-A-I)
- P-triggered (A-A-T)
- QRS-inhibited (AV-I)

AV Sequential Pacing

- Continuous (D-O-O)
- QRS-inhibited (D-V-I)
- P-inhibited atrial pacing, P-triggered ventricular pacing, and QRS-inhibited ventricular pacing (D-D-D)
- **External /Transcutaneous Pacemaker**

Reprinted from Morse D, Steiner RM, and Parsonnet V. A Guide to Cardiac Pacemakers; Philadelphia: FA Davis: 1983: Table 3–1; p. 72

Table 19-6 Pacemaker Malfunction Types

Output Failure

- Generator failure
- Failure to capture

Sensing Failure

- Undersensing
- Oversensing

Common causes of pace sensing failure include a change in the rhythm, such as the development of atrial or ventricular fibrillation, battery depletion, a fractured or dislodged lead, and as previously mentioned, a high depolarization threshold occurs during the first month following implantation.

Pacemaker oversensing occurs when the pacer interprets electrical noise artifact as intrinsic cardiac activity and fails to fire. The ECG will have an abnormally long pause without a pacer spike because movement artifact has been misidentified as intrinsic cardiac activity (Figure 19–29). Other commonly misidentified signals include T or P waves or *myopotentials* generated by chest wall muscle activity.

EVALUATION OF A PATIENT WITH AN ARTIFICIAL PACEMAKER

The presence of an artificial pacemaker does not change the general approach to a patient, the initial evaluation, or treatment. Because modern pacemakers are durable and exremely reliable, they are rarely the cause of a cardiac emergency and a thorough evaluation for other problems is critical.

Normally, if the pacemaker is set to discharge at 60 bpm, the pacemaker will wait one second and will trigger a pacing stimulus if intrinsic activity is not detected (Figure 19–27A). Failure to sense is recognized when a pacer spike occurring in an inappropriate location, such as within or shortly following a P wave or QRS complex—which should have inhibited a properly working pacemaker (Figure 19–27B and 19–28)

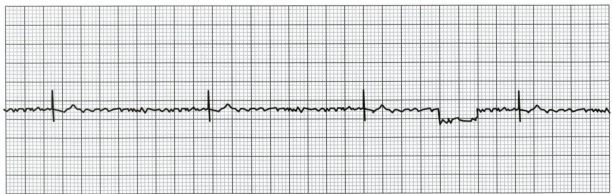

Figure 19–23 This V-V-I pacemaker is not sensing the fine, small amplitude ventricular fibrillation waves and continues to generate pacing spikes without ventricular capture. Fine ventricular fibrillation is often difficult to detect in a single lead and this rhythm strip can be mistaken for pacemaker malfunction in an asystolic patient.

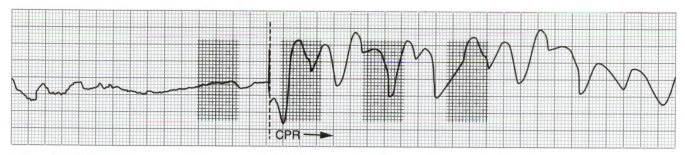

Figure 19–24 Failure to pace. The patient is having an asystolic cardiac arrest, undergoing CPR, and known to have a V-V-I pacemaker. The rhythmic baseline fluctuations are due to CPR artifact (marked: "CPR resumed—>"). Pacing spikes arenot observed when CPR is halted and this rhythm strip is consistent with failure to generate pacing stimulus.

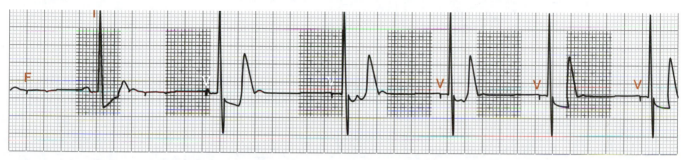

Figure 19–25 Failure to capture. The initial pacemaker spike, labeled "F," fails to generate a ventricular depolarization (capture). The first QRS-T complex is a sinus beat. The remaining complexes are pacemaker-initiated beats (indicated by a "V") with normal capture.

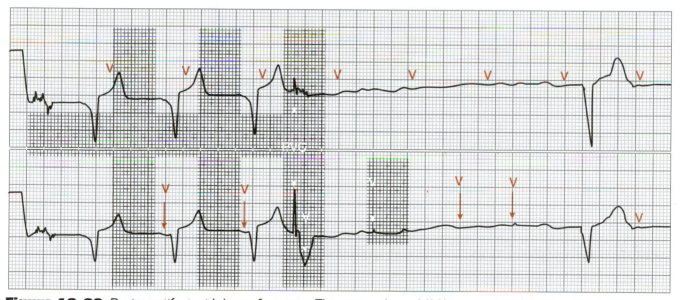

Figure 19–26 Pacing artifact with loss of capture. This patient has a V-V-I pacemaker set at a rate of 85 bpm with intermittent loss of ventricular capture. Ventricular pacing artifact ("V") can be clearly seen only in lead MCL$_5$. The pacemaker also did not sense the native complex or the premature ventricular complex ("PVC") as evidenced by a pacing spike in the T wave.

Clinical History for Pacemaker Patients

In order evaluate a pacemaker, information regarding the type and mode of the pacemaker and the date it was implanted should be obtained. Every patient should carry an identification card containing pacemaker-related information. But when the patient does not, identification of a pacemaker pocket scar and typical chest wall bulge should lead to the following questions, which will likely provide some useful information:

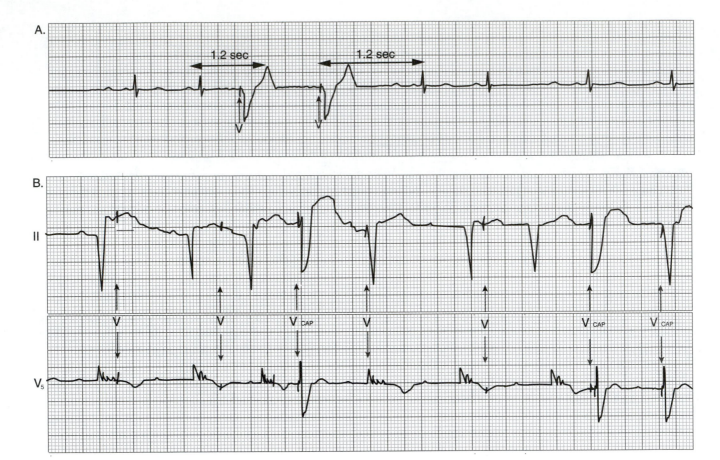

Figure 19-27 Series of ECGs showing normal function in A and failure to sense in B.(A) V-V-I pacemaker with normal sensing. The rhythm is a sick sinus syndrome with a V-V-I pacemaker set a rate of 50 bpm. After a pause of 1.2 seconds during which a QRS is not sensed, a ventricular spike ("V") is seen with normal ventricular capture. (B) V-V-I pacemaker with ventricular undersensing. The rhythm is a sinus rhythm with a first-degree AV block. A V-V-I pacemaker does not sense all of the intrinsic rhythm. Ventricular spikes occur every second (labeled "V") and fall predominantly during the ventricular refractory period, that is, within the QRS, ST segment, or T wave). When a ventricular spike intermittently falls during a nonrefractory period a ventricular capture ("Vcap") results.

- *"Why was the pacemaker inserted?"* The patient may volunteer that syncope, myocardial infarction, heart valve infection or replacement, or a slow heart rate was the reason.

- *"What year was it implanted?"* Older dual-chamber pacemakers had an expected longevity of 4 to 6 years while newer pacemakers last 8 to 12 years. If a pacemaker is near its expected expiration date, battery depletion should be considered as a possible cause of the patient's complaint.

- *"When was the pacemaker last adjusted (reprogrammed or interrogated)?"* Occasionally, a subtle change in the characteristics of a pacemaker can cause a significant malfunction. Typically, patients have their pacemakers evaluated monthly with a complete evaluation or programming once or twice a year depending on whether they are pacemaker dependent and whether the pacemaker is a single- or dual-chamber device.

- *"What is your usual resting pulse rate?"* Patients count and record their pulses each day. This monitoring information is helpful in assessing the patient who presents with an extreme rate change.

Other useful sources of information for pacemaker data include the patient's doctor and the manufacturer of the pacer, if known (Table 19–7).

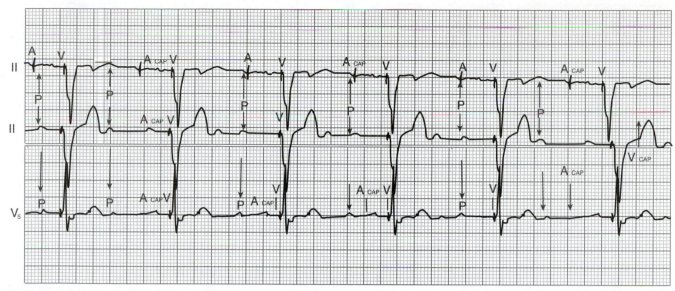

Figure 19–28 D-D-D pacemaker with atrial undersensing. The underlying rhythm is sinus at a rate of 65 to 70 bpm. The P waves ("P"), however, are not sensed and the dual-chamber pacemaker fires atrial ("A") and ventricular ("V") spikes, which intermittently capture the atrium ("Acap") and the ventricle is consistently captured.

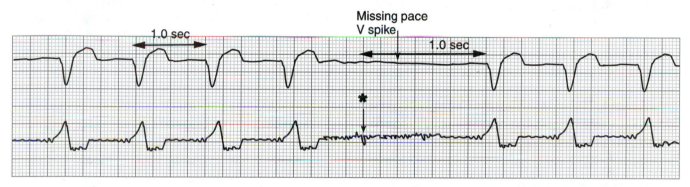

Figure 19–29 Ventricular oversensing. An ECG pause occurs during monitoring of this patient with a V-V-I pacemaker set a rate of 60 bpm. The escape interval is set at a 1 second, yet the asystolic pause is 1.8 seconds so that a paced beat that should have terminated the ECG pause did not occur. Muscular artifact is identified (labeled "*") and the pacemaker "oversensed" these muscle potentials as a ventricular impulse and inhibited the pacemaker.

Evaluation of Artificial Pacemaker Function

Pacing complicates the basic ECG assessment of cardiac rhythm because stimulus spikes are superimposed onto the familiar P-QRS-T complex. An understanding of the basic functions of pacing and sensing is all that is required to decipher the pacemaker function along with the patient's natural rhythm. ECG assessment proceeds as with any tracing:

- *Underlying Rhythm.* The ECG is assessed for the basic underlying rhythm and for the presence of intrinsic cardiac activity (Table 19–8). When the ventricular rate 60/minute or greater, is pacing artifact is not expected.

- *Electrode Location.* If pacemaker artifacts are visible on the ECG tracing, determine if the pacemaker electrode is positioned in the atrium, ventricle, or within both. If atrial *and* ventricular pacing spikes are present, then a dual-chamber pacemaker is present (Figure 19–30). If the pacer spike is followed by a wide QRS complex it is likely a ventricular pacemaker, and if the spike is followed by a P wave, it is an atrial pacemaker.

- *Capture.* Determine if appropriate 1:1 capture follows each pacing artifact. If 1:1 capture is not present, a loss of capture is present.

Table 19–7 Manufacturers' Central Referral Telephone Numbers

Pacesetter	800-423-5611
Medtronic	800-328-2518
Intermedics	800-231-2330
CPI	800-227-3422
Telectronics	800-525-7042 (also Cordis)
ELA Medical	800-352-6466

■ *Sensing*. When the ECG reveals underlying cardiac activity, determine if atrial and/or ventricular activity is being sensed normally? If there are unexpected paced beats, they may be caused by undersensing. When a prolonged pause occurs, oversensing is a common cause. Try to identify if the pacemaker has misidentified a P waves or QRS complex. If no P wave or QRS complexes are present, a "no output" pacing system (pulse generator failure) or oversensing exists.

Table 19–8 Assessment of ECG Pacing Rhythms

■ Assess the underlying rhythm

■ Is intrinsic activity present?

■ Identify pacing spikes

■ Identify atrial, ventricular, or A-V sequential pacing is occurring.

■ Is there appropriate 1:1 capture?

■ Determine if there is appropriate atrial and/or ventricular sensing

■ Is a P wave or QRS absent, as seen with in undersensing?

■ Is there a pause caused by oversensing or failure of output?

Clinical Note *Pacemaker functioning can be tested in the hospital by holding a strong magnet above a patient's chest because the magnetic field closes an "open/close"*

*switch, termed a **"reed" switch** on the pulse generator. When the reed switch is closed, the pacemaker function changes to an asynchronous or non-sensing mode. This converts a pacemaker from a "demand" system to a "fixed rate" system and permits assessment of the pacing and capture function.*

IMPLANTABLE CARDIOVERTER-DEFIBRILLATORS (ICDs)

Between 350,000 and 400,000 Americans die each year from **sudden cardiac death**, the vast majority from ventricular tachycardia and ventricular fibrillation before the patients arrive at the hospital. As increasing numbers of patients survive sudden cardiac death, the use of an implantable cardioverter-defibrillator, or ICD, continues to grow. While 6,000 ICDs were implanted in 1991, currently more than 50,000 patients have ICDs, and around 80,000 ICDs will be implanted worldwide per year by the end of 2000.

The primary goal of an ICD is to detect and treat episodes of life-threatening ventricular tachycardia or fibrillation. Clinical trials have demonstrated an impressive effectiveness of ICDs to abort recurrent ventricular fibrillation and ventricular tachycardia in over 80 percent of cases. Since the first ICD was implanted in 1980, significant advances in technology and the encouraging results of large clinical trials have resulted in widespread acceptance. Because they lack the side effects associated with long-term drug treatment, ICDs are considered as first-line therapy for chronic life-threatening ventricular dysrhythmias. New devices offer a variety of therapies in addition to defibrillation such as antibradycardic pacing.

Indications for ICD INSERTION

Candidates for ICD implantation are those at high risk for sudden cardiac death due to a ventricular tachydysrhythmia. Most patients with ICDs have been resuscitated at least once from a ventricular fibrillation/tachycardia cardiac arrest. Most ICD devices are implanted in patients with significant coronary artery disease and severe left ventricular dysfunction with a markedly diminished cardiac output. Automatic implantable defibrillators have saved numerous patients who have been refractory to or unsuited for antidysrhythmia medication.

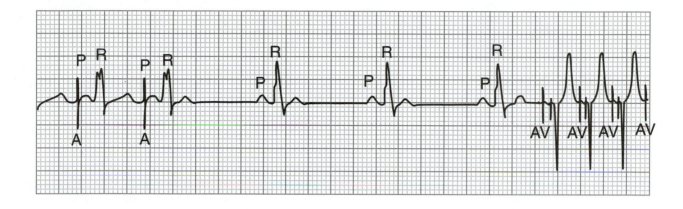

Figure 19–30 Dual-chambered pacemaker ECG rhythm. Atrial and ventricular pacing spikes are seen with this dual-chambered pacemaker rhythm. Three pacing modes are demonstrated: atrial pacing ("A") with normal ventricular conduction ("R"), sinus rhythm ("P") with normal ventricular conduction ("R"), and atrial with ventricular ("AV") sequential pacing during magnet application.

ICD Components

The ICD has three basic parts: the cardioverter/defibrillator generator; ventricular lead electrode; and the cardioversion electrode. The basic design is an extension of pacemaker technology.

ICD generators are larger than pacemaker generators, and originally had to be implanted in the subcutaneous tissues of the upper abdomen (Figure 19–31A) because early models were four times as big as pacemakers and three times as thick. Modern ICDs are less bulky but still weigh considerably more than pacemakers, primarily because large batteries are needed to develop a countershock charge. ICDs are implanted in the same area as pacemakers: within the chest wall's pectoral muscle just below the clavicle, where pacemakers are placed (Figure 19–31B). ICDs rapidly accumulate a large energy charge in holding cells or capacitors for high-energy cardioversion/ defibrillation.

ICDs can deliver **"tiered" antitachycardia pacing,** beginning with low energy electrical discharges of less than 1 joule. If not successful, the ICD follows then sends a series of high-energy shocks ranging from 0.1 to 30 joules in an escalating fashion until the dysrhythmia is terminated. If the rhythm spontaneously converts, the energy is dissipated within the system and the countershock is not delivered.

Early model ICD countershock electrodes required a thoracotomy, or surgical incision into the chest, for placement of epicardial defibrillation patches. A completely transvenous route using the subclavian vein defibrillator system is now used. One patch is affixed to the surface of the superior vena cava while the other barbed electrode is wedged into the muscle of the right ventricle.

ICD Functions

The ICD has two primary functions: dysrhythmia detection and countershock treatment. Some abnormal car-

Once the patient's rhythm disturbance is identified as ventricular tachycardia or fibrillation, an antitachycardic overdrive pacing protocol, using a step-wise increasing energy level countershocks, as well as high-energy unsynchronized defibrillation if required (Figure 19–32).

Evaluation of a Patient Receiving an ICD Counter-shock

As with pacemakers, the implantable cardioverter defibrillator does not alter the overall patient approach, the initial evaluation, or application of the standard emergency cardiac care treatment algorithms. Patients with ICD devices have severe underlying coronary artery disease or cardiomyopathy, and represent a significant clinical challenge. During an emergency situation, determining whether the ICD appropriately detected ventricular tachycardia or fibrillation is critical (Figure 19–33). Some common issues involved in ICD function are:

- *Refractory Ventricular Dysrhythmias.* If ventricular tachycardia or fibrillation continues despite ICD shocks, then standard transthoracic cardioversion or defibrillation should be performed. An alternative paddle position, such as anterior-posterior, may be effective in cases where patients have epicardial patches implanted, as the cardioversion energy may be partially dissipated by these patches.

- *Cardiopulmonary Resuscitation.* Individuals performing chest compressions on a patient with an ICD may receive a relatively low-energy shock, which is harmless. Standard dosing of epinephrine and antidysrhythmics should be given even if the ICD appears to be functioning normally. Standard external cardiac countershock should be done in the event of unsuccessful ICD shocks.

- *Inappropriate Shocks.* If clearly inappropriate shocks are occurring, such as during sinus rhythm in awake patients, placement of a magnet over the defibrillator can temporarily inhibit ICD function until it can be assessed. While this will prevent unneeded shocks, the patient will also no longer be protected against ventricular dysrhythmias.

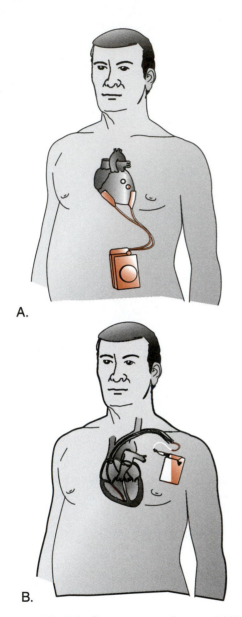

A.

B.

Figure 19–31 Comparison of original (A) and current (B) implantable cardio-defibrillator models. Modern ICDs are placed in the same location as pacemakers, are much lighter than early models, but are still much bulkier.

diac rhythms may meet certain of the criteria stored in the device's computer chip to determine if ventricular tachycardia is present. Rapid dysrhythmias may be due to atrial dysrhythmias, such as paroxysmal supraventricular tachycardia (PSVT) and even sinus tachycardia. To prevent benign dysrhythmias from being cardioverted unnecessarily, the ICD's dysrhythmia assessment algorithms specify the rate in addition to the QRS duration limits and rhythm pattern. The ICD automatically checks the dysrhythmia's rate characteristics against the device's dysrhythmia protocols.

Clinical Note *Magnet application to deactivate an ICD must be done with caution and only when a device is clearly malfunctioning. A standard pacemaker magnet placed over the ICD defibrillator will close the reed switch, as with pacemakers, and temporarily inhibit the detection of arrhythmias and delivery of shocks. In some models such as Ventak® (Cardiac Pacemakers, Inc.), magnet placement will result in a series of beep-ing tones that confirms deactivation of the device. After 30 seconds, a continuous tone will confirm ICD deactivation. Even temporary inhibition of ICD function should be reserved for use by highly experienced in-hospital staff certain of the diagnosis of inappropriate defibrillator shocks and prepared to manage the development of ventricular fibrillation.*

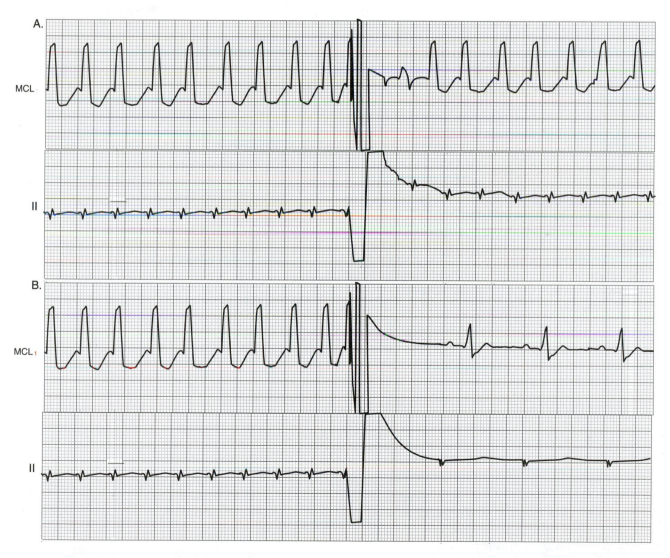

Figure 19–32 Escalating ICD shocks. The ICD senses the wide complex rapid rhythm and initiates a 2-Joule ("2J") cardioversion shock. After this fails to terminate the dysrhythmia, a "5J" cardioversion shock successfully converts the tachycardia to normal sinus rhythm. The cardioversion sequence may take up to 90 seconds to complete three cycles of anti-tachycardia overdrive pacing involving a stepwise increase in cardioversion energy.

2 joule shock ↓

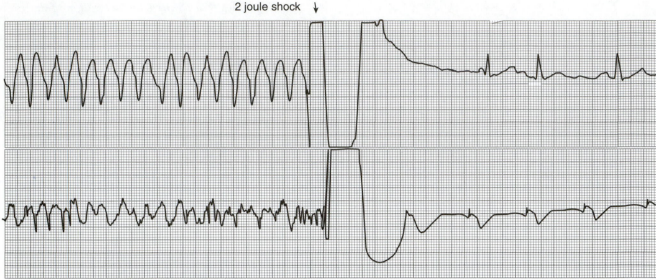

Figure 19-33 Normally functioning ICD. A very rapid, wide-complex tachycardia is appropriately sensed. The ICD delivers a defibrillation pulse of "2J," resulting in the ventricular tachycardia converting to normal sinus rhythm.

Lets Review

1. Artificial pacemakers consist of pulse generators and electrodes that sense intrinsic cardiac activity as well as pace the silent heart. The majority of permanent pacemakers are used to treat symptomatic bradycardia, caused by sick sinus syndrome, sinus block, or third-degree AV heart block.

2. Artificial pacemakers can be used to pace the atria, the ventricles, or both chambers.

3. An ECG with a normally functioning pacemaker system shows a cardiac response described as 1:1 capture, meaning that each pacemaker impulse elicits a cardiac depolarization.

4. Pacemaker impulses appear on the ECG as small spikes that immediately precedes an evoked cardiac complex.

5. A pacemaker that fails to sense, often has an ECG that shows pacemaker spikes superimposed on the intrinsic P-QRS-T complexes. A pacemaker that fails to discharge due to oversensing is often inhibited by ECG artifact.

6. Dual-chamber pacemakers stimulate the atria and ventricles, thereby producing a higher cardiac output than single-chamber devices. AV coordination is maintained with dual-chamber devices but not by single-chamber devices.

7. Pacemakers that activate the atria and the ventricles preserve coordination of atrioventricular activity.

8. The pacing rate or demand rate is the number of spikes per minute that occur if no intrinsic cardiac activity is sensed.

9. The escape interval, also termed the paced interval, refers to the pause before a pacer spike is expected.

10. The automatic interval is the time period between successively paced beats.

11. The paced or escape interval is the period between when a pacemaker senses a spontaneous complex until the paced beat occurs.

12. Asynchronous pacing discharges regardless of the underlying intrinsic cardiac activity, leading to interference. Asynchronous pacing is no longer employed except for external pacing in emergency situations.

13. Permanent pacemakers have a demand pacing function, which means that the pacemaker's discharge is inhibited by intrinsic cardiac activity. The demand mode waits until a preprogrammed ECG pause is detected before discharging.

14. Pacemakers can be identified using a standard three or four letter code that describes the lead location, as well as the pacing modes available for the pulse generator. The code refers to the chamber(s) paced, chamber(s) sensed, response mode, and whether the device is programmable.

15. External transcutaneous pacing is the nondrug therapy of choice to treat unstable bradycardia. Compared with drug therapy, transcutaneous pacing offers greater precision over the heart rate.

16. There are two basic types of pacemaker malfunction: problems with the stimulus output needed to capture the ventricle, and problems with sensing intrinsic cardiac activity.

17. One type of capture failure is caused by an inadequate impulse stimulus strength that does not have enough energy to stimulate the myocardium.

18. Failure to capture is identified when the ECG pattern shows a pacing spike without an associated P wave or QRS-T complex. Failure to capture assumes that the stimulus occurs during a period when it should have caused capture, that is, not during a refractory period.

19. Failure to sense, or undersensing, involves a pacemaker that is not detecting intrinsic cardiac activity.

20. A pacemaker's failure to sense will have pacer spikes within or shortly following a P wave or QRS complex when they should have been inhibited.

21. Common causes for failure to sense include a change in the rhythm, such as the development of atrial or ventricular fibrillation, battery depletion, a fractured or dislodged lead, inappropriate programming, and due to myocardial changes during the month after implantation.

22. The ICD's primary goal is to detect and treat life-threatening ventricular tachycardia or fibrillation. ICDs have considerable success aborting recurrent ventricular fibrillation and ventricular tachycardia (over 80 percent of cases).

23. Candidates for ICD implantation include those at risk for sudden cardiac death due to ventricular tachydysrhythmias. Most patients with ICDs have been resuscitated at least once from a ventricular fibrillation/tachycardia arrest.

24. The ICD's three basic parts include: the cardioverter-defibrillator generator, ventricular lead electrode, and the cardioversion electrode.

25. Presence of an ICD does not alter the overall patient approach, the initial evaluation, or the standard emergency cardiac care treatment algorithm.

Glossary

Artificial pacemaker Device used to treat failure of the heart's electrical conduction system by generating a tiny electrical impulse in order to stimulate the heart.

Artificially paced beat Cardiac complex initiated by an artificial pacemaker.

Asynchronous pacing Electrical discharges occuring at regular intervals regardless of the underlying cardiac activity; also known as fixed rate discharge and rarely used any longer.

Automatic interval Time period between successively paced beats.

Capture Ability of an artificial pacemaker to elicit myocardial depolarization.

Ceiling pacer rate Rate above which a pacemaker cannot discharge; functions as a safety mechanism to prevent cardiac overstimulation.

Demand pacing Pacemaker discharge mode that occurs only after a minimum heart rate (escape interval) is sensed.

Dual-chamber pacemakers Artificial pacemaker that senses and paces the atria and ventricles.

Escape interval Time period between when a pacer senses a spontaneous (intrinsic native) complex and when the succeeding paced beat occurs.

External pacing Same as trancutaneous pacing.

Implantable cardioverter-defibrillator (ICD) Device implanted in a patient's chest wall that constantly monitors the cardiac rhythm and delivers electrical countershocks if unstable tachydysrhythmias are detected.

Internal pacemaker Surgically implanted, permanent pacemaker.

Intrinsic cardiac activity Patient's natural cardiac activity.

Myopotentials Electrical muscle signals produced by muscle activity.

Native complex (beat) Patient's natural cardiac activity.

Paced beat Depolarization resulting from a pulse generator initiated spike.

Pacemaker battery Pacemaker part contained in the pulse generator that provides energy to power the device.

Pacemaker overseeing Pacing sensitivity is set too high and causes artifact to be misread as cardiac activity; pacing does not occur when it should.

Pacemaker reed switch Control switch that regulates the pacemaker activity.

Pacing leads Pacemaker part that senses intrinsic cardiac activity and also transmits the electrical impulse to the heart tissue.

Pacing rate Artificial pacemaker's set number of impulses per minute.

Pacing threshold Minimum amount of pulse generator energy needed to cause consistent cardiac depolarization (capture).

Pulse generator Pacemaker part that contains the battery and produces the electrical discharge.

Rate responsive pacing mode Ability of certain artificial pacemakers to automatically vary it's pacing rate to coordinate with the patient's activity.

Single-chamber pacemaker Artificial pacemaker device type that senses and stimulates only a single cardiac chamber, usually the right ventricle and less frequently the right atrium.

Spike impulse ECG artifact caused by an artificial pacemaker stmulus.

Sudden cardiac death Leading cause of unexpected deaths in patients with coronary artery disease; major mechanism is a ventricular dysrhythmia.

Threshold capture level Minimal amount of

pulse generator energy output (mV) required to cause consistent capture.

Tiered antitachycardia pacing ICDs deliver an escalating series of countershocks to terminate rapid cardiac rhythms.

Transcutaneous pacing (TCP) Pacing current that is applied across the chest wall via large adhesive electrodes; also referred to as transthoracic pacing.

Transthoracic pacing Same as transcutaneous or external pacing.

Artificial Pacemakers and Implantable Cardioverter-Defibrillators—Self-Assessment ECG Tracings

LEARNING OBJECTIVE

Upon completion of this chapter, the reader should be able to:

- *Correctly identify ECG disorders when given a sample of ECG tracings, including artificially paced rhythms and those recorded during cardiac resuscitations.*

SELF-ASSESSMENT ECG TRACINGS

The following ECGs include artificially paced rhythms, artifact rhythms, and cardiac resuscitation tracings. Each ECG tracing should be assessed according to the systematic approach outlined in earlier chapters and an interpretation made. Your answers should be compared with the answers provided in Appendix A. If there is any uncertainty about why an interpretation was selected, the relevant sections in the Chapter 19 should be reviewed.

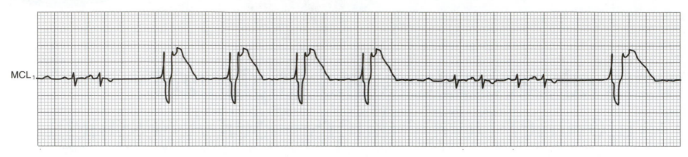

Figure 20-1   Rate _____
Rhythm _____
QRS Duration _____
PR Interval _____
AV Conduction Ratio _____
ST Segment _____
Interpretation _____
Reasoning _____

A.

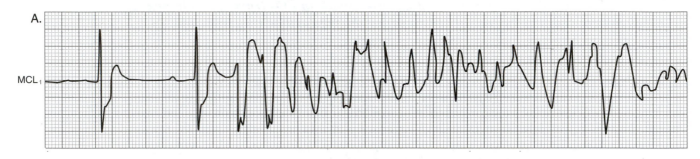

B.

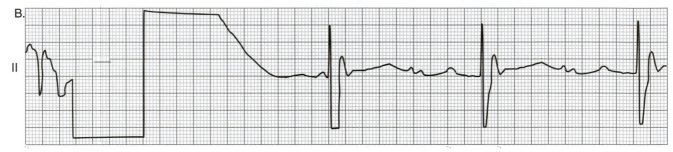

Figure 20-2   Rate _____
Rhythm _____
QRS Duration _____
PR Interval _____
AV Conduction Ratio _____
ST Segment _____
Interpretation _____
Reasoning _____

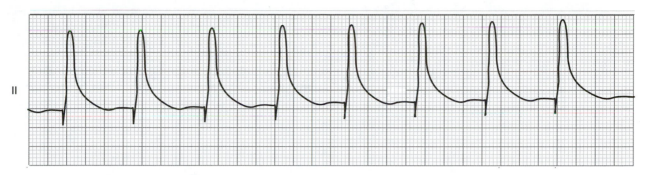

Figure 20-3   Rate _____
Rhythm _____
QRS Duration _____
PR Interval _____
AV Conduction Ratio _____
ST Segment _____
Interpretation _____
Reasoning _____

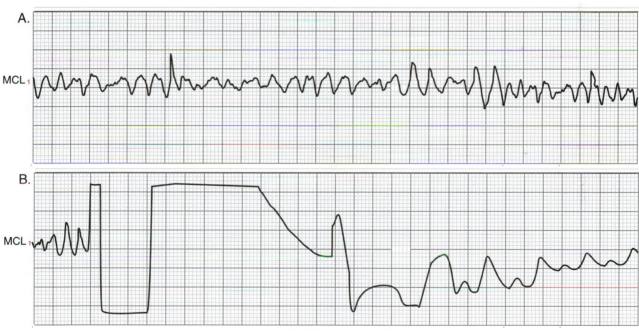

Continuous recording

Figure 20-4   Rate _____
Rhythm _____
QRS Duration _____
PR Interval _____
AV Conduction Ratio _____
ST Segment _____
Interpretation _____
Reasoning _____

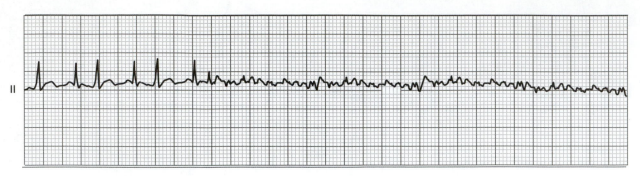

Figure 20–5 Rate _____

Rhythm _____

QRS Duration _____

PR Interval _____

AV Conduction Ratio _____

ST Segment _____

Interpretation _____

Reasoning _____

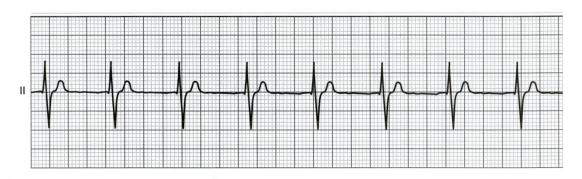

Figure 20–6 Rate _____

Rhythm _____

QRS Duration _____

PR Interval _____

AV Conduction Ratio _____

ST Segment _____

Interpretation _____

Reasoning _____

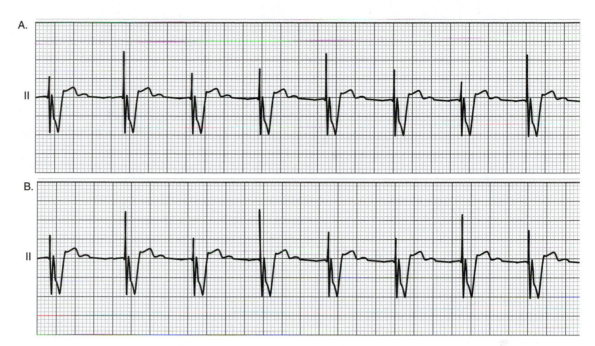

Figure 20–7   Rate _____
Rhythm _____
QRS Duration _____
PR Interval _____
AV Conduction Ratio _____
ST Segment _____
Interpretation _____
Reasoning _____

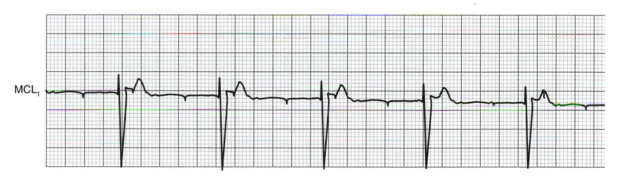

Figure 20–8   Rate _____
Rhythm _____
QRS Duration _____
PR Interval _____
AV Conduction Ratio _____
ST Segment _____
Interpretation _____
Reasoning _____

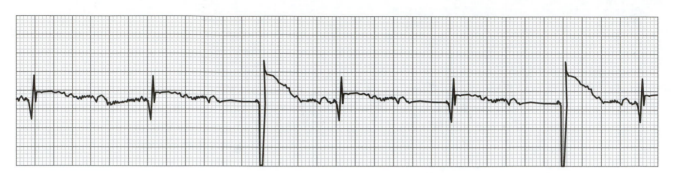

Figure 20-9 Rate _____
Rhythm _____
QRS Duration _____
PR Interval _____
AV Conduction Ratio _____
ST Segment _____
Interpretation _____
Reasoning _____

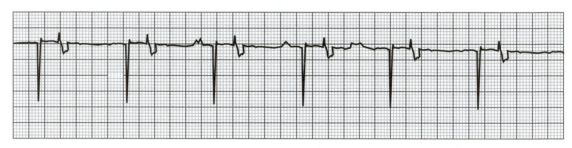

Figure 20-10 Rate _____
Rhythm _____
QRS Duration _____
PR Interval _____
AV Conduction Ratio _____
ST Segment _____
Interpretation _____
Reasoning _____

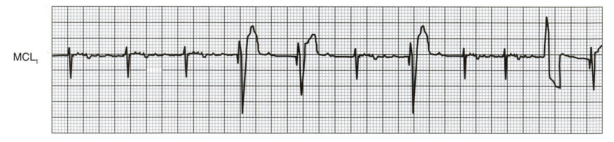

MCL₁

Figure 20-11 Rate _____
Rhythm _____
QRS Duration _____
PR Interval _____
AV Conduction Ratio _____
ST Segment _____
Interpretation _____
Reasoning _____

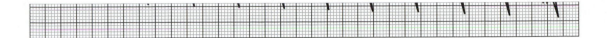

Figure 20.12

Figure 20-12 Rate _____
Rhythm _____
QRS Duration _____
PR Interval _____
AV Conduction Ratio _____
ST Segment _____
Interpretation _____
Reasoning _____

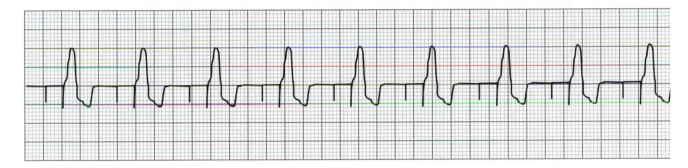

Figure 20-13 Rate _____
Rhythm _____
QRS Duration _____
PR Interval _____
AV Conduction Ratio _____
ST Segment _____
Interpretation _____
Reasoning _____

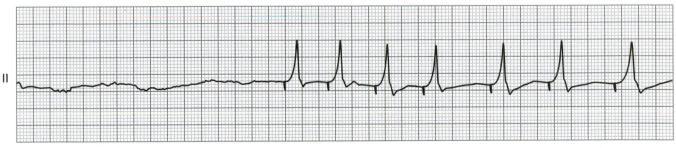

Figure 20-14 Rate _____
Rhythm _____
QRS Duration _____
PR Interval _____
AV Conduction Ratio _____
ST Segment _____
Interpretation _____
Reasoning _____

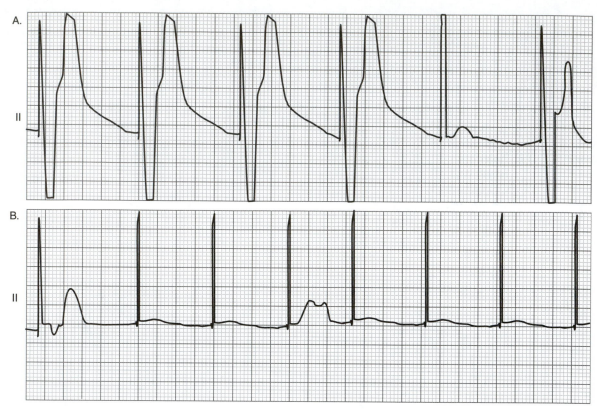

Continuous recording

Figure 20-15 Rate _____
Rhythm _____
QRS Duration _____
PR Interval _____
AV Conduction Ratio _____
ST Segment _____
Interpretation _____
Reasoning _____

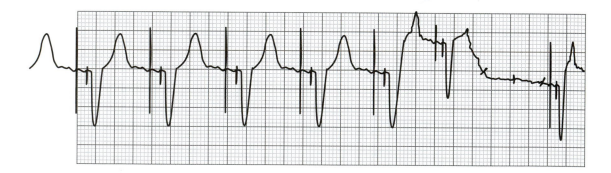

Figure 20-16 Rate _____
Rhythm _____
QRS Duration _____
PR Interval _____
AV Conduction Ratio _____
ST Segment _____
Interpretation _____
Reasoning _____

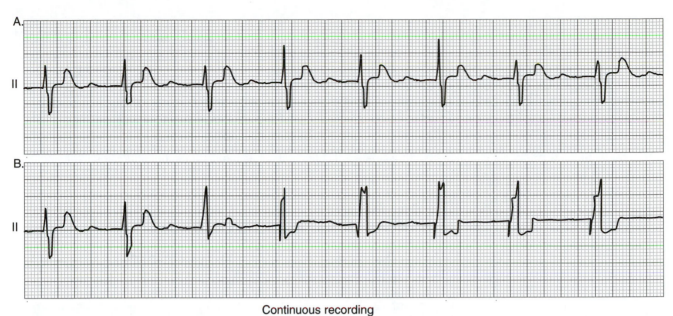

Continuous recording

Figure 20-17   Rate _____
Rhythm _____
QRS Duration _____
PR Interval _____
AV Conduction Ratio _____
ST Segment _____
Interpretation _____
Reasoning _____

A.

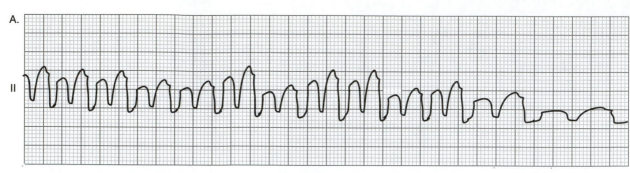

II

B.

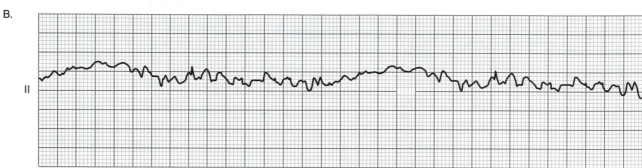

II

Continuous recording

Figure 20–18   Rate _____
Rhythm _____
QRS Duration _____
PR Interval _____
AV Conduction Ratio _____
ST Segment _____
Interpretation _____
Reasoning _____

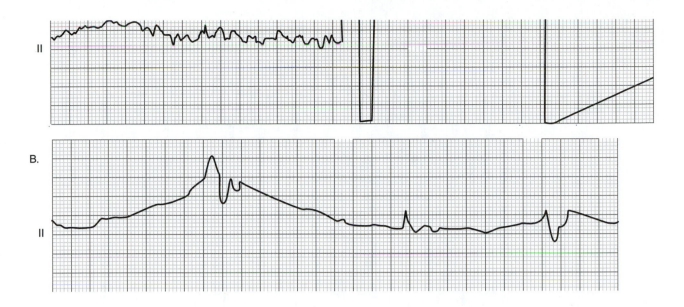

Continuous recording

Figure 20-19 Rate _____
Rhythm _____
QRS Duration _____
PR Interval _____
AV Conduction Ratio _____
ST Segment _____
Interpretation _____
Reasoning _____

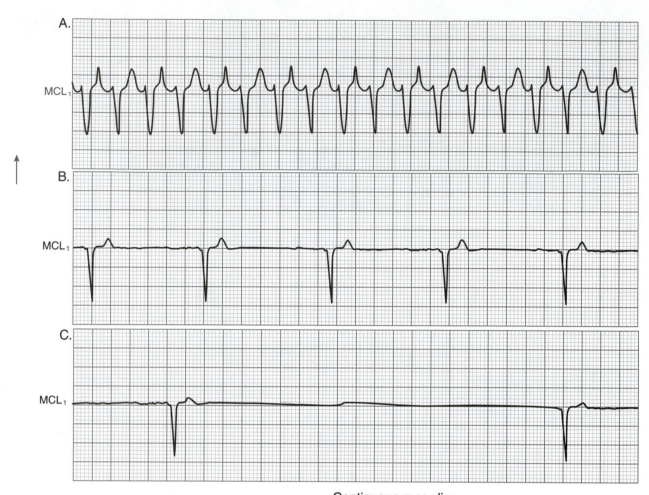

Continuous recording

Figure 20–20   Rate _____
Rhythm _____
QRS Duration _____
PR Interval _____
AV Conduction Ratio _____
ST Segment _____
Interpretation _____
Reasoning _____

chapter ● 21

Approach to Bradycardias and Tachycardias

LEARNING OBJECTIVES

Upon completion of this chapter, the reader should be able to:

■ *Differentiate between various rapid and slow dysrhythmias given sample ECG tracings.*

■ *List the characteristics of the P waves and QRS complexes that allow various bradydysrhythmias to be identified.*

■ *Classify bradydysrhythmias into narrow- or wide-complex disorders based on the QRS duration.*

■ *Describe a condition that would cause atrial fibrillation or atrial flutter to have a bradycardic ventricular response.*

■ *List the relationship between the P waves and QRS complexes that allow various narrow-complex tachydysrhythmias to be identified.*

■ *Classify tachydysrhythmias into narrow- or wide-complex disorders based on the width of QRS duration.*

■ *Describe the emergency cardiac care measures that are indicated when it is not possible to distinguish between SVT with aberrancy from VT.*

CHAPTER OVERVIEW

This chapter will not present new dysrhythmias; it will present an approach that integrates what has already been learned. This chapter will review individual dysrhythmias that were presented in previous chapters but will now divide them into two general groups. When faced with a patient who is not in cardiac arrest, most dysrhythmias can be grouped into the "fast types" or the "slow types". Several rapid and slow rhythms must be quickly recognized because they tend to lead to cardiovascular collapse if not treated. Another group, the irregular cardiac rhythms, are only a problem when they become too fast or too slow.

The fundamentals of interpreting ECGs and the treatment of significant dysrhythmias have already been presented—but as isolated topics: the sinus, junctional, atrial, or ventricular disorders (Figure 21–1). The organization of this book as with all dysrhythmia texts is artificial in the sense that patients with dysrhythmias do not come grouped together with similar disorders. Dysrhythmias will first be divided into bradydysrhythmias or tachydysrhythmias; then they will be subdivided within each group. This approach is useful because of its simplicity and because emergency cardiac care treatment options are also organized according to whether the rhythm is fast or slow.

BRADYDYSRHYTHMIAS

A pulse rate less than 60 bpm in an adult is bradycardic but this does not mean that every slow rate is abnormal or even that the rate is clinically significant. The clinician needs to determine whether the slow heart rate is responsible for the patient's presenting signs and symptoms. Bradycardia may be a normal physiologic finding in the well-conditioned athlete, or pathologic in a patient with heart block that causes dizziness, near-syncope, or hypotension. In contrast, a slow cardiac rate is a therapeutic goal in a patient with an acute ischemic event. A key question is: How slow is *too* slow? A heart rate of 55 bpm never causes hypotension by itself, while a rate of 20 bpm always does. Clinically significant bradycardia depends on individual patient characteristics.

> *Clinical Note* *The influence of the autonomic nervous system is a leading cause of slow heart rates. Increased vagal tone and blocked sympathetic tone, such as due to a beta-adrenergic blocker drug, decreases the heart rate below 60 bpm. Acute damage to the cardiac conduction pathway also leads to bradycardia. The clinical significance of a bradycardic rate must be assessed before choosing whether and how to accelerate the heart rate. The admonition to "treat the patient and not the heart rate" is relevant when evaluating slow rates.*

Patient Evaluation

When deciding whether to treat a specific heart rate, the clinician needs to determine if serious signs and symptoms exist. For hemodynamically unstable patients, immediate resuscitation, including oxygen administration, obtaining IV access, IV medications, and possibly starting external transcutaneous pacing is indicated.

History of Present Illness

The patient's history helps to evaluate a slow cadiac rhythm:

■ Is the patient symptomatic? Bradycardia can lead to inadequate cardiac output, chest discomfort, dyspnea, fatigue, and dizziness. In severe bradycardia, the patient's mental state typically becomes altered. Chest pain may result from a myocardial infarction, which, in turn, causes a slow heart rate.

■ What medication is the patient taking? Many medications, particularly beta-adrenergic blockers, calcium channel blockers, and anti-arrhythmic drugs, such as digitalis, cause bradycardia. Some patients in shock are unable to mount a compensatory tachycardia because their adrenergic nervous system is depressed by medication.

■ Is there a history of hypothyroidism? Low thyroid hormone levels can result in bradycardia because sufficient thyroid hormones must be present in order for the sympathetic nervous system to function properly. Therefore, hypothyroidism may indirectly lead to bradycardia.

■ Is the patient hypothermic or hypoglycemic? Abnormally low body temperature causes sinus node slowing and can induce conduction abnormalities and myocardial irritability. Prolonged hypoglycemia commonly results in significant hypothermia in the range of 92°F to 94°F. Even after the blood glucose level is corrected, several hours are required before the temperature returns to normal.

■ Does the patient have an artificial pacemaker? Pacemakers are often implanted to treat symptomatic bradycardias and conduction abnormalities in sinus and AV nodes. Pacemaker failure will expose the underlying rhythm disturbance.

Differential Diagnosis of Slow Rhythms

There are many types of slow cardiac rhythms, some benign and others quite serious (Figure 21–2). The incidence of various bradydysrhythmias, including bradycardia and AV heart blocks, complicate an MI in 25 and 30 percent of cases.

Sinus Bradycardia

Sinus bradycardia typically results from increased vagal tone, decreased sympathetic tone, and less commonly because of pathologic changes within the sinus node itself (Figure 21–3 and 21-4). Sinus bradycardia is the most common dysrhythmia in patients having an MI, present in 40 percent of cases within the first two hours. Sinus bradycardia can also be caused by increased intracranial pressure, hypothyroidism, hypothermia, severe hypoxia, significant pain, and certain medications, even morphine. Slow rates occur more commonly during inferior wall MIs than with anterior wall MIs, and are usually transient. Sinus bradycardia also develops during myocardial reperfusion with thrombolytics. Sinus bradycardias rarely need treatment but in the event that they do atropine is usually effective owing to the rich parasympathetic innervation of the SA node. Sinus bradycardia can be recognized by the narrow QRS complexes, regular P-QRS-T cycles, and a rate under 60 bpm. If the sinus rhythm is slow enough to allow escape ectopic beats, antidysrhythmia drugs to suppress these ectopic beats should be avoided as they contribute to the cardiac out put (Figure 21–5).

Sinus Block or Sinus Arrest

Sinus block or sinus arrest is recognized when a prolonged sinus activity pause makes the rhythm irregular. Sinus arrest is a very rare dysrhythmia and results in temporary episodes of ventricular asystole if escape pacemakers fail to initiate a rhythm. Brief sinus pauses are of little significance unless they are long enough to cause the patient to become symptomatic, having near-syncope or lightheadedness, or if the escape beats fail to develop. Sinus failure is recognized by absent P-QRS-T complexes and possible escape beats.

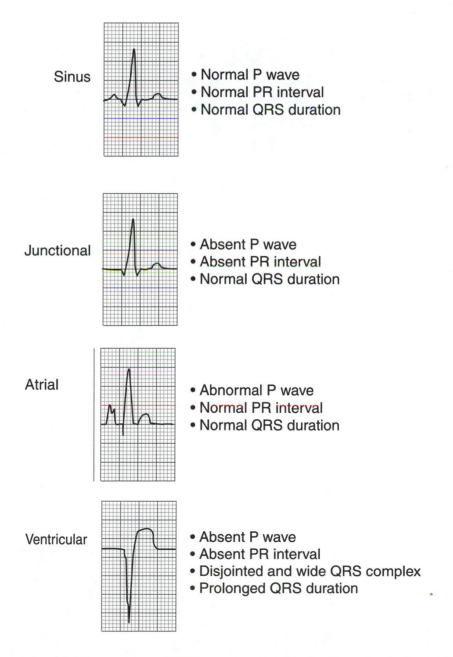

Sinus
- Normal P wave
- Normal PR interval
- Normal QRS duration

Junctional
- Absent P wave
- Absent PR interval
- Normal QRS duration

Atrial
- Abnormal P wave
- Normal PR interval
- Normal QRS duration

Ventricular
- Absent P wave
- Absent PR interval
- Disjointed and wide QRS complex
- Prolonged QRS duration

Figure 21–1 Characteristics of different types of ECG complexes. (Modified from Cecile Hurst. Dysrhythmias,; Table 4–2, p. 91.)

ECG Interpretation Tip *A blocked PAC is frequently misidentified as a sinus arrest. The T wave preceding an ECG pause needs to be scrutinized for a hidden P' wave (Figure 21–6). Nonconducted PAC's occur much more frequently than a sinus arrest. Most ECG pauses are due to blocked PACs, which are benign and not caused by the more serious sinus arrest.*

Junctional Bradycardia

Junctional bradycardia is an escape rhythm that develops as a result of a prolonged sinus arrest (Figures 21–7, 21–8, and 21–9). The AV junction becomes the back-up pacemaker and discharges between 30 and 50 bpm. When patients exhibit significant signs and symptoms, the heart rate should be increased. If the patient is tolerating the slow rhythm, the cause of sinus failure can be addressed and treatment held. Junctional bradycardias can be identified by their narrow QRS complexes and absent or inverted P waves which have a shortened PR interval.

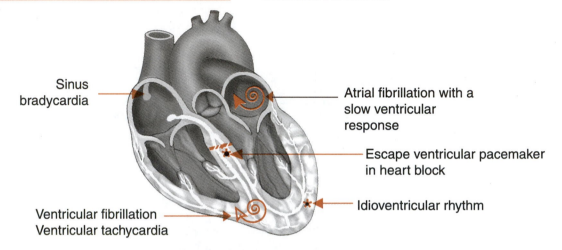

Sinus bradycardia

Atrial fibrillation with a slow ventricular response

Escape ventricular pacemaker in heart block

Idioventricular rhythm

Ventricular fibrillation
Ventricular tachycardia

Figure 21–2 Diagram showing the cardiac locations for various bradycardic dysrhythmias. Note that the ventricular disorders develop below where the AV (His) bundle splits. Escape ventricular pacemakers form below the site of blockage of supraventricular impulse (indicated by cross-hatched strip).

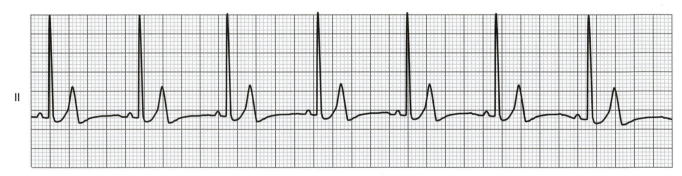

Figure 21–3 Sinus bradycardia at a rate of 38 bpm.

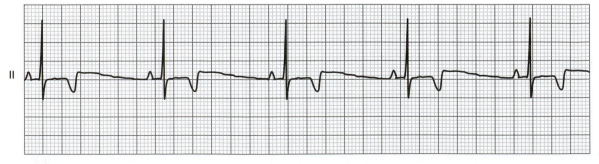

Figure 21–4 Sinus bradycardia at 38 bpm with deeply inverted T waves.

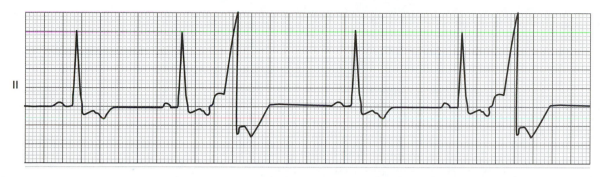

Figure 21-5 Ectopic ventricular beats in the setting of sinus bradycardia. The sinus node is firing at 46 bpm, and the slow rate allows ventricular ectopic beats to develop.

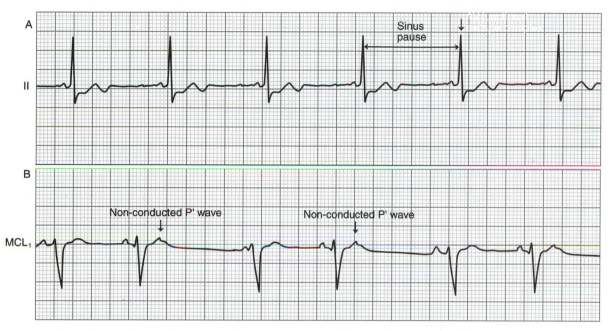

Figure 21-6 Sinus block compared with a nonconducted PAC. In strip A , sinus block develops after the 3rd beat. The sinus pause lasts for 0.44 second (11 large ECG boxes), which corresponds to a heart rate of 27 bpm. An AV junctional escape complex terminates the pause. In tracing B, the T waves of the 2nd and 5th beats are distorted by hidden P' waves of PACs that failed to be conducted because they occurred during the refractory period. Nonconducted PACs are commonly misinterpreted as sinus block.

Sick Sinus Syndrome (SSS)

Sick sinus syndrome applies to a group of dysrhythmias involving the sinoatrial node, including persistent and inappropriate sinus bradycardia, episodes of sinus arrest or sinus block, and a combination of SA or AV node conduction abnormalities. Periods of alternating atrial tachycardias with slow atrial and ventricular rhythms as in tachycardia-bradycardia syndrome occur in sick sinus syndrome. SSS involves a cardiac rhythm that alternates between abrupt slowing and sudden acceleration. The rhythm has narrow QRS complexes unless there are escape ventricular rhythms

Hypersensitive Carotid Sinus Syndrome

Hypersensitive carotid sinus syndrome develops as a result of pressure on the carotid sinus receptor in the neck caused by head turning, necktie compression, tight collars, and the use of an electric razor. Syncope results from stimulation of a hypersensitive carotid sinus leading to asystolic episodes as a result of transient sinus exit block, sinus arrest, or AV blocks. There are two types:

- Cardio-inhibitory carotid sinus hypersensitivity is characterized by periods of asystole

- Vasodepressor carotid sinus hypersensitivity is characterized by a decrease in the systolic blood pres-

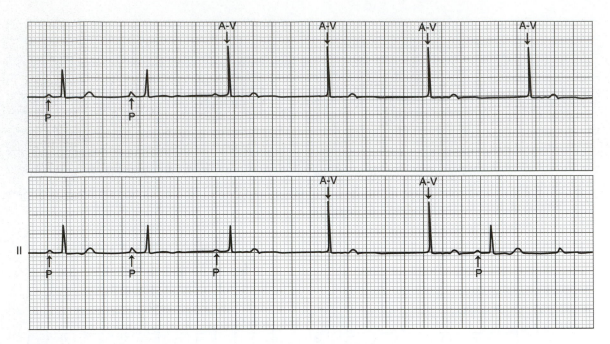

Figure 21–7 AV junctional bradycardia alternating with sinus bradycardia. In this continuous tracing, the rhythm begins as a slow sinus rhythm but a sinus pause after the second beat allows an AV junctional bradycardia to occur during the last four beats in strip A. In tracing B, the sinus node has resumed control for first three beats but the AV junctional escape pacemaker stimulates the 4th and 5th beats. The last beat in strip B is a sinus beat.

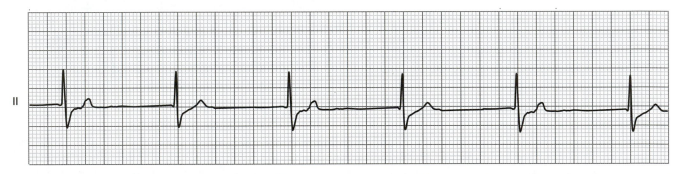

Figure 21–8 AV junctional escape rhythm. The rhythm arises in an AV junctional pacemaker when the sinus node fails to discharge. The QRS complexes are narrow and there are no P waves.

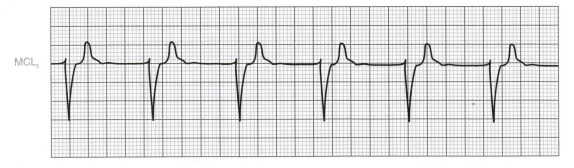

Figure 21–9 AV junctional escape rhythm. The sinus node fails to initiate a rhythm so the AV junction discharges at 38 bpm as the escape pacemaker.

sure of 50 mm Hg or greater without an associated cardiac slowing, or a decrease in the systolic BP of 30 mm Hg with cardiac slowing.

> ***Clinical Note*** *Not all significant bradycardias are due to heart disease or respond to traditional therapy. Two uncommon causes of fatal conduction system failure and cardiovascular collapse involve overdoses of beta-adrenergic blockers and calcium channel blockers. Treating a beta blocker overdose requires high doses of adrenergic agents and glucagon administration along with artificial pacemakers. Calcium channel blocker toxicity partially responds to calcium chloride administration and may require artificial pacing. Blood pressure support using intravenous fluid and a vasopressor medication is indicated.*

AV Blocks

Advanced forms of AV blocks usually result in slow ventricular rhythms depending on the sinus rate and the adequacy of AV conduction (Figures 21–10 and 21–11).

First-degree AV block does not cause bradycardia but does result in a prolonged PR interval that can be associated with a slow rhythm, especially if caused by enhanced vagal tone or beta-adrenergic blockers or calcium channel blocking medication. First-degree AV blocks occur in 15 percent of patients experiencing an MI.

Second-degree AV block Mobitz Type I (Wenckebach block) occurs in about 10 percent of acute MI patients. The number of dropped beats coupled with the sinus rate determines whether the ventricular rate falls below 60 bpm. No treatment is indicated unless the heart rate drops below 50 bpm because Wenckebach usually subsides spontaneously. Mobitz Type I is recognized by a narrow QRS complex, progressive increases in the PR interval prior to dropped QRS, and by grouped beating. Wenckebach is the most common form of second-degree block, present in 90 percent of cases of second-degree block, and is the benign form of Mobitz block. In second-degree AV block, Mobitz Type II, P waves are not consistently conducted, but the PR intervals prior to the dropped beats are constant. Mobitz II block is relatively rare compared with Mobitz Type I (Wenckebach), occurring in only 1 percent of MIs. When it does occur, however, it is likely to quickly progress to third-degree AV block and requires emergent pacemaker use.

Mobitz II block is associated with an increased mortality, generally caused by cardiac pump failure. The QRS complexes are wide (0.12 seconds or greater) because the defect involves the bundle branches. A sinus rate of 90 bpm with an AV conduction ratio of 3:2 will lead to a ventricular rate of 60, while a 3:1 ratio at the same sinus rate will result in a ventricular rate of only 30 bpm.

In third-degree AV block, no atrial activity is conducted to the ventricles so junctional or ventricular bradycardic escape rhythms occur. The most common causes are drug toxicity, intrinsic AV nodal disease, fibrotic degeneration associated with aging, and coronary artery disease. Complete AV block complicates 8 to 15 percent of acute myocardial infarctions. The ventricular rate is solely dependent on the rate of the escape pacemaker because none of the atrial impulses are able to stimulate the ventricles. In 70 percent of cases, the escape rhythm has a narrow QRS complex and the rate is 50 bpm, indicating that it arose from above the AV (His) bundle bifurcation and will be stable at least for the near future (see Figure 21–11A). On the other hand, when the QRS complex is wide and slow, as occurs 30 percent of the time, the impulse arose in a bundle

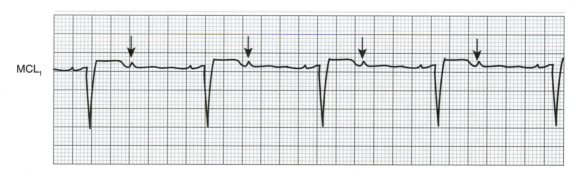

Figure 21–10 Ventricular bradycardia due to an AV block. Because every other P wave is not conducted (indicated by arrows), the ventricular rate of 43 bpm is half of the sinus rate.

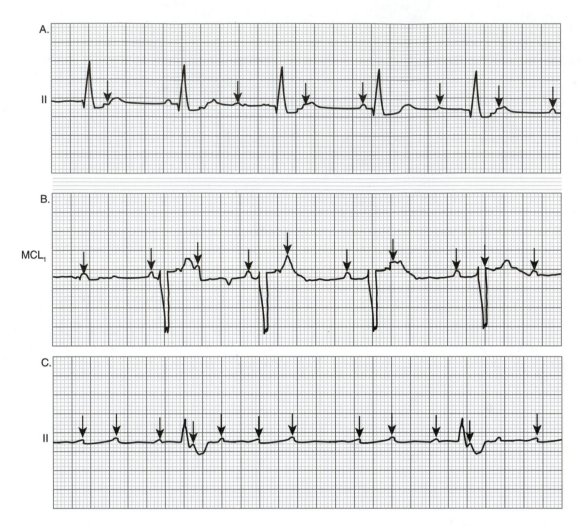

Figure 21-11 Bradycardic ventricular rhythms caused by complete AV heart blocks. The slow ventricular rates are 40 bpm in strips A and B and only 16 bpm in strip C. The nonconducted P waves in each tracing are indicated by arrows.

branch and is not particularly stable (see Figures 21–11B and 21–11C). Artificial pacing will be required.

Idioventricular Escape Rhythm

An idioventricular escape rhythm is chracterized by slow, wide QRS complex rhythms usually occurring in the range of 20 to 40 bpm (Figures 21–12 and 21–13). Escape ventricular rhythms develop to prevent asystole in cases when both the sinus and AV junctional pacemakers fail. Atropine is unlikely to accelerate an idioventricular pacemaker because there are few, if any, parasympathetic fibers in the ventricles. An external pacemaker or an epinephrine infusion is more successful.

Asystole

Asystole can be considered the most extreme form of bradycardia and transiently occurs in 1 percent of MI

patients (Figure 21–14). It results from failure of the SA node or during complete AV block associated with failure of an escape pacemaker (ventricular standstill).

Miscellaneous Rhythms

Untreated atrial fibrillation and flutter have tachycardic ventricular responses in the range of 130 to 150 bpm (Figure 21–15A). With appropriate therapy the ventricular rates stabilize in the range between 70 and 100 bpm (Figure 21–15B). A patient who has been maintained on beta blockers or calcium channel blockers for rate control of chronic atrial fibrillation sometimes presents with a bradycardic ventricular rhythm—sometimes extremely slow (Figure 21–15C). The most likely cause is an excess of medication.

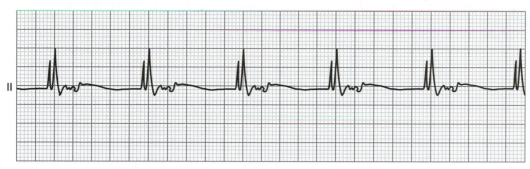

Figure 21-12 Idioventricular escape rhythm. The complex is idioventricular because the QRS complexes are wide and distorted, the rhythm is regular and slow (42 bpm), and P waves are absent.

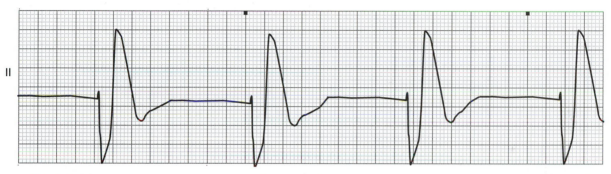

Figure 21-13 Idioventricular escape rhythm. The beats have a bizarre appearance with distorted QRS-T complexes that lack P waves, and they occur at a very slow rate (30 bpm). There is no sign of sinus or AV junctional activity.

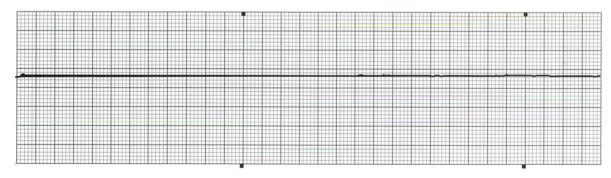

Figure 21-14 Asystole. There is total lack of electical activity without signs of any pacemaker activity. The sinus node, AV junction, and ventricular pacemaker systems have all failed.

TACHYDYSRHYTHMIAS

The patient's presentation often provides an important clue to the type and significance of a tachydysrhythmia. For instance, a narrow complex rhythm occurring in a twenty-year-old female whose only symptom is palpitations is almost certainly a well-tolerated case of PSVT; whereas a wide-complex tachycardia in a fifty-year-old patient recovering from an MI is most likely to be ventricular tachycardia. The significance and treatment of tachycardias vary greatly and are based on whether the rhythm is ventricular or supraventricular.

Heart rates greater than 100 bpm, which define sinus tachycardia in an adult, can represent a physiologic stress response, a compensatory response to acute blood loss or hypoxia, or it can be pathologic—caused by heart disease, drugs, or a cardiomyopathy (myocardial abnormality due to nonischemic causes such as hypertension, alcohol abuse, or a viral illness) (Figure 21-16). The patient who has a heart rate of 110 bpm is

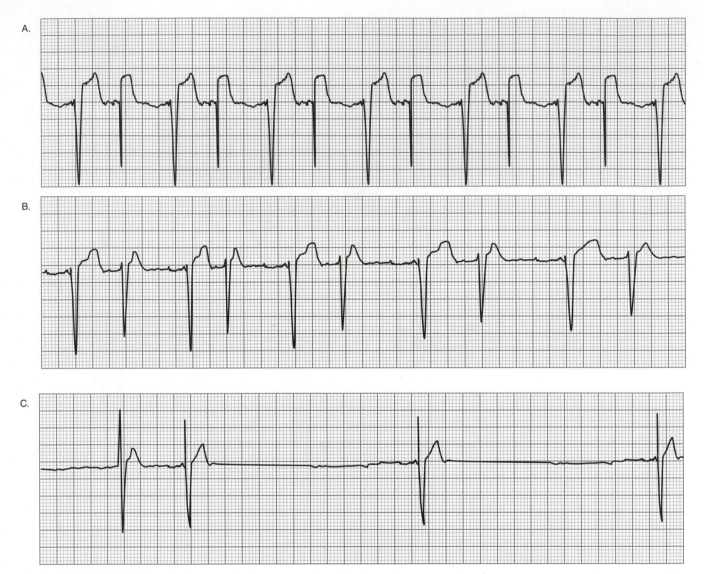

A.

B.

C.

Figure 21-15 Atrial fibrillation with varying ventricular responses. In strip A the ventricular rate is 140 bpm, while it is 75 bpm in strip B. Due to overaggressive medication administration, the bradycardia at a rate of 35 bpm occurs in strip C. Untreated atrial fibrillation has a tachycardic ventricular rate, while atrial fibrillation that has been adequately treated has a rate below 100 bpm.

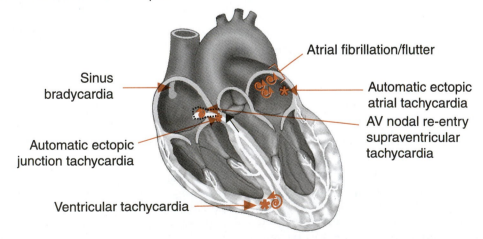

Sinus
bradycardia

Atrial fibrillation/flutter

Automatic ectopic
atrial tachycardia

AV nodal re-entry
supraventricular
tachycardia

Automatic ectopic
junction tachycardia

Ventricular tachycardia

Figure 21-16 Diagragm of the pacemaker sites in various tachycardic rhythms. Note that rapid dysrhythmias can arise from all areas of the heart.

not automatically different from one with a rate of 90 bpm. Knowing only the heart rate is not clinically useful information; important data include the patient's age, past medical history, vital signs, and clinical condition. The clinical significance of a rapid rate also depends on the duration of the tachycardia, the degree of tachycardia, presence of congestive heart failure, and the patient's underlying cardiovascular status.

Patient Evaluation

If the patient is hemodynamically unstable, immediate resuscitation is warranted, including oxygen administration, obtaining IV access, intravenous medications, and electrical cardioversion. If the patient has stable vital signs and is not in shock, there is time for further evaluation before treatment is started. Therapy depends on the underlying cause; for instance, if the tachycardia is a response to hypovolemia, fluid resuscitation and stemming blood loss may be necessary. For instance, if the tachycardia results from a fever, aceteminophen is indicated.

Patient History

The patient's age and the presence of coexisting heart disease can provide clues to the mechanism of the dysrhythmia. Palpitations is the most common complaint in those experiencing tachycardia. The following historical data is important:

- Is the patient symptomatic or displaying signs of inadequate perfusion? Tachycardias may lead to inadequate cardiac output associated with: chest discomfort or pain, dyspnea, fatigue, syncope, or dizziness. Chest pain may result from poor coronary perfusion and myocardial infarction, which can induce tachycardia. True syncope, in contrast to near-syncope, is often used as an indicator for ventricular tachycardia.

- What medication is the patient taking? Many medications, particularly sympathomimetic agents such as albuterol, cocaine use, thyroid treatment, and diuretics can cause a reflex tachycardia secondary to hypovolemia.

- Is there a history of hyperthyroidism? Thyroid hormones cause an increased sensitivity to sympathetic nervous system hormones, thereby leading to tachycardias. Sign and symptoms of hyperthyroidism include heat intolerance, increased sweating, weight loss, insomnia, agitation, and tachycardia.

- Is there a history of heart disease? Patients with valvular heart diseases, artificial heart valves, car-

diomyopathies, or preexcitation syndromes, such as Wolff-Parkinson-White syndrome, often have tachycardia.

- What events preceded the onset of tachycardia? Exercise, pain, emotional stress, fatigue, fever, dyspnea, and acute blood loss are a few examples of conditions that may cause tachycardia. Nicotine, alcohol, and caffeine will also increase the heart rate. If the onset was preceded by ischemic chest pain or followed by syncope, the dysrhythmia is most likely to be ventricular tachycardia.

Differential Diagnosis of Rapid Rhythms

An easy way to divide this large group of dysrhythmias is based on the width of the QRS complex; durations less than 0.12 second are supraventricular, while wider QRS complexes typically represent ventricular tachycardia although some may be supraventicular, which are aberrantly conducted.

Supraventricular (Narrow Complex) Tachycardias

The key ECG finding of a supraventricular tachycardia is a narrow QRS complex (except in the few cases of SVT with a bundle branch block). The only *common irregular* narrow QRS tachycardia is atrial fibrillation. The *very uncommon irregular* narrow QRS complex tachycardia is multifocal atrial tachycardia (MAT). Narrow QRS complex regular tachycardias include sinus tachycardia, atrial flutter, and paroxysmal supraventricular tachycardia (PSVT). Determining which of these three dysrhythmias is present depends on the ventricular rate as well as the shape of the P or P′ wave. The atrial rate and regularity provide a clue. Sinus tachycardia has normal P waves and has a rate of 100 to 150/minute. Untreated atrial flutter can be identified by the precisely regular rate of 150/minute due to 2:1 AV conduction and flutter waves. PSVT is known for its abrupt onset and termination, along with a rate around 200/minute with absent P waves.

Sinus Tachycardia. The sinus node discharges between 100 and 160/minute although it can be even faster with exertion (Figures 21–17 and 21–18). Sinus tachycardia is characterized by a *gradual* onset and a *gradual* slowing, and has a regular rhythm with clearly identifiable P waves. Rapid sinus rates are usually a response to fever, hypotension, anemia, hyperthyroidism, anxiety, exercise, pulmonary embolism, myocardial ischemia, CHF, and drugs such as sympathomimetics, alcohol, caffeine, and nicotine. Selecting an effective therapy must take into account the underlying cause.

Atrial Flutter. The atrial rate is between 250 and 350/minute, most commonly with a 2:1 conduction

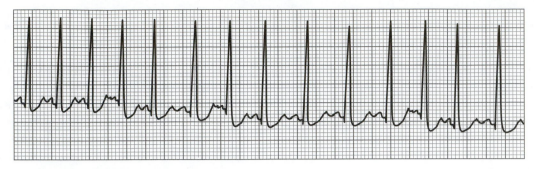

Figure 21-17 Sinus tachycardia. The QRS complexes occur at a rate of 130 bpm, are narrow and each QRS complex is preceded by a P wave.

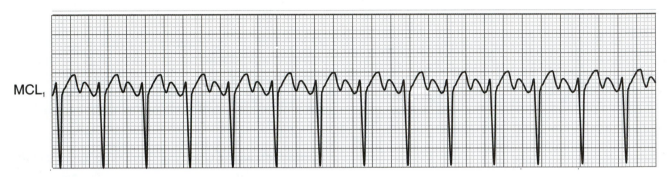

Figure 21-18 Sinus tachycardia at a rate of 130 bpm. P waves are clearly seen before the QRS complexes.

ratio and a ventricular response between 100 and 150 bpm (Figure 21–19). It is the least common dysrhythmia associated with a myocardial infarction, occurring in less than 5 percent of cases. Sharp "F" waves are observed in some leads. Atrial flutter can be an unstable rhythm, but it is usually well tolerated. It often converts spontaneously to atrial fibrillation or NSR. Chronic atrial flutter usually has a well-controlled ventricular rate and is associated with underlying heart disease—mitral or tricuspid valve disease, ischemic heart disease, and cardiomyopathies. Identification of atrial flutter

depends on recognizing the rapid, regular flutter waves, narrow QRS complex, and tachycardic rate.

Atrial Fibrillation (AF). Atrial fibrillation is characterized by disorganized, chaotic atrial activity, associated with "f" waves at a rate of 350 to 600/minute (Figure 21–20). The ventricular response is 130 to 160/minute when the AF recently developed. Chronic AF usually has a rate under 100/minute unless the patient stops taking medication that is used for rate control. AF is a common dysrhythmia, occurring in 1 percent of adults over 60 years of age, and increasing with age.

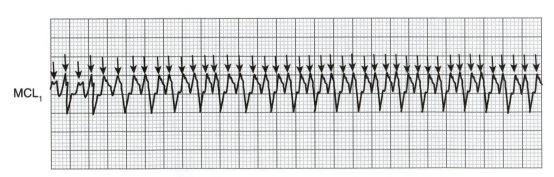

Figure 21-19 Atrial flutter with 2:1 AV conduction. This very fast supraventricular tachydysrhythmia has a ventricular rate of 150 bpm, while the atrial rate is 300 bpm! Atrial fluttter waves are indicated by arrows. The 2nd flutter wave of each pair is superimposed on the T wave. Every other flutter wave is not conducted owing to a normally functioning AV node, which prevents the ventricles from being overstimulated.

Atrial fibrillation occurs much more commonly than atrial flutter and complicates 10 to 15 percent of acute MI cases. Because atrial fibrillation is the most common sustained dysrhythmia, chronic AF cases have a drug-controlled ventricular response rate less than 100 bpm. Most patients with AF have underlying heart disease, including coronary artery disease, hypertensive heart disease, CHF, and cardiomyopathy. Hyperthyroidism is an important cause of new onset atrial fibrillation. The major clues to identify atrial fibrillation are the irregularly irregular rhythm compiled with a narrow QRS complex.

In supraventricular achycardias (SVT), the atrial rate is usually 150 to 200/minute and P waves are usually absent (Figures 21–21 and 21–22). Paroxysmal supraventricular tachycardia (PSVT) is recognized by a sudden onset and termination, narrow QRS complex, and regular rhythm. PSVT is a very commonly encountered dysrhythmia in the emergency department and the pre-hospital phase. PSVT occurs in less than 10 percent of patients having an MI.

In multifocal atrial tachycardia (MAT) atrial rates usually range from 100 to 130/minute and the P waves have at least three different shapes. The rhythm is grossly irregular, as with atrial fibrillation, except that distinct P waves are seen. In essence, MAT is actually sinus tachycardia with frequent multifocal PACs. In MAT the P waves have many different shapes, which cause it to be confused with atrial fibrillation. MAT is an extremely uncommon tachydysrhythmia, seen in less than 1 percent of hospital ECGs. MAT is most commonly seen in elderly patients with chronic obstructive pulmonary disease or CHF.

> ***ECG Interpretation Tip*** *MAT is most frequently confused with atrial fibrillation because of MAT's very irregular rhythm and rapid rate. However, MAT has clear-cut P waves with multiple shapes and does not have nearly as many atrial waves as atrial fibrillation.*

Sick Sinus Syndrome (SSS). SSS is an SA node abnormality that involves sudden episodes of inappropriate sinus bradycardia, sinus arrest or sinus exit block, a combination of SA or AV node conduction anomalies, or periods of paroxysmal atrial tachycardias alternating

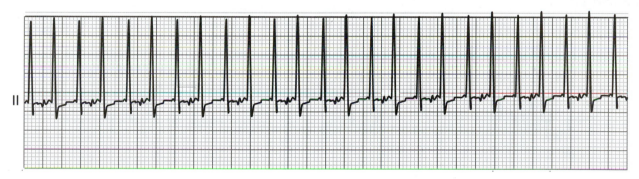

Figure 21–20 Atrial fibrillation at a rate of 160 bpm. The atrial fibrillatory waves are not as clearly seen as in other examples, but the findings of a narrow QRS complex tachydysrhythmia coupled with the irregularly irregular ventricular rhythm (R-R intervals) are hallmark ECG clues of AF. (Lead MCL$_1$ would yield a better view of the fibrillation waves if the interpretation was in doubt.)

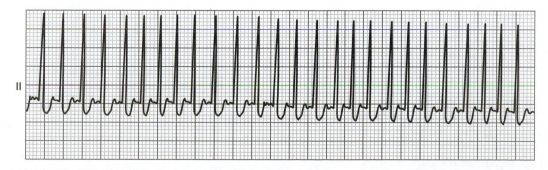

Figure 21–21 Supraventricular tachycardia at a rate over 200 bpm. There are no P waves visible in this rapid and regular narrow complex dysrhythmia. The small positive deflections that are seen between the QRS complexes are T waves—not P waves. (Adenosine coverted the rhythm to the sinus tachycardia found in Figure 21–17.)

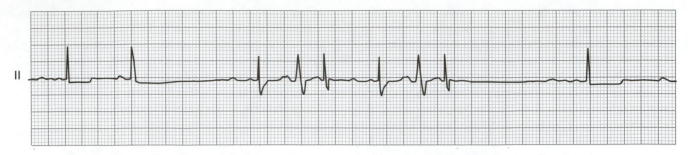

Figure 21–22 Sinus bradycardia at a rate of 56 bpm is disrupted by a 7-beat episode of paroxysmal supraventricular tachycardia at a rate of 150 bpm.

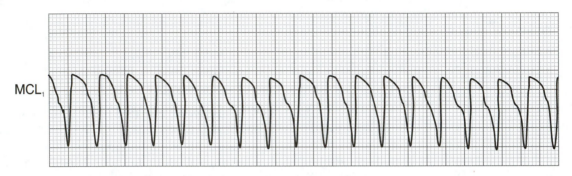

Figure 21–23 Ventricular tachycardia at a rate of 170 bpm. This regular, rapid, wide-complex dysrhythmia lacks clear P waves.

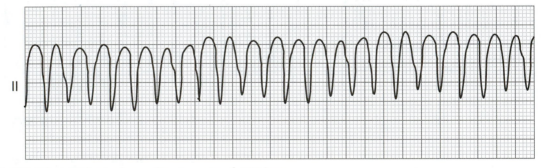

Figure 21–24 Ventricular tachycardia at a rate of 180 bpm.

with slow atrial and ventricular rhythms. SSS can be recognized by dramatically changing rates and rhythms. **Preexcitation Syndrome.** In preexcitation, a normally formed sinus impulse travels along an accessory pathway between the atria and the ventricles, resulting in earlier than expected ventricular activation. Wolff-Parkinson-White (W-P-W) syndrome is the most common form of preexcitation and is characterized by PR intervals less than 0.12 second during NSR, QRS complexes 0.12 second or greater, with a slurred, slowly rising upstroke of the initial QRS portion termed a delta wave. Extremely rapid ventricular rates are possible when impulses are conducted along the accessory pathway because the AV node is bypassed. Atrial fibril-

lation is a particularly dangerous rhythm to be associated with W-P-W because very rapid ventricular rates (greater then 200/minute) can even lead to ventricular fibrillation.

Wide Complex Tachydysrhythmias

In the emergency setting, every case of wide QRS complex tachycardia is best assumed to be—and treated as—ventricular tachycardia because treating such a dysrhythmia as an SVT with aberrancy can lead to sudden cardiac collapse and death. The majority of wide-complex tachycardias in patients who have had a past MI, or when the QRS complex is wider than 0.14 second, are in fact ventricular tachycardias. Some wide-complex tachydysrhythmias do turn out to be abnormally conducted supraventricular tachycardias, but it is safer to treat emergency patients with the therapy for ventricular dysrhythmias because it is often effective in most cases of SVTs and will not precipitate deterioration.

Ventricular Tachycardia (VT) is defined as three or more wide, bizarre QRS complexes (greater then 0.12 second) in a row with a rate over 100/minute (Figures 21–23 and 21–24). VT arises in the lower portions conduction system beyond the bifurcation of the His bundle or in the myocardium. The rate ranges between 120 and 160/minute but can be as fast as 250/minute. The direction of the ST segment and T wave are opposite to the QRS deflection. VT lasting l*ess than 30 seconds* and occurring during the early phase of a myocardial infarction is not associated with a greater mortality rate. However, nonsustained VT occuring more than 48 hours after an MI in patients with depressed left ventricular function is a marker for sudden cardiac death. Sustained VT, lasting *greater than 30 seconds*, or causing hemodynamic compromise needs aggressive therapy because of the tendency to deteriorate into ventricular fibrillation. While it may be difficult to differentiate between VT and an SVT with aberrant conduction, it is prudent to go with the odds: VT is the most common cause of wide QRS complex tachycardia.

Polymorphic Ventricular Tachycardia. Also known as Torsade de Pointes, this much less frequent VT variant is characterized by a cyclical fluctuation in amplitude and direction of the QRS complexes. Sustained Torsade de Pointes following an MI has a 20 percent in-hospital mortality rate. Torsade de Pointes is associated with a prolonged QT interval indicating prolonged ventricular repolarization. Patients taking antiarrhythmics such as procainamide, quinidine, or disopyramide are at risk of developing polymorphic VT.

SVT with Aberrant Conduction. When a patient with a preexisting bundle branch block develops any type of atrial tachycardia, the rhythm will have a wide complex tachycardia that mimics VT. This can happen with rate dependent bundle branch blocks and also when conduction through a bundle branch becomes fatigued from a sustained episode of SVT. In these few cases where there is a prior ECG documenting a wide QRS rhythm, and the patient has not had a past MI, and the patient's condition is not critical, a trial of adenosine or cardizem can be used. For all other cases, they should be treated as VT for the reasons previously mentioned.

Let's Review

1. A useful first step in classifying dysrhythmias is whether they are bradydysrhythmias or tachydysrhythmias.

2. The P wave characteristics and their relationship to QRS complexes is useful in distinguishing among various bradydysrhythmias.

3. The first branch point in the classification of the tachydysrhythmias is determining whether they are narrow- or wide-complex tachydysrhythmias.

4. The characteristics of the P wave and its relationship to QRS complexes is useful in distinguishing among various narrow-complex tachydysrhythmias.

5. Wide-complex tachydysrhythmias can be difficult to distinguish. When it is not possible to quickly differentiate SVT with aberrancy from VT, initial emergency treatment should be directed toward VT because it occurs more commonly and is a more serious disorder.

6. Inadvertently treating a case of VT as if it were a SVT with aberrancy can cause cardiovascular collapse and ventricular fibrillation.

Reference The statistics pertaining to the incidence of various dysrhythmias in the setting of an MI are taken from a chapter by T. Aufderheide, MD, entitled *Arrhythmias Associated with Acute Myocardial Infarction and Thrombolysis* (Emergency Clinics of North America 16. August 1998; No.3: 583–600).

Introduction to Twelve-Lead ECGs and Bundle Branch Blocks

LEARNING OBJECTIVES

Upon completion of this chapter, the reader should be able to:

- *Describe at least two advantages of using a twelve-lead ECG compared with monitoring a single lead.*

- *Contrast the lead placements of a bipolar ECG monitoring system from a unipolar system.*

- *List the electrode positions for the six precordial leads.*

- *State which of the standard ECG leads are: (a) bipolar, (b) unipolar, and (c) precordial.*

- *List the augmented limb leads and describe how they differ from non-augmented limb leads.*

- *Identify the ECG leads that detect electrical activity in the following heart regions: (a) inferior, (b) anterior, (c) posterior, (d) lateral, and (e) right ventricle.*

- *Define the following terms in regard to precordial leads: (a) R wave progression and (b) transition zone.*

- *State the location of the conduction defect in a (R.B.B.B.).*

- *Explain how the right ventricle becomes depolarized in a R.B.B.B.*

- *Name three ECG characteristics of a R.B.B.B.*

- *State the location of the conduction defect in a left bundle branch block (L.B.B.B.).*

- *Explain how the left ventricle becomes depolarized in a L.B.B.B.*

- *Name three ECG characteristics of a left bundle branch block.*

- *Indicate whether a L.B.B.B. or a R.B.B.B. will prevent ECG detection of an acute myocardial infarction.*

CHAPTER OVERVIEW

The twelve-lead ECG is the major tool used to detect myocardial damage caused by insufficient coronary blood flow during an acute coronary syndrome (A.C.S.). Detecting characteristic ECG findings of a myocardial infarction permits prompt use of thrombolytic therapy and emergency cardiac care. The twelve-lead ECG recognition of acute coronary syndromes builds on the ECG principles already learned earlier in this text.

Bundle branch blocks involve a conduction disturbance in one or both bundle branches. A left bundle branch blocks distorts the ECG and obscures the signs of an acute myocardial infarction.

INTRODUCTION TO THE TWELVE-LEAD ECG

Being able to interpret twelve-lead ECGs used to be considered a nice "extra" skill for emergency and critical care nursing clinicians and advanced EMTs to possess, but today, an inability to interpret ECGs is a major clinical handicap. Pre-hospital acquisition of twelve-lead ECGs is routine in many EMS systems. This chapter presents the additional leads beyond the three limb leads and single modified precordial lead that have already been discussed for monitoring purposes. This chapter lays the foundation for the twelve-lead assessment skills that will be presented in Chapter 23. After completing Chapters 23 and 24, myocardial ischemia and injury patterns will be recognized with ease. What advantages are gained by using twelve leads compared with monitoring only one or two leads for dysrhythmia analysis? The main reason that using twelve leads is superior is because *more clinically useful information* can be obtained. While dysrhythmia recognition is adequately done using only leads II and MCL$_1$, they are inadequate for detecting myocardial injury. Additional leads provide more vantage points from which to evaluate cardiac activity (Figure 22–1). ECG rhythm strips are *not* able to identify myocardial ischemia, injury, or infarct patterns, whereas twelve-lead ECGs are able to identify these patterns, as well as gauging cardiac chamber enlargement and detecting bundle branch blockages.

> **Clinical Note** *The vast majority of MIs will be detected with twelve-lead ECGs. Classic ECG findings of ischemia, injury, and infarction, cannot be interpreted with limited monitoring lead systems.*

ECG LEADS

A standard ECG includes six limb leads and six chest leads. Figure 22–2 diagrams the regions of the heart and Figure 22–3 shows the groups of leads that detect cardiac activity from specific heart regions. Traditional ECG recordings use the arms and legs as extensions of the electrical field surrounding the heart.

The ECG leads detect electrical activity in two planes. The limb leads record cardiac activity in the **frontal plane** (Figure 22–4), while the chest leads record action detected in the **horizontal plane** (Figure 22–5). Horizontal chest leads provide information about anterior and posterior cardiac energy flow, as well as rightward and leftward forces. The frontal plane limb leads provide information concerning the energy flow along the inferior and superior heart borders. Modified 12-lead tracings have been developed for EMS use because it is impractical to use the arms and legs. In pre-hospital care, the electrodes are placed as the patient's trunk (torso) as far from the heart as practical.

Limb Leads

Limb leads incorporate a two-electrode and a single-electrode lead system termed bipolar and unipolar, respectively. Bipolar leads link both arms, or an arm to the left leg, to record cardiac activity. These leads are referred to as **bipolar leads** because they record the difference in electrical potential between two limbs in which one electrode is positive while the other is negative. A **unipolar lead**, in contrast, has electrodes that record the electrical potential from a single point. Three of the six limb leads, I, II, and III, are bipolar and have already been discussed in earlier chapters (Figure 22–6). The configuration of the bipolar limb leads are:

■ Lead I uses the left arm as positive (+) and the right arm as negative (−).

■ Lead II uses the left leg as positive (+) and the right arm as negative (−).

■ Lead III uses the left leg as positive (+) and the left arm as negative (−).

Augmented Limb Leads

The three remaining limb leads are unipolar, meaning that each records from a single positive (+) limb electrode while the negative (-) reference site is the central terminal of the ECG machine. The three unipolar limb leads are called **augmented leads** because the size of the deflections are amplified by 50 percent in order to match the ECG sizes obtained with other limb leads (Figure 22–7). For this reason, they are listed as aVR, aVL, and aVF for "augmented right arm," "augmented left arm," and "augmented left leg," respectively. It is

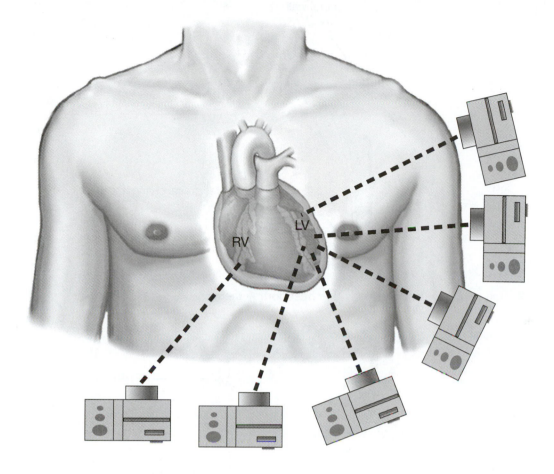

Figure 22–1 Drawing of various "camera" viewing angles in regard to cardiac region viewed by the precordial leads. LV indicates left ventricle and RV indicates the right ventricle.

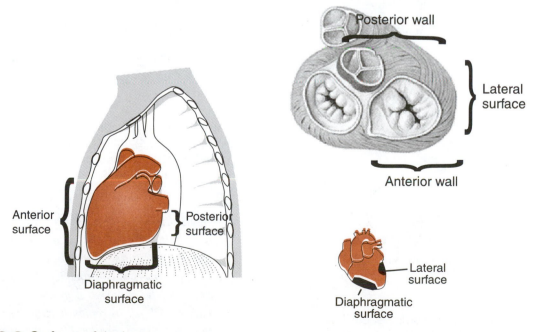

Figure 22–2 Surfaces of the heart.

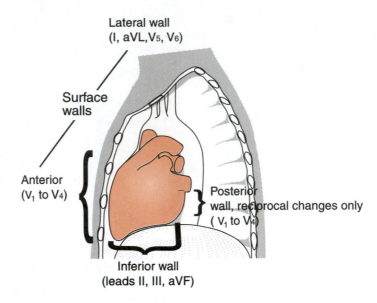

Figure 22-3 Heart surfaces and the leads that best portray them.

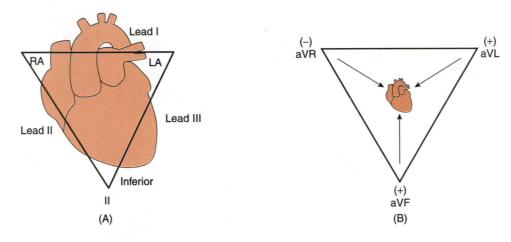

Figure 22-4 Frontal plane electrodes. This schematic represents the relationship of the six extremity leads. [Abbreviations: RA: right arm; LA: left arm; LL: left leg]

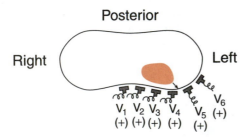

Figure 22-5 Horizontal precordial leads. This schematic [cross-section of chest] represents the relationship of the six chest electrode positions.

interesting to note that lead aVR, which always produces an inverted P-QRS-T complex, is the only lead not used for MI localization and provides little overall useful clinical information.

> ***ECG Application Tip:*** *Each limb lead electrode is assigned a standard color to allow for rapid application: the right arm is white; the left arm is black; the right leg is green and the left leg is red. A mnemonic that may be helpful in remembering these positions is: "Black and white on top; white to the right; and christmas colors below."*

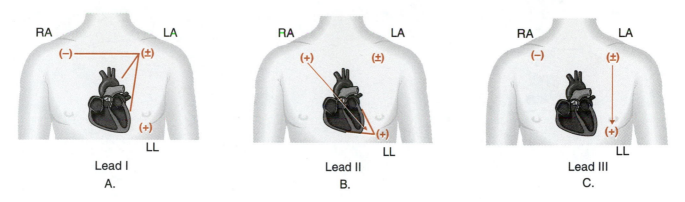

Figure 22–6 Bipolar limb lead locations. One lead is positive and the other negative.

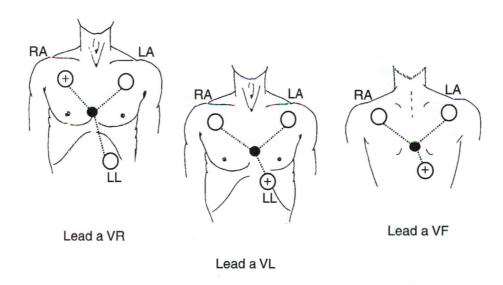

Lead a VR

Lead a VL

Lead a VF

Figure 22–7 Unipolar augmented (aV) limb leads. Augmented leads record the electrical forces between a positive limb electrode and a negative central reference point.

Precordial Leads

Precordial leads are placed on the chest wall so that they wrap around the surface of the left ventricle (Figure 22–8). Leads V_1 through V_6 are unipolar and record heart activity using a single positive precordial chest electrode. Taken together, the information provided by the six precordial leads enables heart damage to be localized.

Precordial Electrode Positions

The six precordial leads are illustrated in Figure 22–9. One lead is located on the right side of the heart (V_1), three are placed across the anterior heart surface (V_2 through V_4), and the remaining two detect activity in the lateral heart area (V_5 and V_6). The anatomic locations of the precordial electrodes are:

- V_1: right 4th intercostal space, just lateral to the sternum

- V_2: left 4th intercostal space, just lateral to the sternum

- V_3: placed midway between the V_3 and V_4 electrode positions

- V_4: midclavicular line in the left 5th intercostal space

- V_5: anterior axillary line at the same level as V_4

- V_6: midaxillary line at the same level as V_4

An example of a precordial lead recording is found in Figure 22–10. Figure 22–11 demonstrates how the chest lead pattern reflects the different surfaces of the myocardium and causes different ECG patterns.

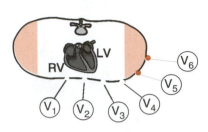

Figure 22-8 Unipolar chest leads. Electrical forces are recorded between a positive chest electrode and a negative central reference point.

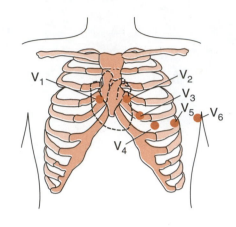

Figure 22-9 Precordial chest lead positions.

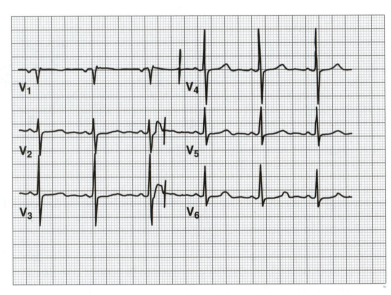

Figure 22-10 Normal precordial R wave progression. The QRS complexes begin primarily as a negative complex in lead V_1, and progress to a positive complex in V_6.

ECG Application Tip: The appearance of the precordial complexes vary when the electrode position is changed. If the electrode positions are changed during serial ECG recordings, the heights of the R waves and Q waves will be altered. When multiple ECGs are anticipated, such as for a patient with an acute myocardial infarction, the electrode positions should be marked as the chest wall or left in place. This will permit accurate tracings despite different ECG machine operators.

Precordial QRS Complex Shape

Three major ventricular events determine the QRS complex shape: septal depolarization, left ventricular depolarization, and right ventricular depolarization (Figure 22–12).

■ *Septal activation.* The initial portion of the QRS complex reflects septal depolarization. The direction of the main electrical vector involved with septal depolarization occurs in a leftward-to-rightward direction. Leads V_1 and V_6 view this cardiac event differently because of their positions are far apart. As Figure 22–13 shows, V_1 depicts septal depolarization as a small positive r wave, while lead V_6 views this as a small negative q wave. The same cardiac activity is recorded differently

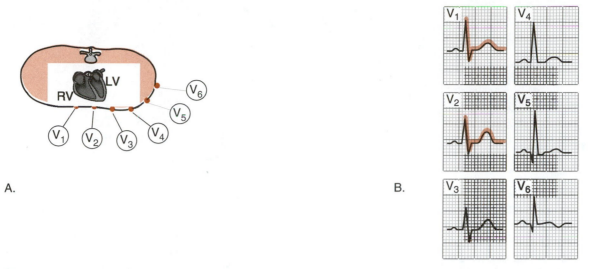

Figure 22-11 R wave progression in relation to precordial electrode position. (Modified with permission from

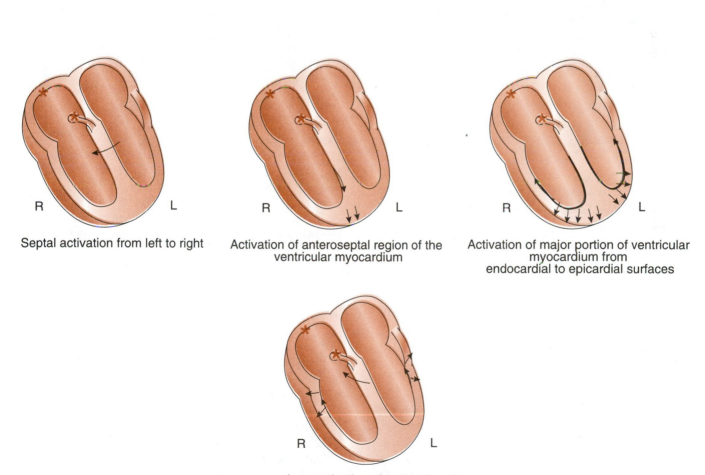

Septal activation from left to right

Activation of anteroseptal region of the ventricular myocardium

Activation of major portion of ventricular myocardium from endocardial to epicardial surfaces

Late activation of posterobasal portion of the left ventricle, the pulmonary conus, and the uppermost portion of the interventricular septum

Figure 22-12 Sequence of ventricular activation.

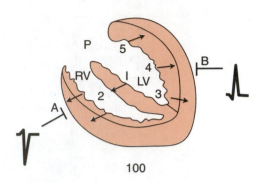

Figure 22-13 Sequence of ventricular depolarization. Septal depolarization occurs first, in a left to right direction indicated by 1. The apical area is activated next (2), followed by most of the ventricular myocardium (3) and uppermost portion of the ventricles (4).

■ *Left and right ventricular activation:* The electrical activity of the septum makes up only a very small portion of QRS complex. The majority of the QRS complex represents activation of the free walls of the ventricles. Because the left ventricle has a much greater mass than the right wall, it contributes a greater proportion to the shape of the QRS complex as indicated in figure 22-17. The precordial electrodes each view and record this activity differently: V_1 is a right-sided lead and views the remainder of ventricular activation as a mainly negative event since the depolarization wave travels away from it, creating a deeply negative S complex. As a result, septal and ventricular wall activation forms an rS complex (Figure 22–14). In contrast, V_6 is a left-sided lead, which sees the same activity as V_1, but views the major energy flow as coming toward it and displays a tall positive R wave. V_6 creates a qR complex formed by the joint activity of the septal and ventricular wall portions (Figure 22–14).

R Wave Progression

Even though the QRS pattern is different in each precordial lead, the *same* cardiac activity is being recorded; however, the electrical events are viewed from slightly different electrode positions. As the QRS complex is recorded across V_1 through V_6, the height of the R wave gradually increases and this typical changing pattern is referred to as the **R wave progression** (Figure 22–15).

The first precordial complex, V_1, begins as a primarily negative QRS complex that gradually becomes mainly positive by the time that V_6 is written. Lead V_1 inscribes

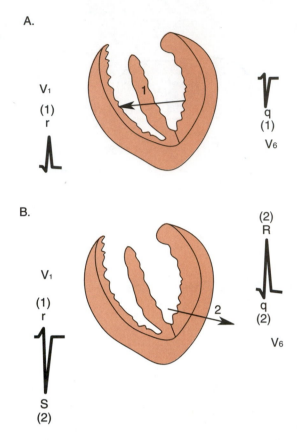

Figure 22-14 Comparison of V_1 and V_6 QRS complexes. The initial portion of the QRS is due to septal depolarization indicated by a 1. Since the left ventricle is much larger than the right, most of the QRS complex is caused by depolarization of the left chamber. This schematic represents the relative contributions of the septum and the left ventricle to the QRS complex.

a small r wave and a large S wave (rS complex), while lead V_6 has a small q wave and a large R wave (qR complex). V_2 through V_5 show QRS complex shapes that are transitions between how V_1 and V_6 appear (Figure 22–20).

R wave progression is important in distinguishing normal from abnormal precordial recordings. For instance, an extensive anterior wall MI causes delayed R wave progression because of loss of R wave height (Figure 22–16). Sometimes, the QRS complex is replaced by a QS complex that totally lacks an R wave, as shown in leads V_1 through V_4. Other conditions, such as *ventricular wall hypertrophy* (abnormally thickened), or right or left ventricular enlargement, as well as chronic obstructive lung disease also alter normal R wave progression.

Specifics of R wave progression

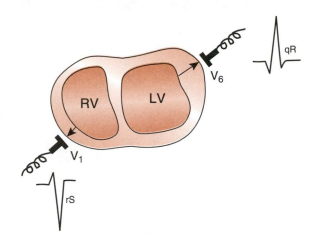

Figure 22–15 Comparison of how V_1 and V_6 represent ventricular depolarization.

Precordial Transition Zone

Midway between V_1 and V_6, an **equiphasic** QRS complex is inscribed at the V_3 electrode position, which has roughly equal positive and negative components. This point is termed the "**zone of transition**" (Figure 22–15A). If an equiphasic QRS complex is not reached or if it occurs much later than the V_3 lead, it is delayed and abnormal (Figure 22–15B). For instance, Figure 22–16 shows an MI in the anterior region, which causes a loss of R wave height in leads V_1 through V_4, and a delayed transition zone—V_5 in this case—as well as "poor R wave progression." An early transition zone can occur because of a posterior wall MI or right ventricular hypertrophy (enlargement), causing the QRS to become mainly positive in V_1 or V_2 (see Figure 22–15C). An early transition zone is also normal in infants and commonly occurs when the precordial electrode positions are misplaced in higher or lower chest position.

BUNDLE BRANCH BLOCKS

Conduction through the ventricles takes place through the AV node, the AV (His) bundle, and the bundle branches, which subdivide until the system ends as tiny Purkinje fibers located throughout the myocardium. Because the left ventricle is thicker, the left bundle branch splits into a left anterior and a left posterior division or fascicle. Normally, the depolarizing impulse travels along each bundle branch simultaneously, thereby ensuring a coordinated ventricular contraction.

Not uncommonly, conduction through a portion of the ventricle is delayed and the QRS complex and ST-T

Normal Chest Lead Patterns

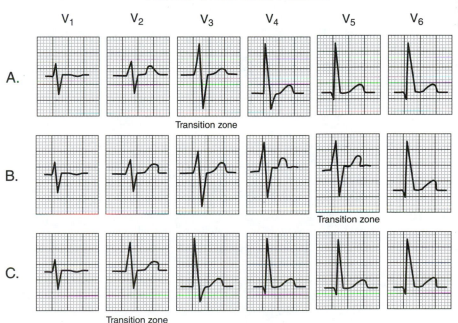

Figure 22–16 Chest lead patterns. The transition zone in pattern A occurs in V_3. The positive and negative portions of the QRS complex are equal in the transition zone. Pattern B shows a delayed transition zone in lead V_5, while C shows an early pattern in V_2.

wave segments become distorted. Bundle branch blocks (BBB) are the most common form of intraventricular conduction disorders that slow down the depolarization impulse. The sequence of events in bundle branch blocks is: impulse travels down unaffected bundle, crosses the septum , and back to the nonfunctioning bundle branch ventricular side. The ventricles are activated sequentially rather than simultaneously in bundle branch blocks and involve abnormal intraventricular conduction.

Right Bundle Branch Block (RBBB)

Right bundle branch block (RBBB) occurs when conduction in the right bundle branch is abnormally delayed or completely blocked. The right bundle is more susceptible to injury and fatigue than is the left bundle branch because of its smaller size. RBBB is a more common finding than left bundle branch block (LBBB). The causes of bundle branch blocks are listed in Table 22–1 and the ECG characteristics are found in Table 22–2.

ECG Characteristics of RBBB

ECG abnormalities result from delayed right ventricular

Table 22–1 Causes of Bundle Branch Blocks
■ May be Normal Variant
■ Coronary Artery Disease
■ Acute Myocardial Infarction
■ Hypertensive Heart Disease
■ Pericarditis and Myocarditis
■ Aortic Valve Disease
■ Degenerative Fibrosis of the Conduction Pathway
■ Mimicked by Wolfe-Parkinson-White (W-P-W) Syndrome

activation (Figure 22–17). As a result, the QRS complex is prolonged, that is, 0.12 seconds or greater, and has an abnormal appeerence. The second r′ wave is caused by the delayed depolarization of the right ventricle (Figure 22–18). As a result, the late portion of the QRS has an abnormal shape. The left-sided leads: I, aVL, V_5, and V_6, display wide, deep S waves because these leads show the delayed right ventricular activation as the last portion of the QRS.

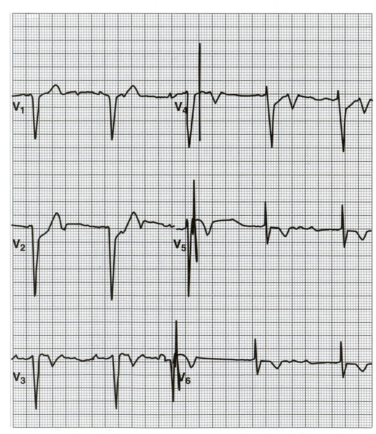

Figure 22-17 Abnormally delayed transition zone due to "poor" R wave progression. An anterior wall MI results in the loss of R wave height and forms mainly QS complexes in V_1 through V_4. The late transition zone occurs in V5. (Note the deeply inverted T waves.)

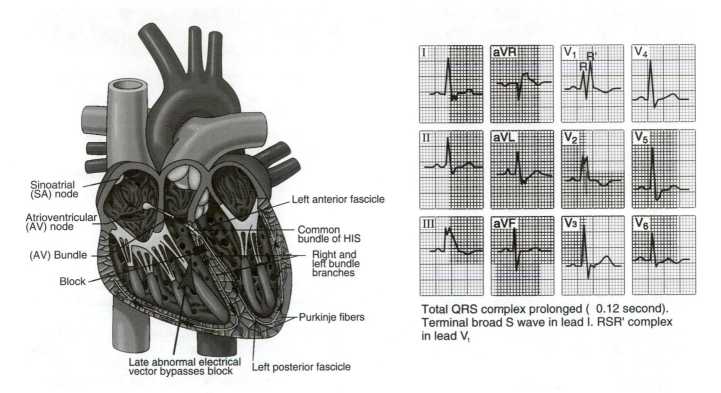

Total QRS complex prolonged (0.12 second). Terminal broad S wave in lead I. RSR' complex in lead V_1

Figure 22–18 Twelve-lead right bundle branch block. Note the wide QRS duration which is best seen in V_1 through V_6 and the rSR complex in V_1. The deep, wide S wave in V_6, I, and a VL is characteristic.

Left Bundle Branch Block (LBBB)

In a left bundle branch block, the impulse initially stimulates the right bundle branch and right ventricle normally, then slowly crosses the interventricular septum to eventually activate the left ventricle in a delayed manner. The depolarization stimulus enters the left ventricle *later than usual* because the septum does not contain conduction fibers, causing a wider than normal QRS complex. QRS widening is more pronounced with

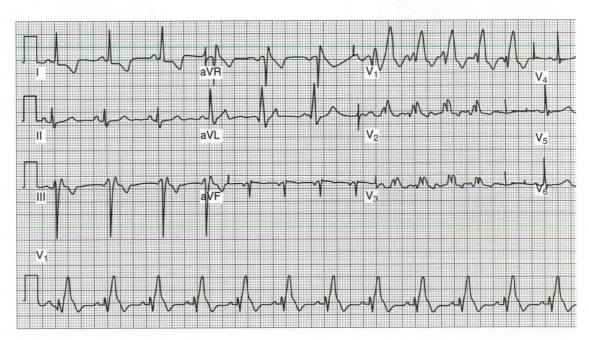

Figure 22–19 Right bundle branch block (RBBB).

Table 22–2 Right Bundle Branch Block ECG Characteristics
■ **Wide QRS complex (0.12 second or greater)**
■ **Distorted QRS complex: r-s-R′ complex in V1 through V2.**
■ **Wide, deep S wave in I, aVL, V5 and V6.**
■ **Abnormal ST segment and inverted T wave in V1 through V2.**

Table 22–3 Left Bundle Branch Block ECG Characteristics
■ **QRS complex is 0.12 second or greater.**
■ **QRS complex is negative (mainly QS) in V1 and V2.**
■ **QRS complex is upright r-s-R′ or QR configuration in V5 and V6.**
■ **There are secondary ST-T wave changes caused by altered depolarization.**

LBBB than with RBBB (Figure 22–19). The abnormal depolarization also causes an altered repolarization process. The ST-T wave complex isabnormal as well. Unlike a right bundle branch block, which can occur in patients without organic heart disease, LBBB always signify heart disease. The most common cause of an acute LBBB is an acute MI. Causes of chronic LBBB include hypertensive and ischemic heart disease (see Table 22–1).

ECG Characteristics of LBBB

Since septal activation causes the R wave formation and is absent in leads V_1 and V_2, the R waves are lost (Table 22–3). The QRS duration becomes at least 0.12 second wide and an abnormal QS complex forms in V_1

and V_2. In the right-sided precordial leads V_5 and V_6, the QRS complex has a wide, notched R wave that lacks a q wave. The ST-T wave complex also becomes abnormal because the altered depolarization leads to repolarization. The ECG changes that occur with a LBBB have important implications about the ability to detect myocardial infarction. A LBBB will mask the signs of an MI, making the ECG unreliable in detecting acute injury patterns. A twelve-lead ECG showing a LBBB is seen in Figure 22–21.

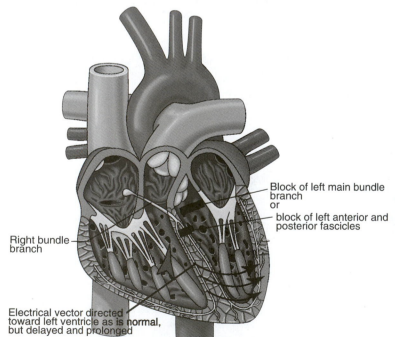

Right bundle branch

Block of left main bundle branch
or
block of left anterior and posterior fascicles

Electrical vector directed toward left ventricle as is normal, but delayed and prolonged

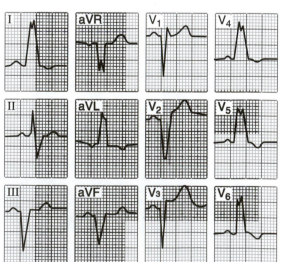

Wide QRS complex prolonged (0.12 second). with ST depressions and inverted T waves, particularly in leads I, aVL, V5 and V6.

Figure 22-20 Twelve-lead ECG with left bundle branch block. Note that the QRS complex is widened and that the ST-T deflection is opposite to the QRS direction. The main electrical impulse (vector) follows a normal direction but is delayed and takes longer than normal.

Clinical Note *When an acute LBBB develops during an MI, the possibility of developing advanced AV heart blocks should be anticipated.*

ECG Interpretation Tip *The most useful leads for identifying bundle branch blocks are V_1 and V_2 along with V_5 and V_6. These leads will distinguish right from left BBBs*

Let's Review

1. Twelve-lead ECGs consist of six limb leads and six precordial leads.

2. Limb leads record cardiac activity in the frontal plane, while chest leads record in the horizontal axis.

3. Twelve-lead ECGs are useful in detecting acute myocardial injury patterns.

4. Augmented limb leads amplify the ECG size to match other limb leads.

5. Left-sided electrodes at the V_5 and V_6 positions are considered lateral leads; right-sided electrodes at the V_1 and V_2 position are called septal leads; and electrodes at the V_3 and V_4 positions are termed mid-precordial or anterior leads.

6. The precordial QRS complex appearance changes from a mainly negative (rS) complex in V_1 to a mainly positive (Rs) complex in V_6.

7. The precordial transition zone is the ECG lead where the QRS complex has equal positive and negative components. The usual transition zone occurs in lead V_3 but may occur earlier or later.

8. Following an anterior wall MI a loss of R wave height occurs and there is a deepening of the Q wave appearance. The result is an abnormally delayed or absent R wave progression across the precordial leads.

9. Right Bundle Branch Block has a widened QRS complex and a r-S-R´ shape in leads V_1 and V_2 while leads V_5 and V_6, I, aVL has deep, slurred S waves.

10. In a LBBB the QRS complex is widened and distorted. V_1 and V_2 has a QS complex while V_5 and V_6 show a tall R wave that lacks a q wave.

11. Repolarization will be altered in bundle branch blocks along with depolarization.

12. LBBB is always indicative of diffuse organic heart disease while RBBB can occur without obvious heart disease.

13. LBBB will mask the ECG findings of an MI while RBBB will not.

Glossary

Acute coronary syndrome (ACS) Ischemic cardiac events, including stable angina, unstable angina, and myocardial infarction.

Augmented lead Limb lead in which the size of the ECG deflections is amplified by 50 percent to match the size of the other leads; the three unipolar limb leads.

Bipolar lead Lead recording the difference in electrical potential between two limb electrodes, one being positive while the other is negative.

Bundle branch block Conduction delay in one or both bundle branches, resulting in delayed ventricular depolarization.

Equiphasic QRS complex ECG complex that has roughly equal positive and negative components.

Frontal plane Area in which the limb leads record cardiac activity; provides information on the energy flow along the inferior and superior heart borders.

Horizontal plane Area in which the chest leads record cardiac activity; provides information on the energy flow anterior and posterior heart regions, as well as rightward and leftward forces.

Left bundle branch block (LBBB) Conduction delay in the left bundle branch that causes a delay in activation of the left ventricle.

Precordial leads Unipolar leads placed on the chest and labeled from V_1 to V_6 based on the position.

R wave progression QRS complex R wave height gradually increases as the precordial leads progress from V_1 through V_6.

Right bundle branch block (RBBB) Conduction delay in the right bundle branch that causes a delay in activation of the right ventricle.

Unipolar lead Lead that records the electrical potential from a single electrode.

Ventricular hypertrophy Abnormally thickened heart wall.

Zone of transition Point during the R wave progression when the QRS complex has roughly equal positive and negative components.

chapter 23

ECG Ischemia, Injury, and Infarction Patterns

LEARNING OBJECTIVES

Upon completion of this chapter, the reader should be able to:

- *List the ECG findings that occur with myocardial ischemia, injury, and infarction.*

- *Explain the reason why recording serial electrocardiograms is useful when an initial ECG is "nondiagnostic" or normal in a patient with a clinical presentation suggestive of cardiac ischemia.*

- *Describe the terms "current of injury" and "acute ST segments."*

- *List at least three descriptive shapes describing pathologic ST segment changes seen during an (AMI) acute myocardial infarction.*

- *List at least three noncoronary conditions that can cause ECG findings that resemble an AMI.*

- *List two causes of primary and secondary T wave changes.*

- *Describe the appearance of reciprocal ECG changes observed during some AMIs and explain their significance.*

- *Distinguish the ECG characteristics of a "non-Q wave" infarction versus a "Q-wave" MI.*

- *Identify those ECG leads that show a myocardial ischemia and injury in the following regions: (a) anterior; (b) inferior; (c) posterior; and (d) right ventricular.*

- *Name the coronary vessel involved during a myocardial infarction that occurs located in the following heart locations: (a) inferior; (b) anterior; (c) posterior; and (d) right ventricular.*

- *Indicate whether there is a higher mortality rate and greater degree of impaired left ventricular function associated with an anterior or an inferior wall MI.*

- *List the ECG criteria for a posterior wall MI.*

CHAPTER OVERVIEW

Inadequate coronary blood flow produces a range of ECG changes—from ischemia to infarction. T wave and ST segment abnormalities, along with the development of pathologic Q wave are indicators of myocardial ischemia and injury. The clinical spectrum resulting from ischemic heart disease is referred to as acute coronary syndromes. Acute coronary syndromes include stable angina pectoris, unstable angina, and myocardial infarction. The twelve-lead ECG is the major diagnostic tool in diagnosing acute myocardial infarctions. The twelve-lead ECG allows the clinician to localize the cardiac abnormality to a specific heart area.

EARLY RECOGNITION OF CARDIAC ISCHEMIA, INJURY, AND INFARCTION PATTERNS

Making a rapid assessment of the cause of chest pain is a daily challenge in emergency care. Large clinical studies of thrombolytic therapy for myocardial infarction have consistently demonstrated that the sooner that coronary blood flow can be reestablished, the better the patients' chance of survival, the fewer complications, and the less impairment of myocardial function. Twelve-lead ECG interpretation remains the cornerstone of detecting an *acute myocardial infarction (AMI)* and instituting thrombolytic therapy. Every emergency care clinician must be able to quickly and accurately interpret the ECG signs of myocardial injury.

Pre-hospital twelve-lead ECG determination, which has been made feasible by the development of compact, portable machines, has proved to significantly diminish the delay in administration of thrombolytic therapy. The ECG changes associated with AMI are straightforward and easy to recognize. Pre-hospital recording of twelve-lead ECGs is practical and has not caused a significant increase in on-scene time, which would have delayed EMS responses to other emergencies. Pre-hospital ECG recordings are digitally transmitted using cellular phone technology to the receiving hospital *prior* to the patient's arrival—permitting staff valuable preparation time. Recently, several studies have shown a benefit from paramedics starting thrombolytic therapy using a bolus dose of tissue plasminogen activator (*t*-PA).

Similarly, ECGs are currently being utilized as part of the initial ED triage process for patients with chest pain at most hospitals. Computerized ECG interpretation programs have been found to be accurate in identifying most infarction patterns—which can now be obtained *before* the patient is even registered. However, computerized interpretation programs are not infallible; clinicians still need to evaluate the ECG in the light of the patient's clinical setting. The benefits of early identification and treatment of an MI highlight how important it is to be able to accurately interpret ECGs.

This chapter will expand ECG evaluation beyond the topic of dysrhythmias and concentrate on recognizing ECG patterns associated with cardiac ischemia and injury. Studying ECG ischemia patterns along with dysrhythmias is a logical approach because both conditions commonly occur together. For instance, the rhythm tracing in Figure 23–1 shows two common dysrhythmias, atrial fibrillation and ventricular tachycardia along with the major finding of an acute injury pattern.

ECG CHANGES DURING ACUTE CORONARY SYNDROMES

There is a spectrum of ECG changes, ranging from T wave changes, altered ST segments, and abnormal Q wave development that happen with acute coronary syndromes. The ECG changes associated with an MI follow a largely predictable sequence. Specific ECG findings that develop during diminished coronary supply depends on whether the coronary artery obstruction is reversible, as with ischemia, or permanent, as during an infarction.

ECG Limitations: Every MI Cannot Be Detected

It is important to recognize that the ECG is not a perfect tool and has limitations in detecting myocardial damage. Sometimes the ECG tracing fails to reflect an AMI because a preexisting ECG abnormality obscures the ischemic pattern or because the cardiac tracing only shows *nonspecific cardiogram changes*. For instance, in the presence of a left bundle branch block, an electronic pacemaker, or in Wolfe-Parkinson-White (WPW) syndrome, the ECG will not show ischemic changes even during advanced myocardial damage (Figure 23–2). The underlying ECG alterations prevent the characteristic MI pattern from developing. Nonspecific ECG changes are minor findings that are not characteristic of an acute coronary syndrome.

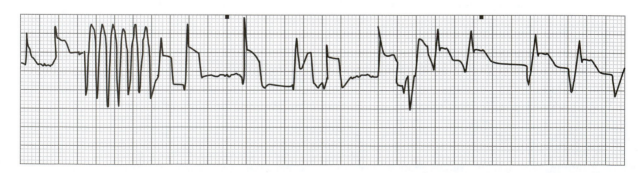

Figure 23–1 ECG tracing displays atrial fibrillation along with acute ST segment elevation and ventricular tachycardia.

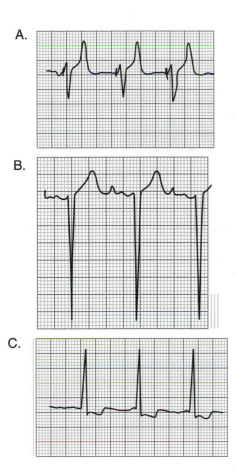

Figure 23–2 Non-ischemic conditions that alter ST segments. Conditions that can mimic an AMI include: (A) artificial pacemaker; (B) left bundle branch block; and (C) Wolfe-Parkinson-White syndrome.

> **Clinical Note** *Patients with a history suggestive of myocardial ischemia—with or without cardiac risk factors—and a normal ECG are a major diagnostic challenge. Despite a normal ECG, a small but significant number of these cases are later found to have acute coronary syndromes, including unstable angina and atypical MIs. Therefore, a normal ECG does not equal normal coronary arteries.*

Nonspecific ECG Changes

In certain cases of ischemia or injury the only ECG signs associated are nonspecific changes, meaning that subtle or unremarkable ECG findings that are not indicative occur—again reinforcing the adage of the importance of "treating the patient and not the ECG tracing." Nonspecific ECG findings commonly involve inverted or biphasic T waves or minor ST segment alterations without clear-cut signs of insufficient coronary artery blood flow.

> **Clinical Note** *A clinical presentation suggestive of an MI but with a left bundle branch block—especially if the block is new—may still be an indication for thrombolytic therapy. Rapid cardiac enzyme or serum maker analysis is a helpful tool if the ECG is nondiagnostic.*

Serial ECG Tracings

One reason that some AMIs are not diagnosed when initially examined is because time is needed for the ECG complexes to reflect myocardial damage. Because ECG changes occur over a period of time, the patient may present to the EMS or ED *before* the ECG becomes diagnostic. Because of this, it is standard practice to record *serial ECGs,* which are typically repeated at half-hour intervals at least three times for cases that have a convincing history but a normal or nondiagnostic ECG. Fortunately, most AMI patients show a classic progression of ECG changes that are straightforward and usually present on the initial tracing.

> **Clinical Note** *A normal ECG never "rules out" myocardial ischemia. The patient is treated with cardiac "precautions" and serial ECG tracings are recorded until the diagnosis is clear.*

CORONARY VESSELS

The heart is supplied by two major vessels, the right and left coronary arteries, which arise from the aorta just beyond the aortic valves (Figure 24–3). Each coronary artery divides and subdivides many times before eventually reaching the myocardial fibers. Except for a very small rim of endocardial heart muscle lying immediately adjacent to the inner wall of the ventricles, oxygen-rich blood within the cardiac chamber does not directly supply myocardial tissue. Myocardial cells depend on receiving a constant blood supply via the two coronary arteries. An obstruction involving either coronary branch will jeopardize myocardial viability. The left atrium and ventricle are dependent on the left coronary artery, while the right side of the heart is mainly served by the right coronary artery. The heart areas served by the two main coronary vessels are largely independent of one another, so that an abrupt occlusion in one branch will cause some myocardial damage. However, when a gradual obstruction occurs, vessels adjacent to the damaged artery are able to slowly dilate and supply additional blood flow. This is referred to as *collateral coronary circulation*, which can compensate to some degree for the diminished vessel flow and limit the heart damage.

Left Coronary Artery

The left coronary artery develops from the aorta immediately beyond where the aortic valves are located and is termed the left main coronary artery. The left main coronary artery extends for a short distance before forming the left anterior descending (LAD) and left circumflex arteries. As the name suggests, the *left anterior descend-*

ing artery travels down along the anterior surface of the ventricle in a groove separating both ventricles. The LAD supplies the anterior and apical portions of the left ventricle. The *circumflex artery* curves around to the back of the heart and flows down along the rear surface, supplying the posterior and inferior left ventricular walls.

Right Coronary Artery

The *right coronary artery* supplies most of the right atria and ventricle, including—in most people—the AV node, interventricular septum, and proximal His bundle. The right coronary artery remains a major vessel without subdivisions. The right coronary artery travels toward the back of the heart and descends within the AV groove, supplying most of the right ventricle and the posterior portion of the left ventricle. In over half of individuals, the right coronary artery supplies the sinus node, via the sinoatrial artery, and in 85 to 90 percent of people forms the AV nodal artery. The inferior wall of

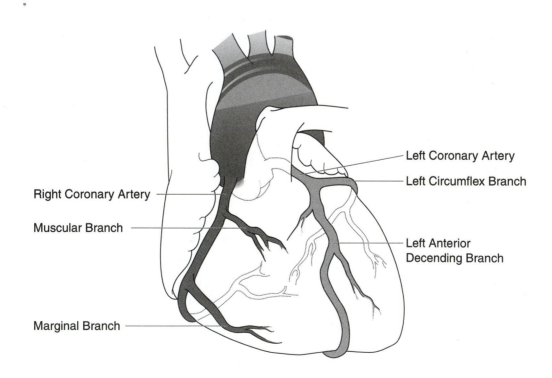

Figure 23-3 Coronary arteries.

the left ventricle—the most common infarct site—is supplied by the right coronary artery in most individuals.

Coronary Veins

Most coronary blood flow returns from myocardial tissue and enters the right atrium via the coronary sinus and anterior coronary veins.

THE SUBENDOCARDIAL REGION

When a coronary artery is occluded, heart damage occurs in stages, beginning in the subendocardial region and progressing outward across the myocardial layers until the outermost layer, the epicardial surface, is affected (Figure 23–4). The *subendocardial region*, is the innermost heart layer closest to the blood in the ventricular chamber. The subendocardial area is most susceptible to compromised blood flow because it experiences the highest pressure forces during contraction.

Coronary blood flow differs dramatically during the contraction and relaxation phases: during myocardial contraction, systolic blood flow virtually ceases as the vessels are compressed in the subendocardial region (Figure 23–6). Most blood flow to the myocardium happens during diastole when the heart muscle is relaxed and the coronary vessels are maximally open. As a result, ischemia affects the subendocardial region first.

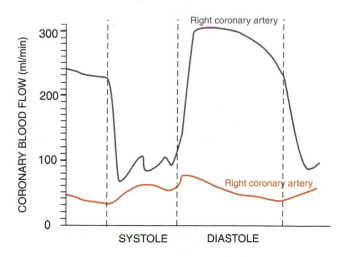

Figure 23–5 Relationship of the relative blood flow through right and left ventricular capillaries to the phases of the cardiac cycle. Coronary blood flow diminishes sharply in the left coronary artery as contraction occurs. (Used with permission from Guyton AC. Textbook of Medical Physiology. 6th ed. Philadelphia: WB Saunders; 1981: Figure 25–2.))

If the ischemia is not corrected, myocardial muscle damage spreads in a wavelike direction beginning in the inner heart region, extending through the thick myocardium, and affecting the epicardium last.

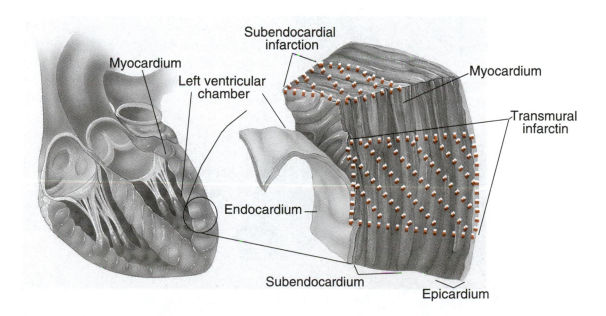

Figure 23–4 Cross-section of the left ventricle showing the area of a non-Q wave (sunbendocardial) infarction and a Q-wave (transmural) infarction. The subendocardial region involves the inner portion of the ventricular wall that is closest to the ventricle, while the transmural region involves all three heart layers.

CORONARY OBSTRUCTION

Two major causes of AMI include coronary thrombosis and coronary vasospasm.

Coronary thrombosis involves an acute blockage, usually of an already narrowed or **stenosed coronary artery**. Coronary thrombosis causes over 90 percent of myocardial infarctions. *Atherosclerosis* is a disease involving the gradual buildup of waste material within the vessel wall, causing narrowing. Atherosclerotic plaque accumulates within the middle layer of the coronary artery wall and contains fatty material, calcium, and cellular debris. The plaque, having accumulated over decades, is covered with a hard fibrous cap that shields it from the blood in the vessel lumen by a thin epithelial intimal layer. As the degree of plaque buildup continues, the vessel finally becomes partially blocked (Figure 23–7).

Plaque rupture with expulsion of the plaque material into the lumen is the initiating event leading to most AMIs (Table 23–1). The body senses the ruptured plaque as damaged tissue that needs repair and acti-

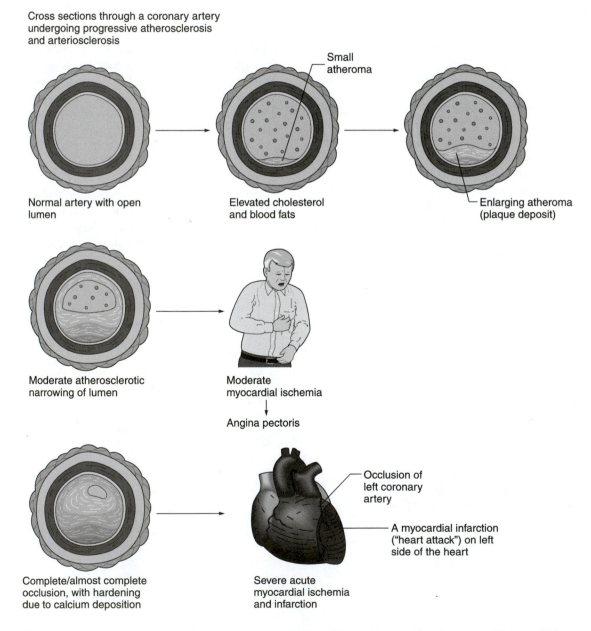

Cross sections through a coronary artery undergoing progressive atherosclerosis and arteriosclerosis

Small atheroma

Normal artery with open lumen

Elevated cholesterol and blood fats

Enlarging atheroma (plaque deposit)

Moderate atherosclerotic narrowing of lumen

Moderate myocardial ischemia

↓

Angina pectoris

Complete/almost complete occlusion, with hardening due to calcium deposition

Severe acute myocardial ischemia and infarction

Occlusion of left coronary artery

A myocardial infarction ("heart attack") on left side of the heart

Figure 23–6 Comparison of a normal coronary artery with a diseased, partially obstructed lumen. The normal portion of lumen is smooth and open, whereas the diseased portion is narrowed due to accumulated cellular debris and proliferation of cellular structures in the intimal region.

Table 23-1 Steps in Coronary Artery Obstruction

- **Formation of atheromatous plaque**
- **Rupture and expulsion of plaque material into vessel lumen**
- **Platelet clumping**
- **Initiation of coagulation process**
- **Fibrin clot formation**
- **Thrombosis formation**
- **Myocardial damage occurs**

vates the coagulation process.

The first step in clot formation begins with platelet clumping at the ruptured plaque site and formation of a fibrin clot. The platelet clot seals the already narrowed vessel lumen and myocardial muscle begins being deprived of blood flow.

Coronary artery spasm refers to the sudden pathologic narrowing of coronary artery due to contraction of smooth muscle found within the wall of the coronary artery. Fewer than 10 percent of MIs are due to coro-nary vasospasm while the majority are due to plaque rupture. *Vasospasm* is often superimposed upon ather-osclerotic vessels but can occur in the absence of plaque. Severe coronary artery constriction deprives heart tissue of circulation. Cocaine use and cigarette smoking are strong mediators of coronary vasoplasm. MIs can occur in patients with cocaine-induced vaso-plasm even in the absence of atherosclerosic plaque. A disorder in the autonomic nervous system innervation can also caused vasospasm.

DYSRHYTHMIAS AS A CAUSE OF ISCHEMIA

Dysrhythmias can decrease cardiac output, which in turn, can compromise coronary blood flow. Ischemia occurs with both rapid and slow rhythm disorders and during supraventricular and ventricular dysrhythmias (Figure 23–7). Shortened diastolic filling times occur with rapid rates and cause a decreased stroke volume. During ventricular tachycardia, for example, coronary artery blood flow can fall by more than half. Bradycardic rates, such as those found with advanced AV heart block, can impair coronary perfusion because cardiac output is determined by the stroke volume and heart rate. So, even a greater than normal stroke volume cannot com-pensate for very slow rates. Even in the absence of coro-nary artery disease, prolonged tachycardic episodes as

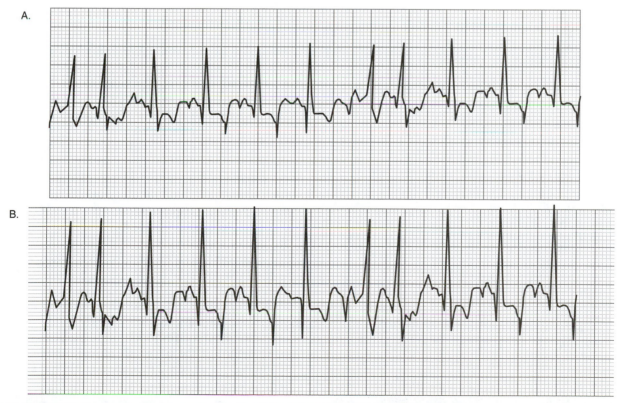

Figure 23–7 Tachydysrhythmias associated with significant ST segment depression.

occurs with PSVT, can lead to ischemic ECG changes, which are usually temporary.

Prolonged hypotension, which can be caused by diverse conditions such as hypovolemia or septic shock, can cause generalized myocardial ischemia, termed **global myocardial ischemia**, if arterial perfusion decreases enough to compromise myocardial perfusion.

ST Segment Abnormalities

Ischemia lowers the cellular resting membrane potential and shortens the action potential duration. This, in turn, causes a difference in energy potential between the injured and normal myocardium which causes an energy current flow between the affected and normal areas. This current of injury results in the ST segment moving away from its isoelectric ECG baseline position and forming an "*acute ST segment*" (Figure 23–8). The ST segment elevation accompanying an AMI occurs *within minutes* of coronary obstruction.

When the myocardial damage involves all three heart layers, the involvement is termed transmural and the ST segment becomes elevated in the ECG leads facing the damaged site. When the injury is limited to the subendocardial layer, ST segment depression and T wave inversion occurs.

Primary and Secondary ST-T Wave Changes

The ST abnormalities caused by ischemia or drugs are termed *primary ST-T wave changes* because these conditions *directly* affect the myocardial fibers. Digoxin usually depresses or "scoops" the ST segment and T wave due to the medication's effect on the heart tissue. These ST-T wave changes are also primary changes.

When ventricular depolarization is abnormal, the repolarization process will also be altered. ST segment alterations due only to abnormal depolarization are termed *secondary ST-T wave changes*. Conditions like W-P-W syndrome, premature ventricular complexes, and bundle branch blocks result in secondary ST-T wave repolarization abnormalities. Secondary ST-T wave changes are caused by an electrical process and are not due to ischemia.

> **Clinical Note** *Primary ST segment changes occur with myocardial injury. Secondary ST segment shifts follow an altered depolarization, as in bundle branch block, PVCs, and left ventricular hypertrophy. Primary ST-T wave changes are clinically significant while secondary changes are not important*

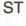
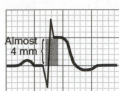

Figure 23–8 ST segment elevation from isoelectric baseline position indicates acute myocardial injury. A pathologic Q wave—wide and deep—is also present.

Ischemic ST Segments

The shape of the ST segment slope is important, in addition to the degree of any ST segment deviation from baseline. Nonischemic ST segments gradually slope upward from the J point as it merges into the T wave.

As described by Goldberger and Goldberger, the ST segments associated with an MI can have one of the four common shapes as shown in Figure 23–9 (1.) plateau appearance with a generalized flattening; (2.) dome shaped, referred to as being concave upward; (3.) obliquely elevated, occurring at a sharp angle relative to the QRS complex; and (4.) a curved or crescent shape with a convex upward appearance. Figure 23–10 shows these ST variations from actual cases.

The plateau or horizontal shape is indicative of an MI but is an uncommon finding. Plateau-shaped ST segments can be inadvertently overlooked when there is minimal ST segment elevation.

A rounded, "dome," or "coving" of the ST segment is the most classical and common appearance of AMI. This change in ST segment characteristics is most commonly noticed in the precordial leads. During an early AMI, oblique elevation or straightening of the ST segment can occur before ST elevation develops. This is the subtlest and earliest clue to an AMI. The "crescent-like" shape has a normally curved ST appearance but the segment is displaced from the ECG baseline. ST segments having the concave downward appearance are one of the most common patterns seen with an MI but it can also be seen with some nonischemic conditions (Table 23–2).

During the recovery phase following an MI, the ST segment returns to baseline. When a thrombolytic agent is successful, the ST segments quickly return to baseline and this often corresponds with resolution of chest pain. Return of the ST segment to a baseline position following thrombolytic therapy is a clinical marker that reperfusion has occurred.

Table 23-2 Nonischemic Causes of ST Segment Changes

- **Pericarditis**
- **Benign Early Repolarization**
- **Ventricular Aneurysm**
- **Cardiac Tamponade**
- **Drugs: Digoxin, Antidysrhythmic Medication**
- **Left Ventricular Hypertrophy**
- **Wolfe-Parkinson-White Syndrome**
- **Left Bundle Branch Block**

Clinical Note More than 25 percent of patients who are later diagnosed with an AMI do not have ST segment elevation when initially seen by EMS or upon arrival in the ED. This illustrates the need to record serial ECGs as an acute coronary syndrome is an ongoing process.

Nonischemic Causes of ST Segment Abnormalities. Elevated and depressed ST segments can also be caused by nonischemic conditions, such as benign early repolarization, pericarditis, and ventricular aneurysms (see Table 23–2). These ST segment elevations may mimic an infarction. Because thrombolytic therapy carries a 3 to 4 percent incidence of serious bleeding, such as gastrointestinal or cerebrovascular bleeding, it is important to be able to distinguish nonischemic from ischemic causes of ST changes. ST elevations in *anatomically contiguous leads* indicate real coronary artery distribution. The patient's clinical presentation determines whether the ECG is compatible with a diagnosis of an AMI.

Benign Early Repolarization. A relatively common cause of nonischemic ST segment elevation (Figure 23–11) occurs in benign early repolarization, which is a common finding in healthy athletic males, especially black teenagers and young men. The ST segment appears diffusely elevated across several ECG leads but is most pronounced in chest leads V_3 through V_5. A helpful clue that benign early repolarization is responsible for ST elevation is that the QRS downstroke shows a small positive deflection referred to as a "notched J point" (Figure 23–13). The ST segment shape retains a normal concave upward slope. Also, the ST segments remain stable over time so a previously recorded ECG would be helpful for comparison. Drugs, such as digoxin, left bundle branch block, and ventricular hypertrophy are other common causes of nonischemic ST segment depression.

Clinical Note ST segment elevation occurs with several common nonischemic conditions. The patient's presentation should be consistent with an acute ischemic coronary syndrome before thrombolytic therapy is considered.

Pathologic Q Waves

Pathologic Q waves indicate that transmural myocardial necrosis has occurred. Pathologic Q waves are deep Q waves that are at least 1/3 the height of the QRS complex and are at least 0.04 second wide (Figures 23–12 and 23–13). Small Q waves may be normal in V_5, V_6, I and aVL. Pathologic Q waves develop after ST segment elevation in a transmural MI. Pathologic Q waves may

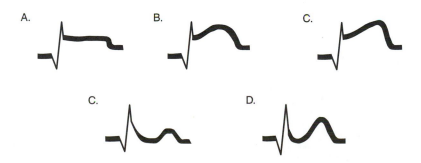

Figure 23-9 Abnormally shaped, elevated ST segments associated with AMI. Example A has a horizontal or plateaued shape; B has a rounded or coved shape; C shows an oblique elevation; and example D shows a crescent shaped ST segment.

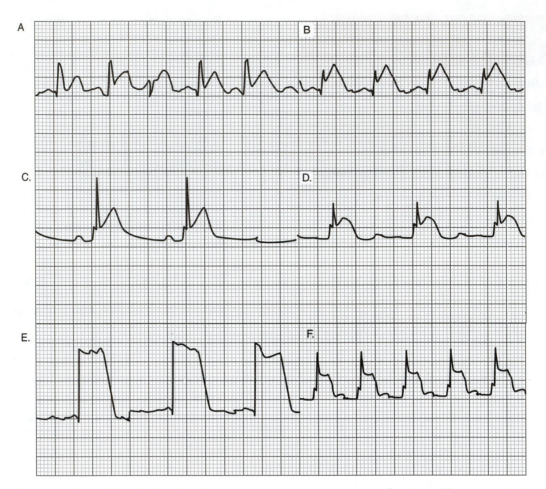

Figure 23–10 ST segment elevations due to acute MIs tracings. A and B show oblique straightening; C and D show a concave upward appearance, E and F show a more horizontal or flattened ST appearance.

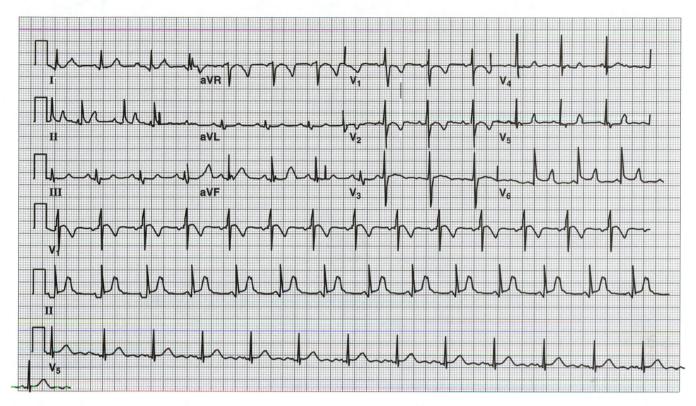

Figure 23–11 Benign early repolarization. Diffuse ST segment elevation occuring across anatomic boundaries, coupled with notching of the QRS downstroke in leads II, III, V₄, and V₅ are clues to this benign ST elevation ECG condition.

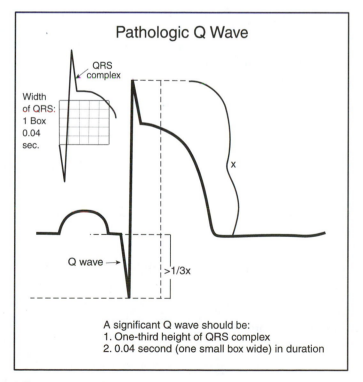

Figure 23–12 Pathologic Q wave.

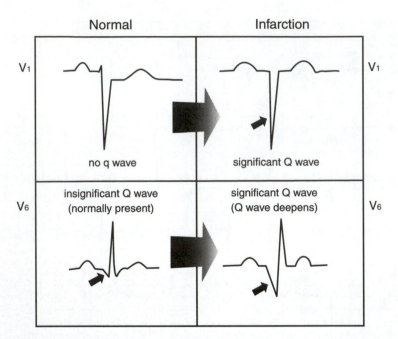

Figure 23–13 Pathologic Q waves. Lead V₁ normally does not have a Q wave, while pathologic Q waves develop following infarction. Lead V₆ normally records a tiny, insignificant Q wave but after an infarction the Q wave becomes deeper and wider.

develop in as little as three hours or take up to 24 hours. Pathologic Q waves often remain as the only ECG finding of an MI, remaining well after the T wave and ST segment changes resolve. During an AMI, the R wave height becomes smaller as the infarcted myocardium loses voltage and is often replaced by a deep "QS" complex (Figures 23–14 and 23–15)

> **ECG Interpretation Tip** *Pathologic Q waves often remain as the only ECG sign that an MI occurred. Abnormal Q waves are an ECG "scar" lasting long after a myocardial injury heals.*

T Wave Abnormalities

T waves, which represent ventricular repolarization, are normally upright in most leads, except in aVR. The following concepts, according to Marriott are important when assessing T wave appearance:

- As a general rule, the T wave direction follows the major deflection of the QRS complex.

- T waves are upright in leads I and II, as well as in the majority of the precordial leads (V₃ through V₆).

- In lead V₁ the T wave may normally be inverted. T wave inversion is abnormal in males if it occurs as

far leftward in the precordial leads as V₃. However, in females shallow inversion in precordial leads to V₃ can be normal.

- The T wave direction is variable in III, aVL, aVF, V₁ and V₂.

- In summary, the T wave direction is variable in leads III, aVF, and aVL, and right precordial leads V₁ and V₂. T waves may appear positive, inverted, biphasic, or flat.

Ischemia causes T waves in leads that are ordinarily upright to become inverted (Figure 23–18). When normally upright T waves invert in several leads during an anginal episode, it is referred to as a *pattern of ischemia* (Figure 23–17). The "flipped" T waves return to their upright position after the ischemia resolves. Ischemic-related T waves are deeply inverted with sharp, pointed tips. During non-Q wave MIs, T wave inversions may be the sole ECG sign that has an appearance that resembles arrowheads.

Hyperacute T waves

One of the earliest ECG findings of an acute MI is "hyperacute" T waves, which refers to unusually tall and pointed T waves. Peaked T waves are best appreciated in leads V₁ through V₃. Although hyperacute T waves are often cited as the earliest AMI finding, it is not a clinically useful finding because by the time that most AMI patients seek assistance, the tall T waves are no longer visible. ST segment coving is a much more

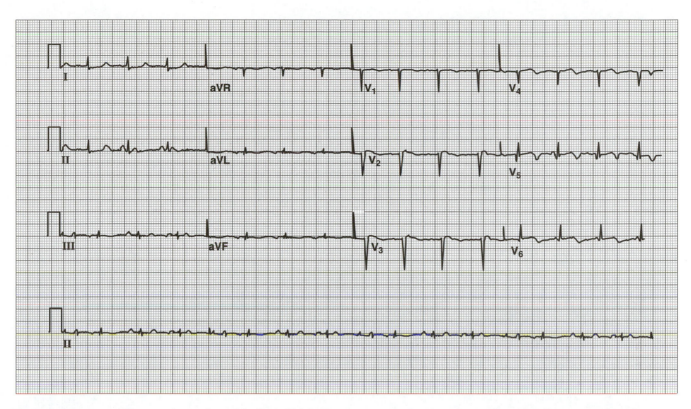

Figure 23-14 QS complexes from V_1 through V_4. T wave inversions coupled with acute ST segments in V_1 through V_4 hint at a semiacute event most likely 24 hours to days old.

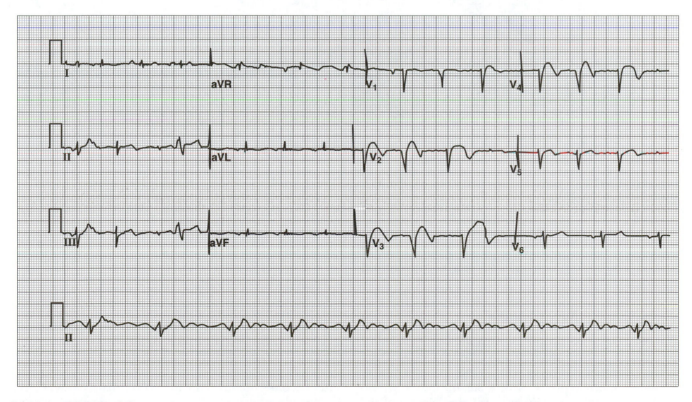

Figure 23-15 QS complexes across leads V_1 through V_4. Elevated ST segments and the coved ST shapes indicates an acute process. The T waves are deeply inverted in leads V_3 through V_6.

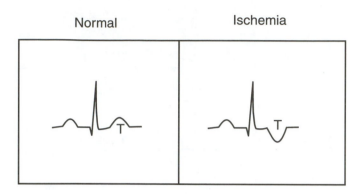

Figure 23-16 Ischemic T wave inversion. Ischemia causes inversion of the normally upright T waves.

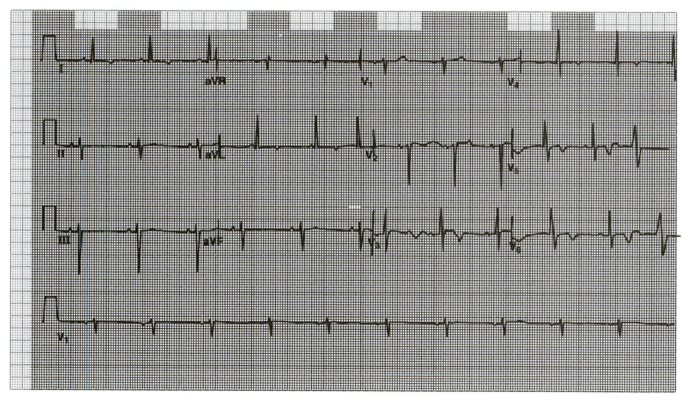

Figure 23-17 T wave inversion in leads V_3 through V_6. These are flat T waves in leads I, II, III, aVR, aVL, and aVF.

helpful and reliable sign. (The most common cause of peaked T waves is hyperkalemia and not myocardial injury.).

Nonischemic T Wave Changes

T wave inversions do not always indicate myocardial ischemia. T waves are normally inverted in aVR and deeply inverted T waves are found in some stroke patients, especially those with a subarachnoid hemorrhage. T wave inversions are also typical in artificial pacemaker rhythms and commonly occur for a brief time after tachycardic episodes.

"Pseudo-normalization" of T Waves

T waves may be chronically inverted in some people (Figure 23–18). Since ischemia alters repolarization, the T waves may become upright compared to the baseline ECG. This paradoxical ECG change is referred to as *pseudo-normalization*, that is, ischemia causes T waves to become upright and mimic normal T waves. The only practical way to recognize pseudo-normalization is to view a prior ECG recording for comparison.

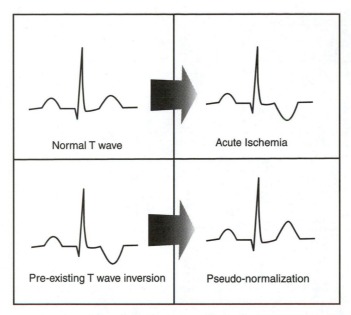

Normal T wave	Acute Ischemia
Pre-existing T wave inversion	Pseudo-normalization

Figure 23-18 "Pseudo-normalization" of an inverted T wave. In patients with chronic T wave inversion, ischemia can cause upright T waves—which subside when the ischemica subsides.

Pseudonormalized T waves revert to their inverted baseline positions when the ischemia resolves.

Reciprocal ST Changes During an AMI

During many AMIs, the ECG will show ST depression in some leads *in addition* to the ST elevation found in other leads. ECG leads *facing* an infarcted heart region show ST elevation, while leads *distant* to the infarcted area show "reciprocal" ST depression (Figure 23–19). For instance, inferior wall MIs show ST segment elevation in leads II, III, and aVF, while the anteriorly placed leads V_1 through V_4, I, and aVL have pronounced ST depression (Figure 23–20).

Clinical Significance of Reciprocal ECG Changes

The clinical significance of reciprocal changes is not certain; they may represent further myocardial ischemia beyond the boundaries of the infarction, or they may reflect an electrical phenomenon. Reciprocal changes are associated with larger myocardial infarctions and the mortality rate is higher than AMIs lacking reciprocal changes. Table 23–3 and Figure 23–21 review the classic ECG characteristics of an infarction.

Reciprocal Changes in Acute MI

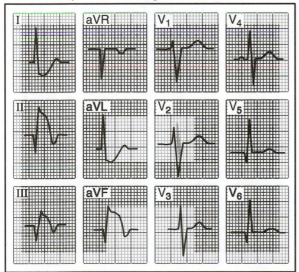

Figure 23-19 Reciprocal changes occur in about 20 percent of MIs. ST segment elevation that is typical of myocardial injury occurs in leads II, III, and aVF. Reciprocal ST depression changes occur in leads I and aVL.

Clinical Note   Nondiagnostic ECGs refer to tracings that do not show characteristic ST segment or T waves changes that are suggestive of ischemia or injury in patients experiencing chest pain. Describing an ECG as nondiagnostic is clinically more useful than describing the tracing as "normal," because a patient with an acute coronary syndrome may have an initial ECG that

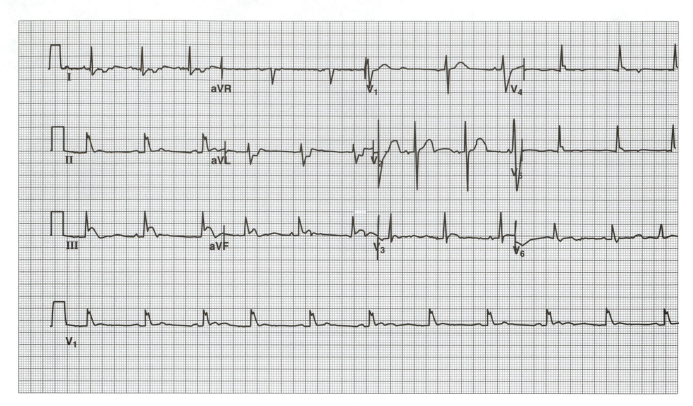

Figure 23–20 Reciprocal ST changes. ST segment elevation exists in II, III, and aVF, while reciprocal ST depression occurs in leads I and aVL.

fails to show pathologic changes, but the term "normal" is falsely reassuring. The ECGs should be repeated at specific intervals—and especially if the patient experiences further chest pain—as an acute coronary syndrome is a changing rather than static event.

"Q-WAVE" VERSUS "NON-Q WAVE" MIs

Traditionally, MIs were classified as either transmural or subendocardial, depending on whether the necrosis involved the full ventricular wall thickness or just partial myocardial thickness. These distinctions were based on the theory that myocardial damage that only extended to the subendocardial area would *not* develop Q waves (Figure 23-24). It had also been believed that Q waves would only develop during transmural damage (Figure 23–24). An example of a Q wave MI is found in Figure 23–23. Subendocardial injury occurs when the coronary vessel occlusion resolves before the entire ventricular wall becomes infarcted. The primary ECG sign of a subendocardial myocardial infarction is deeply inverted T waves (Figure 23–24).

Transmural MIs do occur *without* Q waves developing, while even subendocardial MIs can develop Q waves.

Table 23–3 ECG Ischemia, Injury, and Infarction Patterns
■ **Ischemia**
■ **Symmetrically inverted T waves**
■ **ST segment depressions**
■ **Injury**
■ **ST segment elevation**
■ **Reciprocal ST depression**
■ **Infarction**
■ **Loss of R wave height**
■ **Pathological Q wave formation**

Therefore, it is more accurate to refer to MIs as either "Q wave" or "non-Q wave" rather than transmural or subendocardial (Figure 23–25). Non-Q wave MIs generally cause less myocardial damage than transmural MIs, but non-Q wave MIs have a high risk for subsequent infarction in the subsequent few months. The mortality and complication rates are less with non-Q wave MIs.

Classic Myocardial Infarction

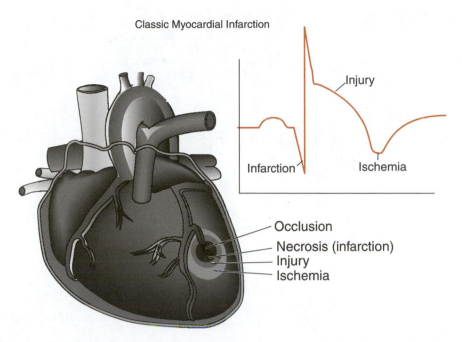

Figure 23–21 Q waves, ST segment elevation, and T wave inversion are found in a typical MI.

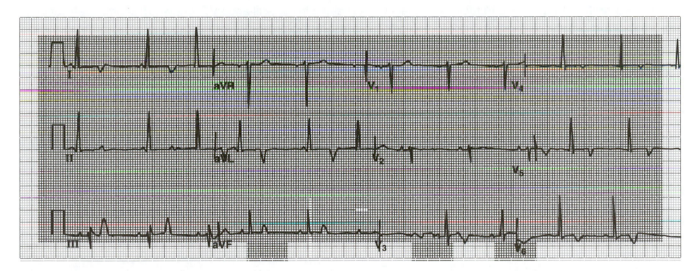

Figure 23–22 Non-Q wave MI. The ECG shows T wave inversion and ST segment straightening in leads V_3 through V_6. Q waves did not develop.

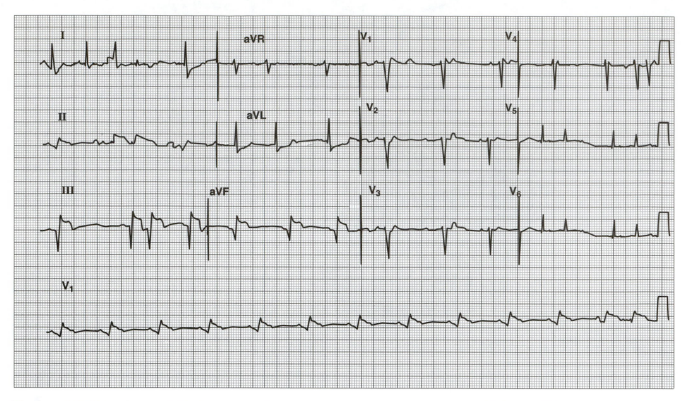

Figure 23–23   "Q wave" MI. Pathologic Q waves are present in leads III and aVF. Acute ST segment elevation is seen in the three inferior (II, III, aVF) leads. The rhythm is irregular because PACs occur.

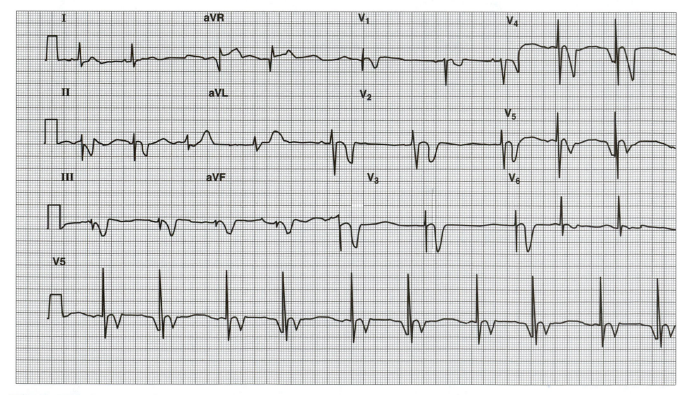

Figure 23–24   "Non-Q wave" MI. Deeply inverted and pointed T waves exist in the inferior (II, III, aVF) and anterior-lateral (V$_1$ through V$_6$) leads. Slight ST segment depression is also present in several of these leads. This pattern is typical of an infarction occuring in the subendocardial regions.

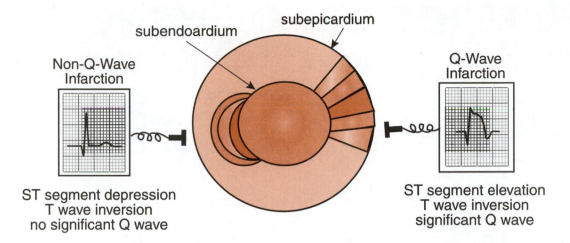

Figure 23–25 Comparison of the appearance of "non-Q wave" and "Q-wave" MIs. (A) In a non-Q wave MI, muscle damage is confined to the subendocardium area. In a Q-wave MI, infarction extends across the full thickness of the myocardium.

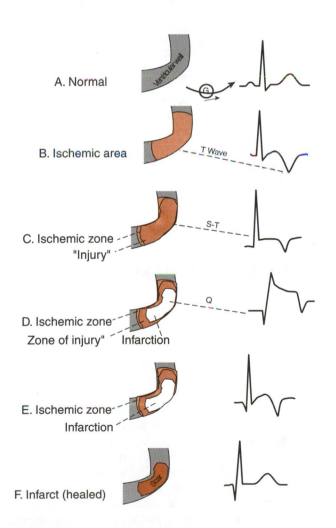

Figure 23–26 Sequence of AMI ECG changes. The ECG changes that evolve during different MI stages is shown.

Stages of ECG Changes During AMI

The following ECG changes occur in several stages, but the sequence in which they develop is variable and all of these findings may not occur (Figure 23–26):

- Hyperacute T waves (tall & peaked) are the earliest ECG change seen during an AMI but they are rarely seen in clinical emergency practice because they are transient and patients delay seeking care.

- ST segment elevation develops within minutes of coronary artery occlusion.

- Pathologic Q waves develop as the height of the R wave diminishes within hours of the obstruction.

- ST segments gradually return to baseline over 24 to 48 hours in a completed MI in the absence of coronary reperfusion.

- T wave inversions occur as the ST segment elevation resolves and can last for weeks.

- Pathologic Q waves remain indefinitely in most patients.

Because the average delay before a typical patient having an AMI seeks medical attention is three hours, by the time patients arrive in the ED or by the time EMS is summoned, most ECGs demonstrate the classic ST elevation pattern. Pathologic Q waves are at least one small ECG box wide and at least one-quarter of the height of the R wave are shown in Figure 23–27.

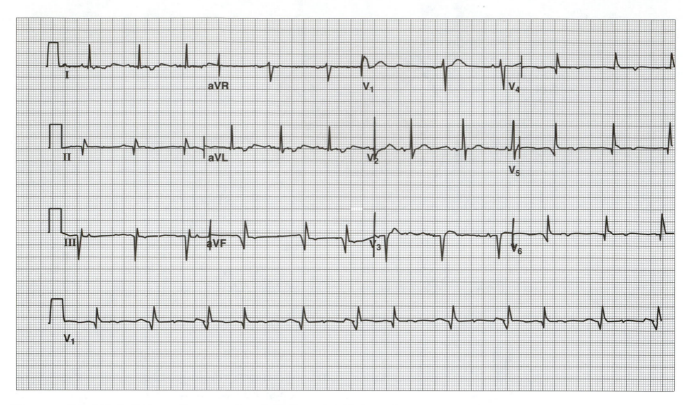

Figure 23–27 Pathologic Q waves. Leads II, III, and aVF show Q waves that are larger than the R waves. Smaller significant Q waves are beginning to form in leads V_4 through V_6.

> *Clinical Note* *Nonspecific ST-T wave changes refers to ECGs that are not completely normal and have minor abnormalities in the appearance of the ECG portions, yet they do not show the characteristic changes found in ischemia, injury, and infarction. ECGs with nonspecific ST-T wave changes are not the same as "normal" ECGs. Nonspecific ECG changes should be considered as suspicious for ischemia in patients with a suggestive history and serial ECGs obtained at specific intervals.*

BUNDLE BRANCH BLOCKS AND AMI DIAGNOSIS

The QRS-T complex is distorted by bundle branch blocks and this can interfere with the ability of the ECG to indicate myocardial injury. Right bundle branch blocks affect the *later phase* of the QRS complex so it does not prevent the development of Q wave so the classical MI ECG findings can still be diagnosed. Left bundle branch block, in contrast, does distort the *early phase* of the QRS-T complex and involves secondary ST-T wave alterations (Figure 23–28). As a result, the ECG with a left BBB will not show the traditional acute MI pattern and makes the diagnosis of AMI difficult.

ECG LOCALIZATION OF AMI

Twelve ECG leads permit identification of the region of the heart experiencing compromised coronary artery blood supply. Coronary obstruction impedes perfusion in specific heart regions, as in the anterior, lateral, or inferior portions. By viewing specific ECG lead groupings, inadequate blood flow can be pinpointed. Anterior and lateral ischemia are best observed in the chest leads V_1 through V_4 and V_5 and V_6 because they overlie the respective heart regions. (Limb leads I and aVL also detect elctrical activity in the lateral heart area.) Inferior wall ischemia is best viewed in the limb leads II, III, and aVF, which face the diaphragmatic heart surface (Table 23–4).

Being able to identify an infarction site is clinically important because it helps predict the relative mortality rates and helps to predict potential AMI complications. For instance, anterior wall MIs are associated with greater myocardial damage than are inferior MIs. The mortality rate is also higher with anterior wall MIs than

Table 23-4 Coronary Arteries Serving Different Cardiac Regions	
■ **Inferior:**	Right Coronary Artery
■ **Lateral:**	Circumflex; Left Anterior Descending
■ **Anterior:**	Left Coronary Artery
■ **Septal:**	Left Anterior Descending
■ **Posterior:**	Right Coronary Artery; Circumflex

Table 23-5 ECG Leads and the Cardiac Regions	
■ **Anterior:**	V_1 through V_4
■ **Lateral:**	V_5 and V_6, I, aVL
■ **Inferior:**	II, III, aVF
■ **Posterior:**	V_1 and V_2 show reciprocal changes: ST depression with abnormally tall R waves
■ **Right Ventricle:**	ST elevation in right-sided precordial leads RV_3 through RV_6

inferior wall MIs. Similarly, a complete AV heart block that develops during an anterior MI is likely to be permanent, while the same AV block developing during an inferior MI often spontaneously subsides. Hypotension that is associated with a right ventricular (RV) infarction is usually responsive to a fluid bolus so the ECG can provide useful information. Table 23–5 shows the heart areas that are detected by various ECG leads.

It is not unusual for myocardial damage to simultaneously occur in several cardiac regions, such as anterior-lateral (V_1 through V_6, I, aVL); inferior-posterior (II, III, aVF, V_1 and V_2) and inferior wall associated with right ventricular infarction (II, III, aVF and Vr_3 through Vr_6). An anterior wall MI affects leads V_1 through V_4, while septal involvement is limited to two of these precordial leads. Knowing these ECG combinations is useful in appreciating which coronary vessels are involved (Figure 23–29).

SPECIFIC MI TYPES

The different types of MIs, the areas affected , and the ECG characteristics associated with each are outlined below.

■ **Anterior Wall MI** is abbreviated as **AWMI** (Figure 23–30).

> **Vessel involved:** occlusion of left anterior descending artery (LAD)
>
> **Area involved:** anterior wall of left ventricle
>
> **ECG leads:** V_1 through V_4
>
> **ECG changes:** Decreased R wave voltage leading to poor R wave progression; ST elevation, QS complexes often develop
>
> **Reciprocal ECG changes:** II, III, aVF

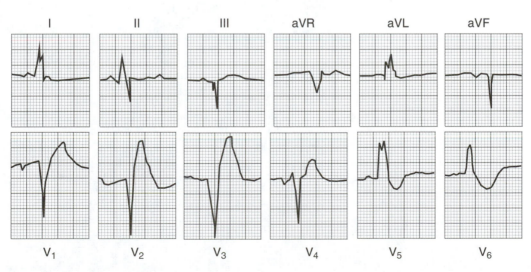

Figure 23–28 Left bundle branch block. This abnormal ECG pattern prevents the ECG interpretation of an AMI because the early part of ventricular activation, where Q waves would usually develop, are distorted and obscure Q waves from forming.

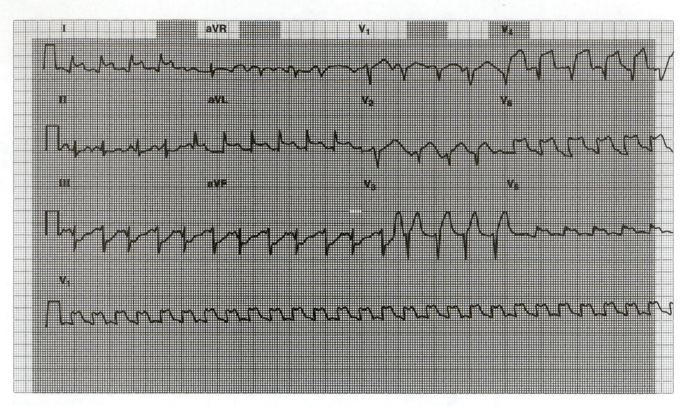

Figure 23-29 Anterior-lateral AMI. Besides acute ST segments in leads V_1 through V_4, elevation exists in leads V_5 through V_6, I, and aVL.

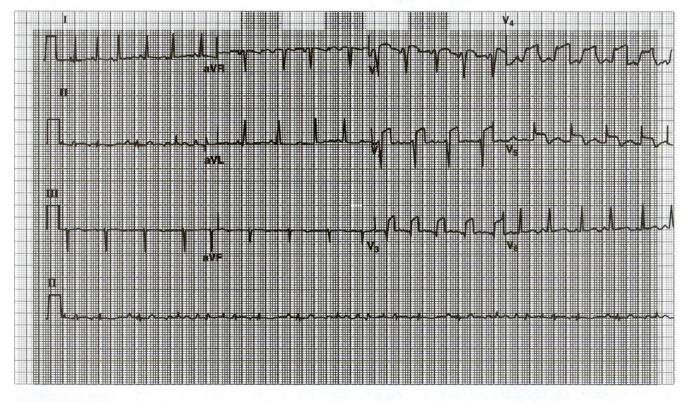

Figure 23-30 Extensive anterior wall AMI. Massive ST elevation and Q wave development occur in the precordial leads (V_1 through V_6).

Associated areas: lateral wall MI (leads V_5 through V_6)

Considerations about AWMI: The AV conduction system may be directly affected by the infarction, causing second-degree AV heart block: Mobitz Type II and requiring pacemaker insertion. There is greater left ventricular impairment, a higher incidence of cardiogenic shock, and a higher mortality rate than with inferior wall MIs.

■ **Lateral Wall MI** (Figure 23–31)

Vessel involved: circumflex coronary artery (less commonly, right CA)

Area involved: lateral wall of left ventricle

ECG leads: V_1 and V_6, I, aVL

Reciprocal ECG changes: II, III, aVF

Consideration about lateral wall MIs: It is rare to have an infarction in only the lateral region; they usually occur in association with anterior or inferior wall MIs.

■ **Inferior Wall MI**, abbreviated as **IWMI** (Figure 23–32)

Vessel involved: right CA or, less commonly, circumflex CA

Area involved: inferior aspect of left ventricle; also termed the diaphragmatic area because the inferior cardiac surface rests on diaphragm

ECG leads: II, III, aVF

Reciprocal ECG changes: I, aVL

Associated areas: In 15 to 25 percent of inferior MIs, the right ventricle is also involved. In 10 to 20 percent of inferior wall MIs, the posterior wall is also involved.

Considerations about IWMIs: Inferior wall MIs are often associated with increased vagal tone, resulting in transient sinus bradycardia and first- or second-degree (Mobitz Type I) AV heart block. There is less impairment of left ventricular function and a lower mortality rate with inferior wall MIs than with anterior wall MIs. Inferior wall MIs occur more frequently than anterior wall MIs. Inferior wall MIs that have lateral or posterior involvement, or when associated with right ventricular infarction are considered "high risk" owing to a higher mortality rate than with isolated inferior MIs.

■ **Right Ventricular MI**, abbreviated **RVMI** (Figure 23–33)

Vessel involved: right CA (same as for inferior MI)

Area involved: right ventricle

Associated areas: A right ventricular MI occurs in association with 15 to 25 percent inferior wall MIs.

ECG leads: right-sided precordial leads: VR_{2-6}

Considerations about RVMIs: The right ventricle is a low pressure/volume-dependent chamber, meaning that it responds with

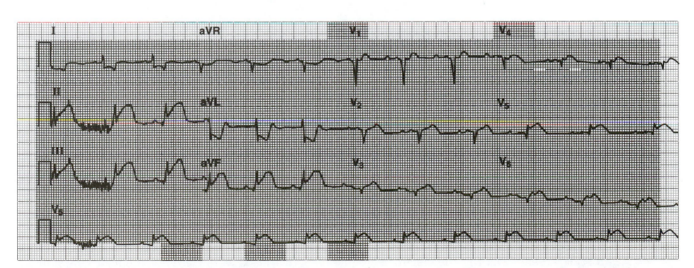

Figure 23–31 Extensive lateral wall AMI associated with inferior infarction. Lateral wall AMIs are most commonly associated with inferior or anterior AMIs.

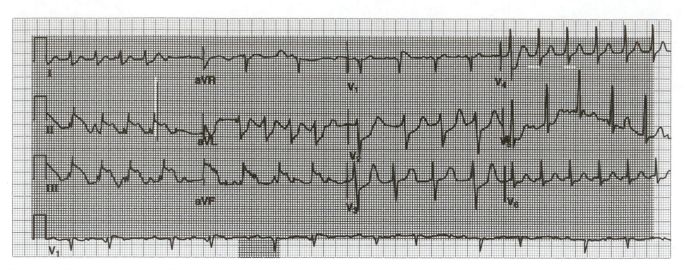

Figure 23-32 Inferior wall MI with reciprocal ST depression. Acute ST segment elevsation is seen in leads II, III, and aVF, while pronounced reciprocal ST depression is found in leads I and aVL.Sinus rhythm with frequent PACs is present.

increased contractility to a greater filling volume. In cases of hypotension caused by a right ventricular infarction, IV fluid boluses can usually raise a low blood pressure.

Standard twelve-lead placement does not record the right ventricle so special right-sided chest leads must be applied. Right ventricular MIs are found in association

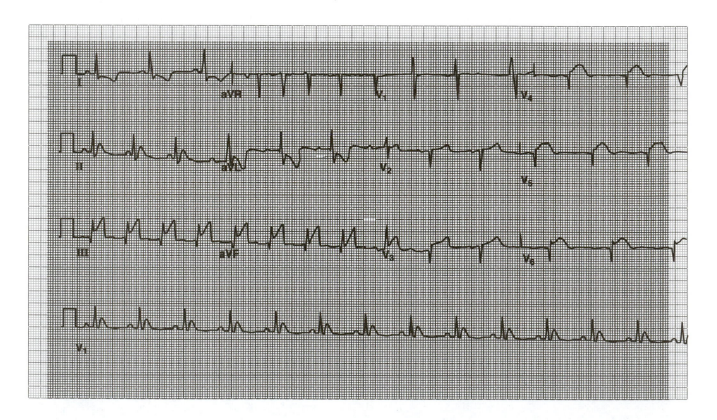

Figure 23-33 Right ventricular MI. The electrodes for the precordial leads were placed on the right side of the chest wall. The right-sided leads show ST elevation in RV_3 to RV_6. In addition, there is an inferior wall MI with reciprocal ST depression in leads I, aVL, and V_6.

with 15 to 25 percent of inferior wall MIs.

■ **Posterior Wall MI**, abbreviated as **PWMI** (Figure 23–34)

Vessel involved: right CA

Area involved: rear portion of ventricle

ECG leads: V_1 and V_2

Considerations about PWMI: Posterior wall MIs are detected by reciprocal ECG changes in the V_1 and V_2 area: tall, prominent R waves and ST depression—these changes are "mirror-images" of deep Q waves and ST elevation. Posterior wall MIs almost never occur alone and are usually seen with inferior wall MI. An isolated posterior MI is rare and occurs when there is distal occlusion of circumflex or right CA. In many posterior MIs, the infarction includes the lateral wall and is seen in lead V_6. Three conditions besides a posterior wall MI can cause tall R waves in leads V_1 and V_2: right bundle branch block, W-P-W syndrome, and right ventricular hypertrophy.

Table 23–6 Summary of ECG Changes in Acute Coronary Syndromes
■ **Ischemia.** ST depression and T waveinversion. Abnormally shaped ST segments involve a horizontal, downsloping, or upsloping appearance.
■ **Injury.** Hallmark finding is ST segment elevation equal to or greater than 1 mm in anatomically contiguous leads. The ST segment appearance may have downsloping ("coving") or upward sloping or have a sharp diagonal slant.
■ **Infarction.** Pathologic Q waves are at least 1 mm wide and at least 1/4 the height of the QRS complex. When combined with ST segment changes and T wave changes, they signify an acute MI. Pathologic Q waves alone point toward an old MI.

The ECG findings that occur during acute coronary syndromes are summarized in Table 23–6

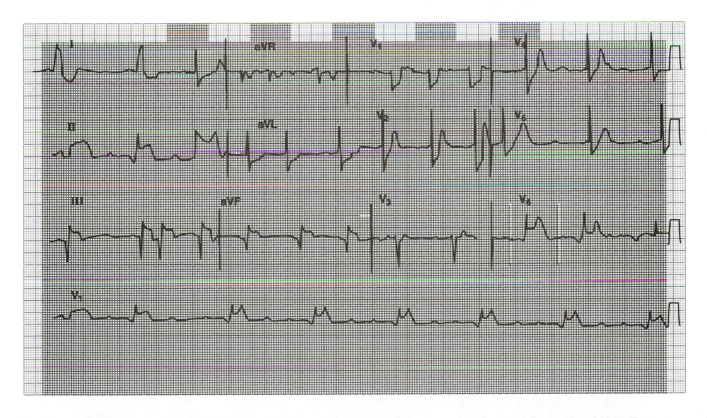

Figure 23–34 Posterior wall MI. Marked ST depression and tall R waves are found in leads V_1 and V_2. There is also an inferior (II, III, aVF)-lateral (V_6) wall MI. The lead II rhythm strip at the bottom of the page shows a second degree AV heart block; Mobitz type I; (wenckebach) block.

Let's Review

1. The coronary circulation is supplied via the left and right coronary arteries. The left main coronary artery forms the left anterior descending (LAD) artery and the circumflex (cfx) artery. The LAD supplies the anterior surface of the left ventricle, while the left circumflex provides blood to the posterior and inferior portions. The right coronary artery (RCA) supplies the right ventricle and the AV conduction system in most people.

2. Coronary blood flow can decrease with both rapid and slow dysrhythmias as well as being caused by atherosclerosis and vasospasm. Global myocardial ischemia affecting the entire heart can result from prolonged hypotensive or shock states.

3. Acute ST segments (currents of injury) occur within minutes of coronary occlusion and reflect myocardial damage. ST segments shift away from the isoelectric ECG baseline because an abnormal electric charge develops across the cell membranes and alters the current flow. Subendocardial injury causes ST depression, while transmural damage leads to ST elevation.

4. ST segment elevation is one of the earliest ECG changes found during an AMI. Hyperacute T waves can precede the ST segment alterations but this finding is not specific for an AMI and are rarely seen.

5. Other common conditions—besides ischemia/injury—can cause ST-T wave alterations. Bundle branch blocks and W-P-W (Wolfe-Parkinson-White) syndrome can cause secondary ST shifts.

6. Pathologic Q waves are wide and deep. They often remain as the only ECG sign that an MI has occurred and last indefinately. These abnormal Q waves are considered as an ECG "scar" lasting after a myocardial injury heals.

7. Reciprocal ECG changes involve ST depression in leads oriented opposite to leads detecting an MI. Reciprocal changes, coupled with acute ST elevation, are a very sensitive marker for AMI. Reciprocal changes are associated with larger infarctions and a higher mortality rate than AMIs without reciprocal changes.

8. Ischemia causes inversion of T waves due to altered ventricular repolarization. However, not all T wave inversions are due to ischemia. T waves that are normally upright become deeply and symmetrically inverted during acute ischemia. In certain cases, T waves that are chronically inverted, become upright during ischemia and is termed "pseudonormalization."

9. Acute ST-T wave changes will subside over several weeks and return to their pre-MI baseline shape. An ECG displaying only abnormal Q waves does not reflect an acute injury. The findings of pathologic Q waves coupled with ST segment elevation and T wave inversions indicate an acute injury

Glossary

Atherosclerosis Disease involving the gradual buildup of waste material within the vessel wall, causing narrowing of the vessel.

Acute coronary syndromes Clinical presentaions associated with ischemic heart disease, including angina, unstable angina, and myocardial infarction.

Acute ST segment changes Characteristic St elevations in ECG leads reflecting an AMI.

Anatomically contiguous leads ECG leads that reflect activity in a cardiac region; i.e. II, III, aVF view the inferior cardiac area.

Benign early repolarization Generalized ST elevation that is a normal variant in healthy young people.

Circumflex artery Coronary artery branch of the left coronary artery that curves along the posterior porion of the heart.

Collateral coronary circulation Vessels adjacent to the damaged artery are able to slowly dilate and supply additional blood flow if the blockage is gradual.

Coronary artery spasm Sudden narrow constriction of the coronary artery due to contraction on smooth muscle found within the wall of the coronary artery; also termed vasospasm.

Coronary thrombosis Acute blockage of an already narrowed artery.

Current of injury Marked ST segment elevation during myocardial injury due to a coronary occlusion.

Global myocardial ischemia Generalized decrease in blood flow to the heart causing ischemia in all regions.

Left anterior descending artery Coronary artery branch of the left coronary artery that travels down along the anterior surface of the left ventricle.

Nondiagnostic ECG Cardiac tracing that has subtle findings which may be significant.

Non-Q wave MI Myocardial infarction in which a pathologic Q wave does not develop.

Nonspecific ECG changes Findings that are subtle or unremarkable.

Nonspecific ECG changes ECG changes that are not normal but do not clearly indicate cardiac ischemia, injury, or infarction.

Patholigic Q waves Deep, wide Q waves that develop following myocardial necrosis.

Pattern of ischemia Pattern in which normally upright T waves become inverted during an anginal episode.

Primary ST-T wave changes Change found in portion of the ECG that directly affects the myocardial fibers.

Pseudonormalization of T waves T waves that are chronically inverted and become upright during ischemia.

Q wave MI Myocardial infarction associated with the development of a pathological Q wave.

Reciprocal AMI ECG changes ST segment depression occurs in some MIs in addition to ST segment elevation.

Right coronary artery Main coronary artery that travels within the AV groove and supplies most of the right atria and ventricle.

Secondary ST-T wave change Change found in portion of the ECG that results from abnormal depolarization and not due to ischemia.

Serial ECGs ECGs repeated at certain intervals (such as every half-hour at least three times) to detect ischemic changes.

Stenosed coronary artery Pathologically narrowed artery causing reduced myocardial blood flow.

Subendocardial injury Partial myocardial damage limited to the area just beyond the endocardium.

Subendocardial region Innermost heart layer closest to the blood in the ventricular chamber that is most susceptible to myocardial ischemia.

Thrombolytic therapy Using a tissue plasminogen activating drug to restore blood flow in a blocked coronary artery.

Tissue plasminogen activator Drug used to restore blood flow in a blocked coronary artery by dissolving the blood clot.

Transmural injury Myocardial damage extending across the full thickness of the ventricle, involving the endocardium, myocardium, and epicardium.

Vasospasm See Coronary artery spasm.

chapter 24

Twelve-Lead ECGs: Self-Assessment Tracings

LEARNING OBJECTIVE

Upon completion of this chapter the reader should be able to:

- *Correctly identify dysrhythmias, myocardial ischemia, injury, and infarction patterns, preexcitation, and bundle branch blocks when presented with sample twelve-lead electrocardiograms.*

INTRODUCTION

The following twenty twelve-lead ECGs present bundle branch blocks, preexcitation, ischemia, injury and infarction patterns, in addition to dysrhythmias for interpretation. Interpretations and the reasoning behind the answers are provided in Appendix A. If any difficulties are encountered, the appropriate sections of Chapters 22 and 23 should be reviewed.

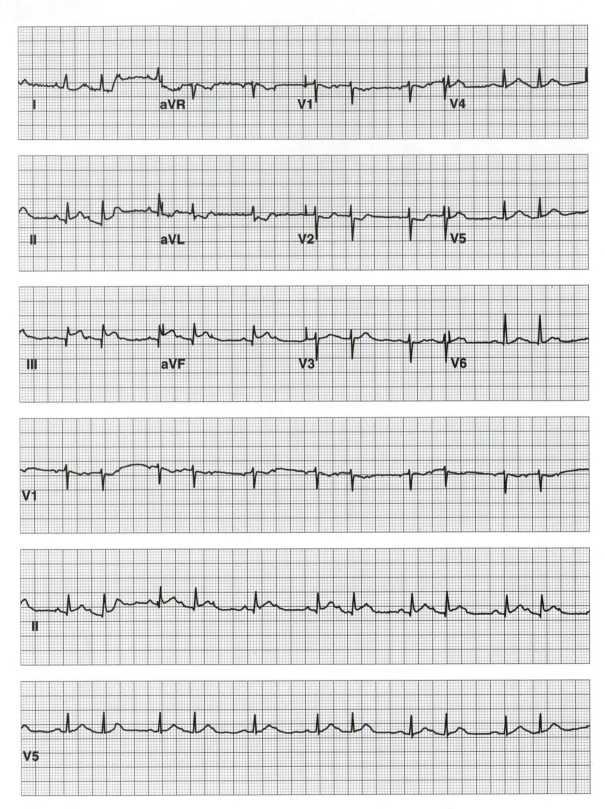

Figure 24-1 Pacemaker _____
Dysrhythmias _____
Interpretation _____
Reasoning _____

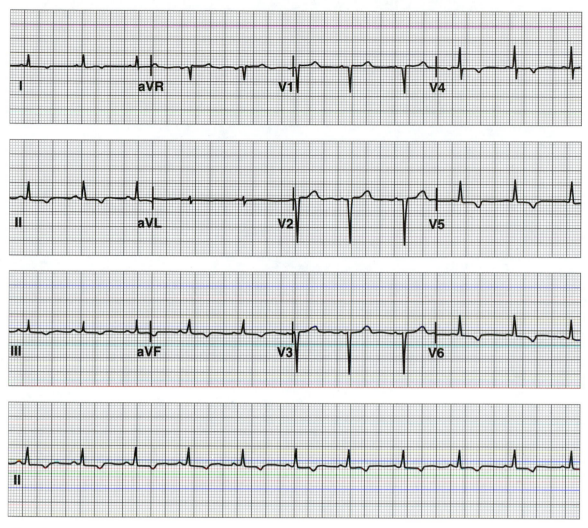

Figure 24-2   Pacemaker _____

Dysrhythmias _____

Interpretation _____

Reasoning _____

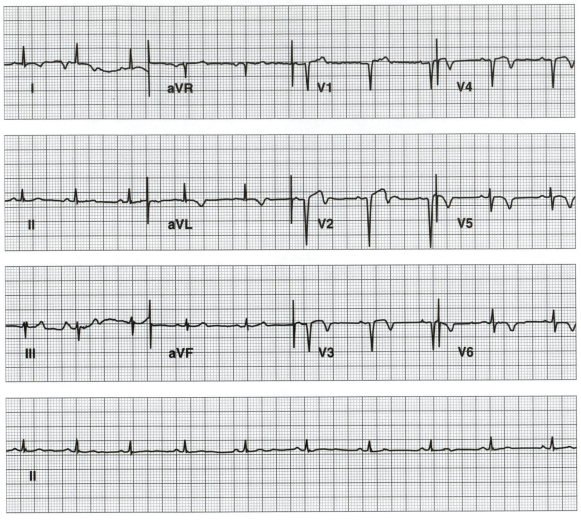

Figure 24-3 Pacemaker _____

Dysrhythmias _____

Interpretation _____

Reasoning _____

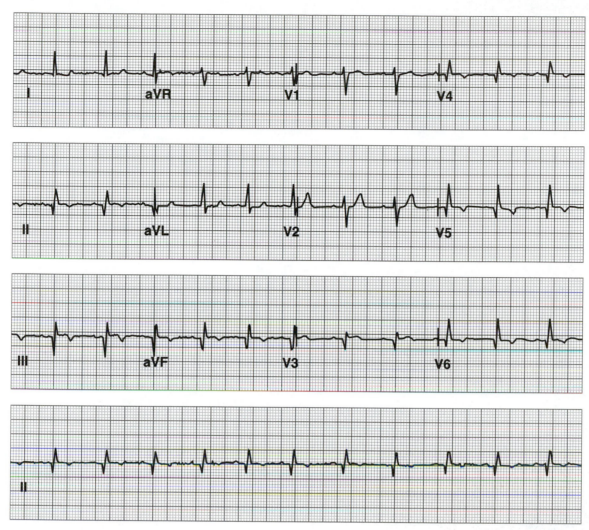

Figure 24-4 Pacemaker _____

Dysrhythmias _____

Interpretation _____

Reasoning _____

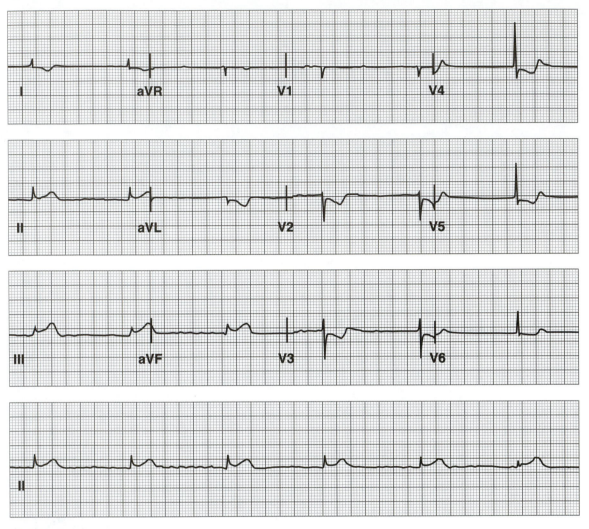

Figure 24-5 Pacemaker _____
Dysrhythmias _____
Interpretation _____
Reasoning _____

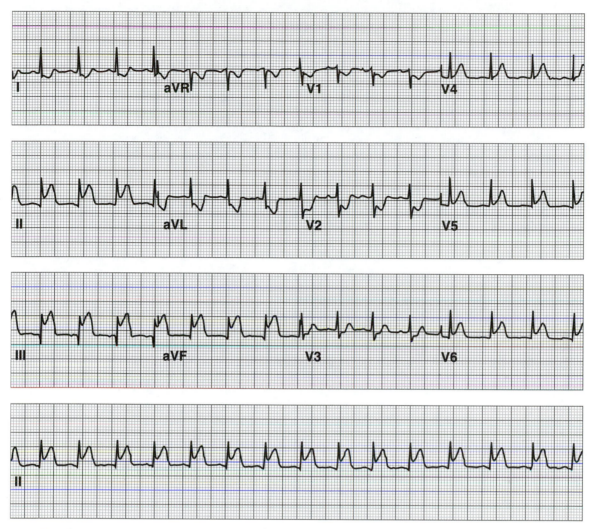

Figure 24-6a Pacemaker _____
Dysrhythmias _____
Interpretation _____
Reasoning _____

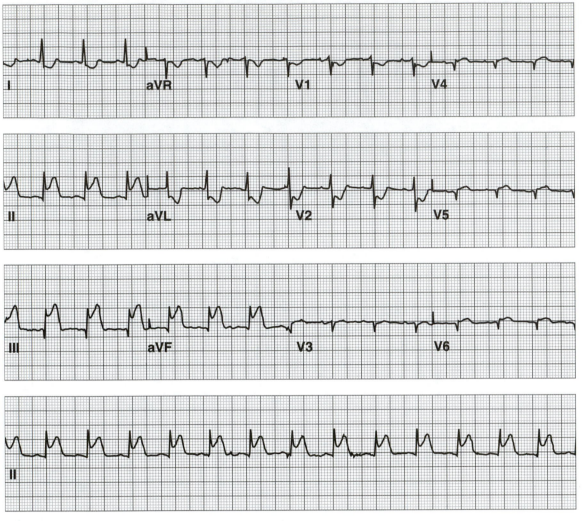

Figure 24-6b Pacemaker _____

Dysrhythmias _____

Interpretation _____

Reasoning _____

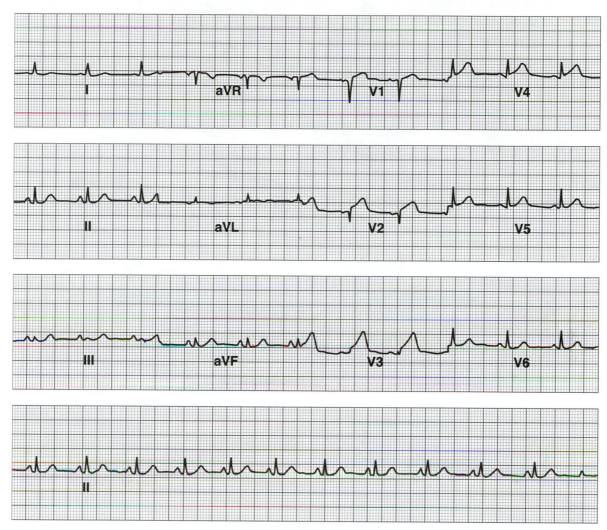

Figure 24-7 Pacemaker _____
Dysrhythmias _____
Interpretation _____
Reasoning _____

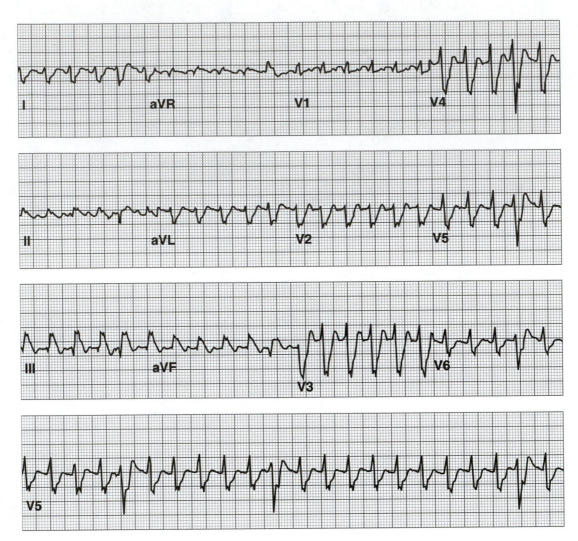

Figure 24-8 Pacemaker _____
Dysrhythmias _____
Interpretation _____
Reasoning _____

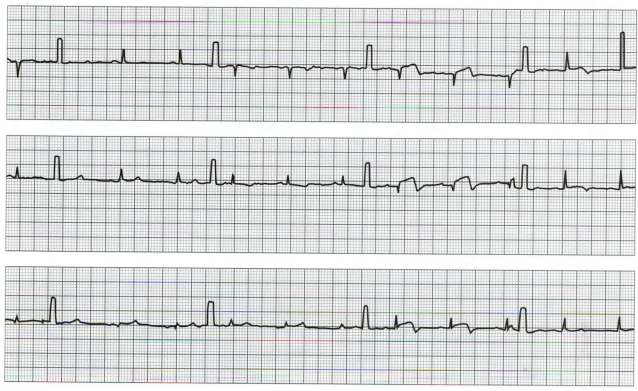

Figure 24-9 Pacemaker _____
Dysrhythmias _____
Interpretation _____
Reasoning _____

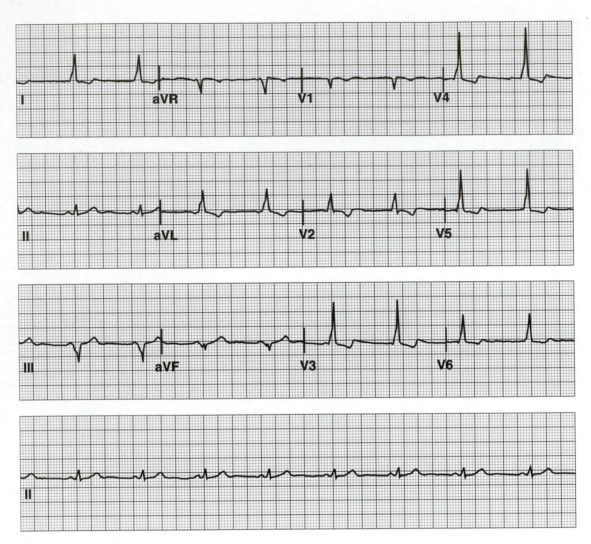

Figure 24-10 Pacemaker _____
Dysrhythmias _____
Interpretation _____
Reasoning _____

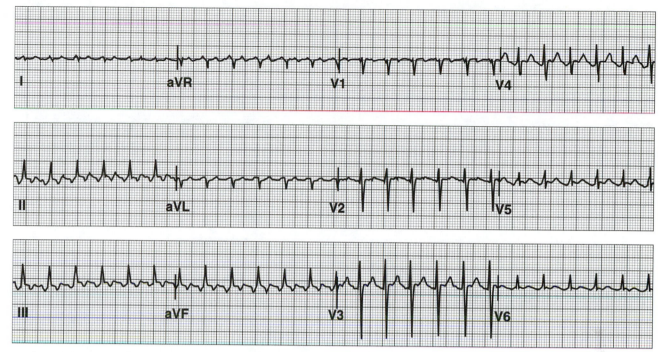

Figure 24-11   Pacemaker _____

Dysrhythmias _____

Interpretation _____

Reasoning _____

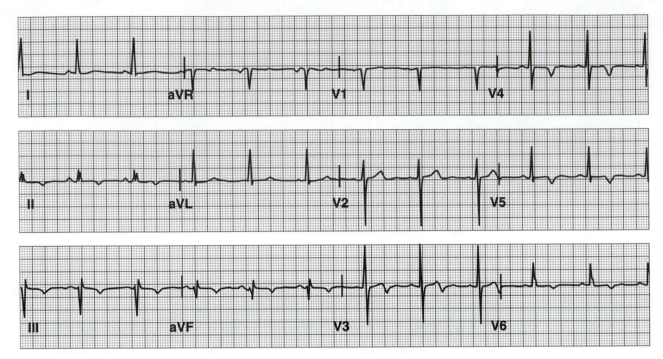

Figure 24-12 Pacemaker _____
Dysrhythmias _____
Interpretation _____
Reasoning _____

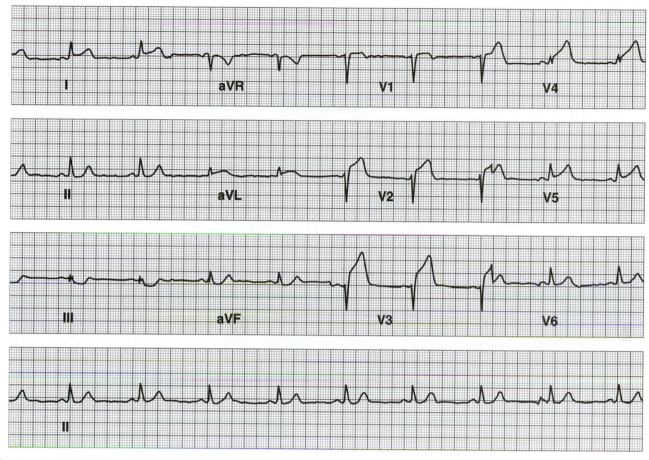

Figure 24-13 Pacemaker _____
Dysrhythmias _____
Interpretation _____
Reasoning _____

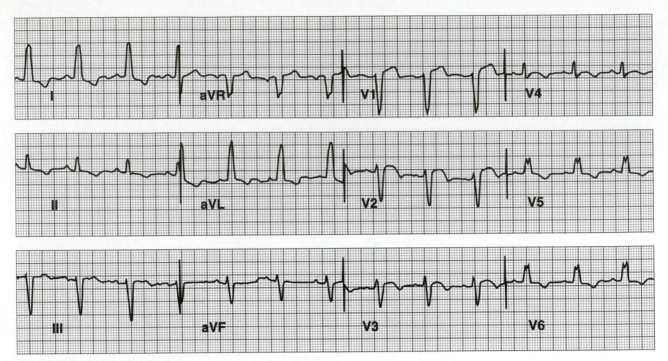

Figure 24-14 Pacemaker _____
Dysrhythmias _____
Interpretation _____
Reasoning _____

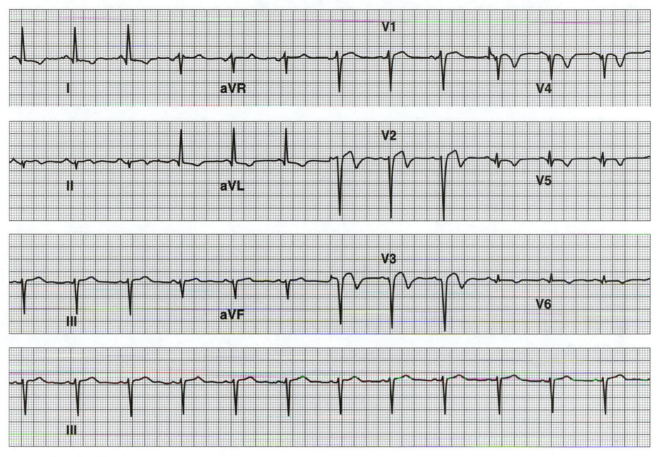

Figure 24-15 Pacemaker _____

Dysrhythmias _____

Interpretation _____

Reasoning _____

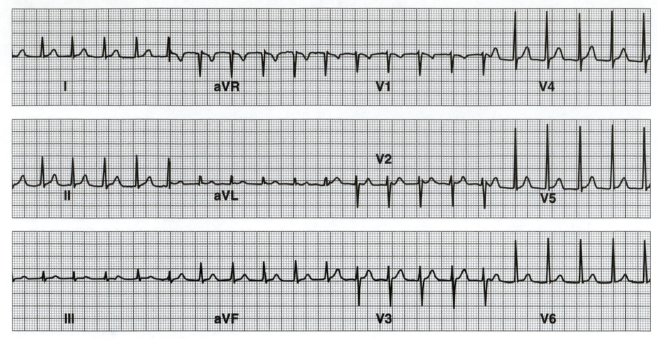

Figure 24-16 Pacemaker _____
Dysrhythmias _____
Interpretation _____
Reasoning _____

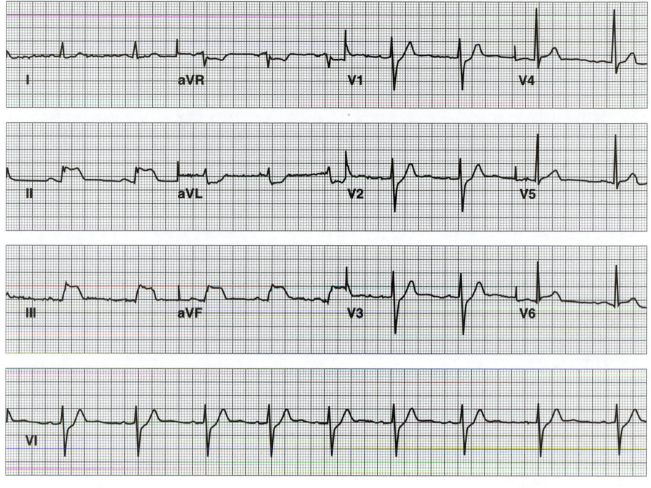

Figure 24-17 Pacemaker _____
Dysrhythmias _____
Interpretation _____
Reasoning _____

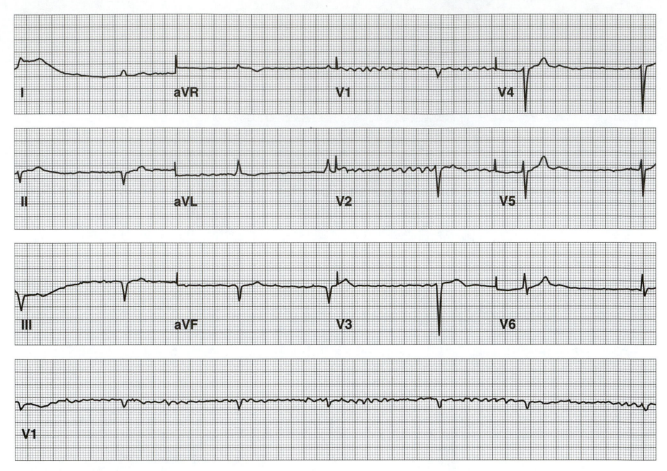

Figure 24-18 Pacemaker _____
Dysrhythmias _____
Interpretation _____
Reasoning _____

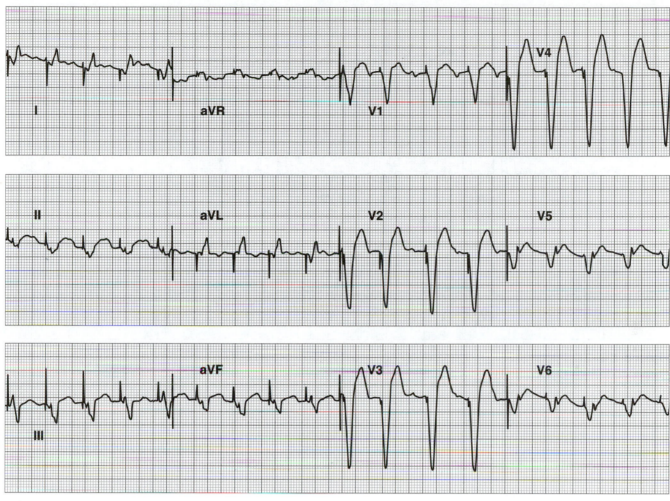

Figure 24-19 Pacemaker _____
Dysrhythmias _____
Interpretation _____
Reasoning _____

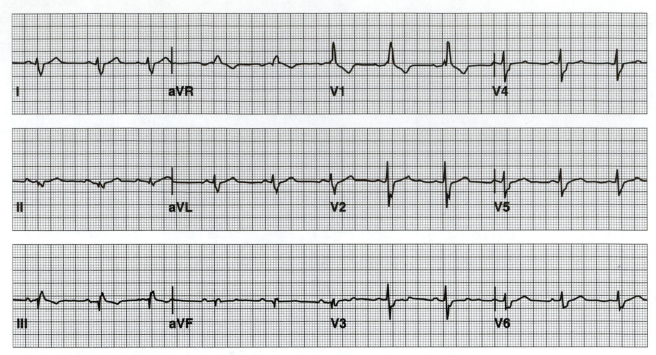

Figure 24-20 Pacemaker _____

Dysrhythmias _____

Interpretation _____

Reasoning _____

Dysrhythmias in Infants and Children

LEARNING OBJECTIVES

Upon completion of this chapter, the reader should be able to:

- *List the two most common dysrhythmias in the pediatric population.*

- *List three common causes of pediatric dysrhythmias and how they differ from adult causes.*

- *Describe how sinus tachycardia in infants and children differs from adults.*

- *Explain the significance of supraventricular tachycardia in infants and children.*

- *List three physical signs that parents commonly describe in nonverbal infants who present with PSVT.*

- *Name two medications that should be avoided when treating PSVT in children younger than one year of age due to the risk of precipitating profound hypotension and cardiovascular collapse.*

- *Explain the significance of atrial fibrillation and atrial flutter in children and describe which cases require emergent treatment.*

- *Explain the significance of ventricular tachycardia in children and describe which cases require emergent treatment.*

- *Describe how sinus bradycardia in infants and children differs from adults.*

- *Name the major form of AV heart block that causes bradycardia in children.*

- *Explain the significance of AV heart block in children and describe which cases require emergent treatment.*

- *Describe the most common causes that require cardiac pacing in infants and children.*

- *Explain the relationship among the ECG PR intervals, QRS intervals, and QT intervals based on age.*

- *Describe the significance of premature atrial and ventricular complexes in children and contrast them to the same findings in adults.*

- *List the emergency cardiac care treatment for asystole and pulseless cardiopulmonary arrest, including pulseless electrical activity (P.E.A.) and electro mechanical activity (E.M.D.).*

CHAPTER OVERVIEW

This chapter is not intended to be all-inclusive because significant dysrhythmias have already been discussed, but will strive to provide information concerning the more commonly encountered pediatric rhythm problems and discuss acute therapy options especially how such rhythm disorders, problems, and treatments differ from adults.

Overall, clinically significant dysrhythmias are fortunately infrequent events in infants and children. Unlike the adult population, pediatric dysrhythmias are rarely caused by ischemia or an acute cardiovascular event. Rather, they result from a variety of non-cardiac conditions. The single most common cardiac cause of pediatric dysrhythmias is congenital heart disease. Treatment of pediatric rhythm disturbances requires a different therapeutic approach than used for adults: one based on cause and significance of the rhythm. Therapies employed in adults cannot simply be applied to the pediatric population because some commonly used drugs in adults can cause cardiovascular collapse in children. Some rhythm disorders that are considered pathological in adults are benign in infants and children. Those dysrhythmia characteristics that differ between adults and children will be highlighted.

INTRODUCTION

Few situations are more anxiety provoking than treating a critically ill child, especially one with an abnormal cardiac rhythm. This chapter focuses on those dysrhythmias that are common in the pediatric age group and which are clinically significant. For instance, of the AV heart blocks, only third degree block will be discussed as it is a leading cause of childhood symptomatic bradycardia.

Pediatric cardiac dysrhythmias are being detected more frequently today and a number of factors are responsible for this: increased utilization of cardiac monitoring in all settings, improved diagnostic techniques, and more surgical procedures for congenital heart anomalies resulting in postsurgical dysrhythmias.

In general, because a cardiovascular-induced cardiac arrest is extremely rare in children, successful treatment of dysrhythmias depends on correcting the underlying causes, including acidosis, hypoxia, sepsis, trauma or hypovolemia. Dysrhythmias in children generally have non-cardiac causes as shown in Table 25–1.

> *Clinical Note* *Pediatric dysrhythmias do not occur as the result of ischemic heart disease. In the very young, the single most common cause is a congenital heart defect. In older pediatric patients, other noncardiac causes should be considered.*

INDICATIONS FOR CARDIAC MONITORING IN INFANTS AND CHILDREN

There are many indications for obtaining pediatric ECGs and using continuous cardiac monitoring. A history of syncope, palpitations, shortness of breath, chest pain, poisoning, or possible drug overdose are common indications because they can alter normal impulse formation, conduction, or repolarization. On physical exam, the discovery of a rapid, slow, or irregular pulse, a previously undetected murmur, cyanosis, or an altered mental status would also indicate the need for an ECG. The most common indications are listed in Table 25–2.

Table 25-1 Common Causes of Pediatric Dysrhythmias

- **Viral or Bacterial Illness**
- **Postsurgical Repair of Congenital Heart Anomalies**
- **Myocardial Contusion**
- **Drug Toxicity, Poisoning, or Overdose**
- **Electrolyte or Metabolic Disturbances**
- **Central Nervous System Dysfunction**
- **Idiopathic (Unknown Cause)**

Table 25-2 Common Indications for Pediatric ECGs

- **Significant Tachycardia**
- **Significant Bradycardia**
- **Irregular Rhythm, Palpitations**
- **Head Trauma or Major/Multiple Trauma**
- **Electrical Shock**
- **Clinical Signs of Heart Failure**
- **Clinical Signs of Pericarditis or Myocarditis**
- **Significant Previously Undetected Heart Murmur**
- **Cyanosis**
- **Altered Mental Status**
- **Syncope**
- **Chest Pain**
- **Electrolyte Disturbances**
- **Toxic Ingestions**
- **During Patient Transfer or Transport**

Clinical Note Asking an adult to lie still or not to talk while recording a twelve-lead ECG is reasonable, whereas the likelihood of being able to convince an anxious child to remain quiet in a strange, unfamiliar, and potentially threatening setting decreases considerably the younger the child's. Having a parent close at hand, a favorite toy, or other distracter has more success.

GENERAL APPROACH TO PEDIATRIC DYSRHYTHMIAS

A brief but systematic approach that focuses first on recognizing a specific pediatric dysrhythmia and then assesses the seriousness of the event or the deterioration of a cardiac rhythm is required. This chapter begins by dividing the clinically significant pediatric dysrhythmias into rapid heart rates, slow heart rates, and irregular cardiac rhythms. To assess whether a rhythm is too fast or slow, the usual ranges of normal cardiac rates based on a child's age are needed (Table 25–3).

ECG Interpretation Tip Clinically significant dysrhythmias in children can be conveniently grouped into the following rhythm types: rapid, slow, and irregular.

FAST HEART RATES

As Table 25–3 illustrates, a "rapid" heart rate is a relative concept based on the child's age and taking into account the clinical setting. By far, the most common dysrhythmia in children is supraventricular tachycardia. Tachydysrhythmias can be difficult to interpret because sinus tachycardia can be unusually rapid in infants and share the rate range typical of SVTs.

Just as for adults, pediatric tachyarrhythmias can be divided into two general groups: those with narrow ventricular QRS complexes and those which are wide (greater than 0.10 second). Rates that generally require rapid intervention in an adult such as 180 bpm may be completely benign in an infant or young child. A narrow QRS complex implies a supraventricular tachycardia which is usually benign when compared with wide complex tachycardias. Distorted QRS complex tachycardias imply a ventricular origin and should be considered to be potentially dangerous with a likelihood of degenerating into ventricular fibrillation.

Clinical Note It is rare for infants and young children to develop heart rates that are so fast as to impair cardiac output. SVTs are the leading cause of tachycardia in this age group and when rates exceed 220/minute, acute congestive heart failure can develop. In such cases, synchronized cardioversion or immediate administration of adenosine is indicated

Table 25-3 Normal Heart Rate Ranges

Age	Heart Rate (bpm)
Newborn	80–180
1 week to 3 months	80–160
3 months to 2 years	80–150
2 years to 10 years	60–110
10 years to adult	50–90

Sinus Tachycardia

The normal sinus node response to fever, anemia, hypovolemia, or any other stress is to increase its depolarization rate, thereby providing a greater cardiac output. The normal upper range for a 3-month-old infant is 160 bpm, but for a severely stressed infant of that age can easily exceed 200 bpm. Correction of the underlying problem will remedy the rapid rate. In cases where an extremely fast sinus tachycardia cannot be differentiated from an SVT, adenosine is helpful because it terminates most SVTs while sinus tachycardias are only slowed for a few seconds.

> **Clinical Note** *The heart rate of an infant and young child is faster than an adult because of the smaller stroke volume and the cardiac reserve is limited. When there is a need for an increased cardiac output in children, the primary mechanism is to increase the heart rate. The heart rate should be faster than normal in children in pain or those with any type of cardiopulmonary stress. Slow or normal heart rates in children in such circumstances may be a warning sign of impending cardiac or respiratory failure.*

Supraventricular Tachycardias

By far, the *single most common cardiac dysrhythmia in the pediatric population is supraventricular tachycardia (SVT)*. On the basis of heart rate alone, there is significant overlap between sinus tachycardia and an abnormal tachycardia (Figure 25–1). *In the case of high fever or severe infection, infants can have sinus rates as high as 240 bpm, young children up to 200 bpm, and teenagers up to 180 bpm.* Heart rates faster than these should raise suspicion that the pacemaker may not be in the sinus node.

Infants often present with SVTs lasting for hours, whereas in older children, it is usually brief and episodic. SVT rarely occurs during sleep for unknown reasons. As in adults, P waves are usually not identifiable, a narrow QRS complex is present, and the SVT rate ranges between 180 and 240 bpm (Figure 25–2). Most infants with SVTs have heart rates at 240 bpm or faster. This narrow-complex (less than 0.08 second) dysrhythmia tends to be a stable rhythm because children can tolerate this rhythm for longer periods than older adults. Clinical deterioration is rare unless the SVT has lasted many hours. Paroxysmal SVT should be considered in any child complaining of palpitations, a "racing heart," or a "thumping" chest sensation. Episodic PSVTs are occasionally detected while children are being monitored in the ED (Figure 25–3) but a holter monitor is usually needed to document the event.

Causes of SVT

Although there are at least sixteen types of SVTs, the vast majority of SVTs result from two causes: an *accessory pathway*, as with Wolff-Parkinson-White syndrome, or an *AV nodal reentry pattern*. The cause coincides with the child's age: in infants only a small percentage of SVT cases are caused by AV node reentry; most are due to the presence of an accessory pathway. In older children accessory pathway mediated tachycardias are twice as common as AV-node reentry dysrhythmias.

Newborns who experience SVTs or infants during the first two months of life will almost all outgrow these episodes before their first birthday. Yet approximately one third of these patients will experience a recurrence at around 8 years of age. If the recurrence of SVT is the result of an accessory pathway and the patient is over the age of 5 years, the episodes are likely to persist into adulthood in nearly 80 percent of cases.

Wolff-Parkinson-White (W-P-W) Syndrome

Wolff-Parkinson-White syndrome and SVT are the single most frequently encountered type of ventricular preexcitation syndrome. Microscopic accessory fibers exist at birth connecting the atria to the ventricles but usually become nonfunctional after 24 hours when the fibers persist, this anatomic short circuit causes preexcitation of the ventricle and results in early depolarization. Males make up more than two thirds of all W-P-W cases, which are usually asymptomatic until the patient experiences the first sudden episode.

Signs and symptoms of W-P-W depend on the child's age: in older children, they include the sudden onset of rapid heart rates frequently accompanied by dizziness, weakness, palpitations, syncope, shortness of breath, and chest discomfort. Syncope is unusual in pediatric SVT but fatigue and generalized weakness are common. In infants and preverbal toddlers, poor feeding, increased respiratory rates, sleepiness, irritability, diaphoresis and pallor are typical.

As with adults, W-P-W is diagnosed by a short PR interval as a result of the impulse bypassing the AV node (Figure 25–4). W-P-W has a wider than normal QRS complex due to the delta wave which refers to the slurred upstroke of the initial portion of the QRS complex. Since most children have QRS complexes less than 0.08 second, the diagnosis of W-P-W may be sub-

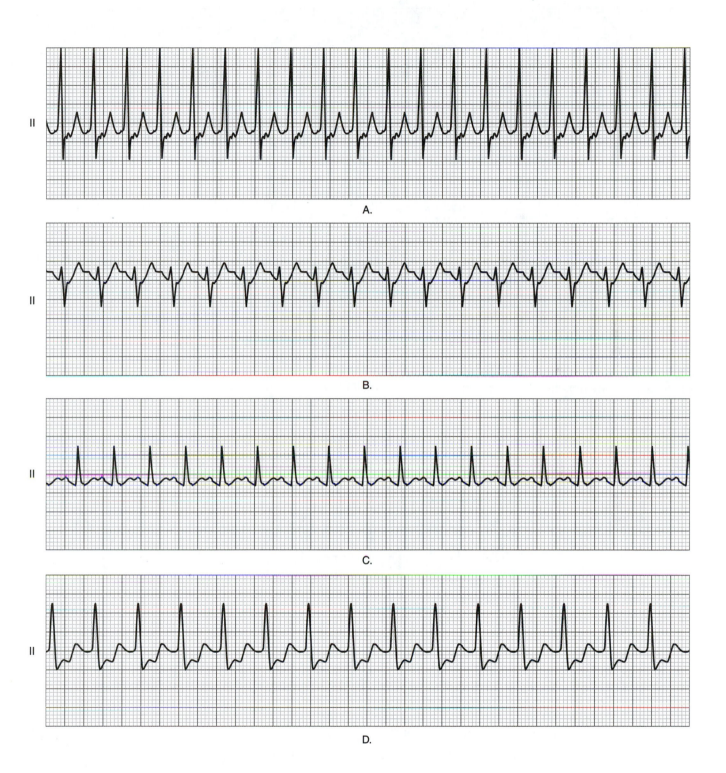

Figure 25–1 Narrow QRS complex tachycardias. Strip A shows a SVT at a rate of 170 bpm. The QRS complexes are narrow yet no P waves are visible. Strip B shows a sinus tachycardia at a rate of 165 bpm since P waves are clearly seen. Strip C also shows a sinus tachycardia at a rate of 170 bpm. In C, the P waves begin to merge with the T waves due to the rapid rate. Strip D shows a SVT at a rate of 150 bpm. No P waves are visible and the QRS complexes are narrow. (There is also considerable ST segment depression.)

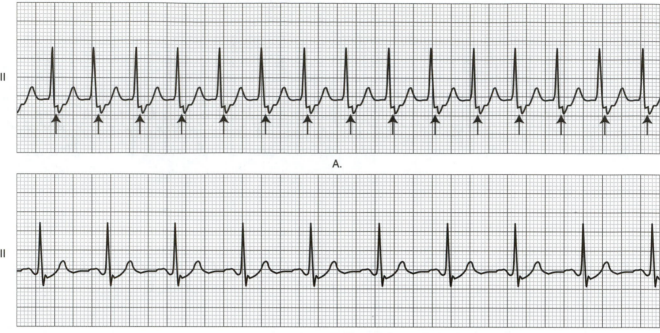

Figure 25–2 SVT at a rate of 165 bpm in Strip A. Strip A shows distinct retrograde P waves (arrows). Strip B shows a sinus rhythm ata rate of 95 bpm and was recorded after adenosine administration.

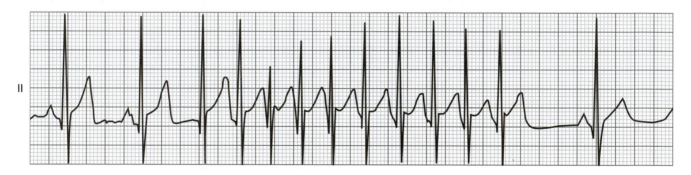

Figure 25–3 Short episode of PSVT at a rate of 180 bpm. The first two beats and the last beat are sinus beats because P waves are clearly visible. The 3rd through the 12th beats have a rapid rate with a narrow QRS complex but they lack P waves so the rhythm is a PSVT. Sinus activity resumes since a P wave is part of the last beat.

tle and even more difficult to diagnose in children than in adults. ECG interpretation is complicated by the higher than normal sinus rates and rapid conduction through the AV node. Variation in the beat-to-beat QRS size is highly indicative of an accessory pathway mediated SVT.

> *ECG Interpretation Tip In children less than 1 year of age, 25 percent of SVT cases will be associated with a wide QRS complex due to fatigue of the bundle branches. The therapeutic approach for infants younger than 1 year old with a wide QRS complex tachycardia is to presume that SVT with abberancy is present until proven otherwise.*

Acute Therapy of SVT

Brief SVT episodes are usually well tolerated and best left untreated; however, episodes lasting more than 30 minutes or associated with significant symptoms require treatment. Carotid sinus massage, sometimes effective in adults, is rarely successful in children. A unique technique limited to very young children involves stimulation of a primitive "diving reflex" by

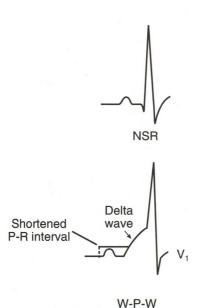

Figure 25–4 W-P-W characteristics are contrasted with a normal P-QRS complex. This preexcitation syndrome has a shortened PR interval and a slurred upstroke of the R wave, termed a "delta" wave.

applying a bag of ice to an infant or young child's face in a monitored setting. The theory behind the ice bag application is that the cold will stimulate an intense vagal reaction that will decrease conduction through the AV node and end the PSVT. It is rarely successful. With the introduction of adenosine, having a half-life of a few seconds and few side effects, the majority of SVTs that are due to a reentry mechanism can easily be treated. Adenosine at a dose of 0.1 mg/kg administered rapidly and followed by a rapid IV fluid bolus, is successful in over 90 percent of pediatric cases.

Other common interventions include procainamide, digoxin, cardioversion, or ultimately, surgical or catheter ablation of bypass tracts. (Other medication usually employed in-hospital after consultation with a pediatric cardiologist include sotalol, amiodarone, propafenone, atenolol, and propranolol.)

Clinical Note *The possibility of a significant base excess (acidosis) should be considered when episodes of SVTs in infants last hours to days, are refractory to cardioversion or adenosine, or convert to sinus rhythm for only a few seconds. In addition to connecting the acidosis, long-acting antidysrhythmic agent and ICU hospitalization are usually necessary for symptomatic SVT cases.*

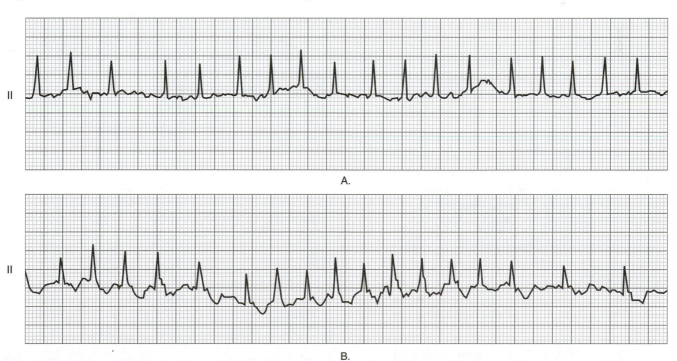

Figure 25–5 Atrial fibrillation with tachycardic ventricular responses. Tracings A and B show the typical variation in the R-R intervals with numerous atrial waves seen. The ventricular rate in untreated atrial fibrillation typically ranges from 140 to 160 bpm.

Atrial Fibrillation (AF)

Other rapid supraventricular tachydysrhythmias, such as atrial fibrillation and flutter are decidedly *uncommon* in children. The characteristics of atrial fibrillation are the same as in adults: a rapid and disorganized atrial activity with atrial rates from 350 bpm to 700 bpm having a variable ventricular response. The typical ECG appearance shows an irregularly irregular ventricular rhythm with atrial waves of varying size (Figure 25–5) .

Causes of Atrial Fibrillation

Although uncommon in children, AF frequently occurs in cases of long-standing rheumatic disease, congenital valvular disease, and hyperthyroidism. AF is more commonly associated with W-P-W in children 12 years of age or older.

Acute Therapy for AF

AF, like atrial flutter, is usually well tolerated by children unless cardiac compromise occurs. Treatment with medication is preferred over synchronized cardioversion for stable patients. A useful emergency cardiac care treatment algorithm for pediatric tachycardias is based on how well the patient tolerates the rapid dysrhythmia: tachycardias with adequate perfusion and poor perfusion are shown in Figures 25–6 and 25–7 respectively.

Ventricular rate control is an early priority while conversion back to a sinus rhythm can be accomplished after the cause is determined and the child's condition stabilized. An acceptable ventricular rate can be obtained by using beta blockers *or* calcium channel antagonists for children *over the age of one*. These two types of drugs should never be used together or severe hypotension and cardiovascular collapse may occur. In children under one year of age, use of either calcium channel blockers or beta-blocking agents are *contraindicated* as their use can precipitate sudden clinical deterioration and death. Digoxin can be used in all cases regardless of age but has a much slower onset of action, often taking hours to be effective.

Clinical Note *Intravenous verapamil or propranolol is contraindicated in children under one year of age because their protracted myocardial depressant effects can precipitate profound and refractory bradycardias along with a rare cardiovascular arrest. Verapamil should also be avoided in children with congestive heart failure or myocardial depression.*

Atrial Flutter

Atrial flutter is *exceedingly rare* in the pediatric patient unless congenital heart disease exists. Atrial flutter is typically seen during the postoperative phase following cardiac surgery but also occurs congenitally or due to unknown reasons (idiopathic).

Atrial flutter is a *sustained* reentry tachycardia that has regular R-R intervals, AV conduction ratios of 2:2 and 3:1, but minor rate variation can occur. The ECG demonstrates a classic "sawtooth" pattern, which can best be seen in leads II and V_1 (Figure 25–8). The atrial rate usually averages 300 bpm during which every other atrial impulse is conducted through the AV node to the ventricles. Higher AV conduction ratios result in ventricular rates of 100 bpm or 75 bpm for 3:1 or 4:1 conduction respectively. Were the AV node to transmit every atrial impulse in 1:1 conduction, ventricular rates in the range of 280 to 320/minute are so fast as to cause profound symptoms, including palpitations, lethargy, poor feeding, dizziness, syncope, hypotension, or acute congestive heart failure.

ECG Interpretation Tip *An elevated heart rate in a postoperative pediatric patient with a narrow-complex tachycardia and congenital heart disease should lead to a search for hidden atrial flutter waves.*

Acute Therapy of Atrial Flutter

The pediatric emergency cardiac care treatment algorithms presented for atrial fibrillation also apply for atrial flutter, as well as any rapid rhythm. Atrial flutter can be treated by *slowing* the ventricular response with a *beta blocker, calcium channel antagonist, or digoxin depending on the patinet's age*. As with atrial fibrillation, beta blockers and calcium channel blockers *must be avoided* in children younger than one year of age.

Restoration of sinus rhythm is usually done after hopitalization while in the intensvie care unit. Useful drugs for in-hospital cardioversion include procainamide, quinidine, flecanide, or amiodarone. Should pharmacologic intervention fail or immediate cardioversion is needed, atrial flutter is the most electrically sensitive dysrhythmia. Cardioversion requires only minimal energy (0.5 joule/kg). If conversion to sinus rhythm does not occur with one or two cardioversion attempts, further attempts should not be tried. As with adults, the longer a patient remains in atrial flutter, the harder it is to convert the dysrhythmia to NSR. A short burst of overdrive transcutaneous pacing has been used successfully to restore sinus activity.

Child and Infant Tachycardia With Adequate Perfusion

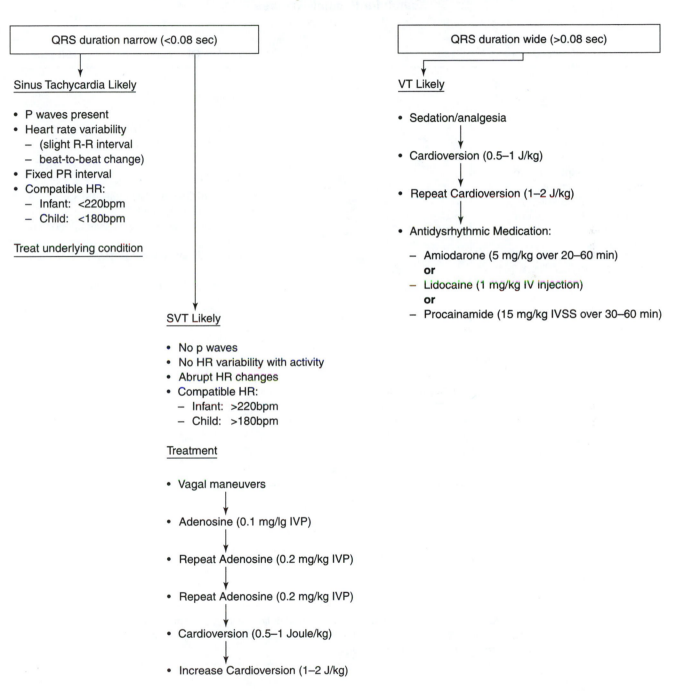

QRS duration narrow (<0.08 sec)

Sinus Tachycardia Likely

- P waves present
- Heart rate variability
  - (slight R-R interval
  - beat-to-beat change)
- Fixed PR interval
- Compatible HR:
  - Infant: <220bpm
  - Child: <180bpm

Treat underlying condition

SVT Likely

- No p waves
- No HR variability with activity
- Abrupt HR changes
- Compatible HR:
  - Infant: >220bpm
  - Child: >180bpm

Treatment

- Vagal maneuvers

- Adenosine (0.1 mg/lg IVP)

- Repeat Adenosine (0.2 mg/kg IVP)

- Repeat Adenosine (0.2 mg/kg IVP)

- Cardioversion (0.5–1 Joule/kg)

- Increase Cardioversion (1–2 J/kg)

QRS duration wide (>0.08 sec)

VT Likely

- Sedation/analgesia

- Cardioversion (0.5–1 J/kg)

- Repeat Cardioversion (1–2 J/kg)

- Antidysrhythmic Medication:
  - Amiodarone (5 mg/kg over 20–60 min)
  or
  - Lidocaine (1 mg/kg IV injection)
  or
  - Procainamide (15 mg/kg IVSS over 30–60 min)

Figure 25–6 Pediatric emergency cardiac care treatment algorithm for tachycardia with poor tissue perfusion. (Continues)

Child and Infant Tachycardia With Poor Perfusion
Search for Possible Causes

Normal QRS duration for age (<0.08 sec)

Probable Sinus Tachycardia

- History consistent
- P waves present
- HR varies with activity
- Constant PR interval with variable RR interval
- Infants: HR <220bpm
- Children: HR <180bpm

Treatment

Treat underlying condition; i.e., hypovolemia, acidosis

Probable SVT

- History consistent
- Absent P waves/abnormal shape
- HR does not vary with activity
- Rate abruptly changes
- Infants: >220bpm
- Children: >180bpm

Treatment

- Vagal maneuvers (as long as this does not delay definitive care)
- Sychronized Cardioversion (0.5–1 J/kg)
  or
- Adenosine (0.1mg/kg IV/IO; 6mg maximum)
- Adenosine (Repeat dose: double 1st dose)
- Adenosine (Repeat again at double 1st dose)

Wide QRS duration for age (>0.08 sec)

Probable VT

- Wide QRS complex with poor profusion is VT until proven otherwise

Treatment

- Electrical Cardioversion (0.5–1 J/kg)
- Alternate Medications:
  - Amiodarone (5mg/kg IV over 20–60min)
    or
  - Procainamide (15mg/kg over 30–60min)
    or
  - Lidocaine (1mg/kg IV bolus)

Pediatric Cardiology Consult

Inadequate perfusion means that shock exists and definitive therapy with electrical cardioversion is indicated. Use of adenosine and vagal maneuvers may be tied as llong as they can be done immediately.

Figure 25-7   Pediatric dysmergency cardiac care treatment algorithm for tachycardia with adequate tissue perfusion. (Continued)

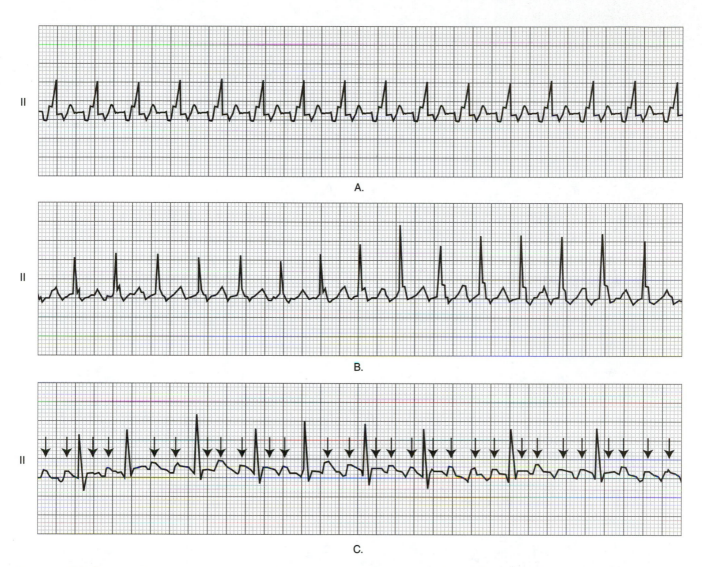

Figure 25–8 Atrial flutter with different A-V conduction ratios. In strips A and B the conduction ratio is 2:1 which results in a ventricular rate of 150 bpm. The atrial rate is precisely 300 flutter waves per minute. In strip C the conduction ratios vary from 2:1 to 4:1 (indicated by arrows), resulting in an average ventricular rate of 95 bpm.

> *Clinical Note Atrial flutter and fibrillation are associated with organic heart disease, whereas SVT occurs without structural cardiac disease. Ventricular rate control is the initial priority for atrial fibrillation and flutter. Restoration of sinus rhythm can be accomplished after the patient's condition has been stabilized. SVT, in contrast, is quickly converted to sinus rhythm with adenosine in most cases.*

is very *uncommon* in pediatric patients and the majority of children who develop it have underlying structural heart disease or prolonged QT intervals.

VT is defined as three or more consecutive ectopic ventricular beats having a rate between 120/bpm and 240/bpm. *Sustained VT* lasts longer than 30 seconds (Figure 25–9). Ventricular tachycardia may be associated with palpitations, chest discomfort, pressure, or tightness, dizziness, shortness of breath, syncope, or even sudden cardiac arrest. In newborns and infants unable to speak, congestive heart failure, lethargy, tachypnea or poor feeding may be the reason medical care is sought.

Ventricular Tachycardia

In stark contrast to adults, ventricular tachycardia (VT)

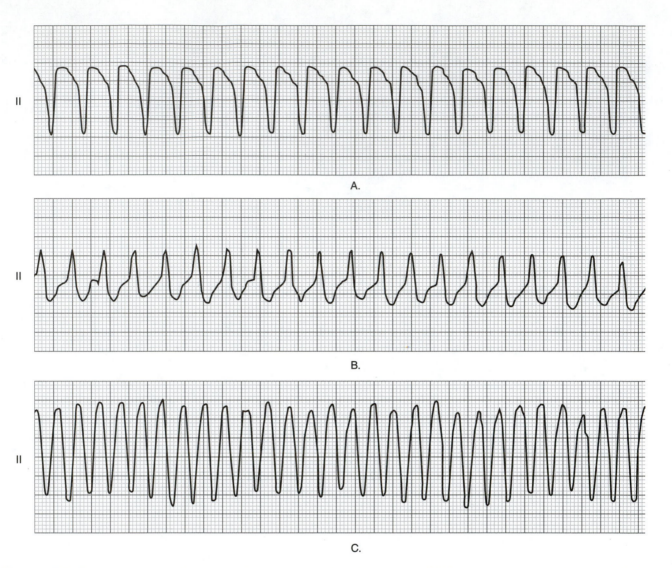

Figure 25-9 Ventricular tachycardias. All three examples show a wide QRS complex tachycardia that lacks clear P waves. In strip C the ventricular rate is 280 bpm and causes the QRS complexes to resemble a smooth sine wave.

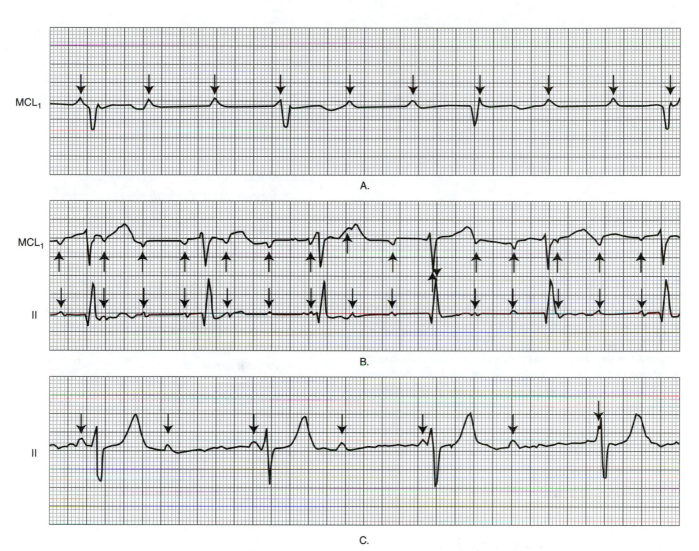

Figure 25–10 Complete AV heart blocks. Arrows point to each nonconducted P wave. The ventricular rates are one half to one third of the atrial rate. In strip B two leads are simultaneously recorded.

Clinical Note *Aberrant ventricular conduction is unlikely in cases of SVT except in infants less than a year old, so previously undiagnosed wide-complex tachycardias in children over one year of age should be treated as VT unless proven otherwise.*

Causes of VT

Ventricular tachycardia is as malignant in children as it is in adults but is fortunately a rare dysrhythmia. In children, ventricular tachycardia (Table 25–4) is most commonly associated with an underlying abnormality of the myocardium, due either to an acquired cardiomyopathy, a congenital heart defect, an acquired or congenital prolonged QT syndrome, Kawasaki-induced coronary artery disease, or exposure to a toxic substance. (Kawasaki disease is a disease unique to pediatric patients of presumed viral cause that results in multiple, small coronary artery aneurysms.)

Acute Therapy for VT

VT is a very serious dysrhythmia that requires emergent evaluation and treatment. Episodic, short bouts of VT and VT that do not cause hemodynamic instability do not require electrical cardioversion. VT is treated with

Table 25-4 Causes of VT in Pediatric Patients

- **Acute Rheumatic Fever**
- **Congenital Heart Disease** (Tetralogy of Fallot, Ventricular Dysplasias)
- **Myocarditis**
- **Hypoxia and Acidosis**
- **Hypertrophic Cardiomyopathy**
- **Electrolyte Disorders** (Hypokalemia, Hyperkalemia, Hypocalcemia)
- **Cardiac Tumors**
- **Cardiac Catheterization and Heart Surgeries**
- **Acquired Prolonged QT Intervals:** Drug Toxicity from Tricyclic Antidepressants and Antidysrhythmia Therapy
- **Congenital Prolonged QT Intervals:** Familial Prolonged QT Intervals

lidocaine, mexiletine, tocainide, phenytoin, and amiodarone, as well as synchronized cardioversion at 0.5 to 1 joule/kg (see Figure 25–6 and 25–7). Correction of any underlying cause, such as hypoxia, acidosis, and electrolyte disorders is important. Although the drugs used to treat this dysrhythmia have potent side effects, the alternative is deterioration into ventricular fibrillation.

Clinical Note *It cannot be over emphasized that ventricular dysrhythmias are extremely rare in children with normal hearts. In contrast to adults, VT in children is not caused by ischemia in contrast to adults. Sudden cardiac death does not occur in children, aside from cases of hypertrophic cardiomyopathy. Metabolic disorders, drug toxicity, and congenital heart structural abnormalities are the major causes of ventricular dysrhythmias.*

Ventricular Fibrillation

Ventricular fibrillation is rare in children, occuring in less than 10% of pediatric cardiac arrests. When it does present, it develops secondary to other conditions such as hypoxia and acidosis. In contrast to adult cardiac arrests where VF is a major rhythm disorder, it occurs during only 10 percent of pediatric codes. Ventricular fibrillation and the more frequently occurring asystole and bradycardia dysrhythmias, are often the final common mechanism of cardiac arrest and represent terminal cardiac rhythms. Initial defibrillation is done at 2 joules/kg and subsequent defibrillations at double the initial charge. The emergency cardiac care treatment algorithm for pulseless arrest (VT/VF) is found in Figure 25–10.

Clinical Note *Cardiac dysrhythmias without a pulse, including pulseless electrical activity (PEA), electromechanical dissociation (EMD), ventricular tachycardia, and ventricular fibrillation are treated essentially the same as for adults. Pulseless VT or VF receives unsynchronized countershocks and epinephrine. A search for reversible causes, such as airway obstruction, hypoxia, hypovolemia or tension pneumothorax, or pericardial tampnoade is done and treatment instituted.*

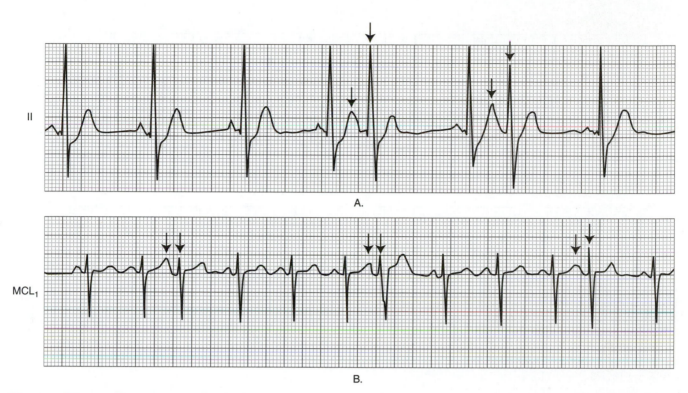

II

A.

MCL₁

B.

Figure 25–11 Premature atrial complexes. The early atrial complexes are indicated by arrows. The hallmark findings of PACs include their narrow QRS complexes, altered P waves, which often are hidden within the T waves of the preceding sinus beats (indicated by arrow heads), and irregular rhythm.

SLOW HEART RATES

In children as in adults, bradycardia refers to an abnormally slow heart rate. Unlike rhythms with rates below 60 bpm which defines *adult* bradycardia, there is no single rate in children because pediatric bradycardia is a relative value. For instance, a heart rate of 120/bpm in a newborn is significantly bradycardic. *Pediatric sinus bradycardia is a rate that falls below the normal range of heart rates based on the patient's age.* It is critical to remember that normal heart rates in children vary widely even in healthy children.

Normal heart rates vary with age, activity level, physical condition and clinical status. Because children, especially neonates, are greatly influenced by vagal stimuli, any increase in parasympathetic tone, such as due to suctioning, may lead to a decreased heart rate. Sinus bradycardia during sleep is common in all ages. Clinically significant bradycardia occurs during severe systemic disease especially those with hypoxemia or central nervous system injuries. The most common cause of permanent bradycardia is damage to the sinoatrial (SA) node following open-heart surgery to repair a congenital heart defect.

Clinical Note *Bradycardia in a critically ill infant or young child commonly signals cardiopulmonary deterioration and should be assumed to be caused by hypoxia and acidosis. Efforts at supporting ventilation and securing a patent airway should be the initial treatment measures. Oxygen is always the first-line drug for symptomatic pediatric bradycardias. In contrast to adults, epinephrine administration, followed by atropine, are the indicated order of drug use.*

Treatment of Pediatric Slow Rhythms

Treatment of bradycardia in children is directed at correcting the underlying condition that caused vagal stimuli, such as suctioning. Figure 25–11 presents the pediatric emergency cardiac care treatment algorithm for symptomatic bradycardias. Epinephrine is given IV or intraosseus (IO) at 0.01mg/kg every 3-5 minutes. In the setting of a symptomatic bradycardia that is associated with hemodynamic compromise and due to increased parasympathetic tone or AV heart block, atropine increases the heart rate and results in an

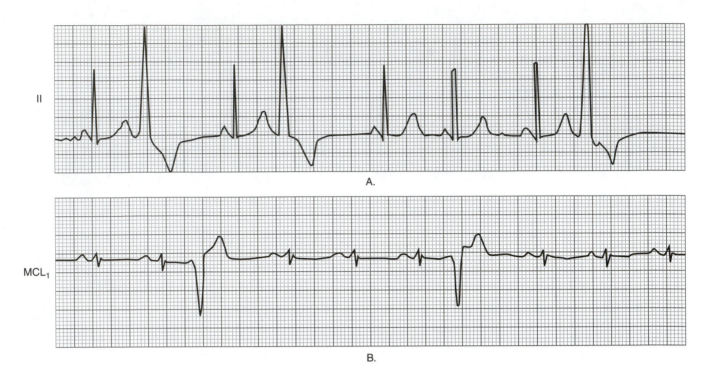

Figure 25–12 PVCs. The 2nd, 4th, and 8th beat is strip A and the 3rd and 7th beat in strip B are premature ventricular complexes.

improved cardiac output. Should the rate fail to increase or does so only briefly, an epinephrine infusion can be used. External cardiac pacing can be considered.

Atrio-Ventricular Heart Blocks

Complete (third degree) AV heart block is the most common cause of significant bradycardia in infants and young children. Atrioventricular heart blocks occur most commonly as a result of a congenital cardiac defect or following surgical repair of such defects. Children have an incredible ability to compensate for a fall in cardiac output caused by a slow heart rate by increasing the amount of blood in each contraction (stroke volume). Severe bradycardia results in hypotension, tachypnea, lethargy, congestive heart failure, and poor feeding, all of which reflect a decreased cardiac output.

In complete AV block the atria and the ventricles continue beating independently without synchronization. P waves appear to march through the QRS-T complexes (Figure 25–12). The ventricular rate is determined by the level of the escape rhythm. In contrast to adults, the ventricular escape rate can be as high as 80 bpm in an infant and as fast as 60 bpm in a teenager. In congenital cases of heart block, the AV junctional escape rate

may be as rapid as 120 bpm in a newborn.

Emergency Treatment for AV Heart Blocks

The emergency cardiac care pediatric bradycardia treatment algorithm is shown in Figure 25–11. Although rarely indicated and only if the patient is symptomatic, an artificial pacemaker is the treatment of choice for profound third-degree heart blocks. Transcutaneous pacing provides a temporary treatment for transient conditions or may serve as a bridge until a permanent pacemaker can be implanted. A single episode of classic *Stokes-Adams syndrome* is considered an indication for a permanent pacemaker.

IRREGULAR HEART RHYTHMS

Sinus dysrhythmia, also known as sinus arrhythmia, is a normal variation of sinus function that is found in adults as well as children but is a *much more common ECG finding in the pediatric population.* This benign irregular rhythm is characterized by variable R-R intervals that follow a pattern corresponding to the respiratory cycle. An irregular rhythm with a variable R-R rhythm is most likely to be sinus dysrhythmia rather than atrial fibrillation because AF is much rarer in children.

> ***Clinical Note*** *Cardiac rhythm disturbances in infants and children are only treated if cardiac output is compromised and symptoms result or if the dysrhythmia has the potential to degenerate into an unstable ECG rhythm.*

Premature Complexes

Premature atrial complexes (PACs) *are one of the most common ECG abnormalities in infants and children* (Figure 25–13). PACs are especially common in newborns and become less common during the first six months of life. Just as in adults, PACs are rarely a cause for concern. Even in the child with congenital heart disease, PACs are only treated if they precipitate frequent bouts of SVT. When frequent PACs are found, a search for underlying precipitants should be undertaken. Caffeine, theophylline, and antihistamines—especially pseudophedrine—can cause PACs.

Premature ventricular complexes (PVCs) in children are recognized as early, wide beats with bizarre QRS complexes (Figure 25–14). PVCs often occur without an identifiable cause in infants and children and are generally benign. In contrast to adults, PVCs are not a sign of myocardial irritability or ischemia. However, in a child with congenital heart disease or congestive heart failure, PVCs may result from a decreased cardiac output and reflect a worsening of the disease. PVCs in children can also be seen during inflammation of the heart muscle (myocarditis), cardiomyopathies, cardiac tumors, and electrolyte disturbances, especially low potassium levels. A child may complain that their "heart skips a beat" or that he is having a strange fluttering chest sensation. PVCs in the pediatric population require treatment only when they lead to ventricular tachycardia. Some emergent, non-cardiac causes of PVCs involve medication overdose and poisonings, especially with tricyclic antidepressants, cocaine, or digitalis.

Atrial Fibrillation, which is the hallmark irregular cardiac rhythm, was already discussed in the section on rapid heart rates, since it is AF's fast ventricular rate that is responsible for most of this dysrhythmia's hemodynamic consequences.

PULELESS ECG RHYTHMS

The absence of a central pulse coupled with apnea identifies all pulseless cardiopulmonary arrests. The underlying ECG rhythm disorder may be asystole, pulseless electrical activity (PEA), including electromechanical dissociation (EMD), and ventricular fibrillation/ pulseless VT. Pulseless VT and VF were discussed earlier in this chapter as a separate topic. The two remaining pulseless dysrhythmias, asystole and PEA will now be mentioned.

Toxic exposures and poisonings are especially dangerous in children and infants and a leading cause of age-related deaths, along with accidents. In all pulseless arrest, the only hope for resuscitation rests with quick identification and treatment of the underlying cause. The various cardiac rhythm mechanisms are not that important as ventricular fibrillation is observed in only one out of ten pediatric arrests.

Asystole

Cardiac electrical activity has ceased. All of the cardiac pacemakers have failed and the ECG resembles a flat line. Asystole is the final (terminal) ECG rhythm of all dying hearts. If the patient has a terminal illness, the more important issue focuses on withholding resuscitation measures. Occasional electrical complexes are commonly seen but these are not associated with a pulse and are signs of a dying heart. The pediatric treatment algorithm was contained with the VF/ Pulseless VT guide in the Pulseless Cardiopulmonary Arrest guide (figure 25-10).

PEA

An organized electrical pattern occurs without a palpable central pulse characterizes pulseless electrical activity. Electrical activity without a pulse excludes VF, VT, and asystole. The treatment and poor prognosis is the same as for asystole unless a reversible cause is discovered (figure 25-10).

Let's Review

1. Treatment of pediatric rhythm disturbances requires a different approach from that of adults. The causes and significance of the rhythmdisturbances vary based on age groups. Therapies used to treat adults with dysrhythmias cannot simply be transferred to children with the same dysrhythmias because some drugs that are safe in adults can result in cardiovascular collapse in kids.

2. Pediatric dysrhythmias do not result from ischemic heart disease in contrast to adults. In the very young, the single most common

cause is congenital heart disease. In older pediatric patients, non-cardiac causes must be considered.

3. The single most common cardiac dysrhythmia in the pediatric population is supraventricular tachycardia (SVT). On the basis of heart rate alone, there is significant overlap between sinus tachycardia and an ectopic atrial tachycardia.

4. Wolff-Parkinson-White (W-P-W) syndrome and SVT are the single most frequently encountered types of ventricular preexcitation syndrome.

5. As many as a quarter of infants less than one year of age who develop SVT will have a wide QRS complex (greater than 0.1 seconds) due to fatigue of the bundle branches.

6. Intravenous verapamil and propranolol are contraindicated in children under one year of age because their protracted calcium and beta-adrenergic blocking effects can precipitate profound and refractory hypotension, bradycardia, and cardiovascular arrest.

7. Carotid sinus massage is rarely successful in treating SVT in children. However, in children five years old or less, application of an ice pack to the child's face is sometimes effective in terminating an SVT through stimulation of a primitive "diving reflex."

8. Atrial flutter is rare in pediatric patients without congenital heart disease. Atrial flutter is typically seen during the postoperative recovery phase after repair of transposition of the great vessels or by a congenital defect.

9. Ventricular rate control is the initial priority in treating atrial fibrillation and flutter in infants and children as it is in adults. Restoration of sinus rhythm can be accomplished after stabilization of the patient's condition.

10. Ventricular dysrhythmias are extremely rare in children with normal hearts. In contrast to adults, VT in children is not caused by ischemia. Metabolic disorders, drug toxicity, and congenital heart abnormalities are the major causes.

11. Ventricular tachycardia is uncommon in the pediatric patient and the majority of cases have underlying structural heart disease or prolonged QT intervals.

12. Ventricular fibrillation is rare in children and is usually secondary to other non-cardiac conditions such as hypoxia and acidosis. Most pediatric cardiac arrest involve brady-asystolic dysrhythmias.

13. Pathological bradycardia occurs during severe systemic disease, especially those associated with hypoxemia or central nervous system injuries. The most common cause of permanent bradycardia is damage to the sinoatrial (SA) node following open-heart surgery to repair a congenital heart defect.

14. Complete (third degree) AV heart block is the most common cause of significant bradycardia in infants and young children. Atrioventricular heart blocks most commonly occur as a result of a congenital cardiac defect or following surgical repair of these defects.

15. Sinus dysrhythmia is characterized by a cyclic variation in the heart rate that is caused by normal respiratory reflexes. This benign dysrhythmia occurs in both adults and children but is often more pronounced in children and requires no treatment.

14. PVCs are not a sign of myocardial irritability or ischemia as in adults. In children with congenital heart disease or congestive heart failure, PVCs may reflect a fall in cardiac output and worsening failure.

15. PACs are especially common in newborns and become less common during the first six months of life. Just as in adults, PACs are rarely a cause for concern.

Glossary

Bradycardia, symptomatic Slow heart rate that results in patient discomfort; such as, light-headedness, dizziness, nausea and vomiting, shortness of breath, easy fatigability and generalized weakness.

Bradycardia, relative Heart rate below the usual heart rate for a patient of a particular age. For instance, a heart rate of below 80 bpm for a newborn would be considered severely bradycardic while the same rate in an adult is normal. This contrasts to bradycardia in adults where a bradycardic rate is defined as a rate below 60 bpm.

Catheter ablation Technique used in the electrophysiology lab to treat SVT by using bursts of sound waves to eliminate the reentry path.

Cardiomyopathy Chronic disorder of the heart muscle leading to impaired contractility.

CHF (congestive heart failure) Inability of the heart to pump an adequate amount of blood to meet the body's needs; associated with pulmonary congestion, jugular venous distension, lower extremity edema ("pitting edema"), shortness of breath, decreased exercise ability, and dyspnea on exertion.

Congenital abnormality Disease or deformity caused during fetal development and present at birth.

Diving reflex Primitive reflex in infants and young children that results in pronounced bradycardia when cold water is applied to the face.

Hemodynamically unstable Patient condition characterized by abnormal vital signs and/or mental status due to diminished tissue perfusion caused by decreased cardiac output.

Ice bag application to face Technique used to stimulate the diving reflex in infants and young children and terminate an SVT.

Idiopathic condition Due to an unknown cause.

Kawasaki Disease Multisystem inflammatory disease, probably due to an infectious agent, affecting blood vessels in children and infants; characterized by rash, conjunctival inflammation, redness of palms or soles, and swollen neck lymph nodes;.

Myocarditis Inflammation of the myocardium which leads to significantly impaired cardiac function.

Non-sustained VT Episode Ventricular tachycardia lasting for less than 30 seconds.

Post-surgery dysrhythmias Abnormal cardiac rhythms that occur during the recovery phase following cardiac surgery.

Stokes-Adams Syndrome Syncope caused by a pause in cardiac stimulation and bradycardia associated with complete AV heart block.

Sustained VT episode Ventricular tachycardia lasting more than 30 seconds and considered more serious than the non-sustained type.

Tetralogy of Fallot Congenital heart defect involving four serious structural abnormalities.

Suggested Reading

Alimurung MM, Joseph LG, Nadas AS, et al. The unipolar, precordial and extremity electrocardiogram in normal infants and children. *Circulation* 4. 1951; 420.

Castaneda AR, Jonas RA, Mayer JE Jr, et al. *Cardiac Surgery of the Neonate and Infant.* Philadelphia: WB Saunders; 1994.

Curley MAQ: Pediatric Cardiac Dysrhythmias. Baltimore, MD: Brady Communications; 1985.

Furman RA, Halloran WR. Electrocardiogram in the first two months of life. *J Pediatr* 39.307, 1951.

Gewitz MH, Vetter VL. Cardiac Emergencies in Textbook of Pediatric Emergency Medicine. 3rd ed. Fleisher GR, Ludwig SW, eds. Baltimore: William & Wilkins; 1993: 533–572.

Gilette PC, Garson A Jr, Crawford F, et al. Dysrhythmias. In: Adams FH, Emmanouilidies GC, Reinmenschneider TA, eds. *Moss' Heart Disease in Infants, Children and Adolescents.* 4th ed. Baltimore: Williams & Wilkins; 1989: 525–539.

Lynch SM, Herman LM. CardioQuandry: Wolff-Parkinson-White syndrome. *Physician Asst* 31. 1997; 168–171.

Morgan BC, Guntheroth WG. Cardiac arrhythmias in normal newborn infants. *J Pediatr* 67. 1965; 1199.

Perry JC, Garson A Jr. Supraventricular tachycardia due to Wolff-Parkinson-White syndrome: Early disappearance and late recurrence. *J Am Coll Cardiol 16.* 1990; 1215–1220.

Perry JC, Giuffre RM, Garson A Jr. Clues to the electrocardiographic diagnosis of subtle Wolff-Parkinson-White syndrome in children. *J Pediatr 117.* 1990; 871–875.

Ross BA. Congenital complete atrioventricular bloc. *Pediatr Clin North Amer 37.* 1990; 69.

Tudbury PB, Atkinson DW: Electrocardiograms of 100 normal infants and young children. *J Pediatr 34.* 1950; 466.

Ziegler RF. *Electrocardiographic studies in normal infants and children.* Springfield, IL: Charles W. Thomas; 1951.

chapter 26

Comprehensive Self-Assessment ECG Tracings

LEARNING OBJECTIVE

Upon completion of this chapter, the reader should be able to:

■ *Correctly identify all types of dysrhythmias given sample ECG tracings, including supraventricular, atrioventricular heart blocks, ventricular dysrhythmias, artificial pacemaker rhythms, and resuscitation dysrhythmias.*

INTRODUCTION

The self-assessment exercises presented so far contained similar grouping of ECG abnormalities; for instance, supraventricular or AV heart blocks. In this chapter the exercises contain *all types* of dysrhythmias presented in random order —just as happens with actual patient encounters. A *variety* of ECG dysrhythmias, including atrial dysrhythmias, atrioventricular blocks, artificial pacemakers, resuscitation tracings, and ventricular disturbances will be presented. The answers and rationales are contained in Appendix A; and if you have any difficulties refer back to the appropriate chapter.

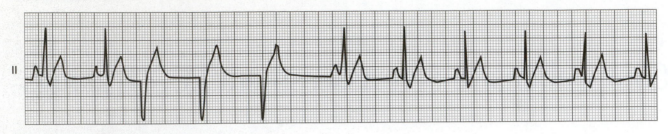

Figure 26-1 Rate _____
Rhythm _____
QRS Duration _____
PR Interval _____
AV Conduction Ratio _____
ST Segment _____
Other Findings _____
Interpretation _____
Reasoning _____

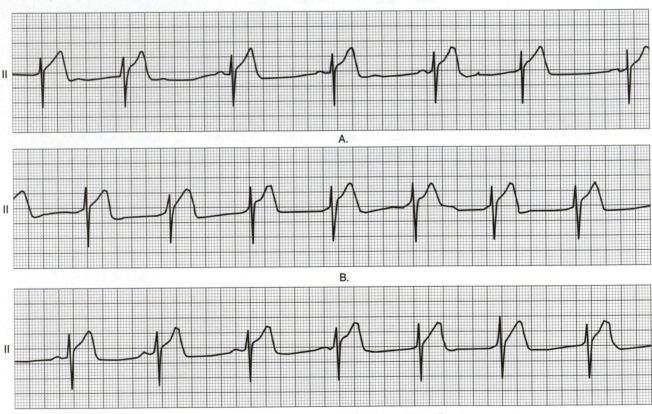

A.

B.

C. Continuous recording

Figure 26-2 Rate _____
Rhythm _____
QRS Duration _____
PR Interval _____
AV Conduction Ratio _____
ST Segment _____
Other Findings _____
Interpretation _____
Reasoning _____

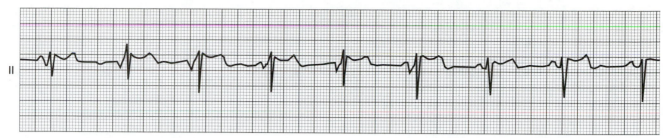

Figure 26-3 Rate _____
Rhythm _____
QRS Duration _____
PR Interval _____
AV Conduction Ratio _____
ST Segment _____
Other Findings _____
Interpretation _____
Reasoning _____

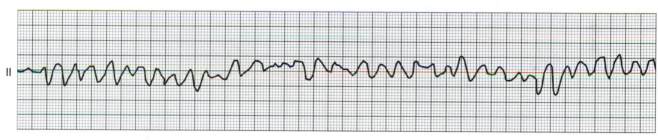

Figure 26-4 Rate _____
Rhythm _____
QRS Duration _____
PR Interval _____
AV Conduction Ratio _____
ST Segment _____
Other Findings _____
Interpretation _____
Reasoning _____

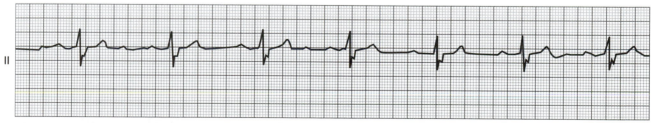

Figure 26-5 Rate _____
Rhythm _____
QRS Duration _____
PR Interval _____
AV Conduction Ratio _____
ST Segment _____
Other Findings _____
Interpretation _____
Reasoning _____

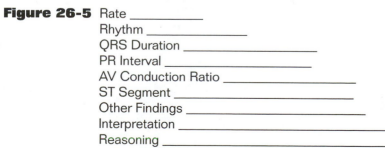

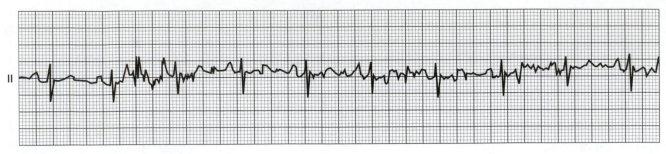

Figure 26-6 Rate _____
Rhythm _____
QRS Duration _____
PR Interval _____
AV Conduction Ratio _____
ST Segment _____
Other Findings _____
Interpretation _____
Reasoning _____

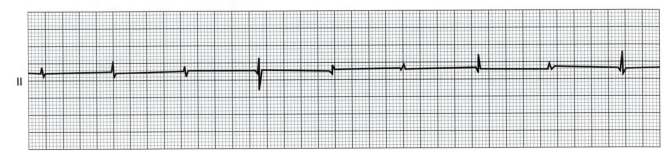

Figure 26-7 Rate _____
Rhythm _____
QRS Duration _____
PR Interval _____
AV Conduction Ratio _____
ST Segment _____
Other Findings _____
Interpretation _____
Reasoning _____

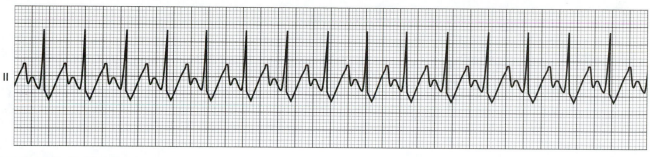

Figure 26-8 Rate _____
Rhythm _____
QRS Duration _____
PR Interval _____
AV Conduction Ratio _____
ST Segment _____
Other Findings _____
Interpretation _____
Reasoning _____

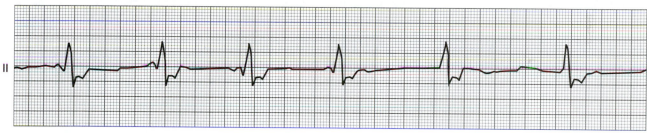

Figure 26-9 Rate _____
Rhythm _____
QRS Duration _____
PR Interval _____
AV Conduction Ratio _____
ST Segment _____
Other Findings _____
Interpretation _____
Reasoning _____

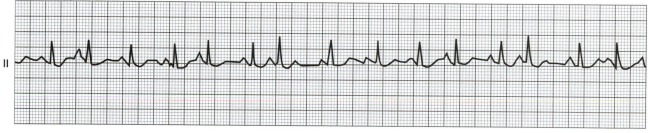

Figure 26-10 Rate _____
Rhythm _____
QRS Duration _____
PR Interval _____
AV Conduction Ratio _____
ST Segment _____
Other Findings _____
Interpretation _____
Reasoning _____

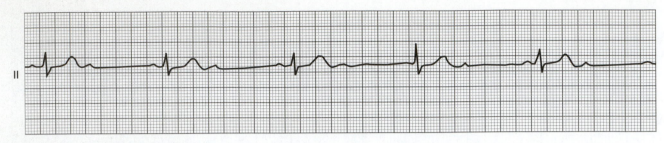

Figure 26-11 Rate _____
Rhythm _____
QRS Duration _____
PR Interval _____
AV Conduction Ratio _____
ST Segment _____
Other Findings _____
Interpretation _____
Reasoning _____

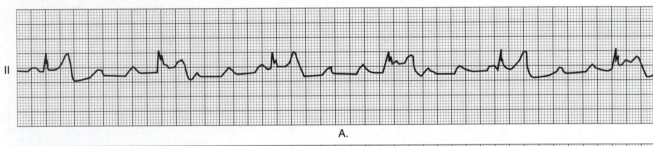

A.

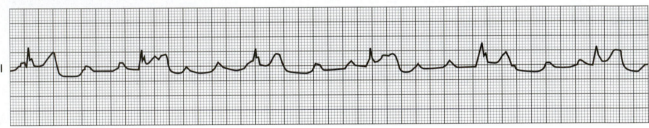

B. Continuous recording

Figure 26-12 Rate _____
Rhythm _____
QRS Duration _____
PR Interval _____
AV Conduction Ratio _____
ST Segment _____
Other Findings _____
Interpretation _____
Reasoning _____

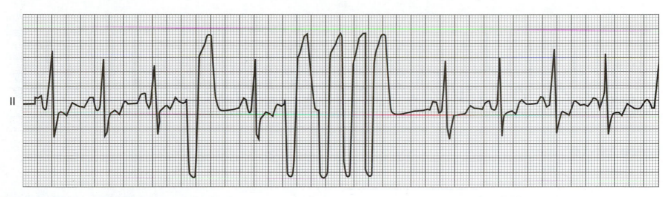

Figure 26-13 Rate _____
Rhythm _____
QRS Duration _____
PR Interval _____
AV Conduction Ratio _____
ST Segment _____
Other Findings _____
Interpretation _____
Reasoning _____

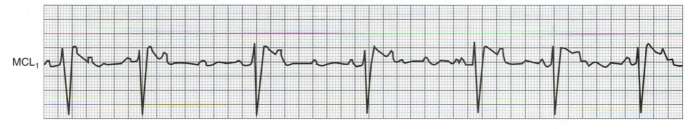

Figure 26-14 Rate _____
Rhythm _____
QRS Duration _____
PR Interval _____
AV Conduction Ratio _____
ST Segment _____
Other Findings _____
Interpretation _____
Reasoning _____

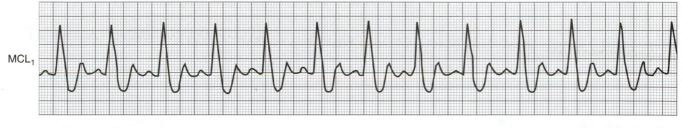

Figure 26-15 Rate _____
Rhythm _____
QRS Duration _____
PR Interval _____
AV Conduction Ratio _____
ST Segment _____
Other Findings _____
Interpretation _____
Reasoning _____

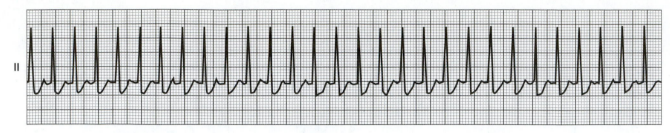

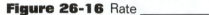

Figure 26-16 Rate _____
Rhythm _____
QRS Duration _____
PR Interval _____
AV Conduction Ratio _____
ST Segment _____
Other Findings _____
Interpretation _____
Reasoning _____

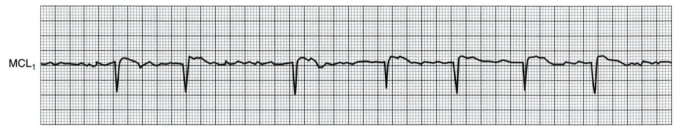

Figure 26-17 Rate _____
Rhythm _____
QRS Duration _____
PR Interval _____
AV Conduction Ratio _____
ST Segment _____
Other Findings _____
Interpretation _____
Reasoning _____

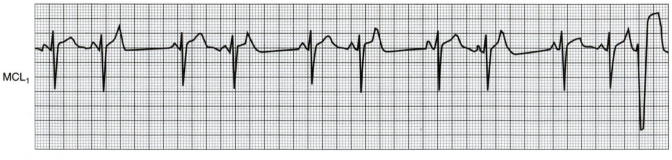

Figure 26-18 Rate _____
Rhythm _____
QRS Duration _____
PR Interval _____
AV Conduction Ratio _____
ST Segment _____
Other Findings _____
Interpretation _____
Reasoning _____

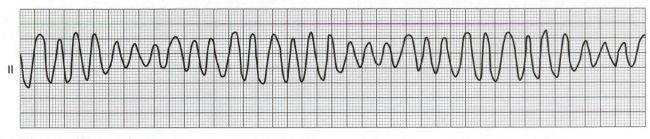

Figure 26-19 Rate _____
Rhythm _____
QRS Duration _____
PR Interval _____
AV Conduction Ratio _____
ST Segment _____
Other Findings _____
Interpretation _____
Reasoning _____

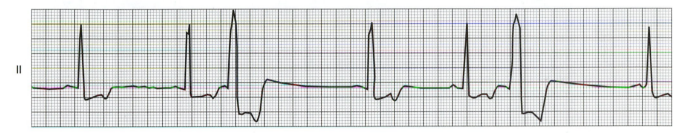

Figure 26-20 Rate _____
Rhythm _____
QRS Duration _____
PR Interval _____
AV Conduction Ratio _____
ST Segment _____
Other Findings _____
Interpretation _____
Reasoning _____

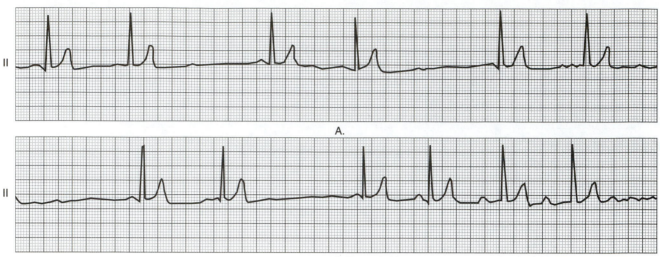

II

A.

II

B. Recorded Later

Figure 26-21 Rate _____
Rhythm _____
QRS Duration _____
PR Interval _____
AV Conduction Ratio _____
ST Segment _____
Other Findings _____
Interpretation _____
Reasoning _____

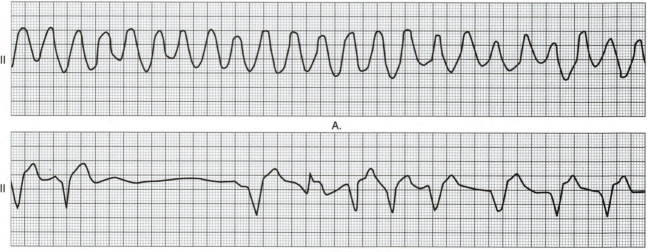

II

A.

II

B. Recorded Later

Figure 26-22 Rate _____
Rhythm _____
QRS Duration _____
PR Interval _____
AV Conduction Ratio _____
ST Segment _____
Other Findings _____
Interpretation _____
Reasoning _____

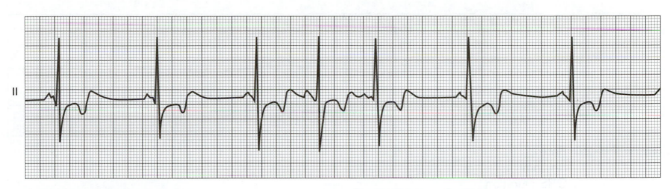

Figure 26-23 Rate _____
Rhythm _____
QRS Duration _____
PR Interval _____
AV Conduction Ratio _____
ST Segment _____
Other Findings _____
Interpretation _____
Reasoning _____

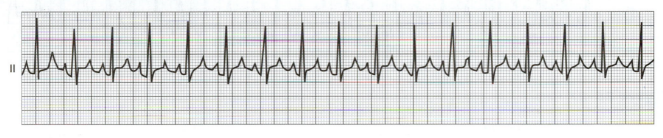

Figure 26-24 Rate _____
Rhythm _____
QRS Duration _____
PR Interval _____
AV Conduction Ratio _____
ST Segment _____
Other Findings _____
Interpretation _____
Reasoning _____

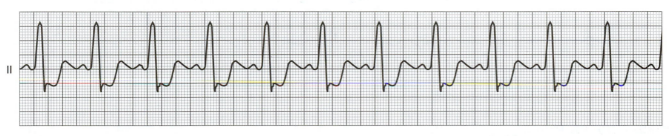

Figure 26-25 Rate _____
Rhythm _____
QRS Duration _____
PR Interval _____
AV Conduction Ratio _____
ST Segment _____
Other Findings _____
Interpretation _____
Reasoning _____

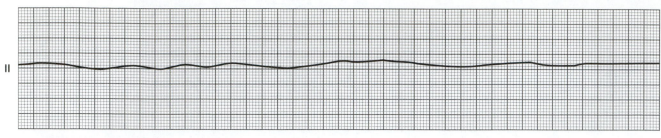

Figure 26-26 Rate _____
Rhythm _____
QRS Duration _____
PR Interval _____
AV Conduction Ratio _____
ST Segment _____
Other Findings _____
Interpretation _____
Reasoning _____

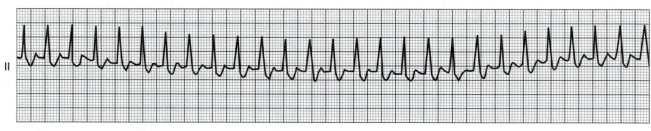

Figure 26-27 Rate _____
Rhythm _____
QRS Duration _____
PR Interval _____
AV Conduction Ratio _____
ST Segment _____
Other Findings _____
Interpretation _____
Reasoning _____

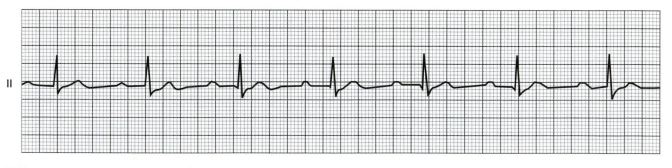

Figure 26-28 Rate _____
Rhythm _____
QRS Duration _____
PR Interval _____
AV Conduction Ratio _____
ST Segment _____
Other Findings _____
Interpretation _____
Reasoning _____

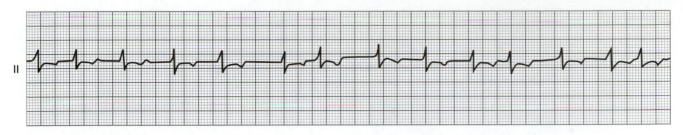

Figure 26-29 Rate _____
Rhythm _____
QRS Duration _____
PR Interval _____
AV Conduction Ratio _____
ST Segment _____
Other Findings _____
Interpretation _____
Reasoning _____

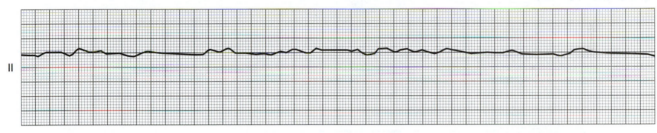

Figure 26-30 Rate _____
Rhythm _____
QRS Duration _____
PR Interval _____
AV Conduction Ratio _____
ST Segment _____
Other Findings _____
Interpretation _____
Reasoning _____

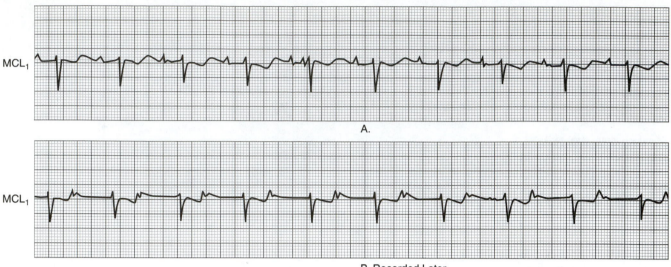

A.

B. Recorded Later

Figure 26-31 Rate _____
Rhythm _____
QRS Duration _____
PR Interval _____
AV Conduction Ratio _____
ST Segment _____
Other Findings _____
Interpretation _____
Reasoning _____

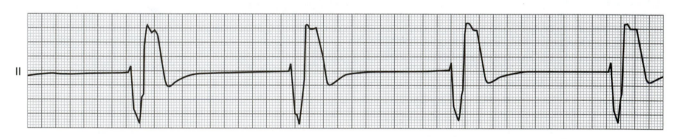

Figure 26-32 Rate _____
Rhythm _____
QRS Duration _____
PR Interval _____
AV Conduction Ratio _____
ST Segment _____
Other Findings _____
Interpretation _____
Reasoning _____

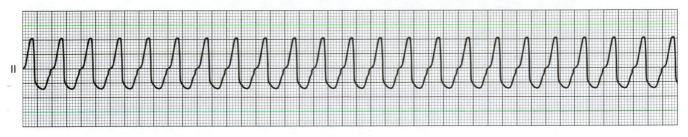

Figure 26-33 Rate _____
Rhythm _____
QRS Duration _____
PR Interval _____
AV Conduction Ratio _____
ST Segment _____
Other Findings _____
Interpretation _____
Reasoning _____

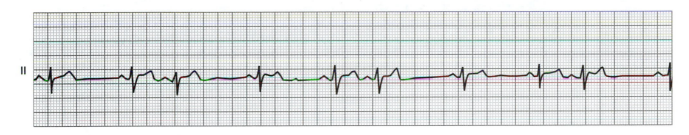

Figure 26-34 Rate _____
Rhythm _____
QRS Duration _____
PR Interval _____
AV Conduction Ratio _____
ST Segment _____
Other Findings _____
Interpretation _____
Reasoning _____

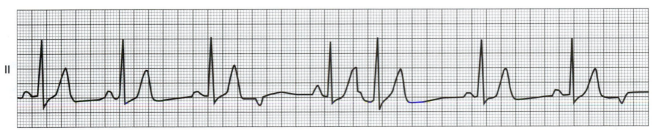

Figure 26-35 Rate _____
Rhythm _____
QRS Duration _____
PR Interval _____
AV Conduction Ratio _____
ST Segment _____
Other Findings _____
Interpretation _____
Reasoning _____

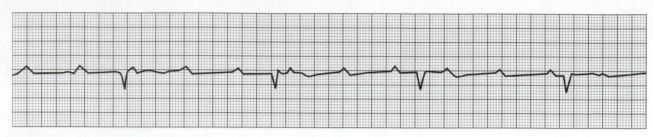

Figure 26-36 Rate _____
Rhythm _____
QRS Duration _____
PR Interval _____
AV Conduction Ratio _____
ST Segment _____
Other Findings _____
Interpretation _____
Reasoning _____

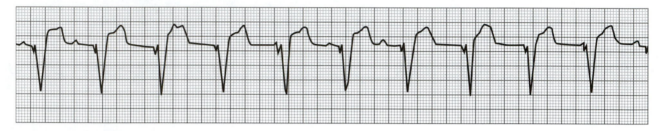

Figure 26-37 Rate _____
Rhythm _____
QRS Duration _____
PR Interval _____
AV Conduction Ratio _____
ST Segment _____
Other Findings _____
Interpretation _____
Reasoning _____

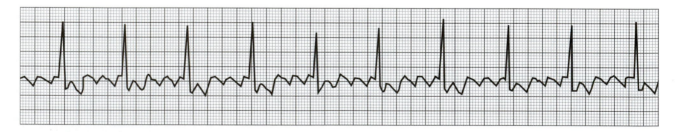

Figure 26-38 Rate _____
Rhythm _____
QRS Duration _____
PR Interval _____
AV Conduction Ratio _____
ST Segment _____
Other Findings _____
Interpretation _____
Reasoning _____

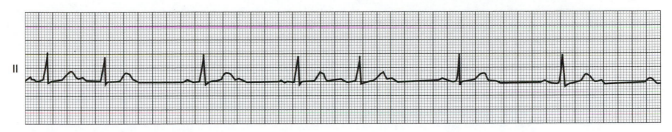

Figure 26-39 Rate _____
Rhythm _____
QRS Duration _____
PR Interval _____
AV Conduction Ratio _____
ST Segment _____
Other Findings _____
Interpretation _____
Reasoning _____

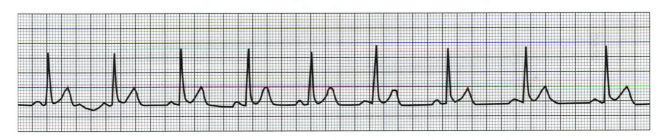

Figure 26-40 Rate _____
Rhythm _____
QRS Duration _____
PR Interval _____
AV Conduction Ratio _____
ST Segment _____
Other Findings _____
Interpretation _____
Reasoning _____

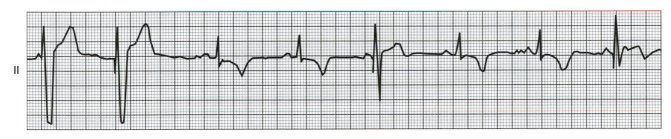

Figure 26-41 Rate _____
Rhythm _____
QRS Duration _____
PR Interval _____
AV Conduction Ratio _____
ST Segment _____
Other Findings _____
Interpretation _____
Reasoning _____

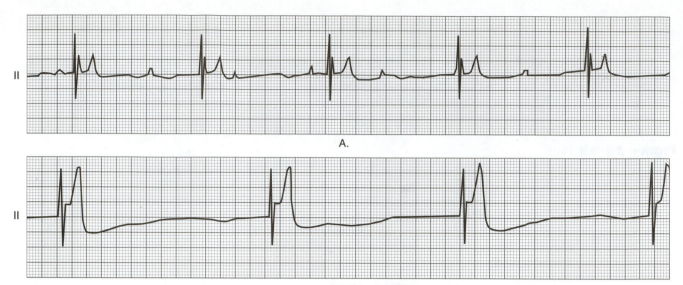

A.

B. Recorded later

Figure 26-42 Rate _____
Rhythm _____
QRS Duration _____
PR Interval _____
AV Conduction Ratio _____
ST Segment _____
Other Findings _____
Interpretation _____
Reasoning _____

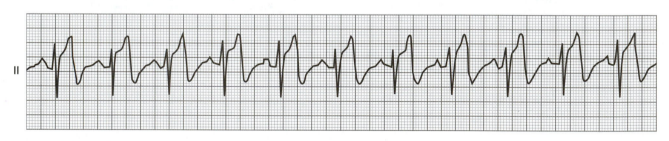

Figure 26-43 Rate _____
Rhythm _____
QRS Duration _____
PR Interval _____
AV Conduction Ratio _____
ST Segment _____
Other Findings _____
Interpretation _____
Reasoning _____

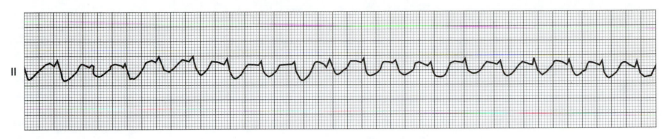

Figure 26-44 Rate _____
Rhythm _____
QRS Duration _____
PR Interval _____
AV Conduction Ratio _____
ST Segment _____
Other Findings _____
Interpretation _____
Reasoning _____

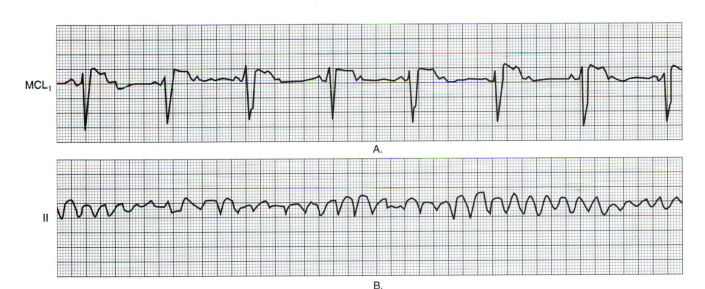

A.

B.

Figure 26-45 Rate _____
Rhythm _____
QRS Duration _____
PR Interval _____
AV Conduction Ratio _____
ST Segment _____
Other Findings _____
Interpretation _____
Reasoning _____

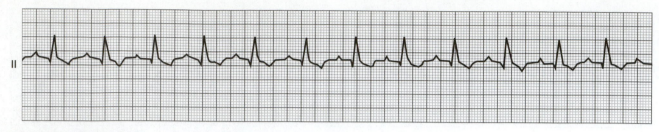

Figure 26-46 Rate _____
Rhythm _____
QRS Duration _____
PR Interval _____
AV Conduction Ratio _____
ST Segment _____
Other Findings _____
Interpretation _____
Reasoning _____

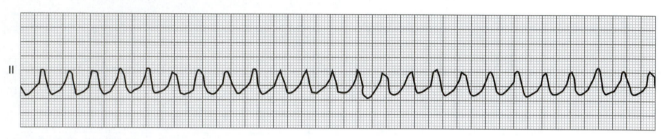

Figure 26-47 Rate _____
Rhythm _____
QRS Duration _____
PR Interval _____
AV Conduction Ratio _____
ST Segment _____
Other Findings _____
Interpretation _____
Reasoning _____

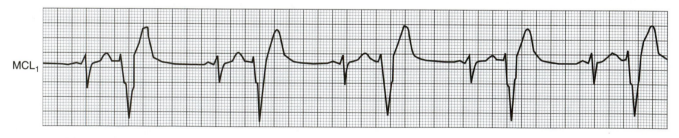

Figure 26-48 Rate _____
Rhythm _____
QRS Duration _____
PR Interval _____
AV Conduction Ratio _____
ST Segment _____
Other Findings _____
Interpretation _____
Reasoning _____

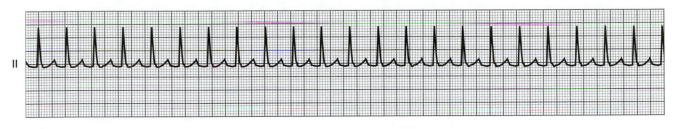
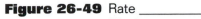

Figure 26-49 Rate _____
Rhythm _____
QRS Duration _____
PR Interval _____
AV Conduction Ratio _____
ST Segment _____
Other Findings _____
Interpretation _____
Reasoning _____

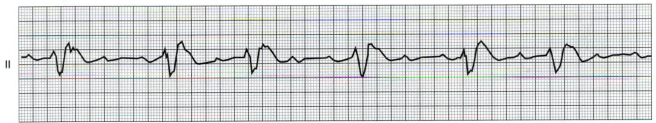

A. Without external pacemaker

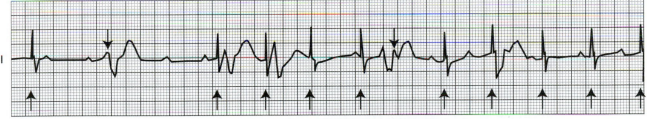

B. With pacemaker

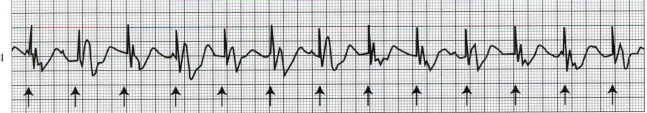

C. With pacemaker recorded one minute after B.

Figure 26-50 Rate _____
Rhythm _____
QRS Duration _____
PR Interval _____
AV Conduction Ratio _____
ST Segment _____
Other Findings _____
Interpretation _____
Reasoning _____

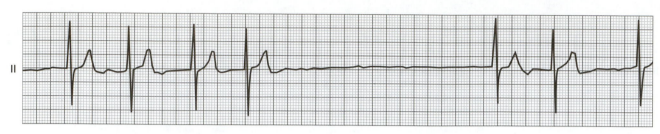

Figure 26-51 Rate _____
Rhythm _____
QRS Duration _____
PR Interval _____
AV Conduction Ratio _____
ST Segment _____
Other Findings _____
Interpretation _____
Reasoning _____

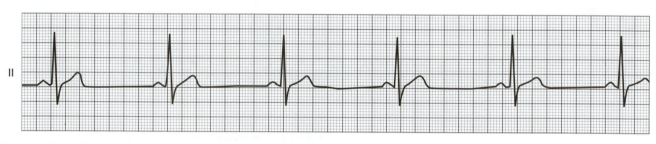

Figure 26-52 Rate _____
Rhythm _____
QRS Duration _____
PR Interval _____
AV Conduction Ratio _____
ST Segment _____
Other Findings _____
Interpretation _____
Reasoning _____

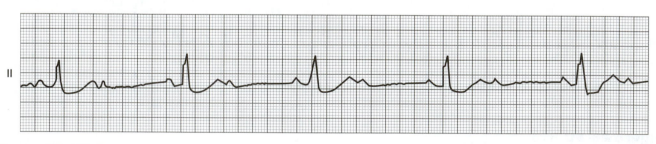

Figure 26-53 Rate _____
Rhythm _____
QRS Duration _____
PR Interval _____
AV Conduction Ratio _____
ST Segment _____
Other Findings _____
Interpretation _____
Reasoning _____

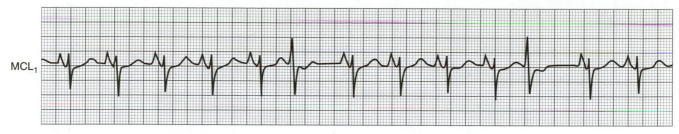

MCL₁

Figure 26-54 Rate _____
Rhythm _____
QRS Duration _____
PR Interval _____
AV Conduction Ratio _____
ST Segment _____
Other Findings _____
Interpretation _____
Reasoning _____

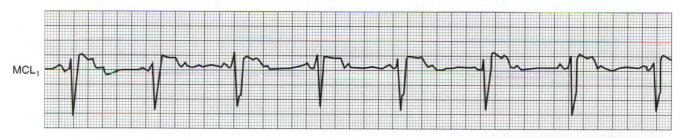

MCL₁

Figure 26-55 Rate _____
Rhythm _____
QRS Duration _____
PR Interval _____
AV Conduction Ratio _____
ST Segment _____
Other Findings _____
Interpretation _____
Reasoning _____

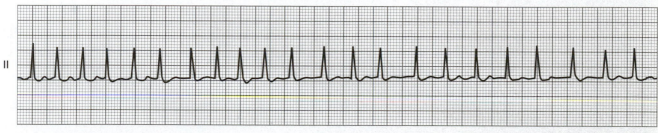

II

Figure 26-56 Rate _____
Rhythm _____
QRS Duration _____
PR Interval _____
AV Conduction Ratio _____
ST Segment _____
Other Findings _____
Interpretation _____
Reasoning _____

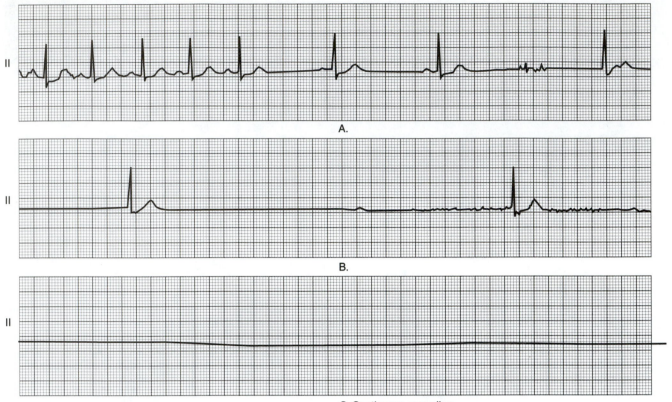

A.

B.

C. Continuous recording

Figure 26-57 Rate _____
Rhythm _____
QRS Duration _____
PR Interval _____
AV Conduction Ratio _____
ST Segment _____
Other Findings _____
Interpretation _____
Reasoning _____

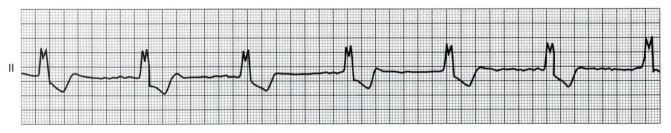

Figure 26-58 Rate _____
Rhythm _____
QRS Duration _____
PR Interval _____
AV Conduction Ratio _____
ST Segment _____
Other Findings _____
Interpretation _____
Reasoning _____

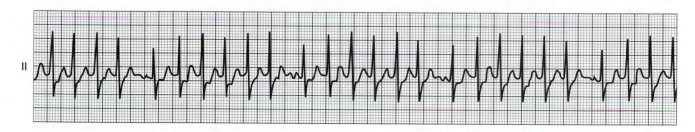

Figure 26-59 Rate _____
Rhythm _____
QRS Duration _____
PR Interval _____
AV Conduction Ratio _____
ST Segment _____
Other Findings _____
Interpretation _____
Reasoning _____

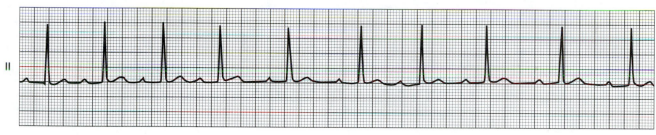

Figure 26-60 Rate _____
Rhythm _____
QRS Duration _____
PR Interval _____
AV Conduction Ratio _____
ST Segment _____
Other Findings _____
Interpretation _____
Reasoning _____

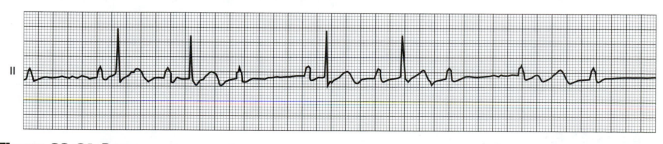

Figure 26-61 Rate _____
Rhythm _____
QRS Duration _____
PR Interval _____
AV Conduction Ratio _____
ST Segment _____
Other Findings _____
Interpretation _____
Reasoning _____

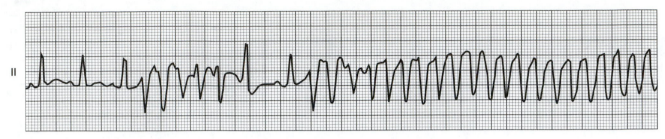

Figure 26-62 Rate _____
Rhythm _____
QRS Duration _____
PR Interval _____
AV Conduction Ratio _____
ST Segment _____
Other Findings _____
Interpretation _____
Reasoning _____

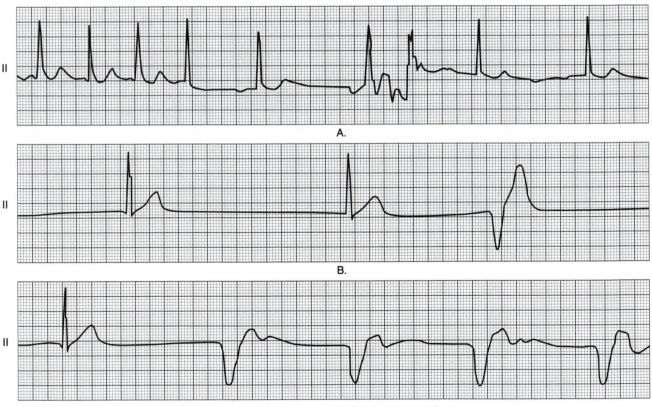

A.

B.

C. Continuous recording

Figure 26-63 Rate _____
Rhythm _____
QRS Duration _____
PR Interval _____
AV Conduction Ratio _____
ST Segment _____
Other Findings _____
Interpretation _____
Reasoning _____

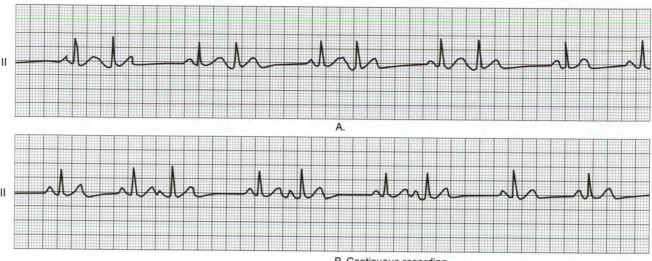

A.

B. Continuous recording

Figure 26-64 Rate _____
Rhythm _____
QRS Duration _____
PR Interval _____
AV Conduction Ratio _____
ST Segment _____
Other Findings _____
Interpretation _____
Reasoning _____

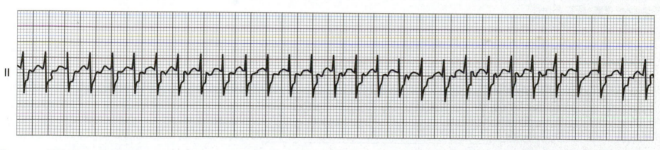

Figure 26-65 Rate _____
Rhythm _____
QRS Duration _____
PR Interval _____
AV Conduction Ratio _____
ST Segment _____
Other Findings _____
Interpretation _____
Reasoning _____

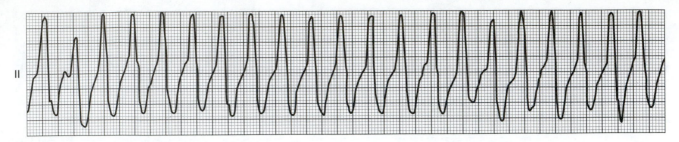

Figure 26-66 Rate _____
Rhythm _____
QRS Duration _____
PR Interval _____
AV Conduction Ratio _____
ST Segment _____
Other Findings _____
Interpretation _____
Reasoning _____

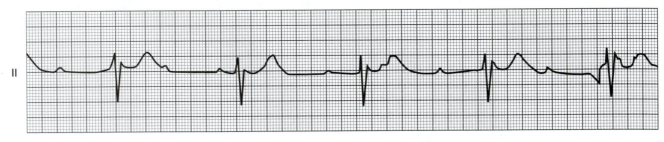

Figure 26-67 Rate _____
Rhythm _____
QRS Duration _____
PR Interval _____
AV Conduction Ratio _____
ST Segment _____
Other Findings _____
Interpretation _____
Reasoning _____

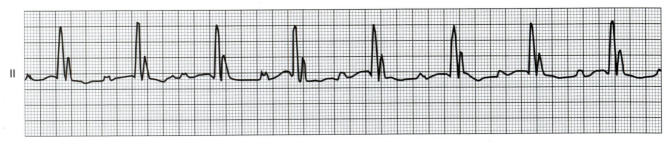

Figure 26-68 Rate _____
Rhythm _____
QRS Duration _____
PR Interval _____
AV Conduction Ratio _____
ST Segment _____
Other Findings _____
Interpretation _____
Reasoning _____

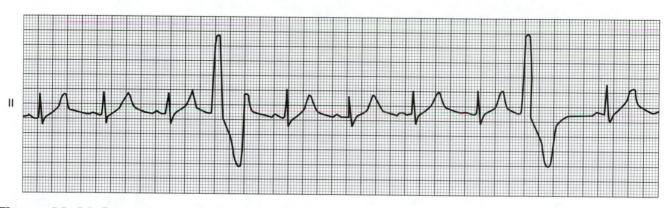

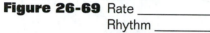

Figure 26-69 Rate _____
Rhythm _____
QRS Duration _____
PR Interval _____
AV Conduction Ratio _____
ST Segment _____
Other Findings _____
Interpretation _____
Reasoning _____

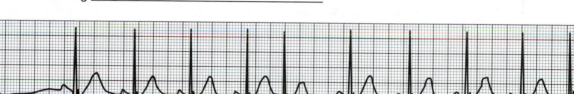

Figure 26-70 Rate _____
Rhythm _____
QRS Duration _____
PR Interval _____
AV Conduction Ratio _____
ST Segment _____
Other Findings _____
Interpretation _____
Reasoning _____

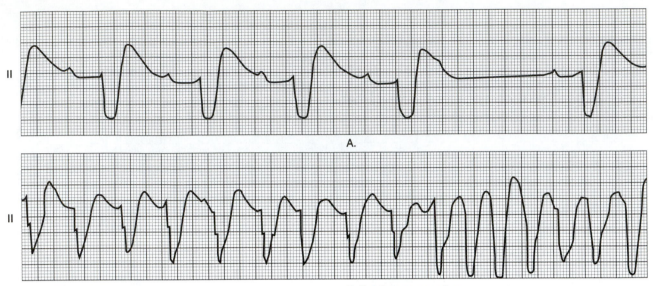

A.

B. Continuous recording

Figure 26-71　Rate _____

Rhythm _____

QRS Duration _____

PR Interval _____

AV Conduction Ratio _____

ST Segment _____

Other Findings _____

Interpretation _____

Reasoning _____

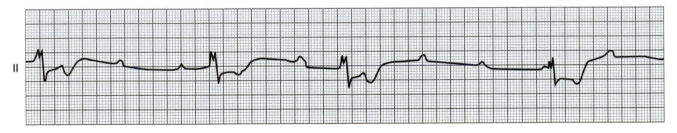

Figure 26-72　Rate _____

Rhythm _____

QRS Duration _____

PR Interval _____

AV Conduction Ratio _____

ST Segment _____

Other Findings _____

Interpretation _____

Reasoning _____

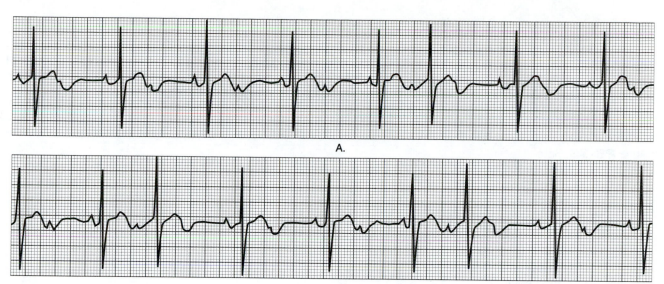

A.

B. Continuous recording

Figure 26-73 Rate _____
Rhythm _____
QRS Duration _____
PR Interval _____
AV Conduction Ratio _____
ST Segment _____
Other Findings _____
Interpretation _____
Reasoning _____

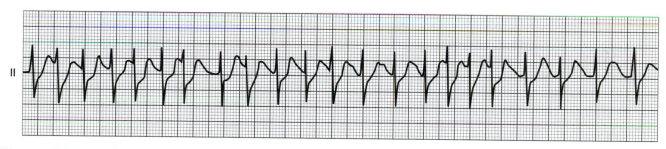

Figure 26-74 Rate _____
Rhythm _____
QRS Duration _____
PR Interval _____
AV Conduction Ratio _____
ST Segment _____
Other Findings _____
Interpretation _____
Reasoning _____

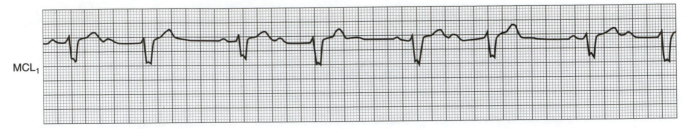

Figure 26-75 Rate _____
Rhythm _____
QRS Duration _____
PR Interval _____
AV Conduction Ratio _____
ST Segment _____
Other Findings _____
Interpretation _____
Reasoning _____

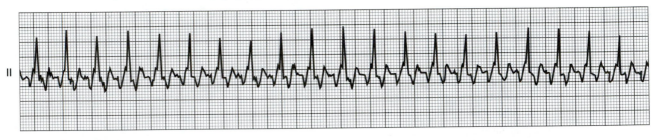

Figure 26-76 Rate _____
Rhythm _____
QRS Duration _____
PR Interval _____
AV Conduction Ratio _____
ST Segment _____
Other Findings _____
Interpretation _____
Reasoning _____

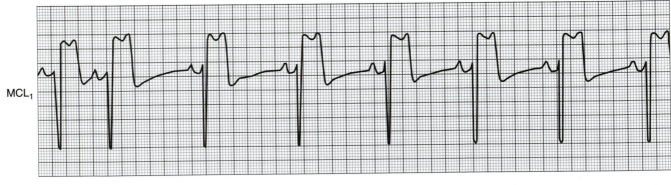

Figure 26-77 Rate _____
Rhythm _____
QRS Duration _____
PR Interval _____
AV Conduction Ratio _____
ST Segment _____
Other Findings _____
Interpretation _____
Reasoning _____

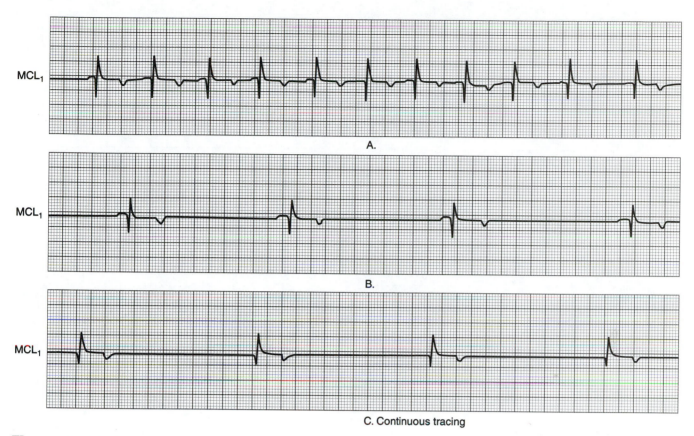

A.

B.

C. Continuous tracing

Figure 26-78 Rate _____

Rhythm _____

QRS Duration _____

PR Interval _____

AV Conduction Ratio _____

ST Segment _____

Other Findings _____

Interpretation _____

Reasoning _____

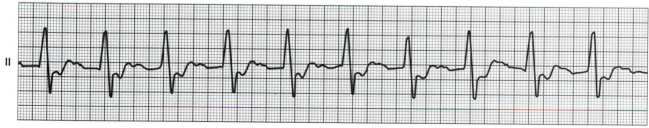

Figure 26-79 Rate _____

Rhythm _____

QRS Duration _____

PR Interval _____

AV Conduction Ratio _____

ST Segment _____

Other Findings _____

Interpretation _____

Reasoning _____

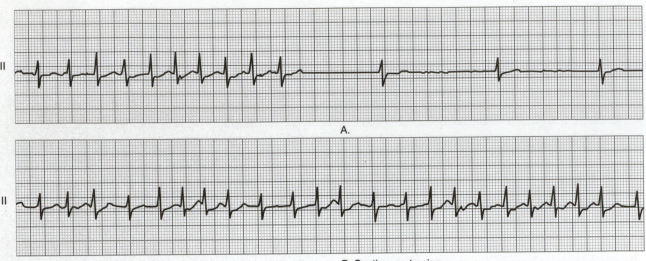

A.

B. Continuous tracing

Figure 26-80 Rate _____
Rhythm _____
QRS Duration _____
PR Interval _____
AV Conduction Ratio _____
ST Segment _____
Other Findings _____
Interpretation _____
Reasoning _____

Answers for Self-Assessment Tracings

Interpretations are included in parentheses for later reference.

Answers for Chapter 7 ECG Tracings

FIGURE 7–6

The ventricular rhythm is regular and the QRS complexes have a normal appearance. The rate of the P-QRS-T complexes is 50/minute, which is slower than defined for NSR (between 60 and 100/minute). Atrial activity is regular and the P waves have a normal shape. The AV conduction ratio is 1:1 and the PR interval is normal at 0.16 second. (This tracing shows a sinus bradycardia.)

FIGURE 7–7

The ventricular rhythm is regular and the QRS complexes have a normal shape and QRS duration. The PR interval is prolonged well past 0.20 second and measures 0.32 to 0.34 second. The AV conduction ratio is 1:1. This dysrhythmia is sinus rhythm with first-degree AV heart block.

FIGURE 7–8

The ventricular rhythm is irregular and the ventricular rate is 90/minute. Atrial activity consists of numerous waves at a rate of about 300/minute. P waves are missing so the sinus node cannot be the pacemaker. A fixed AV conduction ratio is not present because two, three, four, or five atrial waves exist for each QRS. The AV conduction ratios would be described as 2:1, 3:1, 4:1, and 5:1, respectively. (The dysrhythmia is atrial flutter with variable AV conduction.)

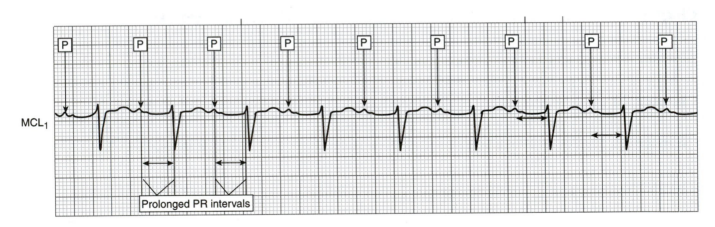

Figure 7–7 Answer

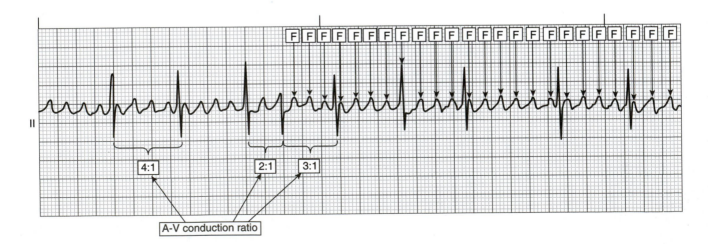

Figure 7–8 Answer

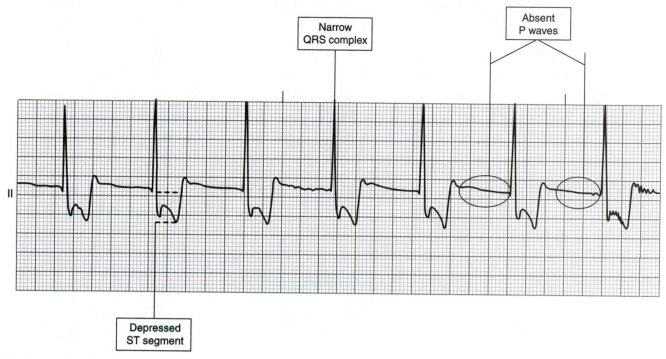

Figure 7–9 Answer

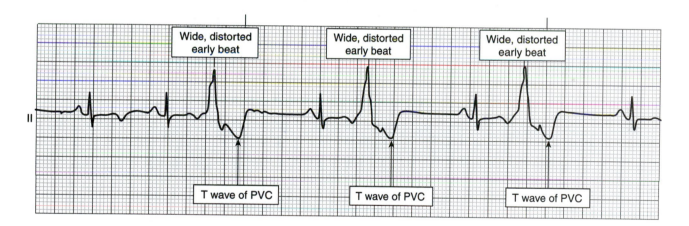

Figure 7–10 Answer

FIGURE 7–9

Ventricular activity consists of narrow QRS complexes with regular R-R intervals. The ventricular rate is 65/minute. There are no P waves or other atrial waves so an AV conduction ratio cannot be calculated. The ST segments are markedly depressed below the ECG baseline. (An AV junctional rhythm exists because sinus node activity has failed.)

FIGURE 7–10

After the two initial normal beats occur, the first wide and distorted QRS complex is seen. The 3rd, 5th, and 7th beats are abnormal because they lack P waves and occur early in the R-R cycle. Each of the abnormal beats is followed by a pause before the next sinus beat occurs. The ventricular rate is 75/minute. The atrial rhythm is irregular and the P waves are identical. Aside from the wide QRS beats, the rest of the beats have an AV conduction ratio of 1:1 and the PR interval is 0.16 second. (This dysrhythmia is a sinus rhythm with three premature ventricular complexes.)

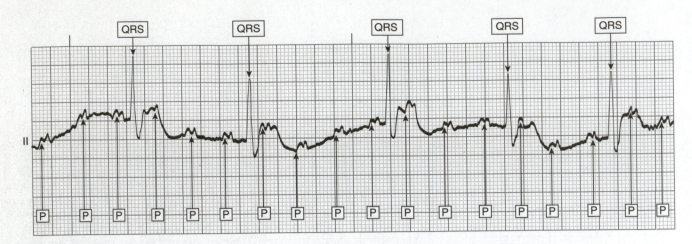

Figure 7–12 Answer

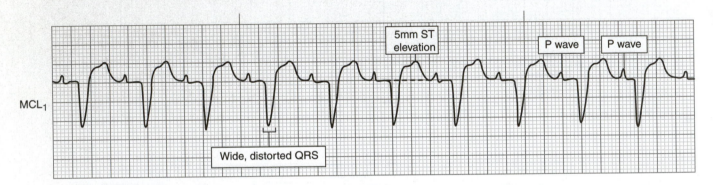

Figure 7–13 Answer

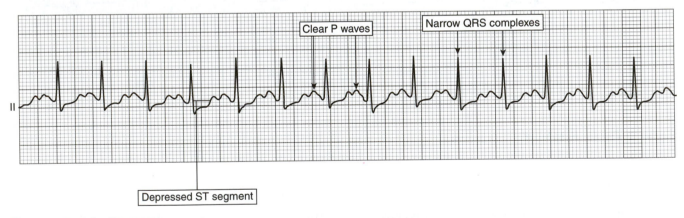

Figure 7–14 Answer

FIGURE 7–11

The ventricular activity consists of narrow QRS complexes with a regular R-R interval. The atrial activity has normal appearing P waves with regular P-P intervals. The PR intervals are normal and the same for each beat. AV conduction is normal (1:1). Everything appears normal: the ventricular activity, the atrial activity, and the AV conduction ratio. Therefore normal sinus rhythm is present.

FIGURE 7–12

The ventricular rate is about 45/minute and the QRS duration is slightly prolonged at 0.12 second. The P waves are wide and notched and the P-P intervals are regular. The atrial rate is about 140/minute, which is much faster than the ventricular rate of 45/minute. Numerous P waves exist before each QRS complex. Many of the P waves are *not* associated with QRS complexes. The PR intervals for the QRS complexes that are preceded by a P wave change. The PR intervals vary from 0.16 second to 0.32 second. Instead of a single P wave linked to each QRS as in NSR, many P waves exist for each QRS complex. Since most of the P waves are not followed by QRS complexes some type of conduction problem exists. The ST segments are abnormally elevated about three small boxes from the ECG baseline. (This is a sinus tachycardia with third-degree AV heart block.)

FIGURE 7–13

The QRS duration of 0.12 second is wider than normal. Normal QRS complexes should be 0.11 second or less. The ventricular rhythm is regular. The PR interval of 0.22 second is slightly longer than normal (0.20 second). There is also a 5 mm ST segment elevation. (The tracing shows a sinus rhythm with first-degree AV block, ST segment elevation, and a wide QRS complex.)

FIGURE 7–14

The ventricular activity is regular with narrow QRS complexes. The ventricular rate is faster than found with a NSR (60-100 per minute) at 115 per minute. The atrial rhythm is regular and the P waves have a consistent shape. The AV conduction ratio is 1:1 and the PR interval is 0.16 second. Aside from the rapid rate, the tracing resembles NSR. (The dysrhythmia is sinus tachycardia.)

FIGURE 7–15

The ventricular rate is 200/minute—dramatically faster than the range for NSR which is 60 to 100/minute. The QRS complexes are narrow and have a normal appearance. It is difficult to know whether the positive waves between the QRS complexes are atrial waves or T waves. Assessing AV conduction is not possible since clear atrial waves are absent. The narrow QRS complexes indicate that a supraventricular pacemaker—located in either the atria, sinus node, or AV junction—is present. Since the ventricular rate is over 100/minute the rhythm is tachycardic. (This dysrhythmia is supraventricular tachycardia.)

FIGURE 7–16

The QRS complex duration is 0.16 second, which is much wider than the upper limit of normal, which is 0.11 second. The ventricular complexes have a distorted appearance because their are slurred waves instead of sharp QRS waves that appear in NSR. The ventricular rate is just below 150/minute, which is much faster than in NSR. P waves are not visible so an AV conduction ratio cannot be assessed. (This serious dysrhythmia is ventricular tachycardia.)

FIGURE 7–17

The ventricular rate is less than 60/minute, which is the lower rate limit for NSR. The QRS complexes are narrow and look normal except that they lack P waves. P waves should precede the QRS's if this were a sinus rhythm. Since atrial activity is lacking, it is not possible

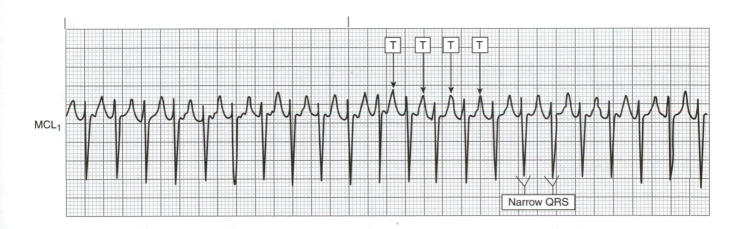

Figure 7–15 Answer

to calculate an AV conduction ratio. In summary, the narrow QRS complex bradycardia lacks P waves so it could not have arisen in the SA node. However, the narrow QRS complex rules out the possibility of a ventricular pacemaker. A normal QRS complex (duration of less than 0.12 second) indicates that pacemaker must have arisen in a supraventricular site: either the sinus node, atria, or AV junction. (The dysrhythmia is an AV junctional escape rhythm that arises when sinus node functioning is depressed.)

FIGURE 7–18

The ventricular activity has regular R-R intervals and narrow QRS complexes (duration of 0.04 to 0.06 second). The ventricular rate is 200 per minute. The upper limit before NSR is 150/minute. Regular atrial activity is not visible; the small positive waves in the middle of the R-R intervals are actually T waves. An AV conduction ratio is not able to be assessed. The narrow QRS complex eliminates the possibility of a ventricular pacemaker. (The dysrhythmia is a supraventricular tachycardia.)

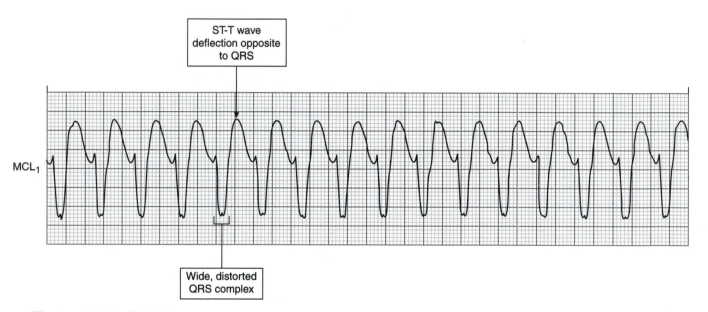

ST-T wave deflection opposite to QRS

MCL₁

Wide, distorted QRS complex

Figure 7–16 Answer

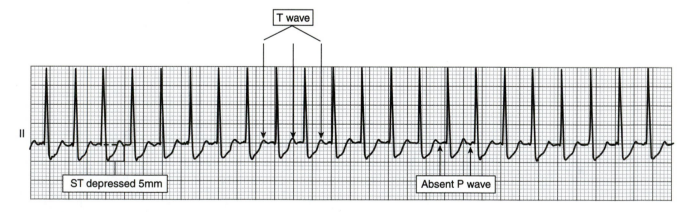

T wave

II

ST depressed 5mm

Absent P wave

Figure 7–18 Answer

Answers for Chapter 10 ECG Tracings

FIGURE 10–1

DATA:

- Rate: 65/minute

- Rhythm: regular

- QRS Duration: 0.06 second

- PR Interval: 0.18 second

- AV Conduction Ratio: 1:1

- ST Segment: 1 mm depression with "scooped out" appearance

Interpretation: Normal sinus rhythm (NSR)

Reasoning: The ventricular activity is normal and regular, which is also true for atrial activity. The P waves have a consistent shape with a positive deflection in lead II. The PR interval has a normal duration of 0.20 second or less. Each P wave is immediately followed by a QRS complex and every QRS is preceded by a single P wave. The pacemaker is located in the sinus node and no conduction delays or rhythm disturbances are noted.

> **ECG Interpretation Tip** When the ST segments appear "scooped out" along with flattened T waves in several leads, consider digitalis effect, hypokalemia, and diffuse ischemia as they all affect ventricular repolarization.

FIGURE 10–2

DATA:

- Rate: (A) 30; (B) 94/minute

- Rhythm: (A) irregular

- Rhythm: (B) regular

- QRS Duration: (A) 0.08 second; (B) 0.08–0.10 second

- PR Interval: (A) 0.18 second; (B) 0.18 second

- AV Conduction Ratio: (A and B) 1:1

- ST Segment: Normal

Interpretation: Sinus block with pronounced asystolic pauses which are terminated by junctional escape complexes

Reasoning: *Strip A:* The first beat in Strip A clearly arises within the sinus node because it consists of a normal P-QRS-T complex. A delay of almost 4 seconds follows the first sinus beat. The pause is terminated by a narrow QRS complex beat, which lacks a P wave. Therefore, the second beat must be a supraventricular beat, having originated in an escape pacemaker site located above the ventricles. This back-up pacemaker fortunately terminates a long period of electrical and cardiac silence. The isoelectric ECG phases represents the part of the cardiac cycle when no activity is occurring, that is, when complete P-QRS-T complexes are missing. Cardiac output ceases during these asystolic periods, often resulting in a loss of consciousness. In sinus block the impulse from the SA node fails to develop or fails to be conducted to the area. After the third complex, another period of sinus block occurs.

Strip B was recorded soon after 1 mg of intravenous atropine was administered and it shows the resumption of normal sinus rhythm. In strip B the ventricular and atrial activity are normal. The AV conduction ratio is 1:1, meaning that each P wave is conducted. The sinus rate accelerates to just below 100/minute.

FIGURE 10–3

DATA:

- Rate: 60/minute

- Rhythm: regularly irregular

- QRS Duration: 0.08 second

- PR Interval: 0.16 second

- AV Conduction Ratio: 1:1

- ST Segment: normal

Interpretation: Sinus arrhythmia

Reasoning: This tracing shows sinus nodal activity, which varies in relation to the phases of ventilation. The ventricular rhythm is regularly irregular since the R-R interval waxes and wanes, as does the atrial rhythm. There is no clinical difference between sinus arrhythmia and NSR, aside from the altered sinus rhythm.

FIGURE 10–4

DATA:

■ Rate: 38/minute

■ Rhythm: regular

■ QRS Duration: 0.12 second

■ PR Interval: 0.16 second

■ AV Conduction Ratio: 1:1

■ ST Segment: markedly elevated (4 mm) from baseline with an acute injury pattern

Interpretation: **Sinus bradycardia at 40/minute**

Reasoning: The ECG baseline is slightly distorted by artifact but not enough to prevent an accurate interpretation. Ventricular activity is slow but regular. The QRS duration is normal but the shapes of the QRS complexes have been altered by the upward slope of the elevated ST segments. P waves occur immediately before the QRS complexes at a constant PR interval. AV conduction is normal. The major way that this tracing differs from NSR is that the sinus discharges slower than 60/minute. Since the rate of 38/minute is within the range expected for an AV junctional pacemaker as well as an idioventricular escape pacemaker, the area immediately ahead of the QRS's is inspected to confirm that atrial activity exists and that this is a sinus rhythm.

> ***ECG Interpretation Tip*** *ST segment elevation is found in many conditions such as acute myocardial injury, inflammation of the heart, termed myocarditis, and inflammation of the pericardial sac, termed pericarditis, as well as a normal variant called benign early repolarization (B.E.R.).*

FIGURE 10–5

DATA:

■ Rate: 140/minute

■ Rhythm: regular

■ QRS Duration: 0.08 second

■ PR Interval: 0.12 second

■ AV Conduction Ratio: 1:1

■ ST Segment: depressed 5 mm below the baseline

Interpretation: **Sinus tachycardia at 140/minute**

Reasoning: Ventricular activity appears normal: the QRS complexes are sharp, regular, and narrow. P waves have a constant shape, are upright, and precede every QRS complex. AV conduction is also normal. The significant variation from NSR is that the sinus node is discharging at a rate faster than 100/minute, which is the upper limit of a normal sinus rhythm.

FIGURE 10–6

DATA:

■ Rate: 56/minute

■ Rhythm: regular

■ QRS Duration: 0.08 second

■ PR Interval: absent

■ AV Conduction Ratio: absent

■ ST segment: 1 to 2 mm depression below the ECG baseline

Interpretation: **AV junctional escapte rhythm at 56/ minute due to sinus block**

Reasoning: The QRS complexes are narrow and have a normal shape, yet there is no atrial activity. Since the P waves are absent, an AV conduction ratio cannot exist. Since P waves are absent the sinus node cannot be setting the heart rate. The rhythm must have originated within the AV junction for several reasons: (1) the QRS duration is within the expected range for a supraventricular pacemaker site, that is, less than 0.12 second; (2) the ventricular rate is between 40 and 60/minute; and (3) P waves are absent.

FIGURE 10–7

DATA:

■ Rate: (A) 110/minute; (B) 30/minute

■ Rhythm: (A and B) irregular

■ QRS Duration: (A and B) 0.16 second

■ PR Interval: (A) 0.20 second; (B) Beat number 1: 0.20 second; Beats number 2 and 3: absent

■ AV Conduction Ratio: (A) 1:1 ; (B) Beat number 1: 1:1; Beats number 2 and 3: absent

■ ST Segment: markedly depressed 4 mm from the ECG baseline

Interpretation: **Tachycardia-bradycardia (tachy-brady) syndrome with a 5 second period of sinus arrest and a ventricular escape rhythm**

Reasoning: *Strip A* shows sinus tachycardia at 110/minute, which abruptly slows. The rate decreases further during the early portion of strip B. After the first QRS complex in tracing B the sinus node fails for 5 seconds. The second and third QRS complexes in B are escape pacemakers, which emerge to rescue the silent heart. The escape pacemaker beats lack P waves but have QRSs that are identical to surrounding sinus complexes. They arose from either an AV junctional site or a ventricular focus. Despite the distorted shapes they appear identical to the sinus beats. Even the escape AV junction's pacing ability is unreliable. The rather slow rate of junctional pacing at 33/minute is slower than expected for a healthy AV junction. An artificial pacemaker is needed to stabilize the cardiac rhythm. In fact, sick sinus syndrome is the leading cause of pacemaker insertion.

FIGURE 10–8

DATA:

■ Rate: 40/minute

■ Rhythm: irregular

■ QRS Duration: 0.06 second

■ PR Interval: 0.20 second

■ AV Conduction Ratio: 1:1

■ ST Segment: 1mm depression below the ECG baseline

■ Other Findings: inverted T waves

Interpretation: **Sinus bradycardia at 40/minute with a sinus arhythmia**

Reasoning: The ventricular rhythm is irregular as reflected by the varying R-R intervals. The QRS complexes are normal, narrow, and have identical shapes. The atrial rhythm is irregular but each P wave has a normal shape. The PR interval is 0.20 second, which is the upper limit of normal. The P-P intervals are irregular in exactly the same way as the R-R intervals. AV conduction is normal with constant PR intervals. A sinus arrhythmia is present because the rhythm is irregular with normal P waves. The P-QRS-T rate is well below 60/minute, which is the normal lower limit for adults. Of the two findings, bradycardia is the main clinical concern in evaluating this patient—not the irregular rhythm which is benign and has no clinical significance. Note that the ST segments are depressed and the T waves are inverted, suggesting myocardial ischemia.

FIGURE 10–9

DATA:

■ Rate: 50/minute

■ Rhythm: regular

■ QRS Duration: 0.08 second

■ PR Interval: 0.12 second

■ AV Conduction Ratio: 1:1

■ ST Segment: abnormal curve but no deviation from baseline

Interpretation: **Sinus bradycardia at a rate of 50/minute with a sinus dysrhythmia**

Reasoning: The ventricular complexes are normal but the rhythm is irregular. Toward the end of the tracing, the complexes are spaced closer together. Atrial activity consists of normal P waves. The atrial rhythm is irregular and the P waves also are closer together toward the end of the tracing. The sinus rate is below 60/minute. The AV conduction ratio has a normal 1:1 relationship. The ST segments have a sharp take-off from the baseline instead of the normal gradual merge with the T waves. This may be suggestive of myocardial ischemia so a twelve-lead ECG should be done to evaluate the ST segments in all the standard leads.

FIGURE 10–10

DATA:

■ Rate: (A) 45/minute; (B) 25/minute

■ Rhythm: (A) regular; (B) irregular

■ QRS Duration: (A and B) 0.12 to 0.14 second

■ PR Interval: (A) 0.20 second; (B) Beats number 1,4, and 5: 0.20 second; Beats number 2 and 3: absent

■ AV Conduction Ratio: (A) 1:1; (B) 1:1 except beats number 2 and 3: absent

■ ST Segment: 1 mm elevation from ECG baseline

Interpretation: **Sinus bradycardia at 45/minute with a period of sinus depression that allows an AV junctional escape rhythm to discharge**

Reasoning: The slow rhythm in strip A consists of regular but slow P-QRS-T cycles. The QRS complexes are wider than normal and their shapes are slightly distorted due to an intraventricular conduction decay (bundle branch block). All ventricular complexes in A are preceded by P waves having a consistent shape and a fixed, normal PR interval. In strip B a 2-second pause follows the first beat. The beat that terminates the pause does not have a P wave but the QRS complex is identical to the sinus beats in strip A. In contrast to strip A, however, the atrial activity differs markedly; beats number 2 and 3 are not preceded by P waves. The similarity of the QRS complexes in strips A and B indicates that ventricular depolarization follows the same intraventricular conduction pathway as the sinus beats. Beats number 2 and 3 are escape pacemaker complexes that discharge at a very slow rate and arose from the ventricle or AV junction. The last two beats have P waves that have a fixed association with the QRS-T complexes, thereby confirming that sinus activity has resumed.

FIGURE 10–11

DATA:

- Rate: 50/minute

- Rhythm: regularly irregular

- QRS Duration: 0.06 second

- PR Interval: 0.16 second

- AV Conduction Ratio: 1:1

- ST Segment: 1 to 2 mm depression from the ECG baseline

Interpretation: **Sinus bradycardia at 50/minute with a sinus arrhythmia**

Reasoning: The ventricular activity is irregular and consists of normal QRS complexes. Atrial activity consists of a single upright P wave before each QRS complex. The P-P intervals are irregular in the same manner as the R-R intervals. The PR intervals and AV conduction ratios are normal. This tracing differs from NSR in that the rhythm is noticeably irregular and the rate is below 60/minute. The rate is as slow as 38/minute at one point but later increases to 60/minute. The slow rate makes the irregular rhythm more apparent. The irregular sinus activity corresponds to the respiratory cycle

FIGURE 10–12

DATA:

- Rate: 136/minute

- Rhythm: regular

- PR Interval: 0.20 second

- QRS Duration: 0.06 second

- AV Conduction Ratio: 1:1

- ST Segment: normal

- Other Findings: The P and T waves begin to merge together

Interpretation: **Sinus tachycardia at 136/minute**

Reasoning: The ventricular complexes have a regular rhythm and a narrow shape. The atrial rhythm consists of regular P waves all with the same shape. The sinus rate is well over 100/minute. The PR interval and AV conduction ratios are both normal. As the cardiac rate exceeds 100/minute, portions of the ECG complexes begin to merge together: the P waves meet the T waves of the previous beats. However, individual waves can still be identified, but if the rate became faster, this might not be the case.

FIGURE 10–13

DATA:

- Rate: 60/minute

- Rhythm: regular

- PR Interval: 0.18 second

- AV Conduction Ratio: normal

- ST Segment: 1 to 2 mm depression from the ECG baseline

- Other Findings: T wave inversion

Interpretation: **Normal sinus rhythm**

Reasoning: Ventricular activity consists of narrow complexes and a regular rhythm. The QRS complexes have a mostly negative deflection because lead MCL_1 is being recorded. The P waves are extremely tall and are sharply pointed which is partly due to the MCL_1 lead. Another possible cause is that the right atrium is enlarged. The T waves are inverted, but this is typical in this lead. The PR intervals and the AV conduction ratios are normal. Even though this tracing's appearance differs from how NSR appears in a lead II, it is still sinus rhythm.

FIGURE 10–14

DATA:

- Rate: 43/minute
- Rhythm: regular
- QRS Duration: 0.10 second
- PR Interval: Beat number 1: 0.16 second; Beat number 2: 0.12 second and Beat number 3: 0.08 second
- AV Conduction Ratio: absent for most beats (see explanation)
- ST Segment: normal
- Other Findings: T wave shapes vary

Interpretation: Sinus bradycardia with an AV junctional escape rhythm at 43/minute

Reasoning: The ventricular rhythm is composed of narrow and regular QRS complexes. Atrial activity is only seen before some QRS complexes. While the first few beats have P waves they do not occur in a fixed relationship to the QRS complexes. The first beat has a normal P wave and PR interval, but the P waves of the next two beats (beats number 2 and 3) have changing PR intervals. The P waves of beats number 2 and 3 appear to merge into the adjoining QRS complexes. Aside from the first beat, the QRS complexes of most beats probably represent AV junctional escape beats. An escape pacemaker fires because the sinus node fails to stimulate the heart. The ST segments and T waves have a variable appearance, which is caused by hidden P waves.

FIGURE 10–15

DATA:

- Rate: 120/minute
- Rhythm: Regular
- QRS Duration: 0.08 second
- PR Interval: 0.16 second
- AV Conduction Ratio: 1:1
- ST Segment: 3 mm elevation from the ECG baseline
- Other Findings: T waves are very tall and peaked

Interpretation: Sinus tachycardia at 120/minute

Reasoning: The QRS complexes are normal and the ventricular rhythm is regular. When faced with a nar-row QRS complex tachycardic rhythm, the challenge is to determine whether the rhythm originated in the sinus node or from an ectopic location, such as in the AV junction or an atrial site. If the pacemaker arose from outside the sinus node, there should be a missing or altered P wave shape. In the present case, the P waves have tall, pointy, upright shapes, and are therefore sinus. A normal AV conduction ratio of 1:1 and a normal PR interval of less than 0.20 second is present.

> **ECG Interpretation Tip** The T waves are over 10 mm tall, which is referred to as hyperacute. Normally, the upper limit for T wave height in a properly calibrated ECG machine is 10 mm in the limb leads. Two common conditions that cause taller than normal T waves are hyperkalemia (high serum potassium level) and early myocardial injury. Continuous ECG monitoring is indicated for both conditions as dysrhythmias are common..

FIGURE 10–16

DATA:

- Rate: averages 70/minute but ranges from 50 to 100/minute
- Rhythm: irregular
- PR Interval: 0.16 second except for beat number 5 and 6
- AV Conduction Ratio: 1:1 except for beats number 5 and 6. Beat number 5 lacks a P wave, while beat number 6 has an extremely short PR interval
- ST Segment: normal

Interpretation: Sinus block and AV junctional escape beats (beat number 5 and 6)

Reasoning: The ECG tracing shows a markedly irregular rhythm. Toward the beginning and end of the tracing, beats appear clustered together, while in the center of the strip, the beats are spread apart. Every ventricular complex has a narrow and uniformly shaped QRS complex. The P waves have a notched shape and not every QRS has a P wave associated with it. A pause in cardiac activity follows beat number 4 that lasts longer than one second. The fifth beat terminates the pause but QRS lacks a P wave. The QRS of beat number 5 has the same shape as do the sinus beats so beat number 5 must have arisen from an AV junctional focus since its QRS is normal yet it lacks a P wave. Beat number 5 "escapes" after the pause in order to rescue the heart from asystole.

Beat number 6's P wave differs from the shape of other beats and it has an extremely short PR interval. These findings indicate that beat number 6 is also an AV junctional escape complex that began at almost exactly the same time that the next scheduled sinus P wave developed. As a result, the distorted P wave and abnormal QRS represents a fusion complex. The remainder of the beats (number 7 to 11) are sinus beats.

FIGURE 10–17

DATA:

- Rate: 50/minute
- Rhythm: regular
- QRS Duration: 0.10 second
- PR Interval: 0.16 second
- AV Conduction Ratio: 1:1
- ST Segment: 2 mm elevation from the ECG baseline

Interpretation: **Sinus bradycardia at 50/minute**

Reasoning: This ECG tracing appears identical to NSR except that the sinus rate is below 60/minute. Otherwise, the ventricular rhythm, atrial rhythm, PR intervals, and AV conduction are normal.

FIGURE 10–18

DATA:

- Rate: 80/minute
- Rhythm: irregular
- QRS Duration: 0.08 second
- PR Interval: 0.16 second
- AV Conduction Ratio: 1:1
- ST Segment: Marked 6 mm elevation from the ECG baseline
- Other Findings: hyperacute T waves

Interpretation: **Sinus rhythm with a sinus arrhythmia**

Reasoning: The cardiac rhythm is markedly irregular. As the rate begins to slow toward the end of the strip, the ECG complexes appear to spread apart. The cardiac slowing corresponds to exhalation. The QRS complex-

es are narrow with a normal shape. The sinus rhythm variability corresponds with the change in ventricular rhythm. The PR interval is fixed and is within a normal range between 0.12 and 0.20 second. A normal 1:1 AV conduction ratio exists.

Discussion: The markedly elevated ST segment has a normal upward deflection and could represent several serious conditions such as myocardial injury, myocardial inflammation, or a ventricular aneurysm. The T waves are 15 mm in height. In a properly standardized ECG machine (1 mV equals 10 mm of stylus elevation), T waves should not exceed 10 mm. T waves taller than 10 mm are described as hyperacute is one of the earliest ECG signs of myocardial infarction.

FIGURE 10–19

DATA:

- Rate: 50/minute
- Rhythm: regular
- QRS Duration: 0.06 second
- PR Interval: 0.16 second
- AV Conduction Ratio: 1:1
- ST Segment: 1.5 mm elevation from the ECG baseline
- Other Findings: P wave inversion and deep, wide Q waves

Interpretation: **Sinus bradycardia at 50/minute**

Reasoning: The ventricular complexes are narrow and occur regularly. The P waves are inverted, which is a normal finding in lead MCL_1. The PR intervals are normal, as is the 1:1 AV conduction ratio. The rate is slower than normal (60/minute) and the Q waves are pathologic and occur with myocardial infarction. There is straightening and elevation of the ST segment. These findings suggest a recent myocardial infarction.

FIGURE 10–20

DATA:

- Rate: 125/minute
- Rhythm: regular
- QRS Duration: 0.08 second
- PR Interval: 0.16 second
- AV Conduction Ratio: 1:1
- ST Segment: 1 mm depression from the ECG baseline

Interpretation: Sinus tachycardia at 125/minute

Reasoning: This ECG tracing looks like a NSR rhythm except that the sinus node is discharging much faster than expected. The ventricular rhythm, QRS complexes, atrial rhythm, P waves, PR intervals, and AV conduction are otherwise normal. Accelerated sinus node discharge occurs in normal and pathologic conditions. The clinical significance of rapid sinus rates can only be assessed by correlating the ECG finding to the patient's condition.

Discussion: Increased sinus node depolarization is usually caused by enhanced sympathetic tone or diminished parasympathetic tone. Sinus tachycardia is not a primary dysrhythmia; it occurs secondary to another condition. For instance, anxiety, dehydration, hypovolemia, or anti-cholinergic drugs such as diphenhydramine (Benadryl ®) increase the heart rate. Therapy for sinus tachycardia, therefore, must be directed at correcting the underlying disorder rather than simply administering a drug to slow the heart.

FIGURE 10–21

DATA:

- Rate: 52/minute

- Rhythm: regular

- QRS Duration: 0.12 second

- PR Interval: 0.16 second

- AV Conduction Ratio: 1:1

- ST Segment: markedly elevated 5 mm

- Other Findings: Hyperacute T waves

Interpretation: Sinus bradycardia at 52/minute with an acute injury patterns

Reasoning: The ECG rate is slightly below 60/minute. The ST segment is strikingly elevated. Otherwise, the remaining ventricular rhythm, QRS complexes, atrial rhythm, P waves, PR intervals, and AV conduction ratio are all normal. (This tracing was recorded from a patient having an acute myocardial infarction.) One of the earliest nonspecific signs of an MI is hyperacute T waves. The ST segments are markedly elevated and the ST segments have a sharp take-off rather than the normal gradual slope.

FIGURE 10–22

DATA:

- Rate: 62/minute

- Rhythm: regular

- QRS Duration: 0.12 second

- PR Interval: 0.14 second

- AV Conduction Ratio: 1:1

- ST Segment: marked (7 mm) depression

Interpretation: Normal sinus rhythm

Reasoning: Aside from the marked depression of the ST segments, the remainder of the ECG tracing looks normal. The ventricular and atrial activity, along with the PR intervals and AV conduction are normal. The marked ST segment depression may indicate ischemia or be secondary to hypertrophy of the left ventricle. The significance of ST segment depression must be assessed by evaluating a twelve-lead ECG and correlating it to the patient's clinical condition.

FIGURE 10–23

DATA:

- Rate: 135/minute

- Rhythm: regular

- QRS Duration: 0.08 second

- PR Interval: 0.16 second

- AV Conduction Ratio: 1:1

- ST Segment: normal

Interpretation: Sinus tachycardia at 135/minute

Reasoning: Atrial and ventricular activity is normal. The AV conduction and PR intervals are also normal. The rate is considerably faster than the upper limit of 100/minute seen in NSR. The T waves and the P waves begin to merge at such rapid rates. Sinus tachycardia results from increased sympathetic nervous system activity such as fever, adrenergic mediation such as epinephrine, exercise, or hypovolemia.

FIGURE 10–24

DATA:

- Rate 40/minute
- Rhythm: irregular
- QRS Duration: 0.08 second
- PR Interval: 0.16 second
- AV Conduction: 1:1
- ST Segment: normal

Interpretation: Sinus bradycardia at 40/minute with a sinus arrhythmia

Reasoning: The cardiac rate is slow and the rhythm is irregular. Ventricular activity has narrow QRS complexes and normal T waves. Atrial activity is also irregular and the P waves are normally shaped. AV conduction and the PR intervals are normal. The regular waxing and waning rhythm is caused by the ventilatory cycle's changing vagal tone. As the patient inspires, the cardiac rate increases while the opposite occurs during exhalation. Slow heart rates further exaggerate the variability of sinus function.

FIGURE 10–25

DATA:

- Rate: 45/minute
- Rhythm: regular
- QRS Duration: 0.06 second
- PR Interval: 0.20 second
- AV Conduction Ratio: 1:1
- ST Segment: 1 mm depression below the ECG baseline
- Other Findings: T waves have a biphasic appearance and the P waves are notched

Interpretation: Sinus bradycardia at 45/minute

Reasoning: The ventricular complexes are narrow and have a regular rhythm. The atrial complexes have widened and notched P waves, which reflect consecutive—rather than simultaneous—depolarization of both atria. AV conduction and the PR intervals are normal. The T wave appears biphasic, meaning that there is a positive as well as a negative component. The biphasic T waves and ST segments depression are nonspecific findings which may or may not indicate a pathologic condition such as myocardial ischemia. A repeat ECG in 30 to 60 minutes or comparison with an old ECG may help to clarify such findings.

Answers for Chapter 13 ECG Tracings

FIGURE 13–01

DATA:

- Rate: 170/minute

- Rhythm: regular

- QRS Duration: 0.10 second

- PR Interval: absent

- AV Conduction Ratio: not measurable

- Other Findings: QRS complexes are notched

- ST Segment: 1.5 mm depression

Interpretation: **Supraventricular tachycardia (SVT) at 170/minute**

Reasoning: The ventricular rhythm is regular and the QRS complexes have normal duration (less than 0.12 second). The shape of the QRS complexes is slightly altered from NSR because the downslope of the R wave shows an additional positive deflection termed a small r´. The QRS configuration is labeled as an RSr´ complex. P waves or atrial waves are absent so determining a PR interval or AV relationship cannot be done. Although the sinus node can discharge as fast as 170 times per minute in some circumstances, the rapid rate in this tracing is too fast to be caused by a sinus pacemaker. An ectopic pacemaker must be stimulating the heart. Since the QRS duration and shape are normal, the dysrhythmia must have originated above the His bundle bifurcation—that is, from a supraventricular focus. A QRS duration of 0.10 second or less can only occur when intraventricular depolarization is normal. Had the pacemaker arisen from a ventricular site, the QRS would have been wide and abnormally shaped.

FIGURE 13–02

DATA:

- Rate: 140/minute

- Rhythm: irregular

- QRS Duration: 0.10 second

- PR Interval: absent

- AV Conduction Ratio: random conduction

- ST Segment: 1.5 mm depression

Interpretation: **Atrial fibrillation with a ventricular rate of 120/minute**

Reasoning: The ventricular rhythm does not have a set pattern. Because the rapid ventricular rate causes the QRS complexes to crowd together, the R-R intervals variability is not so apparent. The QRS complexes are narrow, less than 0.12 second, which indicates a supraventricular pacemaker. Instead of P or atrial waves, the baseline between R waves is flattened. The irregular rhythm, absent P waves, narrow QRS complexes, and tachycardic rate provide the evidence that atrial fibrillation is present.

Based on laboratory studies involving atrial fibrillation, the atria are depolarizing between 350 and 600/minute. Individual atrial waves are not visible because organized atrial activity is lacking. Lead I does not detect atrial activity well, and atrial fibrillation commonly appears with a fine wavy or flat baseline. By switching to another lead, such as MCL$_1$ or lead II, the fibrillatory waves become much more apparent. However, despite lacking classical "f" waves, the correct interpretation is still possible by noting the tachycardic rate, narrow QRS complexes, and the irregularly irregular rhythm. A grossly irregular rhythm is associated with only two dysrhythmias: atrial fibrillation and multifocal atrial tachycardia (MAT). Since atrial fibrillation is much more common, it should be considered first.

FIGURE 13–03

DATA:

- Rate: 46/minute

- Rhythm: regular

- QRS Duration: 0.06 second

- PR Interval: absent

- AV Conduction Ratio: absent

- ST Segment: 2 mm depression

Interpretation: **An escape AV junctional rhythm at 46/minute caused by sinus arrest**

Reasoning: The ventricular rhythm is regular and the QRS complexes are narrow. Atrial activity is not present so an AV relationship or a PR interval cannot be determined. The absence of P waves in the face of a slow, escape junctional rhythm indicates failure of the sinus node. The hallmark findings of an escape AV junctional rhythm are:

- Missing or altered P´ waves (inverted and seen before or after the QRS)

- Narrow QRS complexes

- Regular R-R intervals

- Rate between 40 and 60/minute (usually averaging 50/minute)

FIGURE 13–04

DATA:

- Rate: atrial 300/minute

- Rhythm: atrial and ventricular: regular

- QRS Duration: 0.12 second

- PR Interval: absent

- AV Conduction Ratio: 4:1

- ST Segment: Normal

- Other Findings: ECG baseline has numerous positive deflections

Interpretation: Atrial flutter with a ventricular response of 70/minute

Reasoning: The ventricular rhythm is regular but the QRS complexes appear distorted due to the rapid atrial waves. The narrow ventricular complexes indicate a supraventricular focus. The atrial rate of 300/minute is extremely fast. The atrial waves lack the smooth, rounded outline normally associated with sinus P waves. The "F" or flutter waves represent rapid, regular atrial activity. The AV conduction ratio is approximately 4:1, indicating that one of every four atrial waves is conducted through the AV node. Another way of looking at the conduction ratio is that the AV node blocks three out of every four F waves (75%) from overstimulating the ventricles.

Discussion: In this case, failure of the AV node to conduct some rapid atrial impulses is not due to a pathologic block. Rather, the relatively long refractory period of the AV node serves as a safety mechanism to prevent the ventricles from being overstimulated. The ventricles could not tolerate a rate of 300/minute. The node functions similar to a filter that limits the conduction to a reasonable number—70/minute in this case. The 4:1 conduction in this example produces a near-normal rate of 70/minute.

FIGURE 13–05

DATA:

- Rate: 65/minute

- Rhythm: irregular

- QRS Duration: 0.06 second

- PR Interval: 0.14 second

- AV Conduction Ratio: 1:1

- ST Segment: normal

Interpretation: Sinus rhythm with frequent non-conducted and one aberrantly conducted PACs

Reasoning: The QRS complexes are narrow and, aside from beat number 8, have an identical appearance. Each QRS is preceded by a P wave—again, except for beat number 8 and the first beat, which was cut off during the ECG mounting process. The PR intervals and AV conduction ratios are normal. Abnormal T waves are seen immediately prior to the pauses. Beats number 1, 3, and 5, provide an important clue to the dysrhythmia's identity. The T waves of beats number 1, 3, and 5 appear tall and pointy compared to the T waves of the beats not followed by pauses. The reason is because non-conducted P' waves are hidden in the abnormally shaped T waves.

The PACs occur so early during the R-R cycle that they encounter an AV node that is still refractory from the previous beat. As a result, PACs are not conducted. The only sign of the missing P-QRS-T complexes—aside from the pauses—is the taller than normal T waves. Beat number 8 is also a PAC that it is abnormally conducted due to partial refractoriness of the AV node.

FIGURE 13–06

DATA:

- Rate: (A) 75/minute; (B) 40 to 50/minute

- Rhythm: (A) regular; (B) irregular

- QRS Duration: (A and B) 0.08 second

- PR Interval: (A) 0.16 second; (B) 0.20 second

- AV Conduction Ratio: (A) 4:1; (B) variable (see below)

- ST Segment: 4 mm elevation

Interpretation: Strip A: Atrial flutter with a regular ventricular response of 75/minute. Strip B: (Recorded a short time later): Atrial flutter with a much slower ventricular response averaging 40 to 50/minute.

Reasoning: Ventricular activity consists of narrow QRS complexes, typical of supraventricular beats, occurring at regular intervals in a regular rhythm. The "sawtooth" pattern of the atrial waves is characteristic of atrial flutter. The atrial rate is much faster than the ventricular rate. The ratio of 300 "F" waves to 75 QRS complexes yields a 4:1 AV conduction ratio in strip A. AV nodal refractoriness produces a physiologic "block" that fails to conduct 75 percent of the atrial waves, which is beneficial for the patient because it results in a near normal ventricular rate. In strip B, however, the ventricular rate slows significantly, owing to increased AV nodal refractoriness. The conduction ratio becomes variable, producing an irregular, bradycardic ventricular response. The decreased AV conduction which can also be expressed as higher conduction ratios, results from excessive medication administered to slow the ventricular rate.

Discussion: A bradycardic ventricular response in the setting of atrial flutter is always secondary to medication or carotid sinus massage. The conduction ratio of 4:1 ratio seen in strip A changes to conduction ratios of 8:1, 6:1, and 10:1. The previous physiologic 4:1 AV conduction becomes a pathologic blockage. When the ventricular rate slows to 40 to 50/minute patients become symptomatic as the bradycardia diminishes cardiac output.

FIGURE 13–07

DATA:

- Rate: 230/minute

- Rhythm: regular

- QRS Duration: 0.08 second

- PR Interval: absent

- AV Conduction Ratio: absent

- ST Segment: 2 mm depression

Interpretation: Supraventricular tachycardia at 230/minute

Reasoning: The dysrhythmia is an SVT because it has:

- regular and narrow QRS complexes

- a ventricular rate much faster than expected for a sinus tachycardia rate (100 to 150/minute)

- a ventricular rate that falls within the usual range expected for an SVT (150 to 250/minute)

- absent P waves

- a ventricular rhythm that is precisely regular

FIGURE 13–08

DATA:

- Rate: 55/minute

- Rhythm: regular

- QRS Duration: 0.06 second

- PR Interval: absent

- AV Conduction Ratio: absent

- ST Segment: 2 mm depression

Interpretation: AV junctional escape rhythm at 55/minute secondary to sinus node failure

Reasoning: The ventricular rhythm is regular and the QRS complexes are narrow, as expected for a supraventricular rhythm. Since atrial activity is missing, the sinus node cannot be the pacemaker. An AV relationship is also absent because there are no P waves. The ventricular rate is slower than expected for a sinus rhythm (60 to 100/minute) and falls within the range for a junctional escape pacemaker, 40 to 60/minute.

FIGURE 13–09

DATA:

- Rate 120/minute

- Rhythm: irregular

- QRS Duration: 0.10 second

- PR Interval: absent

- AV Conduction Ratio: variable

- ST Segment: normal

Interpretation: Atrial fibrillation with a ventricular response of 120/minute

Reasoning: The ventricular pattern is irregularly irregular and small fibrillatory "f" waves have replaced P waves. A fine, wavy baseline exists between the QRS complexes. A fixed AV conduction ratio does not exist; instead, random AV conduction of atrial impulses causes the irregular ventricular rhythm. Key features of atrial fibrillation include:

- grossly irregular R-R intervals

- narrow QRS complexes (unless there is a preexisting conduction disturbance)

- absent P waves

- tachycardiac ventricular rate over 100/minute, usually 140 to 150/minute if untreated

- Controlled ventricular rate less than 100/minute if treated

FIGURE 13–10

DATA:

- Rate: 80/minute
- Rhythm: grossly irregular
- QRS Duration: 0.08 second
- PR Interval: absent
- AV Conduction Ratio: variable
- ST Segment: 1 to 2 mm depression
- Other Findings: wavy ECG baseline

Interpretation: **Atrial fibrillation with a ventricular response of 80/minute**

Reasoning: The ventricular rhythm does not have a fixed pattern. The R-R intervals are irregularly irregular. The QRS complexes have similar shapes and a normal QRS duration. P waves have been replaced by fibrillatory "f" waves, which represent chaotic atrial activity. Fibrillation waves cause the baseline to have a wavy appearance.

Clinical Note The major determinant of how well a patient tolerates an atrial dysrhythmia mainly depends on the ventricular rate and the presence of other preexisting medical conditions. For instance, rapid supraventricular tachydysrhythmias, such as atrial fibrillation at a tachycardic rate will tax a patient's cardiac function more than an identical dysrhythmia but with a controlled ventricular response. This is because rapid rates shorten the diastolic filling period so that the ventricles are not able to fill completely before contraction occurs. The ventricular rate of 80/minute seen in Figure 13-10 is within the range expected for a normal sinus rhythm and should be better tolerated. Also, a heart rate of 80/minute requires considerably less oxygen than one contracting at 120/minute because it is doing less cardiac work.

FIGURE 13–11

DATA:

- Rate: 90/minute
- Rhythm: regularly irregular
- QRS Duration: 0.06 to 0.08 second
- PR Interval: varies (sinus beats: 0.12 second; PAC: 0.10 second)
- AV Conduction Ratio: 1:1
- ST Segment: 1 mm depression

Interpretation: **Sinus rhythm with atrial trigeminy, every third beat (Beats number 3, 6, 9, and 12) is a premature atrial complex.**

Reasoning: The ventricular rhythm is regularly irregular and the R-R intervals vary in a regular pattern: two normal beats are followed by one early beat. Atrial and ventricular activity has a correspondingly irregular rate. The P wave shapes vary in shape and height, indicating that they arose from different sites. The PACs (beats number 3, 6, 9, and 12) have P´ waves that are smaller and somewhat flatter than the P waves of sinus beats. The QRS complexes of the PACs and the sinus beats have identical shapes.

FIGURE 13–12

DATA:

- Rate: atrial 300/minute; ventricular 75/minute
- Rhythm: regular
- QRS Duration: 0.08 second
- PR Interval: absent
- AV Conduction Ratio: 4:1
- ST Segment: 2 mm depression

Interpretation: **Atrial flutter with a controlled ventricular response of 75/minute**

Reasoning: The ventricular rhythm is regular and the QRS duration is normal. QRS complexes have a normal and constant shape. P waves have been replaced by rapid atrial "F" (flutter) waves which shows a flattened sawtooth pattern. The usual atrial rate found during atrial flutter is exactly 300/minute—one flutter wave occurs for every large ECG box—as seen in this case, although the rate can range between 240 and 350/minute. The AV conduction ratio is 4:1, that is, four "F" waves occur for each QRS complex. By failing to respond to most atrial impulses, the AV node protects

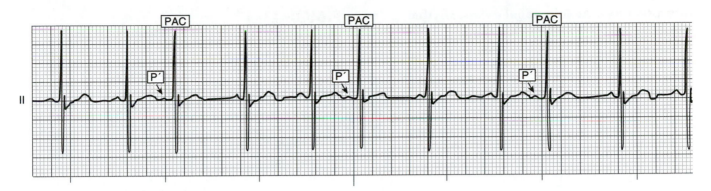

Figure 13-11 Answer

the ventricles from being activated too rapidly. The ventricular rate is 75/minute in this example and falls within the range expected for a sinus rhythm (60 to 100/minute).

FIGURE 13-13

DATA:

- Rate: 63/minute

- Rhythm: regularly irregular

- QRS Duration: 0.08 second

- PR Interval: varies; sinus: 0.16 second; PACs: 0.12 second

- AV Conduction Ratio: 1:1

- ST Segment: 1 mm depression

Interpretation: Sinus rhythm with atrial trigeminy—every third beat is a premature atrial complex (beat number 2, 5, 8, and 11).

Reasoning: The ventricular and atrial rhythms show a regular irregularity: the third P-QRS-T complex of each set of grouped beats occur early. The sinus beats have normal P-QRS-T complexes. PACs have the following features:

- prematurity (occur early during the P-P interval)

- abnormal P′ waves

- short PR intervals

- QRS complexes that are identical to sinus beats

FIGURE 13-14

DATA:

- Rate: 140/minute

- Rhythm: irregularly irregular

- QRS Duration: 0.08 second

- PR Interval: absent

- AV Conduction Ratio: variable

- ST Segment: normal

Interpretation: Atrial fibrillation with a ventricular rate of 140/minute

Reasoning: The rapid ventricular rhythm is irregularly irregular with narrow QRS complexes. P waves are absent, having been replaced by a wavy baseline consisting of "f" waves. The narrow QRS complexes—seen with supraventricular complexes—have a tachycardic rate and an irregularly irregular rhythm. These are hallmark findings of atrial fibrillation. Because the ventricular rate is so fast, the R-R interval variability is not as obvious as it would be if the rate was slower.

FIGURE 13-15

DATA:

- Rate: 60/minute

- Rhythm: regular

- QRS Duration: 0.10 second

- PR Interval: absent

- AV Conduction Ratio: absent

- ST Segment: 4 mm elevation

- Other Findings: rSR′ complex

Interpretation: **AV junctional escape rhythm secondary to SA nodal block**

Reasoning: The ventricular rhythm is regular, consisting of narrow QRS complexes that lack P waves, indicating that they arose from an ectopic supraventricular site. The cardiac rate is within the range expected for an AV junctional escape pacemaker: 40 to 60/minute. Absent P waves, a regular rhythm, and normal QRS complexes are characteristic findings of AV junctional rhythms. Elevated ST segments distort the ends of the QRS complexes. The QRS complexes have an rSR´ configuration, which indicates altered ventricular depolarization.

FIGURE 13–16

DATA:

- Rate: 180/minute

- Rhythm: regular

- QRS Duration: 0.08 second

- PR Interval: absent

- AV Conduction Ratio: absent

- ST Segment: 1.5 mm depression

Interpretation: **Supraventricular tachycardia at 180/minute**

Reasoning: The regular ventricular activity is very rapid. Narrow QRS complexes indicate a supraventricular pacemaker site, while the absence of P waves excludes a sinus node origin. The rate is too fast to be a sinus rhythm because the SA node does not usually discharge at rates above 160/minute in adults. P waves are absent during most SVTs because the reentry circuit involves the AV node.

> ***Clinical Note*** *Treating SVTs with vagal maneuvers, such as the Valsalva maneuver, and applying carotid sinus massage are much more effective in children than adults. Application of an ice-water bag to the face of an infant for 10 to 15 seconds stimulates a primitive diving reflex, that activates the vagal nervous system and terminate the SVT by slowing AV conduction. In adults most clinicians do not bother with vagal maneuvers and proceed directly to adenosine (Adenocard®).*

FIGURE 13–17

DATA:

- Rate: atrial 300/minute; ventricular 100/minute

- Rhythm: regular

- QRS Duration: 0.10-0.12 second

- PR Interval: absent

- AV Conduction Ratio: 3:1

- ST Segment: distorted by flutter waves

Interpretation: **Atrial flutter with 4:1 AV conduction and a ventricular rate of 75/minute**

Reasoning: Ventricular activity consists of regular R-R intervals and narrow QRS complexes. Atrial activity shows rapid flutter (F) waves occurring at an rate of 300/minute while the ventricular rate is only 75. The AV conduction relationship is 4:1, that is, four F waves for each QRS complex.

FIGURE 13–18

DATA:

- Rate: 107/minute

- Rhythm: regularly irregular

- QRS Duration: 0.10 second

- PR Interval: sinus: 0.16 second; PAC: 0.12 second

- AV Conduction Ratio: 1:1

- ST Segment: 1 mm depression

- Other Findings: notched P waves

Interpretation: **Sinus rhythm with frequent PACs**

Reasoning: Beats number 3, 6, 13, and 17 are premature and consist of QRS complexes that are identical (except for some alteration in beat number 17) to the sinus beats. The PACs occur early during the sinus R-R cycles. The sizes and shapes of the P´ waves in the PACs—as well the direction of their deflection—varies from sinus beats. Some of the P´ waves are inverted, indicating that depolarization started low in the atrium and moving upward to stimulate the rest of the atria.

The early beats have altered P´ waves and PR intervals. The PACs are termed "multiformed" or multifocal because they have two or more shapes, reflecting more than one depolarization path. Even the P waves of sinus beats are notched, representing consecutive activation of each atria rather than normal simultaneous depolarization. Although P wave notching is an interesting finding, it is not clinically important.

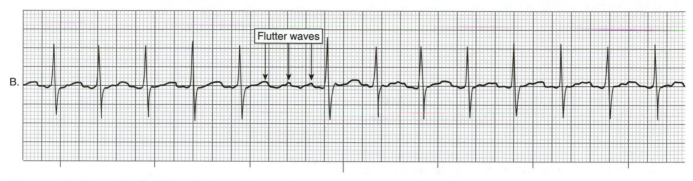

Figure 13–19 Answer

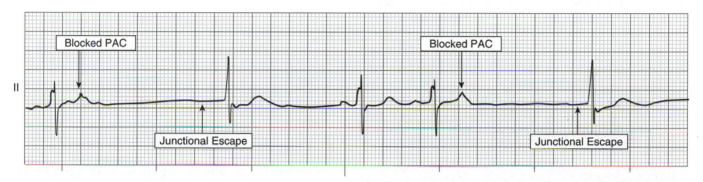

Figure 13–20 Answer

FIGURE 13–19

DATA:

- Rate: 130/minute

- Rhythm: (A) regular; (B) irregular

- QRS Duration: (A and B) 0.06 second

- PR Interval: absent

- AV Conduction Ratio: variable (see "reasoning" section below)

- ST Segment: normal

Interpretation: **Atrial flutter with variable AV conduction: AV conduction in tracing A and most of strip B is 2:1.**

Reasoning: Tracing A shows a regular rhythm with narrow complexes that initially appears to be a sinus tachycardia. During strip B, however, atrial flutter is unmasked when carotid sinus massage (CSM) increases vagal tone and causes decreased AV conduction. Until CSM was done, the rhythm had been assumed to be a sinus tachycardia because the flutter waves are not pronounced. The QRS complexes are 0.08 second in duration and have a normal appearance. When CSM is applied in strip B three flutter waves are seen following the 5th and 15th beats at a rate of 300/minute.

ECG Interpretation Tip *Hidden atrial waves should be sought in cases of sustained, unexplained narrow QRS complex tachycardias. Narrow QRS complex tachycardias occurring at 150/minute could be sinus tachycardia, PSVT, or atrial flutter with 2:1 conduction. Vagal maneuvers and adenosine (Adenocard®) administration usually expose the true cause of the rapid rhythm. In the case of PSVT, adenosine will also usually restore NSR, but not within atial flutter.*

FIGURE 13–20

DATA:

- Rate: 45/minute

- Rhythm: irregular

- QRS Duration: 0.08 to 0.10 second

- PR Interval: 0.20 second

- AV Conduction Ratio: 1:1

■ ST Segment: 1 mm depression for beats number 2 and 5

■ Other Findings: QRS complexes with different shapes

Interpretation: Sinus rhythm with two blocked PACs, each is followed by an AV junctional escape beat (Beats number 2 and 5)

Reasoning: The ventricular rhythm is irregular and consists of two differently shaped QRS complexes. Beats number 2 and 5 have mainly positive QRS complexes while the other beats have equal positive and negative components. The pauses that occur after beats number 1 and 4 are due to nonconducted PACs. The pauses are terminated by AV junctional escape beats (number 2 and 5). The T waves that occur just before the pauses are abnormally tall and pointy because they are caused by the hidden early P´ waves. The P waves of the sinus beats are notched (number 1,3,4,6, and 7). Beats number 2 and 5, on the other hand, have no associated P waves because they originate in the AV junction.

> *ECG Interpretation Tip Whenever a pause in cardiac activity is found, inspect the: (a) T wave just prior to the pause, and (b) beat terminating the pause. These findings will provide useful clues about the cause of the cardiac pause and whether there are escape beats.*

FIGURE 13–21

DATA:

■ Rate: atrial: 300/minute; ventricular: 70/minute

■ Rhythm: irregular

■ QRS Duration: 0.10 second

■ PR Interval: absent

■ AV Conduction Ratio: variable

■ ST Segment: distorted by the flutter waves

Interpretation: Atrial flutter with variable AV conduction and a ventricular rate of 70/minute

Reasoning: The QRS complexes are narrow and the ventricular rhythm is regular except at the end of the tracing. Atrial activity consists of very fast flutter waves at a rate of 300/minute. It is easy to see why the atrial

complex appearance is commonly described as resembling a sawtooth or picket fence. The AV conduction ratio varies from 4:1 for the majority of the tracing but changes to 3:1 toward the end. Variable AV conduction only occurs following treatment that slows AV conduction.

FIGURE 13–22

DATA:

■ Rate: 170/minute in the first half tracing; 80/minute during the second half of tracing.

■ Rhythm: irregular

■ QRS Duration: 0.10 second

■ PR Interval: 0.16 second for the second half of tracing; absent for first half of tracing

■ AV Conduction Ratio: 1:1 for the second half of tracing

■ ST Segment: normal

■ Other Findings: abrupt rate decrease in second half of tracing

Interpretation: Paroxysmal supraventricular tachycardia (PSVT) abruptly converting to NSR

Reasoning: The QRS complexes have the same appearance at the start and at end of the tracing. In the first half, the ventricular rate is 155/minute but this abruptly slows to 85/minute towards the tracing's end. The rhythm in the first half of the tracing is regular. No P waves are associated with QRSs during the rapid rate but are clearly seen at the end of the strip. The dramatic rate change occurs suddenly when the rate slows to 85/minute. As the rate slows, P waves appear and the beats have a PR interval of 0.16 second and a 1:1 AV conduction ratio. These findings indicate that sinus activity has resumed The first part of the tracing is a PSVT because of:

■ absent P waves

■ narrow QRS complexes

■ tachycardic rate between 150 and 250/minute

■ abrupt dysrhythmia termination and initiation

FIGURE 13–23

DATA:

- Rate: 45/minute

- Rhythm: regular

- QRS Duration: 0.10 second

- PR Interval: absent

- AV Conduction Ratio: absent

- ST Segment: normal

- Other Findings: fluctuating, choppy baseline

Interpretation: **Atrial fibrillation with complete AV block and an AV junctional escape rhythm**

Reasoning: The ventricular rate is 45/minute and the QRS complexes are narrow (less than 0.12 second). This is not a *typical* case of atrial fibrillation because the ventricular rhythm is regular. The hallmark finding of atrial fibrillation is an **irregularly irregular** R-R rhythm due to the random AV conduction. The atrial activity, typical of atrial fibrillation, consists of hundreds of small f waves. For a regular ventricular rhythm to exist with atrial fibrillation, the ventricles must be paced by an independent pacemaker below the AV node. AV conduction has been totally interrupted and an escape AV junctional rhythm develops.

> *Clinical Note Drug toxicity should be considered in cases of atrial fibrillation when there is a slow regular ventricular rhythm. Digitalis drugs, beta-blockers, and calcium channel blockers are common offending agents causing complete AV heart block in the setting of atrial fibrillation.*

FIGURE 13–24

DATA:

- Rate: 85/minute

- Rhythm: irregular

- QRS Duration: 0.08 second

- PR Interval: 0.14 second

- AV Conduction Ratio: 1:1

- ST Segment: 2 mm elevation

- Other Findings: tall pointy T waves

Interpretation: **Sinus rhythm with frequent nonconducted (blocked) PACs**

Reasoning: The ventricular rhythm is irregular, consisting of groups of normal P-QRS-T complexes separated by brief pauses. Every QRS complex is narrow and has sharp, clear waves. Each QRS complex is preceded by a P wave. Atrial activity consists of sharp, somewhat pointy P waves, which is typical for lead MCL_1. A major clue pointing toward the presence of nonconducted PACs concerns the shapes of the T waves before the pauses. The T waves of beats number 2, 5, and 7 have shapes that differ from other T waves: they are especially tall and pointy, being much higher than surrounding T waves (Figure 13–24 ans.). The tall T waves are hiding the P´ waves from the nonconducted PACs. The PACs are not conducted because they occur so early during the cardiac cycle that the ventricles have not had time to become fully repolarized following the sinus beat. Because the ventricular tissue is still partially refractory, the PAC is not conducted.

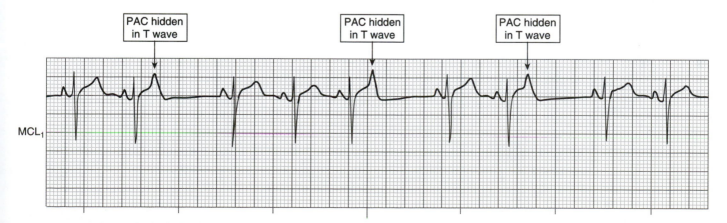

MCL₁

Figure 13-24 Answer

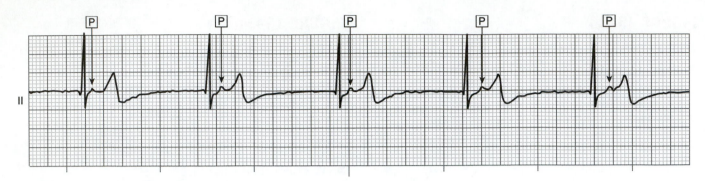

Figure 13-25 Answer

FIGURE 13–25

DATA:

■ Rate: 43/minute

■ Rhythm: regular

■ QRS Duration: 0.08 second

■ PR Interval: absent

■ AV Conduction Ratio: absent

■ ST Segment: normal; except for positive notch, which distorts it

Interpretation: Sinus block with a junctional escape rhythm at 50/minute

Reasoning: Ventricular activity consists of regularly occurring narrow QRS complexes at a bradycardic rate of 50/minute. No P waves are found before any of the QRS complexes as would be expected for sinus beats. However, some P´ waves are seen but they occur just **after** the QRS complexes—buried in the early part of the ST segment (Figure 13–25 ans.). The P' waves follow ventricular depolarization—which is opposite to the normal activation sequence—because the atria are stimulated in a retrograde (backward travelling) impulses from the AV junction.

Answers for Chapter 15 ECG Tracings

FIGURE 15–01

DATA:

- Rate: sinus: 40/minute; ventricular: 20/minute

- Rhythm: regular

- QRS Duration: 0.10 second

- PR Interval: 0.40 second

- AV Conduction Ratio: 2:1

- ST Segment: 2 mm depression

Interpretation: **First- and second-degree AV heart block with 2:1 AV conduction and a severely bradycardic ventricular rate of 20/minute**

Reasoning: The slow ventricular rhythm consists of narrow QRS complexes. The atrial rhythm has twice as many P waves as QRS complexes. The PR intervals of the conducted P waves (number 1, 3, and 5) show a fixed delay of 0.40 second (Figure 15-1 Answer). Every other P wave is not conducted, resulting in half the QRS-T complexes being dropped. Since the sinus rate is only 40/minute, 2:1 AV conduction results in a ventricular rate of only 20/minute and inadequate perfusion.

Discussion: Is this 2:1 AV conduction rhythm due to a Mobitz Type I (Wenckebach) or a Mobitz Type II form of second-degree AV block? It is not possible to determine with certainty which Mobitz Type block exists because at least two consecutively conducted P waves must occur in order to determine if the PR intervals

increase or remain constant. In the case of 2:1 conduction it is possible that Wenckebach is present and the second P wave has a prolonged PR interval but the second PR interval is not visible as the QRS complex is dropped but, we cannot be certain.

Some clues help to determine whether Mobitz Type I or II is likely in 2:1 AV conduction disorders. Figure 15-1 is probably a Type I (Wenckebach) block because the PR interval for each set of grouped beats is prolonged and yet the QRS complex is narrow, suggesting an **intra**nodal delay. Wenckebach block usually occurs within the AV node. Mobitz Type II, in contrast, has normal PR intervals and wide QRS complexes. AV nodal conduction is normal in Mobitz Type II and the block occurs below the AV node.

FIGURE 15–02

DATA:

- Rate: A: 55/minute; B: 65/minute

- Rhythm: irregular

- QRS Duration: 0.08 second

- PR Interval: progressively increases: 0.30 second, 0.32 second, 0.34 second, 0.36 second, and 0.40 second

- AV Conduction Ratio: varies between 6:5 and 11:10

- ST Segment: 1–2 mm depression

Interpretation: **Second-degree AV block; Mobitz Type I (Wenckebach), with an average ventricular rate between 55 and 65/minute**

Reasoning: The ventricular rhythm is irregular when pauses in ventricular activity occur after beats number 2, 7, and 16. Atrial activity is regular with constant P-P intervals, indicating that sinus activity is normal. The AV conduction ratio is not 1:1, however, suggesting that

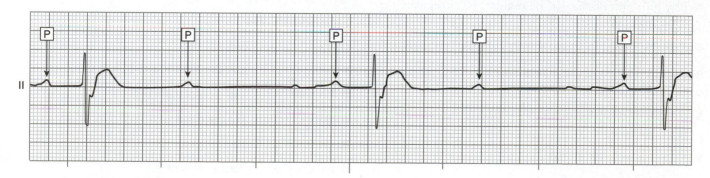

Figure 15–1 Answer

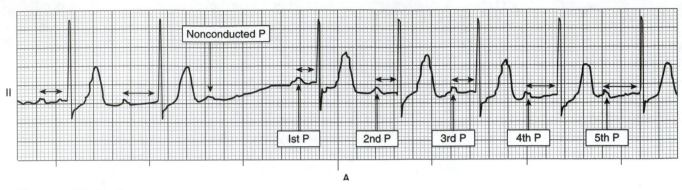

Figure 15-2 Answer

some P waves are not being conducted. Some type of second-degree block must be present. (Had this been a third-degree block, complete AV dissociation would occur. Also, had this been a first-degree block, every P wave would have been associated with a QRS-T complex.)

The PR intervals are examined to determine if the AV block is a Type I or II form. Since the PR intervals are not constant, as they gradually increase until a P wave is not conducted, a Wenckebach block exists. Figure 15–2 shows the increasing PR intervals with double arrows. During the first complete cycle of beats, the AV conduction ratio is 6:5 (numbered in Figure 15–2 Answer) while for the second group it is 11:10. These very high AV conduction ratios are not typical findings in Wenckebach and are caused by medication to slow AV conduction. More common ratios are 4:3 and 3:2.

FIGURE 15–03

DATA:

- Rate: ventricular: (A-B) 30/minute; (C) 10–15/minute; (D) absent

    Arial: (A-B) 60/minute; (C-D): 50/minute

- Rhythm: ventricular: (A-B) regular; (C) irregular; (D) absent

- QRS Duration: (A-C) 0.08-0.12 second; (D) absent

- PR Interval: (A and B) 0.28 second; (C) 0.32 second; (D) absent

- AV Conduction Ratio: (A) 4:3; (B) 3:2; 4:3; (C) 5:4; (D) absent

- ST Segment: 4 mm elevation

Interpretation: Tracings A–C show the lethal progression of second-degree heart block (Mobitz

Type II) into third-degree AV block. Ventricular standstill occurs in tracing D owing to the failure of an escape idioventricular rhythm.

Reasoning: The QRS activity is irregular and has unusually narrow complexes for such a slow rhythm. The atrial activity has notched P waves occurring at a regular rate of 60/minute. The AV relationship has many more P waves than QRS-T complexes. The PR intervals of the conducted beats are prolonged. Every QRS complex is preceded by one P wave at a fixed distance *but not every P wave is followed by a QRS*. This is the main feature of an incomplete type of AV block.

The conduction ratio varies between 2:1 and 3:1 and this is termed a *high-degree form* of heart block because two or more consecutive P waves are blocked (Figure 15-3 Answer). Tracing C, which was recorded a few minutes after A and B, shows a worsening block because most P waves fail to be conducted. Conduction ratios of 5:1 mean that only 1 of every 5 P waves is conducted. For instance, if the sinus rate were 100/minute, the ventricular rate would only be 20/minute. Two minutes later, final tracing D was obtained that shows third-degree AV block with ventricular standstill. Escape ventricular pacemakers fail to discharge and asystole results. Artificial pacing was not effective.

FIGURE 15–04

DATA:

- Rate: sinus 75/minute; ventricular 30/minute

- Rhythm: atrial and ventricular: regular

- QRS Duration: 0.12 second

- PR Interval: absent

- AV Conduction Ratio: absent

- ST Segment: 1 mm elevation

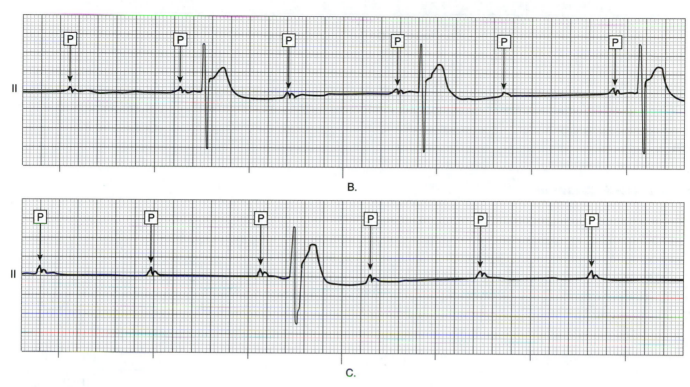

Figure 15-3 Answer

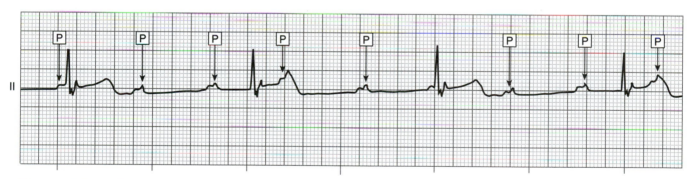

Figure 15-4 Answer

Interpretation: Complete (third-degree) AV heart block with a ventricular rate of 30/minute

Reasoning: Ventricular activity is slow, consisting of regularly occurring QRS complexes that are 0.12 second in duration. The QRS complexes have a relatively normal appearance and indicate that an escape focus is discharging within the AV bundle. The notched and widened P waves mean that there is a conduction disturbance exists in atrial depolarization as well as in AV conduction. Many more P waves than QRS complexes exist. Some P waves are hidden in the T waves of the 2nd and 4th QRS complexes, distorting their shapes (Figure 15-4 Answer).

A fixed AV relationship is absent and results in complete dissociation that gives the appearance that the P waves are "marching through" the QRS complexes. The atria are paced at a faster rate by the sinus node, while the ventricles are plodding along at a much slower rate due to an escape pacemaker. The key features of third-degree AV block are:

- regular P-P intervals;

- regular R-R intervals; and

- no relationship between the Ps and the QRSs.

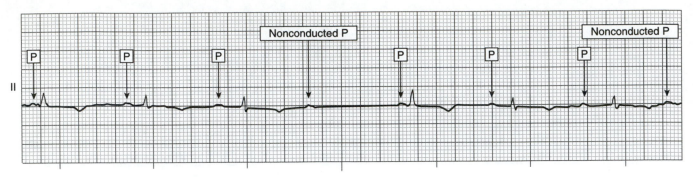

Figure 15-5 Answer

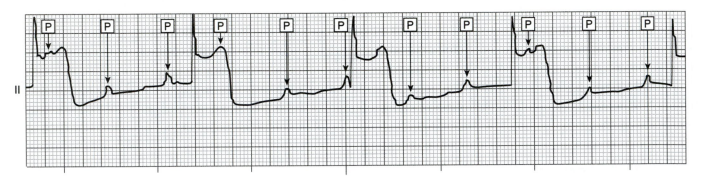

Figure 15-6 Answer

FIGURE 15–05

DATA:

- Rate: ventricular: 45/minute; sinus: 60/minute

- Rhythm: regularly irregular QRS-T complexes

- Duration: 0.10 second

- PR Interval: 0.16, 0.24, 0.36 second, dropped beat

- AV Conduction Ratio: 4:3

- ST Segment: 1 mm depression

Interpretation: Second-degree AV heart block Mobitz Type I with an AV conduction ratio of 4:3 and a ventricular rate of 45/minute

Reasoning: The tracing illustrates the following characteristics of a Wenckebach form of second-degree AV block (Mobitz Type I):

- grouped QRS beating ("periods") (Figure 15-5 Answer);

- PR intervals that increase prior to the dropped QRS-T complexes; and

- ECG pauses that contain the dropped beat are *less than twice the length* of the last cycle of the group without the dropped beats.

Because the sinus rate is only 60/minute and the conduction ratio is 4:3, the resulting ventricular rate is 45/minute. Had the sinus rate been 100/minute, a 4:3 conduction ratio would yield a more tolerable rate of 75/minute.

FIGURE 15–06

DATA:

- Rate: sinus 100/minute

- Rhythm: atrial and sinus: regular

- QRS Duration: 0.10 second

- PR Interval: absent/ dissociated

- AV Conduction Ratio: absent/dissociated

- ST Segment: 8 mm ST segment elevation with an acute myocardial injury pattern

Interpretation: Third-degree (complete) AV heart block with a ventricular rate of 35/minute

Reasoning: No fixed relationship exists between the P waves and the ventricular complexes. P waves appear to "march through" the QRS complexes, forming a random pattern (Figure 15-6 Answer). Nonconducted P waves occur at a more rapid rate than the QRS-T complexes. The atrial rate is 100/minute while the ventricles

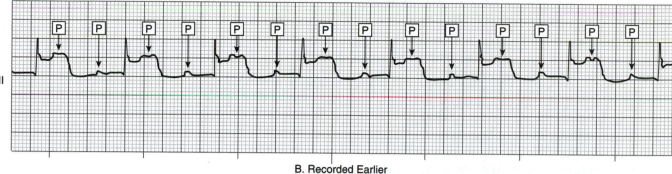

B. Recorded Earlier

Figure 15-7 Answer

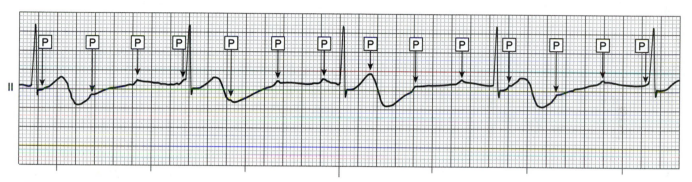

Figure 15-8 Answer

are beating at only 36/minute. The ventricular rhythm is regular but the QRS complexes are distorted owing to the elevated ST segments. A permanent pacemaker was implanted (after initial stabilization with an external pacemaker) that provided good myocardial capture. The ST segments are elevated owing to an inferior wall myocardial infarction.

FIGURE 15–07

Data:

■ Rate: Tracing (A) sinus: 125/min; ventricular: 50/minute, Tracing (B) sinus: 120/minute; ventricular: 60/minute

■ Rhythm: (A-B) sinus and ventricular: regular

■ QRS Duration: (A-B) 0.08 second (appears somewhat distorted due to elevated ST segment)

■ PR Interval: (A) absent; (B) 0.36 second

■ AV Conduction Ratio: (A) absent; (B) 2:1

■ ST Segment: 4 mm elevation with an acute injury pattern consistent with acute myocardial injury

Interpretation: Tracing A: Third-degree AV block. Tracing B: First-degree AV block and a second-degree AV block with 2:1 AV conduction ratio

Reasoning: In Tracing A both the atrial and ventricular rhythms are regular but they lack a fixed relationship to each other (Figure 15-7 Answer). Following the administration of atropine in tracing B, the ventricular rhythm becomes regular with two P waves for every QRS complex. A fixed 2:1 AV conduction is present in tracing B but the second P wave for each QRS-T complex is hidden within the ST segments. Despite atropine's ability to change the third-degree block to a second-degree block, AV conduction remains unstable and an artificial pacemaker is needed. The elevated ST segments are caused by an inferior wall MI.

FIGURE 15–08

DATA:

■ Rate: sinus: 100/minute; ventricular: 30/minute

■ Rhythm: sinus: ventricular: regular

■ QRS Duration: 0.10 second

■ PR Interval: absent/dissociated

■ AV Conduction Ratio: absent/dissociated

■ ST Segment: 2 mm depression

■ Other Findings: large biphasic T waves

Interpretation: **Complete (third-degree) AV heart block with a ventricular rate of 30/minute**

Reasoning: The R-R intervals are regular and the ventricular rate is very slow at 30/minute yet the QRS complexes look remarkably normal. The atrial rate of 100/minute is three times faster than the ventricular rate. Many P waves are hidden among the QRS-T complexes. No fixed relationship exists between the P waves and the QRS complexes indicating that complete AV dissociation exists (Figure 15–8 Answer). The narrow QRS complexes indicate that the escape ventricular pacemaker is located within the AV junction because it has such a narrow QRS duration and normal appearance.

FIGURE 15–09

DATA:

■ Rate: ventricular: 52/minute; sinus: 120/minute

■ Rhythm: ventricular: regular; sinus: regular

■ QRS Duration: 0.16 second

■ PR Interval: absent

■ AV Conduction Ratio: absent

■ ST Segment: distorted and elevated

Interpretation: **Third-degree AV block with a ventricular rate of 50/minute**

Reasoning: The atria are paced at 120/minute by the sinus node while an escape focus in the ventricles beats at only 52/minute. Third-degree block is recognized by the P waves that "march through" the ventricular complexes (Figure 15-9 Answer). Some ST segments are distorted by P waves that are hidden within. This occurs because the upper and lower heart chambers are being paced independently. The atrial pacemaker depolarizes more rapidly than the ventricular rhythm, causing there to be more P waves than QRS complex-

es. The atrial rate is about 2 1/2 times faster than the ventricles.

FIGURE 15–10

DATA:

■ Rate: ventricular and atrial: 64/minute

■ Rhythm: regular

■ QRS Duration: 0.12 second

■ PR Interval: 0.24 second

■ AV Conduction Ratio: 1:1

■ ST Segment: 3 mm depression

Interpretation: **Sinus rhythm with first-degree AV block**

Reasoning: Ventricular and atrial activity is normal. The AV conduction ratio is 1:1. The only conduction disturbance is the prolonged PR interval. First-degree AV block is the only type of heart block where all QRS complexes are conducted. Aside from the prolonged PR intervals, the ECG tracing meets the criteria for NSR.

FIGURE 15–11

DATA:

■ Rate: ventricular: 35/minute; sinus: 94/minute

■ Rhythm: ventricular and sinus: regular

■ QRS Duration: 0.16 second

■ PR Interval: absent/dissociated

■ AV Conduction Ratio: absent/dissociated

■ ST Segment: 1 mm depression

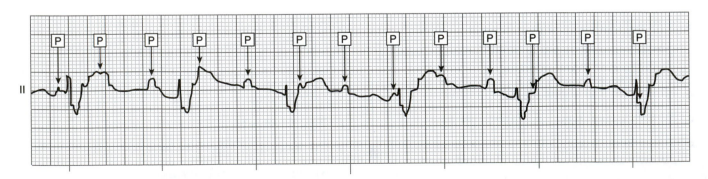

Figure 15-9 Answer

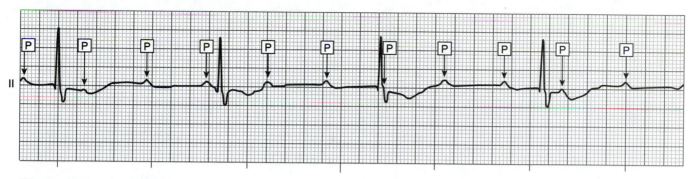

Figure 15-11 Answer

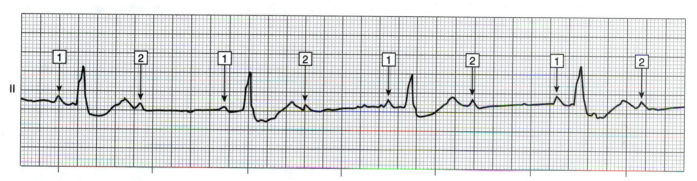

Figure 15-12 Answer

Interpretation: Sinus rhythm with third-degree (complete) AV heart block and a ventricular rate of 35/minute

Reasoning: The ventricular and atrial rhythm are regular. However, no relationship exists between the P waves and the QRS complexes (Figure 15-11 Answer). This is a case of complete AV dissociation, in which there are two independent pacemakers. The atria are being stimulated by the sinus node at a much faster rate than the ventricles. An idioventricular pacemaker, which arose within the His bundle, results in QRS complexes that are only slightly wider than normal. The loss of coordination between the atria and ventricles, coupled with the slow ventricular rate, cause a significant fall in cardiac output.

FIGURE 15–12

DATA:

- Rate: ventricular: 33/minute; sinus: 66/minute

- Rhythm: ventricular and atrial: regular

- QRS Duration: 0.12 second

- PR Interval: 0.20 second for conducted beats

- AV Conduction Ratio: 2:1

- ST Segment: 3 mm depression

Interpretation: Sinus rhythm with 2:1 AV heart block and a ventricular rate at 33/minute

Reasoning: The slow ventricular rhythm consists of wide but regular QRS-T complexes. Atrial activity is composed of regular, normal appearing P waves at twice the ventricular rate. Two P waves are present for each QRS-T complexes, the second of which has a fixed PR interval (Figure 15-12 Answer). When the AV conduction ratio is greater than 1:1, either a second-degree or a third-degree AV block exists. In order to narrow down these possibilities, the relationship of the P waves to the QRS-T complexes must be evaluated. If there is *no fixed relationship* between the Ps and the QRS-T complexes, then complete AV block is present. On the other hand, if there is a set pattern between the P waves and the QRS-T complexes—but not all of the P waves are conducted—a second-degree AV block must exist. The last step in evaluating which type of block is present, involves assessing the PR intervals that occur immediately before the dropped beats.

ECG Interpretation Tip *If the second P wave of each pair of P waves were mistaken for U waves, this tracing might have been incorrectly interpreted as a sinus bradycardia. However, P waves have identical shapes and the P-P intervals are constant.*

FIGURE 15–13

DATA:

- Rate: ventricular and atrial: 60/minute
- Rhythm: ventricular and atrial: regular
- QRS Duration: 0.12 second
- PR Interval: 0.52 second (significantly prolonged)
- AV Conduction Ratio: 1:1
- Other Findings: 5 mm ST segment elevation

Interpretation: Sinus rhythm with first-degree AV heart block

Reasoning: The ventricular activity consists of wide QRS-T complexes and has a regular rhythm. The atrial activity has normally appearing P waves and a regular rhythm. The AV relationship has a single P wave for each QRS-T complex but the PR intervals are very prolonged.

FIGURE 15–14

DATA:

- Rate: ventricular: 50/minute; atrial: 75/minute
- Rhythm: ventricular: regularly irregular; atrial: regular
- QRS Duration: 0.16 second
- PR Interval: changes between: 0.20 second, 0.52 second, a dropped beat, from the pattern repeats
- AV Conduction Ratio: 3:2
- ST Segment: 1 mm elevation
- Other Findings: widen and distorted QRS complexes

Interpretation: Second-degree AV heart block; Mobitz Type One (Wenckebach) with a 3:2 AV conduction and a ventricular rate of 40/minute

Reasoning: This tracing contains the hallmark findings of Wenckebach (Mobitz Type I):

- regular P-P intervals
- grouped beating with changing R-R intervals
- gradual prolongation of the PR intervals
- R-R intervals that include the dropped beat measure less than two R-R cycles that do not have the dropped beat.

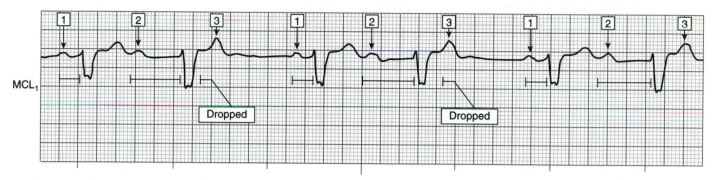

Figure 15-14 Answer

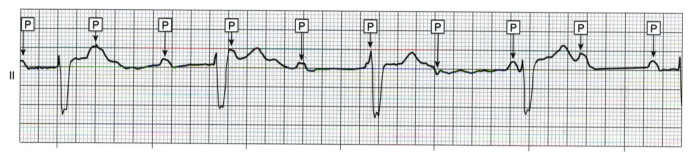

Figure 15-15 Answer

- progressive decrease in the R-R intervals as the QRS-T complexes fall further behind the P waves

- AV conduction ratio greater than 1:1

The third P wave of each cycle is difficult to see because it is hidden within the last T wave of each group, as diagrammed in Figure 15–14 Answer. The signs of Wenckebach help to identify this dysrhythmia even when the above findings have been partially obscured, such as by hidden P waves in the ST-T segment or in the case of atrial fibrillation. The QRS complexes are wider than normal and have a distorted shape, which is due to a preexisting bundle branch block.

FIGURE 15–15

DATA:

- Rate: ventricular: 42/minute; atrial: 90/minute

- Rhythm: ventricular: regular; atrial: regular

- QRS Duration: 0.16 second

- PR Interval: none/ dissociated

- AV Conduction Ratio: none/ dissociated

- ST Segment: 2 mm elevation

- Other Findings: mild baseline artifact

Interpretation: Third-degree AV heart block with a ventricular escape pacemaker rhythm of 42/minute

Reasoning: There are considerably fewer QRS-T complexes than P waves. Ventricular activity is regular and composed of wide QRS complexes occurring at a bradycardic rate (Figure 15-15 Answer). Atrial activity is regular and consists of normally shaped P waves. The sinus node remains in control of the atria while the ventricles are paced by an escape pacemaker from somewhere below the blocked AV conduction.

FIGURE 15–16

DATA:

- Rate: ventricular: absent; atrial: 50/minute

- Rhythm: ventricular: absent; atrial: regular

- QRS Duration: absent

- PR Interval: absent

- AV Conduction Ratio: absent

- ST Segment: absent

- Other Findings: total absence of QRS-T complexes

Interpretation: **Third-degree AV heart block with ventricular standstill due to failure of the escape pacemaker mechanism**

Reasoning: There is no ventricular activity. Atrial activity is strikingly normal, yet none of the P waves generate an associated QRS-T complex (Figure 15-6 Answer). As a result of the failure of atrial activity to be conducted into the ventricles—and failure of an escape pacemaker to develop—the ventricles remain in asystole. This is a terminal ECG rhythm.

Discussion: Ventricular asystole reflects widespread failure of the entire escape impulse formation system in addition to the failure of the conduction pathway.

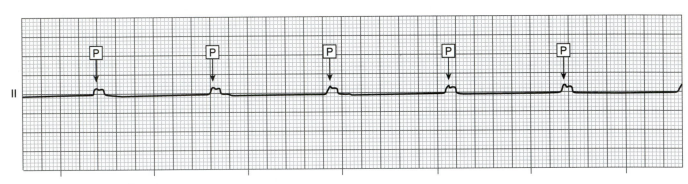

Figure 15-16 Answer

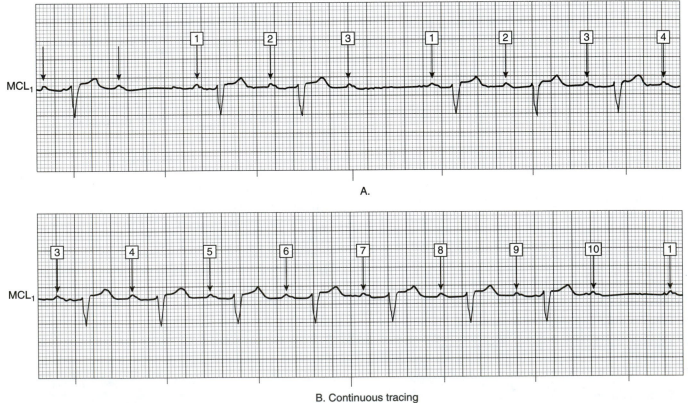

A.

B. Continuous tracing

Figure 15-17 Answer

Fortunately, ventricular asystole during third-degree block is rare. In most cases of third-degree block, an escape pacemaker quickly develops after a pause to stimulate the ventricles. In this case, neither the AV junction, AV bundle, bundle branches, or the Purkinje fibers spontaneously depolarize. The only therapy that might be effective would be an external pacemaker.

FIGURE 15–17

DATA:

■ Rate: ventricular: ranges 55–75/minute; atrial: 75/minute

■ Rhythm: ventricular: irregular; atrial: regular

■ QRS Duration: 0.08 second

■ PR Interval: varies: 0.24 second, 0.34 second, 0.38 second dropped QRS

■ AV Conduction Ratio: varies: 3:2, 4:3, and 10:9

■ ST Segment: Normal

Interpretation: Second-degree AV heart block; Mobitz Type I (Wenckebach) with varying AV conduction and an average ventricular rate of 65/minute

Reasoning: This is an interesting example of Wenckebach because the varying AV conduction ratios yield an irregularly irregular pattern. Most cases of Wenckebach have a fixed conduction ratio, such as a 3:2 or 4:3 AV ratio which results in a cyclical pattern (Figure 15-17 Answer). The ventricular activity consists of narrow QRS complexes while the atrial activity is regular. The P waves in the grouped beats encounter an increasingly refractory AV node until a QRS-T complex is eventually dropped. The cycle then begins again with the first beat having the shortest PR interval of the group.

The first PR interval of each Wenckebach cycle has a prolonged PR interval of 0.24 second. An associated first-degree AV block is a common finding in Wenckebach. The 10:9 conduction ratio is an especially long cycle. Most Wenckebach conduction ratios involve a 3:2 or a 4:3 sequence. High AV conduction ratios, such as seen in this ECG, result in many fewer QRS-T complexes being dropped than does 3:2 or 4:3 AV conduction.

FIGURE 15–18

DATA:

■ Rate: ventricular: 30/minute; atrial: 65/min

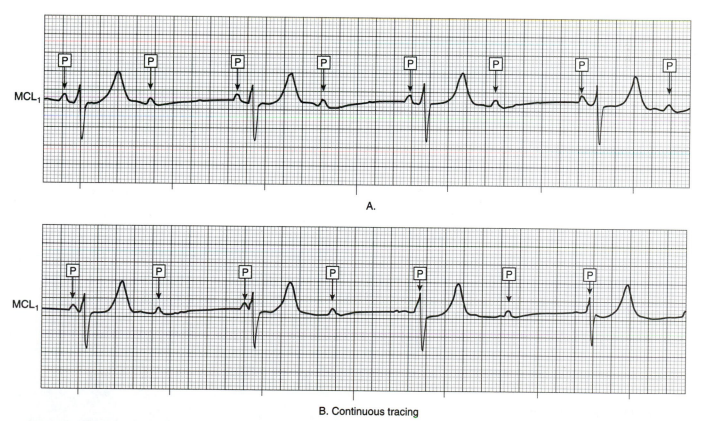

A.

B. Continuous tracing

Figure 15-18 Answer

- Rhythm: ventricular: regular; atrial: regular

- QRS Duration: 0.16 second

- PR Interval: none/dissociated

- AV Conduction Ratio: none/dissociated

- ST Segment: normal

- Other Findings: peaked (10 mm tall) and pointy T waves

Interpretation: Complete AV heart block with a ventricular rate of 30/minute

Reasoning: The slow ventricular activity consists of wide, distorted QRS-T complexes. Atrial activity involves normal appearing P waves that occur regularly. An atrial-ventricular relationship does not exist as all PR intervals show a random association (Figure 15-18 Answer). The ventricular rhythm is regular but the QRS complexes are totally unrelated to the P waves. Tall and pointy T waves are most often caused by hyperkalemia so a serum potassium level should be assessed. Hypokalemia can also cause ventricular dysrhythmias.

FIGURE 15–19

DATA:

- Rate: ventricular and atrial: 50/minute

- Rhythm: ventricular and atrial: regular

- QRS Duration: 0.08 second

- PR Interval: 0.28 second

- AV Conduction Ratio: 1:1

- ST Segment: normal

Interpretation: Sinus bradycardia with prolonged PR intervals

Reasoning: The ventricular activity is regular but

slow, while the atrial activity is normal appearing and has a regular rhythm. The fixed PR intervals are prolonged well beyond 0.20 second. The only deviation from NSR involves a slow heart rate and delayed AV conduction. These two findings suggest that increased parasympathetic tone is the cause as vagus nerve stimulation slows sinus node activity and AV conduction velocity.

Discussion: Why is this tracing not termed a first-degree AV block? In order for the prolonged PR interval to be considered abnormal, the heart rate must be at least 60/minute. This is because many sinus bradycardias also have prolonged PR intervals that quickly shorten to normal when the heart rate increases. Vagal tone can be decreased by atropine administration if clinically needed, although this is rarely required.

FIGURE 15–20

DATA:

- Rate: ventricular: 25/minute; atrial: 80/minute

- Rhythm: ventricular: slightly irregular; atrial: regular

- QRS Duration: 0.12 second

- PR Interval: no fixed intervals

- AV Conduction Ratio: dissociated

- ST Segment: normal

- Other Findings: deeply and symmetrically inverted T waves

Interpretation: Third-degree AV heart block with a ventricular escape pacemaker rhythm of 25/minute

Reasoning: The R-R intervals are slightly irregular and the ventricular rate is very slow. Atrial activity consists of notched P waves that lack associated QRS-T com-

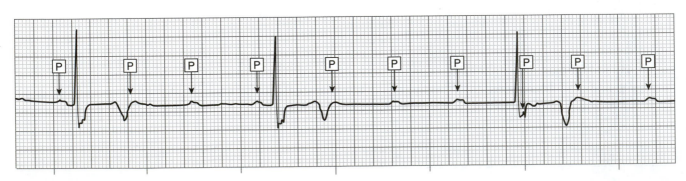

Figure 15-20 Answer

plexes (Figure 15-20 Answer). This ECG tracing meets the criteria for third-degree AV block:

- bradycardic ventricular rate (45/minute or less);

- many more P waves than QRS-T complexes; and

- absent AV conduction (random PR intervals).

These conditions must be present in order to label a rhythm complete heart block because AV dissociation can occur even with normal AV conduction. Periods of AV dissociation can develop if the ventricular rate accelerates or the sinus node significantly slows leading to an interference in the coordinated AV relationship. ECG tracings that meet the three requirements listed above allow ample opportunity for AV conduction to take place so if dissociation is present it is due to a complete AV heart block.

> **ECG Interpretation Tip** *Deeply inverted T waves, especially when the shape is symmetrical and form an "arrowhead" appearance, indicates myocardial injury. Although Tracing 15-20 suggests injury, a twelve-lead ECG is needed to see if the T wave abnormalities are present in an anatomically related group of leads (such as, in an inferior, anterior, or lateral distribution).*

FIGURE 15–21

DATA:

- Rate: ventricular: 40/minute; atrial: 80/minute

- Rhythm: ventricular and atrial: regular

- QRS Duration: 0.16 second

- PR Interval: 0.20 second

- AV Conduction Ratio: 2:1

- ST Segment: 10 mm elevation

- Other Findings: The QRS complexes are wide and distorted

Interpretation: **Sinus rhythm with second-degree AV heart block with 2:1 AV conduction and a ventricular rate of 40/minute**

Reasoning: The bradycardic ventricular activity has a wide and bizarre QRS shape. The atrial activity appears at exactly twice the ventricular rate because two P waves are present for each QRS-T complex (Figure 15-21 Answer). The second P wave could easily have been overlooked unless the ST-T complexes were carefully scrutinized. The partially hidden second P waves are clearly present within the downslope portion of the T waves (Figure 15-21 Answer).

Discussion: Wide QRS complexes coupled with normal PR intervals strongly point toward an infranodal conduction problem. In this case, third-degree block developed a short time later, as expected for Mobitz Type II. (Mobitz Type I, in contrast, has prolonged PR intervals and narrow QRS-T complexes because it is caused by an AV nodal conduction defect. Also, Mobitz Type I rarely progresses to complete AV block.)

> **ECG Interpretation Tip** *Second P waves should always be suspected when bradycardic rhythms occur during a myocardial infarction, especially if the ST segments and the T waves are distorted. A major clue pointing to hidden P waves is changing shapes of the ST segments or T waves from beat-to-beat in the same ECG lead.*

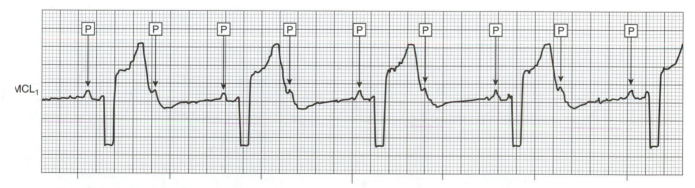

Figure 15-21 Answer

FIGURE 15–22

DATA:

- Rate: ventricular: 60/minute; atrial: 75/minute

- Rhythm: ventricular: irregular; atrial: regular

- QRS Duration: 0.12 second

- PR Interval: gradually increasing cycle: 0.20 second, 0.32 second, dropped QRS

- AV Conduction Ratio: 3:2

- ST Segment: 4 mm depression

- Other Findings: the 3rd and 6th QRS-T complexes are escape beats

Interpretation: Sinus rhythm with second-degree AV heart block; Mobitz Type I (Wenckebach); 3:2 AV conduction with a ventricular rate of 55/minute

Reasoning: The ventricular rhythm is irregular and the QRS complexes are wider than normal. Atrial activity consists of regular and normally shaped P waves. The PR intervals change according to a pattern: the duration gradually increases until the third P wave of each group is not conducted (Figure 15-22 Answer). The

pause in cardiac activity after the blocked P wave allows the ventricles to briefly initiate their own rhythm: QRS number 3 and 6 lack P waves and arise following a delay, lasting six large boxes which correspond to an intrinsic rate of 50/minute. The P waves occurring after beats number 3 and 6 are not conducted and are buried within the ST segments.

FIGURE 15–23

DATA:

- Rate: ventricular: 25/minute; atrial: 110/minute

- Rhythm: ventricular: irregular; atrial: regular

- QRS Duration: 0.16 second

- PR Interval: 0.18 second for the conducted beats

- AV Conduction Ratio: 2:1 for first three beats; 5:1 for last two beats

- ST Segment: 5 mm elevation

- Other Findings: long pauses in cardiac activity and numerous P waves

Interpretation: Sinus rhythm with a second-degree AV block (2:1) developing into a high

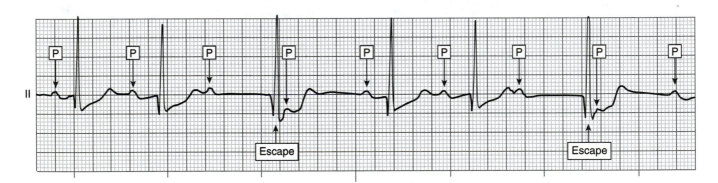

Figure 15-22 Answer

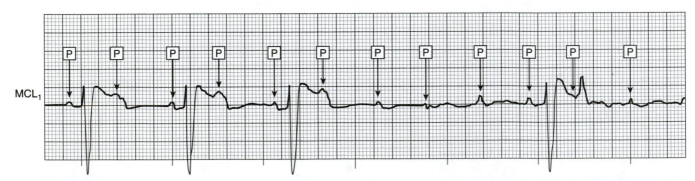

Figure 15-23 Answer

grade AV block with a ventricular rate of 25/minute

Reasoning: The ventricular rhythm is irregular and the beats are wide and bizarre. The P waves are upright and have a regular rhythm. The P wave that immediately precedes each QRS complex has a fixed PR interval. However, every P wave is *not* followed by a QRS-T complex, indicating that an AV heart block exists (Figure 15-23 Answer). The first three QRS-T complexes have a 2:1 AV conduction during which the second P wave for each of the three QRS-T complexes is partially hidden within the ST segment. After the third P-QRS-T complex, conduction abruptly changes so that just one of every five P waves is transmitted. The term "high grade" AV block is applied to such cases when two or more consecutive P waves are not conducted. High grade AV blocks indicate that an advanced form of heart block is present and that abrupt progression to third-degree block should be anticipated.

FIGURE 15–24

DATA:

- Rate: ventricular: 40/minute; atrial: 50/minute

- Rhythm: ventricular: irregular; atrial: 50/minute

- QRS Duration: 0.08 second

- PR Interval: progressive changes: 0.20 second, 0.22 second, 0.26, dropped QRS

- AV Conduction Ratio: 4:3

- ST Segment:

- Other Findings: very tall and pointy T waves

Interpretation: Sinus rhythm with second-degree AV heart block; Mobitz Type I (Wenckebach) with 4:3 AV conduction and a ventricular rate of 50/minute

Reasoning: The ventricular rhythm is irregular while the atrial rhythm is regular. The PR interval lengths gradually increase. The fourth QRS-T complex lacks a P wave because it is an escape beat (Figure 15-24 Answer). The pause in cardiac activity following the third QRS-T complex is ended by an escape AV junctional beat (fourth complex). The shapes of the QRS complexes of the escape beat and other beats have the same shape: narrow and normal appearing.

FIGURE 15–25

DATA:

- Rate: ventricular: 75/minute, atrial: 75/minute

- Rhythm: ventricular and atrial: regular

- QRS Duration: 0.12 second

- PR Interval: 0.36 second

- AV Conduction Ratio: 1:1

- ST Segment: normal

- Other Findings: notched P waves

Interpretation: Sinus rhythm with a first-degree AV heart block

Reasoning: The ventricular and atrial activity have normal configurations and the rhythm is regular. Every P wave is conducted following a considerable delay of 0.36 second. First-degree AV block involves a delay in conduction but—unlike all other forms of AV heart block—every P wave is eventually conducted. First-degree block is usually a benign condition that does not adversely affect cardiac output; however, the severe prolongation should prompt a search for its cause and continuous cardiac monitoring should be done to observe for development of a more advanced heart block.

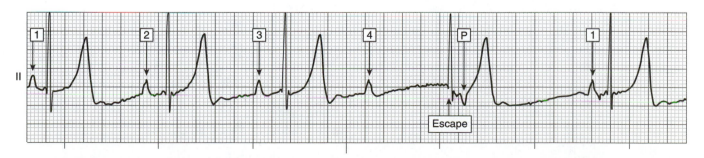

Figure 15-24 Answer

Answers for Chapter 18 ECG Tracings

FIGURE 18–01

DATA:

- Rate: 40/minute
- Rhythm: regular
- QRS Duration: 0.20 second
- PR Interval: absent
- AV Conduction Ratio: absent
- ST Segment: normal
- Other Findings: none

Interpretation: **Escape idioventricular ventricular rhythm at 40/minute caused by sinus node block**

Reasoning: The distorted and wide QRS complexes have a regular rhythm. Atrial activity is absent because P waves cannot be seen, so an AV relationship does not exist. The slow ventricular rate is within the range expected for a spontaneously discharging idioventricular focus (20 to 40/minute). The wide QRS complexes indicate an abnormal ventricular activation. Only QRS durations that are less than 0.12 second are certain to be supraventricular beats, that is, having originated above the His bundle branch point and been normally conducted. Impulses formed below the His bundle result in distorted QRS complexes because they follow an abnormal path. Instead of both bundle branches being simultaneously activated, the right and left ventricles are sequentially stimulated (one ventrical after the other). Because of this abnormal activation, conduction velocity is slowed, and the QRS duration is prolonged to 0.12 second or more.

FIGURE 18–02

DATA:

- Rate: 210/minute
- Rhythm: irregular
- QRS Duration: 0.16–0.24 second
- PR Interval: absent
- AV Conduction Ratio: absent
- ST Segment: distorted
- Other Findings: the QRS complexes vary greatly in size and shape

Interpretation: **Torsade de Pointes (TdP) polymorphic ventricular tachycardia**

Reasoning: The ventricular complexes are distorted, with variable R-R intervals, and have a rate exceeding 200/minute. Regular atrial activity is missing; therefore, an AV relationship cannot be determined. Polymorphic VT consists of a series of consecutive PVCs whose height and shape regularly wax and wane. Toward the center of this ECG tracing, the complexes decrease in size and then gradually begin to widen and increase in size. If left untreated, Torsade de Pointes often degenerates into ventricular fibrillation. Some TdP cases occur intermittently and spontaneously convert to sinus rhythm. The causes and treatment of polymorphic ventricular tachycardia differs from the much more common monomorphic type of VT.

> **ECG Interpretation Tip** At first glance, this tracing looked as if it were ventricular fibrillation. But a careful analysis will show that there is a repetitive pattern: waxing and waning rhythm with wide QRS complexes.

FIGURE 18–03

DATA:

- Rate: 94/minute
- Rhythm: regularly irregular
- QRS Duration: PVC: 0.16 second; sinus 0.6 second
- PR Interval: sinus 0.16 second
- AV Conduction Ratio: 1:1
- ST Segment: 2 mm depression

■ Other Findings: sinus beats have QS configuration

Interpretation: Sinus rhythm and unifocal PVCs every fourth beat; also known as ventricular quintigeminy

Reasoning: The ST segments of the sinus beats are displaced below the ECG baseline, distorting the QRS-T complexes. The PVCs (beats number 5, 10, and 15) can be recognized by the following characteristics:

■ wide and distorted QRS complexes;

■ prematurity, occurring early during the R-R interval;

■ absent P waves;

■ T waves opposite in direction to the abnormal R wave; and

■ constant coupling intervals to the preceding sinus beats.

FIGURE 18–04

DATA:

■ Rate: absent

■ Rhythm: absent

■ QRS Duration: absent

■ PR Interval: absent

■ AV Conduction Ratio: absent

Interpretation: Asystole with several isolated low voltage complexes, that are possibly isolated P waves or artifact

Reasoning: Except for the few small positive deflections, the baseline is flat because electrical activity is largely absent. Occasional baseline fluctuations are seen, which may represent occasional P waves or cable movement artifact. It is important to monitor one additional lead that is oriented perpendicular to the original lead when asystole is detected to eliminate the possibility that low voltage ventricular fibrillation is present but not detected in the original lead.

FIGURE 18–05

DATA:

■ Rate: 106/minute

■ Rhythm: irregular

■ QRS Duration: PVC: 0.16 second; sinus: 0.06 second

■ PR Interval: 0.16 second

■ AV Conduction Ratio: 1:1

■ ST Segment: normal

■ Other Findings: none

Interpretation: Sinus tachycardia with two unifocal PVCs

Reasoning: The rhythm is regular except for two early, wide QRS complexes (beats number 2 and 9). The remainder of the tracing shows sinus activity because regular P-QRS-T complexes occur at a rate slightly over 100/minute. Both ectopic beats have the same shape and are wide and distorted. The early beats lack P waves and are followed by compensatory pauses.

The shapes of the ectopic beats differ from typical PVCs: the T waves are not opposite to the deflection of the QRS complexes and they are not taller than the surrounding normal beats. However, there are no signs that the beats are supraventricular complexes that were aberrantly conducted, although that remains a possibility. Another interesting finding is that the coupling intervals of the PVCs to the preceding sinus beats are variable. Variable coupling intervals are suggestive of an independent ventricular ectopic focus. Most PVCs result from a reentry mechanism rather than an automatic ectopic focus.

FIGURE 18–06

DATA:

■ Rate: absent

■ Rhythm: absent

■ QRS Duration: absent

■ PR Interval: absent

■ AV Conduction Ratio: absent

■ ST Segment: absent

■ Other Findings: chaotic rhythm

Interpretation: Coarse ventricular fibrillation

Reasoning: The disorganized ventricular waves have an amplitude of at least 5 mm. Findings that indicate ventricular fibrillation include:

■ chaotic ventricular activity

■ absent atrial activity

■ absent AV conduction

Discussion: The pacemaker mechanism involves a chaotic reentry pattern within the ventricles which may result from an R-on-T phenomenon. Organized cardiac activity is absent because of electrical disorganization. Effective cardiac contractions can only follow an orderly sequence of electrical stimulation. If an electrical countershock is unable to restore sinus activity, the fibrillatory waves will become finer and finer until asystole develops.

FIGURE 18–07

DATA:

- Rate: 155/minute
- Rhythm: regular
- QRS Duration: 0.40 second
- PR Interval: absent
- AV Conduction Ratio: absent
- ST Segment: absent

Interpretation: Ventricular tachycardia at 155/minute

Reasoning: Regular ventricular activity is present, consisting of very wide (0.40 second) and bizarre QRS complexes. The QRS-T complexes are not preceded by regular atrial activity. Since atrial activity cannot be seen, an AV relationship is not present.

Discussion: This dysrhythmia originates from a rapid reentry circuit within the His-Purkinje conduction system. VT severely depresses cardiac output and impairs tissue perfusion. VT can suddenly deteriorate into ventricular fibrillation. In the pulseless form of ventricular tachycardia, cardiac output is absent. Except for cases of nonsustained VT, this dysrhythmia must be aggressively treated.

FIGURE 18–08

DATA:

- Rate: 20/minute
- Rhythm: regular
- QRS Duration: 0.36 second
- PR Interval: absent
- AV Conduction Ratio: absent
- ST Segment: massive elevation; merges with QRS complexes
- Other Findings: bizarre, distorted QRS-T complexes

Interpretation: Idioventricular (agonal) rhythm at 20/minute

Reasoning: The infrequent ventricular activity consists of large, bizarre QRS complexes that lack P waves. The extremely slow rate of 20/minute is within the range expected for a low ventricular focus depolarization, which ranges from 20 to 30/minute. The distorted ventricular complexes, coupled with the prolonged QRS duration, confirm the abnormal ventricular activation. Slow idioventricular pacemakers are unstable and unreliable. The term "agonal" is applied to such dysrhythmias because they usually occur just prior to death and degenerate to asystole within minutes.

FIGURE 18–09

DATA:

- Rhythm: absent
- Rate: occasional beat
- QRS Duration: 0.28 second
- PR Interval: absent
- AV Conduction Ratio: absent
- ST Segment: massive elevation in the single complex
- Other Finding: flat baseline

Interpretation: Asystole with a single agonal idioventricular complex

Reasoning: Ventricular activity is absent aside from the lone very wide and distorted QRS complex that lacks a P wave. The rest of the ECG tracing is flat because there is no electrical activity. Asystole occurs in a dying heart and resuscitation attempts are almost always unsuccessful.

FIGURE 18–10

DATA:

- Rate: 100/minute
- Rhythm: irregular
- QRS Duration: sinus 0.10 second; PVC: 0.16 second
- PR Interval: 0.16 second
- AV Conduction Ratio: 1:1
- ST Segment: normal

Interpretation: Sinus rhythm with multifocal PVCs. The first PVC is a fusion complex.

Reasoning: Aside from the PVC beats, sinus rhythm exists with regular and normal P-QRS-T complexes. The three premature beats (number 1, 8, and 11) have distorted QRS complexes, which appear somewhat different from each other. The PVCs lack P waves except for the first beat, which is a fusion complex.

Discussion: Fusion complexes share some of the characteristics of two pacemakers: P waves plus distorted QRS complexes. A fusion complex results when a pacemaker originates in the sinus node at the same time as another forms in the ventricles. A PVC occurs, while almost simultaneously, the SA node also begins depolarizing. Both depolarization waves meet somewhere in between causing the ECG complex to have portions of both waves. As a result, a somewhat distorted QRS complex appears to be preceded by a P wave but these events are actually unrelated.

FIGURE 18–11

DATA:

- Rate: 200/minute

- Rhythm: regular

- QRS Duration: 0.24 second

- PR Interval: absent

- AV Conduction Ratio: absent

- ST Segment: massively displaced from baseline

- Other Findings: regular, wide complex, rapid rhythm

Interpretation: Ventricular tachycardia at 200/minute

Reasoning: The ventricular activity consists of rapid, wide, and bizarre QRS complexes. P waves and an AV relationship are absent. VT is an unstable rhythm that is likely to deteriorate into ventricular fibrillation unless quickly and aggressively treated. Individuals are unable to tolerate VT for very long before cardiac output falls due to diminished diastolic filling, decreased coronary artery perfusion, and increased myocardial workload.

Clinical Note Ventricular tachycardia is one type of a group of related rhythm disturbances termed tachydysrhythmias. Tachydysrhythmias pertain to rhythms with a ventricular rate over 100/minute—regardless of where the pacemaker is located. The tachydysrhythmia group includes: sinus, AV junctional, PSVTs, atrial fibrillation, and atrial flutter with a rapid ventricular response, as well as those of ventricular origin, including polymorphic (Torsades de Pointes) and monomorphic ventricular tachycardia.

FIGURE 18–12

DATA:

- Rate: 100/minute

- Rhythm: irregular

- QRS Duration: sinus: 0.12 second; PVC: 0.16 second

- PR Interval: 0.20 second

- AV Conduction Ratio: 1:1 for sinus beats

- ST Segment: sinus: 3 mm depression

- Other Findings: PVCs have the same shape

Interpretation: Sinus rhythm with frequent uniformed PVCs, two of which occur as a couplet

Reasoning: The rhythm of the sinus beats is disrupted by frequent PVCs. The third and fourth beats are consecutive PVCs, which are termed a ventricular couplet. Couplets serve as a warning that a more sustained ventricular tachycardia rhythm may follow. The third PVC is beat number 13. Every PVC has a wide and distorted QRS complex, while the sinus beats have narrow QRS durations with normal shapes. PVCs exhibit the following characteristics: taller than sinus beats, ST segments and T waves that occur in a direction opposite to that of the QRS complexes, and they are followed by a compensatory pause.

FIGURE 18–13

DATA:

- Rate: 45/minute

- Rhythm: irregular

- QRS Duration: 0.28 second

- PR Interval: absent

- AV Conduction Ratio: absent

- ST segment: 3 mm "scooped out" depression

- Other Findings: slow, bizarre complexes

Interpretation: Idioventricular rhythm at 45/minute

Reasoning: The ventricular activity is irregular. The QRS complexes are wide and distorted. T waves are missing because the ST segments and T waves have merged with the QRS complexes to form slurred and widened complexes. Cardiac activity is controlled by a pacemaker originating low within the ventricles, probably emerging from the His-Purkinje fibers to stimulate a dying heart. Notoriously unreliable, idioventricular pacemakers are prone to sudden failure.

FIGURE 18–14

DATA:

- Rate: 63/minute

- Rhythm: irregular

- QRS Duration: PVC : 0.16 second; sinus: 0.04 second

- PR Interval: 0.16 second

- AV Conduction Ratio: 1:1

- ST Segment: sinus: 5 mm depression

Interpretation: Sinus rhythm with a PVC (beat number 3)

Reasoning: The ventricular rhythm is disturbed by an early, wide QRS complex. Sinus activity consists of normal P-QRS-T complexes. The fourth beat is a junctional complex that lacks a P wave but has a QRS similar to the sinus beats. A fully compensatory pause is *not* observed because the long R-R intervals caused by the slow heart rate allows the junctional escape complex to end the pause.

FIGURE 18–15

DATA:

- Rate: absent

- Rhythm: chaotically irregular

- QRS Duration: absent

- PR Interval: absent

- AV Conduction Ratio: absent

- ST segment: absent

Interpretation: Coarse ventricular fibrillation

Reasoning: No organized electrical activity exists, only a distorted zig-zagging baseline. The ECG tracing does not have P waves, QRS complexes, or T waves. The dysrhythmia is described as coarse because the size of the complexes is at least 5 mm. Coarse fibrillation has a greater chance of being successfully converted to NSR than does fine VF.

FIGURE 18–16

DATA:

- Rate: 50/minute

- Rhythm: occasionally irregular

- QRS Duration: PVC: 0.16 second; sinus: 0.06 second

- PR Interval: sinus: 0.16 second

- AV Conduction Ratio: 1:1

- ST Segment: 2 mm depressed

Interpretation: Sinus bradycardia at 50/minute with one PVC striking the T wave in an "R-on-T" fashion

Reasoning: Sinus rhythm occurs at a bradycardic rate. The sinus beats have normal P-QRS-T configurations, while the PVC has a wide QRS complex and the T wave's direction is opposite to that of the abnormal QRS complex. The PVC (beat number 5) occurs prematurely, landing precisely during the T wave of the prior sinus beat. Such early PVCs have a greater likelihood of causing ventricular fibrillation because the ventricular repolarization phase is not uniform.

FIGURE 18–17

DATA:

- Rate: absent

- Rhythm: absent

- QRS Duration: absent

- PR Interval: absent

- AV Conduction Ratio: absent

- ST Segment: absent

Interpretation: **Ventricular tachycardia changes to ventricular fibrillation.**

Reasoning: Organized ventricular activity is absent. It is difficult to distinguish ventricular fibrillation from ventricular tachycardia. Because organized atrial activity is absent, an atrioventricular relationship does not exist. A chaotic ECG baseline is present. During this dysrhythmia cardiac output ceases.

FIGURE 18–18

DATA:

- Rate: 94/minute

- Rhythm: regularly irregular

- QRS Duration: PVC: 0.24 second; sinus: 0.04 second

- PR Interval: 0.20 second

- AV Conduction Ratio: 1:1

- ST Segment: PVC: depressed 10 mm; sinus: normal

- Other Findings: every fourth beat is wide and distorted

Interpretation: **Sinus rhythm with ventricular quadrageminy**

Reasoning: Beats number 3, 7, and 11 show the characteristic PVC findings: wide, distorted QRS complexes, absent P waves, and T waves that slope in the direction opposite to the QRS complex. The ECG pattern of a PVC after every three sinus beats causes a "grouped beating" cycle, typical of a regular PVC pattern. The sinus beats have normal P-QRS-T waves and 1:1 AV conduction.

FIGURE 18–19

DATA:

- Rate: 180/minute

- Rhythm: regular

- QRS Duration: 0.28 second

- PR Interval: absent

- AV Conduction Ratio: absent

- ST Segment: absent

- Other Findings: very wide, abnormally shaped tachycardia

Interpretation: **Ventricular tachycardia at 180/minute**

Reasoning: The dysrhythmia is VT because:

- the rate is tachycardic (greater than 100/minute);

- the complexes are wide (0.12 second or greater) and distorted; and

- regular atrial activity is lacking.

This rapid regular ventricular rhythm must be treated aggressively to prevent sudden deterioration into ventricular fibrillation. In this case, the patient was receiving thrombolytic therapy for a myocardial infarction and the dysrhythmia only lasted for several minutes until being converted to NSR with lidocaine.

FIGURE 18–20

DATA:

- Rate: 42/minute

- Rhythm: regular

- QRS Duration: 0.36 second

- PR Interval: absent

- AV Conduction Ratio: absent

- ST Segment: 7 mm elevation

- Other Findings: ST segments merge with the QRS complexes and T waves to form wide distorted QRS-T complex

Interpretation: **Idioventricular rhythm at 40/minute**

Reasoning: The QRS complexes are distorted and occur at a bradycardic rate. Their bizarre shapes do not have the sharp deflections typical of sinus-initiated ventricular complexes. P waves are absent so an AV relationship cannot be determined.

Discussion: Even a slow idioventricular rhythm provides temporary assistance when higher pacemakers fail. Idioventricular rhythms produce a significantly diminished cardiac output due to their slow rate and lack of synchronized atrioventricular function. Idioventricular rhythms prevent asystole when sinus and junctional pacemakers fail. An idioventricular rhythm should be stabilized by a transcutaneous or transvenous artificial pacemaker as soon as possible.

FIGURE 18–21

DATA:

- Rate: 84/minute

- Rhythm: regularly irregular

- QRS Duration: PVC 0.16 second; sinus: 0.06 second

- PR Interval: 0.20 second

- AV Conduction Ratio: 1:1

- ST Segment: PVCs: depressed 6 mm.; sinus: normal

- Other Findings: R-R rhythm has a regularly occurring long-short pattern

Interpretation: **Sinus rhythm with ventricular bigeminy**

Reasoning: The ventricular rhythm is regularly irregular and the ECG pattern has grouped beating. A pattern of long-short-long-short R-R intervals happens when a PVC is coupled to a preceding sinus beat and followed by a compensatory pause. The QRS complexes of the sinus beats are narrow, while the PVCs are wide.

FIGURE 18–22

DATA:

- Rate: 5–10/minute

- Rhythm: irregular

- QRS Duration: 0.40–0.56 second

- PR Interval: absent

- AV Conduction Ratio: absent

- ST Segment: 5 mm depression

- Other Findings: agonal, slow beats

Interpretation: **Asystole with occasional idioventricular complexes**

Reasoning: The rhythm is mainly asystole but a few distorted idioventricular complexes are formed between the long pauses. The ventricular activity is characterized by wide and bizarre QRS complexes that occur at an extremely slow rate. The ST-T waves merge together and distort the complex. This pattern is commonly seen at the end of cardiac resuscitation efforts when a few isolated idioventricular fibers depolarize but are not able to stimulate the dying myocardium. Scattered idioventricular complexes are not able to generate a cardiac output.

FIGURE 18–23

DATA:

- Rate: 60/minute

- Rhythm: irregular

- QRS Duration: sinus: 0.04 second; idioventricular: 0.20 second

- PR Interval: sinus: 0.16 second

- AV Conduction Ratio: sinus: 1:1

- ST Segment: sinus: 1.5 mm elevation with downward coving pattern

Interpretation: **Sinus rhythm with brief episodes of accelerated idioventricular rhythm (beats number 3 through 5, 9, and 10)**

Reasoning: The ECG tracing shows a sinus rhythm which is interrupted at two points by a slow, wide complex rhythm. The wide complexes involved in the three beat episodes (beats number 3 through 5) resemble PVCs. These ectopic beats occur at a faster rate than expected for an escape ventricular pacemaker

(20–40/minute). The rhythm is also slower than for ventricular tachycardia (100/minute). Since it is faster than expected for an *escape* idioventricular rhythm, it is termed an "*accelerated*" idioventricular rhythm.

FIGURE 18–24

DATA:

- Rate: absent

- Rhythm: absent

- QRS Duration: absent

- PR Interval: absent

- AV Conduction Ratio: absent

- ST Segment: absent

Interpretation: Asystole

Reasoning: This is the easiest dysrhythmia to recognize because cardiac activity is absent and the ECG resembles a flat line. Asystole is also the most difficult dysrhythmia to treat because it results from a widespread failure of cardiac electrical activity.

FIGURE 18–25

DATA:

- Rate: 250/minute

- Rhythm: regular

- QRS Duration: 0.20 second

- PR Interval: absent

- AV Conduction Ratio: absent

- ST Segment: absent

- Other Findings: appearance resembles a sine wave

Interpretation: Very rapid ventricular tachycardia (sometimes termed ventricular flutter)

Reasoning: The ventricular rhythm is regular and composed of wide and distorted QRS complexes. As the rate increases well above 200/minute, VT resembles a distorted sine wave—no longer having recognizable QRS complexes and T waves. Very rapid cases of ventricular tachycardia are termed ventricular flutter. Within moments, ventricular fibrillation occurred.

Answers for Chapter 20 ECG Tracings

vals of at least 0.84 second, which corresponds to a rate of 72/minute. Sinus activity resumes after the fourth paced beat. The second group of artificial pacemaker beats also occurs after a pause in sinus activity following the 10th beat.

FIGURE 20–01

DATA:

■ Rate: sinus: 85/minute; paced rhythm: 72/minute

■ Rhythm: irregular

■ QRS Duration: sinus: 0.08 second; paced rhythm: 0.16 second

■ PR Interval: 0.24 second

■ AV Conduction Ratio: sinus: 1:1

■ ST Segment: Elevated for paced beats: number 3–6, 11

Interpretation: Sinus rhythm with first-degree AV block. A pause in sinus activity permits an artificially paced rhythm to develop.

Reasoning: The underlying rhythm is sinus with a first-degree AV block. An artificial pacemaker rhythm with 1:1 capture—that is, every spike is followed by a QRS complex—occurs at two points: beats number 3 to 6, and 11. The artificial pacemaker discharges when long R-R intervals develop due to slowing of the SA node. The pacing device constantly monitors the beat-to-beat ventricular activity and its sensor activates the pacing mode when the rate drops under 73/minute. When the sinus node discharges above the threshold rate, the artificial pacemaker remains in standby. Two types of ventricular activity are seen: some are tall and wide (the paced beats) while others are short and narrow (the sinus beats). The first artificial pacemaker spike begins with beat number 3 and follows R-R inter-

FIGURE 20–02

DATA:

■ Rate: sinus (first two beats only): 30/minute

■ Rhythm: grossly irregular for most of tracing

■ QRS Duration: sinus: 0.12 second

■ PR Interval: sinus 0.32 send

■ AV Conduction Ratio: sinus: 1:1

■ ST Segment: 5 mm depression for first two beats.

Interpretation: Sinus bradycardia with a first-degree AV heart block that changes to ventricular fibrillation following two consecutive PVCs after beat number 2

Reasoning: The first two beats in strip A are sinus because their QRS complexes are narrow and preceded by upright P waves, which have the same fixed interval. A rate of 30/minute is extremely slow for the SA node to continue as the pacemaker because escape atrial, junctional, or ventricular pacemakers usually become active. The PR interval of 0.32 second indicates slowed conduction velocity through the AV node. Two wide and aberrant beats (PVCs) appear after the second sinus beat which leads to ventricular fibrillation-tachycardia. The dysrhythmia in strip B is terminated quickly by successful application of electrical countershock. Defibrillation converts the rhythm to a slow narrow complex rhythm.

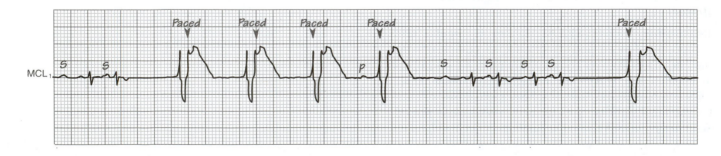

Figure 20-1 Answer

FIGURE 20–03

DATA:

- QRS complexes: absent; pacemaker spikes: 72/minute

- Rhythm: absent

- QRS Duration: absent

- PR Interval: absent

- AV Conduction Ratio: absent

- ST Segment: absent

Interpretation: Noncapturing artificial pacemaker rhythm. No atrial or ventricular activity is associated with pacemaker spikes. The patient's underlying rhythm is asystole

Reasoning: No ventricular or atrial complexes are present. A pacemaker was inserted during cardiac resuscitation efforts. Each pacemaker complex begins with a sharp initial negative deflection. The pulse generator is discharging at a fixed rate of 72 impulses per minute, but the heart muscle is not responding. When the heart fails to respond to an artificial pacer, it is termed "non-capture" or "failure to capture."

FIGURE 20–04

DATA:

- Rate: absent

- Rhythm: chaotic; absent organized rhythm

- QRS Duration: absent

- PR Interval: absent

- AV Conduction Ratio: absent

- ST Segment: absent

Interpretation: Coarse ventricular fibrillation refractory to electrical countershock

Reasoning: Regular cardiac activity is absent in strip A; instead, a chaotic baseline without organized complexes is seen that is typical of ventricular fibrillation. An attempt to terminate the ventricular fibrillation with an electrical countershock causes a sudden deflection of the stylus off the ECG paper with a slow return to midline. The defibrillation is unsuccessful and ventricular fibrillation persists in strip B.

FIGURE 20–05

DATA:

- Rate: initial seven beats: 135/minute; rest of tracing: absent

- Rhythm: initial seven beats: irregular; remainder: absent

- QRS Duration: initial seven beats: 0.10 second

- PR Interval: absent

- AV Conduction Ratio: initial seven beats: 1:1; remainder: absent

- ST Segment: initial seven beats: normal

- Other Findings: abrupt change in rhythm after first seven beats

Interpretation: Sinus tachycardia abruptly changes to ventricular fibrillation after a PVC strikes the T wave of a sinus beat.

Reasoning: Sinus rhythm is present in the first seven beats because P waves are seen, the QRS complexes are narrow, and the PR intervals are fixed. The rhythm is disrupted by a ventricular ectopic beat, which strikes the T wave of the last sinus beat. Ventricular fibrillation resulted and was unsuccessfully countershocked.

FIGURE 20–06

DATA:

- Rate: 60/minute

- Rhythm: regular

- QRS Duration: 0.20 second

- PR Interval: absent

- AV Conduction Ratio: absent

- ST Segment: normal

Interpretation: Artificially paced rhythm is present at 60/minute with 1:1 capture

REASONING: The ventricular rhythm is regular. Each negatively deflected, wide QRS complex is preceded by a tall, upright pacer spike. Atrial activity is missing. Each pacer stimulus results in an associated QRS-T complex and is referred to as 1:1 capture.

FIGURE 20–07

DATA:

- Rate: 74/minute

- Rhythm: regular

- QRS Duration: 0.20 second

- PR Interval: absent

- AV Conduction Ratio: absent

- ST Segment: altered by the pacemaker complex

- Other Findings: varying QRS complex shapes

Interpretation: **Artificially paced rhythm with 1:1 capture. Many nonconducted P waves are visible, indicating an underlying AV heart block**

Reasoning: The ventricular rhythm is regular but the QRS complexes have varying shapes. The QRS complexes are preceded by biphasic pacemaker spikes, that is, a spike that is above and below the baseline. P waves are observed, but they are not associated with (conducted) QRS complexes. Each pacemaker spike is associated with a QRS complex, so there is 1:1 pacemaker capture.

FIGURE 20–08

DATA:

- Rate: ventricular: 42/minute

- Rhythm: ventricular: regular

- QRS Duration: 0.20 second

- PR Interval: absent

- AV Conduction Ratio: absent

- ST Segment: 3 mm elevation

- Other Findings: small negative spikes distort

baseline

Interpretation: **Sinus arrest with a bradycardic ventricular escape rhythm at 42/minute exists. An artificial pacemaker discharges but fails to capture or sense.**

Reasoning: The ventricular rhythm is slow but regular. P waves are absent so AV conduction does not occur. Sinus arrest is the primary ECG disorder, along with failure of the patient's artificial pacemaker. Pacemaker capture is absent, meaning that none of the spikes (labeled "V") cause the myocardium to depolarize. The pacemaker's sensing function is also defective as spikes occur immediately after intrinsic ventricular activity. If the sensor was working properly, it would have been inhibited by the intrinsic heart activity. Three of the spikes in Figure 20–8 Answer can be seen within the ST-T wave complexes of beats number 1, 3, and 6, confirming the device's failure to sense intrinsic cardiac activity.

FIGURE 20–09

DATA:

- Rate: 70/minute

- Rhythm: irregular

- QRS Duration: sinus: 0.08 second; paced beats: greater then 0.20 second

- AV Conduction: 3:2

- PR Interval: sinus beats: 0.20 second, 0.26 second

- ST Segment: sinus: 3 mm elevation; paced beats: 10 mm elevation

- Other Findings: Pattern of two sinus beats followed by an artificially paced beat.

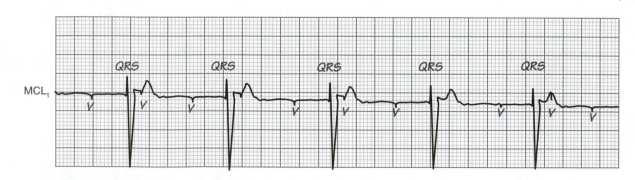

Figure 20-8 Answer

Interpretation: Sinus rhythm with second-degree AV heart block: Mobitz Type I (Wenckebach). An artificial pacemaker detects the pauses and discharges

Reasoning: The ventricular activity is composed of two types of QRS complexes: narrow sinus complexes (beats number 1, 2, 4, 5, 7, and 8) and distorted, artificially paced complexes (beats number 3, 6, and 9—labeled "V"). The AV relationship shows progressive prolongation of the PR intervals before the dropped QRS complexes (Figure 20-9 Answer). Non-conducted P waves are indicated.

Clinical Note There are two dysrhythmias occurring: an underlying heart block and an artificial pacer rhythm. It is important to be able to determine if the pacemaker is properly sensing and capturing and in this case the answer is yes. The artificial pacemaker remains inactive (on standby mode) when the ventricles are stimulated naturally. The artificial pacer functions exactly like a escape pacemaker, which is only activated when higher pacemakers fail to discharge and a pause in cardiac activity is sensed.

FIGURE 20–10

DATA:

- Rate atrial: 70/minute; ventricular: 47/minute; pacer: 46/minute

- Rhythm: regular

- QRS Duration: ventricular escape: 0.20 second

- PR Interval: absent

- AV Conduction Ratio: absent

- ST Segment: escape ventricular beats: 5 mm depression

Interpretation: Complete AV heart block with a bradycardic ventricular escape rhythm at 47/minute. An artificial pacemaker fails to capture the ventricles.

Reasoning: The intrinsic ventricular rhythm is slow at 47/minute, consisting of small, wide QRS complexes (0.16 second). Atrial activity consists of notched P waves occurring at 66/minute. No AV conduction exists since all atrial impulses are blocked. Regular pacemaker spikes are evident at 46/minute but they are *not* associated with QRS-T complexes (Figure 20-10

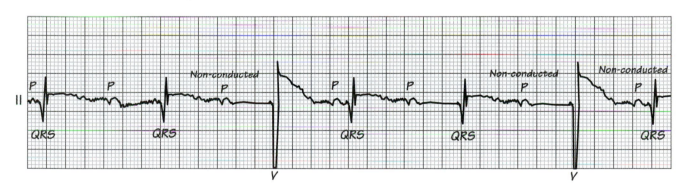

Figure 20-9 Answer

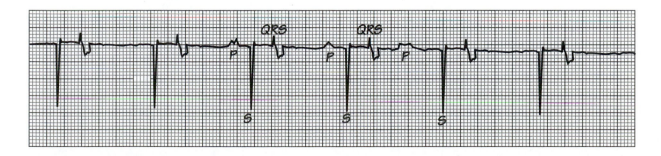

Figure 20-10 Answer

Answer). Failure of the pacer to stimulate (capture) the ventricle is apparent because the large negative pacer spikes are not followed by ventricular complexes.

FIGURE 20–11

DATA:

- Rate: 75/minute

- Rhythm: irregularly irregular

- QRS Duration: conducted beats: 0.18 second; paced beats: 0.20 second

- PR Interval: absent

- AV Conduction: absent

- ST Segment: paced beats: 5 mm elevation

Interpretation: **Atrial fibrillation with a controlled ventricular response. There are also artificially paced beats and an aberrantly conducted atrial beat (beat number 11).**

Reasoning: Ventricular activity consists of at least three differently shaped QRS complexes. The majority of the beats have narrow QRS complexes because they

result from normally conducted atrial fibrillatory waves (beats number 1–3, 6, and 8–9). Complex number 10 is an aberrantly conducted atrial beat with a wide QRS complex. Artificially paced beats (labeled "V") occur whenever the pause after the last QRS reaches 0.88 second. As long as the ventricles are stimulated by the conducted atrial fibrillation waves within the 0.88-second period, the pacer only senses but does not discharge.

FIGURE 20–12

DATA:

- Rate: paced: 79/minute

- Rhythm: regular

- QRS Duration: 0.20 second

- PR Interval: 0.16 second

- AV Conduction Ratio: 1:1

- ST Segment: 2 mm elevation

- Other Findings: multiple pacer spikes with each QRS complex

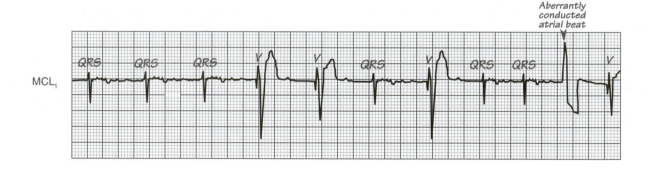

Figure 20-11 Answer

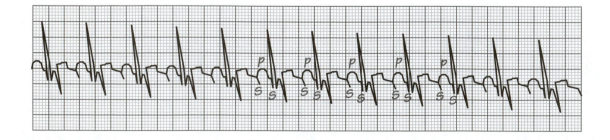

Figure 20-12 Answer

Interpretation: **Artificial AV sequential pacemaker rhythm with 1:1 capture**

Reasoning: The ECG rhythm differs markedly from NSR. The distorted ventricular activity includes a tall, positive spike that is part of the wide QRS complex. The QRS duration is prolonged to about 0.16 second. Regular atrial activity occurs before each QRS complex and consists of a typical, rounded upright P wave—but it differs from NSR in that it is preceded by a large, negative pacer spike. The pacer stimulates the atria when it does not sense regular atrial activity. After 0.20 second, the ventricular pacemaker fires if an intrinsic ventricular depolarization is not detected. The ventricular pacemaker is set to discharge at a fixed interval following the atrial spike because this simulates the natural sequence of heart activation. The AV conduction pattern is normal (1:1) and the PR interval is fixed.

Discussion: The advantages of an AV sequential pacemaker over a single ventricular pacing lead is that a more normal atrioventricular action is simulate because atrial contraction precedes the ventricular contraction. The improved chamber coordination allows the ventricles to more completely fill before contracting. In comparison to single-chamber pacemakers, AV sequential types are more complex and cause more of a battery drain. AV sequential pacemakers are best suited for active individuals who need the added "atrial kick" contribution to stroke volume.

FIGURE 20–13

DATA:

- Rate: paced: 74/minute

- Rhythm: regular

- QRS Duration: 0.20 second

- PR Interval: absent.

- AV Conduction Ratio: absent

- ST Segment: 3 mm elevation

- Other Findings: two pacemaker spikes before each QRS complex

Interpretation: **An artificial AV sequential pacemaker rhythm with failure of the atrial lead to capture while ventricular capture is 1:1.**

Reasoning: The ventricular rhythm is regular and consists of wide and bizarre QRS complexes, which include two pacer spikes for each complex. Each cardiac complex has a *pair* of pacer spikes. The first pacer spike is generated by an atrial lead but it fails to stimulate atrial depolarization. The non-capturing atrial spike occurs before the QRS complex at a distance of 5 mm which corresponds to 0.20 second. P waves are absent because the atrial electrode has lost contact with the right atrial endocardium.

FIGURE 20–14

DATA:

- Rate: pacer: 93/minute

- Rhythm: regular

- QRS Duration: 0.20 second

- PR Interval: absent

- AV Conduction Ratio: absent

- ST Segment: 3 mm depression

Interpretation: **Asystole during the first half of the tracing is followed by an artificially paced rhythm with 1:1 capture.**

Reasoning: The initial half of the ECG tracing shows a flat line without electrical activity. Ventricular activity exists during the latter half of the tracing and is reflected by wide, distorted QRS-T complexes. Each cardiac complex is preceded by a small negatively deflected pacer spike. Atrial activity is missing. This ECG tracing was recorded during a resuscitation effort for asystole, which was not responsive to medication. Despite the presence of adequate capture complexes, pulses were not detected. This reinforces the need to assess the patient—rather than relying solely on what the ECG tracing displays—whenever a rhythm changes during a resuscitation.

FIGURE 20–15

DATA:

- Rate: 72/minute

- Rhythm: irregular

- QRS Duration: intrinsic: 0.08 second; paced: 0.24 second

- PR Interval: absent

- AV Conduction Ratio: 1:1

- ST Segment: 12 mm elevation

Interpretation: Artificially paced rhythm in strip A with 1:1 capture. The ninth beat is a normally conducted natural beat. Strip B was recorded several minutes later and shows only pacer spikes with two agonal idioventricular complexes.

Reasoning: In strip A, every pacemaker spike is followed by QRS-T complex; whereas in strip B, none of the spikes stimulate the ventricles. The myocardium is damaged and cannot respond. Two intrinsic agonal beats that arose from a ventricular focus are noted in the second tracing.

> **Clinical Note** *Two reasons for pacemaker failure involve: (a) the pacemaker electrode does not adequately contact the cardiac tissue, or (b) the electrodes make good contact but the myocardium is diseased and unresponsive. Scar tissue can form around the pacemaker tip and prevent an adequate stimulus strength.*

FIGURE 20–16

DATA:

- Rate: 75/minute

- Rhythm: irregular during the last third of the tracing

- QRS Duration: 0.16 second

- PR Interval: absent

- AV Conduction Ratio: absent

- ST Segment: 2 mm elevation

- Other Findings: ECG baseline is chaotic during the last third of tracing

Interpretation: Artificially paced rhythm with an episode of lost capture

Reasoning: The overall rhythm looks grossly irregular, but aside from the last third of the tracing, the rhythm is regular. The QRS complexes are wide and distorted. Pacemaker spikes appear throughout the tracing—even when there are no associated QRS complexes. When pacemaker spikes (labeled "V") occur without ventricular capture, it is termed "loss of ventricular capture." In this case, pacemaker failure could have occurred for several reasons: loss of electrode contact with the ventricle, inadequate pulse generator output, or increased myocardium resistance, as occurs after the first month of pacing. The underlying rhythm, which is seen during the period of pacer failure, is atrial fibrillation.

FIGURE 20–17

DATA:

- Rate: sinus: 70–75/minute; pacer rhythm: 72/minute

- Rhythm: regular

- QRS Duration: sinus: 0.10 second; paced beats: 0.20 second

- PR Interval: sinus: 0.16 second

- AV Conduction Ratio: sinus: 1:1

- ST Segment: sinus: normal; paced beats: 5 mm depression

Interpretation: NSR at 75/minute which slows slightly, allowing an artificially paced rhythm at a rate of 72/minute to discharge

Reasoning: There are narrow as well as wide QRS complexes. The narrow complexes are sinus paced

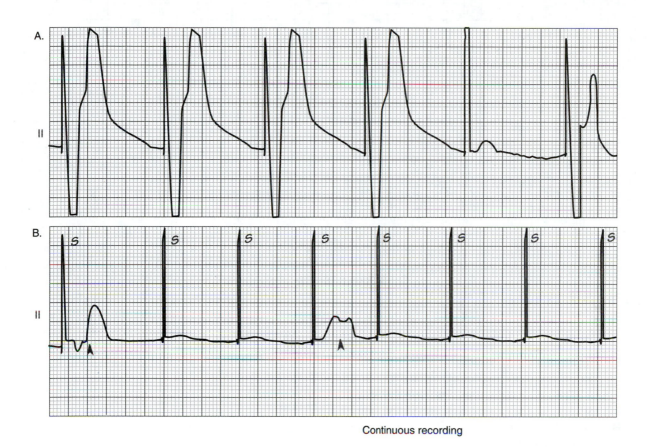

Continuous recording

Figure 20-15 Answer

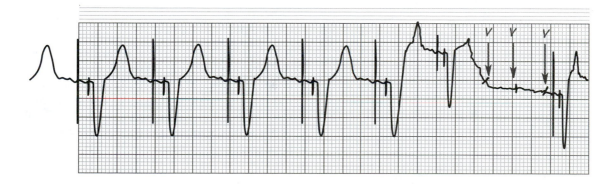

Figure 20-16 Answer

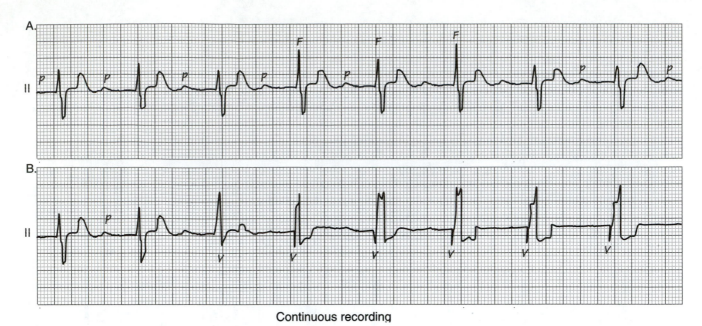

Figure 20-17 Answer

beats. The wide complex rhythm (labeled "V") is a paced rhythm. The AV conduction ratio for the sinus beats is 1:1. Several of the complexes are fusion complexes (labeled "F"), having both sinus and artificially paced complex characteristics.

Clinical Note If the presence of the pacemaker spikes had not been appreciated, the paced rhythm might have been mistaken for an accelerated idioventricular rhythm, because the rhythm arises suddenly and is a wide QRS complex rhythm that lacks P waves.

FIGURE 20–18

DATA:

- Rate: strip A: 150/min

- Rhythm: strip A: regular except at end

- QRS Duration: 0.36 second

- PR Interval: absent

- AV Conduction Ration: absent

- ST Segment: massively distorted

Interpretation: **Ventricular tachycardia at 150/minute that deteriorates suddenly into ventricular fibrillation.**

Reasoning: The rhythm is regular during most of strip A. The complexes are wide and distorted and occur at a rate well over 100/minute. Toward the end of strip A, the rhythm suddenly changes to a very irregular pattern. Strip B has classic signs of ventricular fibrillation: absence of organized cardiac complexes and a chaotic baseline.

FIGURE 20–19

DATA:

- Rate: absent

- Rhythm: chaotic

- QRS Duration: 0.20 second

- PR Interval: absent

- AV Conduction Ratio: absent

- ST Segment: absent

Interpretation: **Strip A displays ventricular fibrillation with defibrillation artifact**

Reasoning: Ventricular activity consists of a wavy baseline but there are no organized complexes. Atrial activity is missing. After the two defibrillations, the rhythm remains asystolic for nine seconds until three isolated, distorted QRS complexes are seen in strip B.

FIGURE 20–20

DATA:

- Rate: A: 150/minute; B: 55/minute; C: occasional complexes

- Rhythm: regular

- QRS Duration: 0.8 second

- PR Interval: absent

- AV Conduction Ratio: absent

- ST Segment: normal

- Other Findings: bradycardia-tachycardia pattern

Interpretation: **Supraventricular tachycardia at 150/minute. The rate slows to 50/minute in strip B and asystole is present in strip C.**

Reasoning: Ventricular activity is composed of narrow QRS complexes. P waves are missing in all strips. The rate of the ventricular complexes changes dramatically. The ventricular rhythm suddenly slows beginning in strip B and essentially stops in strip C. Only irregular and occasional ventricular complexes are seen in strip C. Asystole represents failure of the sinus pacemaker along with any escape pacemakers.

Answers for Chapter 24 ECG Tracings

FIGURE 24–1

■ **Pacemaker:** Sinus

■ **Dysrhythmias: Second-degree AV heart block; Mobitz Type I Wenckebach; 3:2 AV conduction. The ventricular rate is 100/minute.**

Interpretation: Acute inferior wall myocardial infarction with second-degree AV block; Mobitz Type I

Reasoning: The ventricular rhythm is irregular and there are acute ST segments in leads II, III, and aVF. The ST segments are elevated 4 mm from the baseline in leads III and a VF. The ST segments have a sharp take-off angle from the QRS complex merging with the T waves. Reciprocal ST depression is present in leads I and aVL. A Wenckebach AV heart block exists based on the presence of the following findings:

■ irregular ventricular rhythm;

■ grouped beating (two P-QRS-T complexes followed by a pause);

■ regular P-P intervals; and

■ progressive increase of the PR intervals for two beats, followed by a dropped QRS-T complex.

FIGURE 24–2

■ **Pacemaker:** Sinus

■ **Dysrhythmias:** None

Interpretation: Sinus rhythm with inferior-lateral ischemia and prior anterior wall MI

Reasoning: T waves are inverted in leads II, III, and aVF (which are the inferior leads) as well as leads V_4 through V_6, which view the lateral heart surface. The T waves are symmetrically inverted 3 mm in the lateral leads. The T wave abnormalities occur in a distinct anatomic pattern and suggest ischemia. QS complexes are seen in leads V_1 through V_3 indicating a past anterior wall MI. It is not possible to determine how long in the past the MI occurred but there are no signs of an acute process because the ST segments are not elevated or depressed and the T waves remain upright. The QS complexes seen in the first three precordial leads causes what is termed "poor R wave progression," this is caused by the loss of R wave height due to the past MI and results in QS complexes without R waves.

FIGURE 24–3

Pacemaker: Sinus
Dysrhythmias: None

Interpretation: Sinus rhythm with acute anterior wall MI and lateral wall ischemia

Reasoning: Pathologic QS complexes exist in precordial leads V_1 through V_4 along with ST segment elevation that shows an acutely rounded "coving" shape. The ECG appearance of elevated ST segments with abnormally shaped ST segments happen during an acute MI. The ST segments are beginning to return to baseline but the T waves remain inverted in all precordial leads along with leads I and aVL. These findings are consistent with acute ischemia of the lateral heart wall.

FIGURE 24–4

■ **Pacemaker:** Sinus

■ **Dysrhythmias:** None

Interpretation: Sinus rhythm with semi-acute inferior-lateral MI

Reasoning: Pathologic Q waves are seen in leads II, III, and aVF (inferior) as well as leads V_3 through V_6 (lateral). Pathological Q waves indicate transmural (full thickness) myocardial damage. There is some suggestion that a recent MI has occurred since 1 mm ST segment elevation still exists in leads V_3, III, and aVF.

FIGURE 24–5

■ **Pacemaker:** AV junctional escape

■ **Dysrhythmias:** Sinus arrest

Interpretation: AV junctional escape rhythm at 38/minute with an acute inferior wall MI with posterior wall extension and lateral reciprocal ST depression

Reasoning: P waves are not visible. A narrow QRS complex bradycardic rhythm exists. The ST segments in the inferior leads of II, III, and aVF are elevated 3 mm from the ECG baseline, signifying an acute process. Reciprocal ST segment 4 mm depression occurs across the precordial leads of (V_2 through V_6) along with lateral leads of I and aVL. Posterior wall MIs have R waves and ST depression in leads V_1 to V_3. These are "mirror" image findings rather than the usual ST elevation and Q waves.

FIGURE 24–6

- **Pacemaker:** Sinus

- **Dysrhythmias:** None

Interpretation: Acute inferior-lateral-posterior wall MI

Reasoning: Acute ST segments are massively elevated (7 to 8 mm) in the inferior leads II, III, and aVF. There is also 2 mm ST elevation in the lateral leads V_6 and V_6. ST depression in leads V_1 and V_2 coupled with prominent R waves is indicative of a posterior wall MI, which complicates 10 to 20 percent of inferior wall MIs. Posterior wall injury patterns occur in leads V_1 through V_3 and show what is termed "mirror" images of other heart areas. Instead of pathologic Q waves and ST elevation, R waves and ST depression appear instead. Right-sided chest leads show an associated right ventricular MI (Figure 24–6B). ST elevation is found in right precordial leads VR_4 through VR_6. Reciprocal ST segment depression occurs in leads I, aVL, and V_1, to V_3.

FIGURE 24–7

- **Pacemaker:** Sinus

- **Dysrhythmias:** None

Interpretation: Acute anterior wall MI

Reasoning: The ST segments in leads V_1 through V_3, which face the anterior surface of the heart, are elevated in an acute injury pattern. QS complexes are present in the chest leads V_1 and V_2. QS complexes develop when transmural myocardial damage causes the loss of R wave height while pathologic Q waves form. The remaining R wave in V_3 is only 1-2 mm tall. The ST segment shape in leads V_1 through V_3 is abnormal because it forms an acute oblique path after leaving the QRS complex. The sharp ST segment take-off is indicative of acute injury and may happen even before ST elevation begins. The T waves are tall and peaked in leads V_2 through V_4.

FIGURE 24–8

- **Pacemaker:** Sinus

- **Dysrhythmias:** Sinus tachycardia and PACs with abberancy

Interpretation: Sinus tachycardia at 140/minute with an acute inferior wall MI and anterior-lateral ischemia

Reasoning: The massively elevated ST segments in leads II, III, and aVF indicate acute myocardial injury. A pathological Q wave in lead III indicates transmural myocardial damage. Marked reciprocal ST depression exists across all precordial leads along with leads I and aVL.

FIGURE 24–9

- **Pacemaker:** Sinus

- **Dysrhythmias:** None

Interpretation: Sinus rhythm with an anterior wall MI. This tracing was recorded 24 hours after the acute event.

Reasoning: The ST segments are elevated in anterior leads V_1 through V_4. The ST segment shapes that show "coving" or a horizontal takeoff are abnormal in leads V_1 through V_5. T wave inversions are present in the same leads. R waves have been lost in leads V_1 and V_2 while QS complexes have developed, indicating transmural damage.

FIGURE 24–10

- **Pacemaker:** Sinus

- **Dysrhythmias:** Sinus bradycardia

Interpretation: Sinus rhythm with Wolff-Parkinson-White (W-P-W) syndrome

Reasoning: ST depression is present in leads I, aVL, and V_3 through V_5 due to W-P-W syndrome. The QRS complexes appear wider than normal due to the slurred upstrokes, which are termed "delta" waves. The PR intervals appear shortened, which is also secondary to the delta waves caused by ventricular preexcitation. W-P-W involves a congenital accessory bypass tract that links the atria and ventricles.

Discussion: The main problem associated with W-P-W is that rapid atrial impulses bypass the AV node and overstimulate the ventricles. W-P-W also obscures the diagnosis of an MI because the delta wave prevents Q wave development and the ST segments are chronically distorted. The ST segments are distorted in leads I, aVL, and V_2 to V_3 .

FIGURE 24–11

- **Pacemaker:** Atrial reentry

■ **Dysrhythmias:** Atrial flutter

Interpretation: Atrial flutter with a ventricular response of 150/minute

Reasoning: The rhythm is a narrow QRS complex tachycardia. P´ waves have been replaced by flutter waves: regular, rapid P waves that have a constant shape. The lead II rhythm strip at the bottom of the page shows the classical sawtooth or picket-fence pattern of atrial waves that distorts the ECG baseline. The AV conduction ratio is 2:1 leading to the ventricular rate of 150/minute because the atrial rate in flutter is always 300/minute.

FIGURE 24–12

■ **Pacemaker:** Sinus

■ **Dysrhythmias:** None

Interpretation: Sinus rhythm with an inferior-lateral wall MI of undetermined age

Reasoning: Pathologic Q waves are present in the inferior leads III and aVF. T wave inversion exists in leads II, III, aVF, and in the lateral leads V_3 through V_6. While the ST segments in leads II, III, and aVF have an abnormally flat appearance, ST segment elevation is not present.

FIGURE 24–13

■ **Pacemaker:** Sinus

■ **Dysrhythmias:** None

Interpretation: Normal sinus rhythm with an acute anterior-lateral myocardial infarction.

Reasoning: There is significant ST segment elevation in the anterior leads V_2 through V_5, and the lateral leads I and aVL. R waves height has been lost in the precordial leads. The T waves are peaked in leads V_2 and V_3 averaging a striking 13 mm in lead V_3. Reciprocal ST segment depression occurs in leads III and aVF.

FIGURE 24–14

■ **Pacemaker:** Sinus

■ **Dysrhythmias:** None

Interpretation: Sinus rhythm with a left bundle branch block (LBBB)

Reasoning: The QRS complexes are wide and distorted. The T waves are directed opposite to the QRS complexes. The QS complex is caused by the deep, slurred S waves in lead V_1 and poor R wave progression, The rSR´ ventricular complexes in V_6 are typical of a left bundle branch block. Tall and widened R waves with a slurred upstroke are present in leads I, aVL, and V_5 and V_6. ST depression occurs in leads I, aVL, and V_5 and V_6, while ST elevation occurs in leads V_1 through V_3 in a LBBB. The rhythm is regular and the wide QRS complexes are preceded by P waves indicating a sinus rhythm.

Discussion. A Left bundle branch block always indicates a diseased heart. While an acute left BB block can occur during an MI, most cases are chronic conditions. Hypertensive and coronary artery diseases are the most common causes of left bundle branch block. Acute causes involve myocardial infarction, congestive heart failure, and inflammation of the pericardial sac or myocardium (pericarditis and myocarditis). Left bundle branch blocks obscure the diagnosis of a myocardial infarction because Q waves cannot develop and the ST segments are already distorted.

FIGURE 24–15

■ **Pacemaker:** Sinus

■ **Dysrhythmias:** None

Interpretation: A recent (subacute) anterior-lateral wall MI.

Reasoning: The anterior surface of the heart is reflected in the precordial leads which show 2 mm ST elevation in leads V_2 and V_3 with deeply inverted T waves in V_2 through V_6. There are also minor T wave inversions in leads I and aVL. The ECG findings suggest that an MI happened one to several days ago. It takes several days for the ST segments to return to baseline after an MI, while the T wave inversion may remain for weeks.

FIGURE 24–16

■ **Pacemaker:** AV junctional re-entry

■ **Dysrhythmias:** Supraventricular tachycardia

Interpretation: Supraventricular tachycardia (SVT)

Reasoning: The ventricular activity consists of narrow QRS-T wave complexes that lack clear P waves. There are no ECG signs of an acute ischemic condition because there are no ST segment elevations or T wave inversions. The sinus node is no longer the pacemaker since P waves are lacking. Since the QRS durations are 0.10 second or less, the rhythm had to have arisen from a supraventricular site. Because there are no flutter or fibrillation waves and the rhythm is regular, the dysrhythmia must be a SVT, which most likely originated in the AV node via a re-entry circuit

FIGURE 24–17

■ **Pacemaker:** Sinus

■ **Dysrhythmias:** None

Interpretation: Acute inferior wall MI.

Reasoning: The QRS complexes in the inferior leads of II, III, and aVF look very wide because the ST segments are massively elevated in an acute myocardial injury pattern. Reciprocal ST segment depression is present in leads aVL and aVR.

FIGURE 24–18

■ **Pacemaker:** Atrial

■ **Dysrhythmias:** Atrial fibrillation with a bradycardic ventricular response

Interpretation: Atrial fibrillation with a bradycardic ventricular response of 30-40/minute. A prior inferior wall MI is noted.

Reasoning: The QRS complexes are narrow, indicating a supraventricular pacemaker. The ventricular rate is very slow. Fibrillation (f) waves are clearly seen in leads V_1 and V_2 and the lead II rhythm strip. There are no ST segment changes or T wave inversions. Since atrial fibrillation is characterized as a tachydysrhythmia, a bradycardic ventricular rate results from overtreatment. The medication, probably a calcium channel blocker or beta blocker has decreased AV node conduction. The QRS complexes leads II, III, and aVF signify a past MI but there are no acute ST segment elevations so the MI happened in the past.

FIGURE 24–19

■ **Pacemaker:** Artificial

■ **Dysrhythmias:** None

Interpretation: Artificial pacemaker rhythm with 1:1 capture

Reasoning: The QRS complexes are wide and distorted. There are no P waves. A pacemaker spike immediately precedes each QRS complex. The pacemaker is functioning properly.

FIGURE 24–20

■ **Pacemaker:** Sinus

■ **Dysrhythmias:** None

Interpretation: Sinus rhythm with a right bundle branch block (RBBB)

Reasoning: The QRS complexes are wide and show a notched configuration. The findings of an rSR´ complex in V_1 and a broad S wave in V_6, I, and aVL are indicative of a right bundle branch block. During a RBBB, the right ventricle is not activated directly by the right bundle branch. Instead, the left bundle branch activates the left ventricle in the normal fashion and then crosses the septum to reach the right ventricle. Because the right bundle branch becomes activated later than normal, the QRS duration will be prolonged. The QRS complex will have an abnormal appearance, usually a rSR´ since the impulse travels across the septum from the left ventricle. The QRS complex in RBBB is at least 0.11 second and has a triphasic appearance (r-S-R´ components). The T wave also shows secondary changes (inversion) related to the altered depolarization process in lead V_1.

Answers for Chapter 26 ECG Tracings

FIGURE 26–1

DATA:

- Rate: 70/minute

- Rhythm: irregular (beats number 3 to 5 disrupt an otherwise regular rhythm)

- QRS Duration: sinus: 0.06 second; ventricular 0.14 second

- PR Interval: 0.16 second

- AV Conduction Ratio: 1:1

- ST Segment: normal

- Other Findings: pointed T waves

Interpretation: **Sinus rhythm with a three-beat episode of accelerated idioventricular rhythm (AIVR)**

Reasoning: Aside from the aberrant beats (number 3, 4, and 5), the rhythm has normal sinus beats. The three consecutive aberrant beats show typical ventricular characteristics:

- wide QRS complexes

- lack of P waves

- T wave deflections in a direction opposite to the major QRS complex (discordant T waves)

The ectopic beats occur at a rate of 70/minute, which is less than the 100/minute that would have classified this dysrhythmia as ventricular tachycardia. The T waves are peaked which is usually associated with high serum potassium levels. Accelerated idioventricular rhythms commonly develop the first or second day following a myocardial infarction. Even before the use of thrombolytic therapy, this was frequently observed during an MI. Accelerated idioventricular rhythms are common during myocardial reperfusion and this benign dysrhythmia subsides spontaneously.

FIGURE 26–2

DATA:

- Rate: sinus and junctional escape: 40/minute

- Rhythm: irregular

- QRS Duration: 0.08 second

- PR Interval: 0.20 second

- AV Conduction Ratio: 1:1

- ST Segment: 1.5 mm elevation

Interpretation: **Sinus bradycardia shifting to an AV junctional escape rhythm due to sinus block**

Reasoning: The QRS complexes of both the sinus and junctional rhythms are identical, confirming that both pacemakers originated in a supraventricular pacemaker site. Many junctional complexes lack atrial activity. When P waves are seen, they appear just ahead of the QRS complexes, as expected for sinus beats. The main finding that indicates a changing pacemaker site rests with the configuration of P waves. P waves are clearly present for some of the beats, while they are absent for other ventricular complexes.

Discussion: It is not uncommon to see backup pacemakers discharge when sinus node activity is depressed—or fails completely—and an escape focus emerges. Enhanced vagal tone is a common cause of sinus depression. The automaticity range of the AV junction is between 40 and 60 per minute; while the normal range for sinus activity is 60 to 100/minute. Junctional escape paced rhythms are transient and subside as soon as the sinus node resumes control.

FIGURE 26–3

DATA:

- Rate: 64/minute

- Rhythm: irregular

- QRS Duration: 0.08 second

- PR Interval: atrial: 0.02 second; sinus: 0.16 second

- AV Conduction Ratio: 1:1

- ST Segment: 3 mm elevation

- Other Findings: changing P wave shapes

Interpretation: **Sinus rhythm with a wandering atrial pacemaker (WAP)**

Reasoning: The ventricular complexes are normal and have identical shapes regardless of the pacemaker's origin. Beats number 1, 7, 8, and 9 are sinus complexes, while beats number 2 through 6 arise from an ectopic atrial focus and have biphasic P waves. Each QRS complex is preceded by a P wave, but the shapes of the atrial waves differ. Beat numbers 4 and 6 have P waves that develop from the fusion activity of two pacemakers: they start off having a rounded shape as the atria are stimulated by the sinus node while they are simultaneously activated by a lower atrial focus. The simultaneous depolarization of joint pacemakers results in a P wave that has an initial rounded portion as well as a sharp, inverted part. Along with varying P wave sizes, the ectopic beats have different PR intervals yet AV conduction ratio remains 1:1.

> ***ECG Interpretation Tip*** *A wandering atrial pacemaker (WAP) is sometimes confused with the emergence of an escape rhythm caused by sinus depression. In escape rhythms, the ectopic pacemaker emerges after a pause that is longer than the normal R-R interval and represents a backup system to stimulate the heart. In contrast, during WAP the sinus rate is adequate but there is a transient shift and competition between supraventricular pacemakers.*

FIGURE 26–4

DATA:

- Rate: absent
- Rhythm: absent
- QRS Duration: absent
- PR Interval: absent
- AV Conduction Ratio: absent
- ST Segment: absent
- Other Findings: there is a total lack of an organized rhythm

Interpretation: **Coarse ventricular fibrillation (VF)**

Reasoning: Organized QRS complexes or P waves do not exist. The erratic tracing reflects chaotic ventricular activity. The rhythm is characterized as coarse because the size of the waves ae at least 5 mm tall.

FIGURE 26–5

DATA:

- Rate: 47/minute
- Rhythm: regular
- QRS Duration: 0.12 second
- PR Interval: 0.32 second
- AV Conduction Ratio: 1:1
- ST Segment: normal
- Other Findings: mild baseline artifact

Interpretation: **Sinus bradycardia at a rate of 47/minute with a prolonged PR interval**

Reasoning: The ventricular and atrial activity are normal. The key differences from normal sinus rhythm include a PR interval beyond 0.20 second and a slow sinus rate. Both characteristics result from increased vagal tone, which decreases conduction velocity and slows sinus node activity. After a significant delay, each P wave eventually passes through the AV node.

> ***ECG Interpretation Tip*** *The tracing was not labeled as "first-degree AV block" because the sinus rate is bradycardic. For a prolonged PR interval to be accurately termed a first-degree AV block, the rate must be at least 60/minute.*

FIGURE 26–6

DATA:

- Rate: 75/minute
- Rhythm: regular
- QRS Duration: 0.08 second
- PR Interval: 0.16 second
- AV Conduction Ratio: 1:1
- ST Segment: normal (based on the first beat)
- Other Findings: baseline is distorted

Interpretation: **Normal sinus rhythm is disguised by artifact caused by patient movement**

Reasoning: Artifact distorts the baseline and makes it difficult to see the P and T waves for most of the strip. The QRS complexes, however, can still be identified.

Artifact causes the wavy baseline to superficially mimic atrial fibrillation. Unlike true atrial fibrillation, however, the R-R interval remains constant and P waves can be seen as part of several complexes.

FIGURE 26–7

DATA:

■ Rate: absent

■ Rhythm: absent complexes; regular pacemaker spikes

■ QRS Duration: absent

■ PR Intervals: absent

■ AV Conduction Ratio: absent

■ ST Segment: absent

■ Other Findings: regular pacemaker spikes are not associated with cardiac complexes

Interpretation: **Pacemaker rhythm without cardiac capture. Asystole is the underlying rhythm.**

Reasoning: The spike artifact is created by the pacemaker's pulse generator. Pacemaker spikes without capture are recognized by the small sharp baseline deflections. The spikes are not accompanied by a single myocardial capture. The heart is electrically silent because the myocardium is too diseased to respond to external stimulation.

FIGURE 26–8

DATA:

■ Rate: 132/minute

■ Rhythm: regular

■ QRS Duration: 0.08 second

■ PR Interval: 0.16 second

■ AV Conduction Ratio: 1:1

■ ST Segment: 1.5 mm depression

■ Other Findings: rapid narrow-complex tachycardia

Interpretation: **Sinus tachycardia at a rate of 132/minute**

Reasoning: This tracing is a sinus tachycardia because:

■ ventricular activity is regular with normally shaped QRS complexes;

■ regular R-R intervals and consistent P waves shapes;

■ normal AV conduction; and

■ the rate is over 100/minute.

FIGURE 26–9

DATA:

■ Rate: 46/minute

■ Rhythm: irregular

■ QRS Duration: 0.16 second

■ PR Interval: 0.16 second

■ AV Conduction Ratio: 1:1 for sinus beats

■ ST Segment: 4 mm depression

■ Other Findings: biphasic T waves

Interpretation: **Sinus bradycardia at a rate of 46/minute shifting to an AV junctional escape rhythm at a rate of 40/minute**

Reasoning: Ventricular activity consists of wide QRS complexes—even for beats number 1 through 4, which have clearly associated P waves. The last three beats do not have P waves and must have arisen within the AV junction because the QRS complexes are identical to those of the sinus beats. The escape pacemaker activity of the AV junction discharges only when the ventricles fail to be stimulated.

FIGURE 26–10

DATA:

■ Rate: 114/minute

■ Rhythm: irregular

■ QRS Duration: 0.08 second

■ PR Interval: 0.16 second

■ AV Conduction Ratio: 1:1

■ ST Segment: "scooped-out" appearance

■ Other Findings: QRS complexes have varying sizes

Interpretation: Sinus tachycardia with frequent PACs. This dysrhythmia is also termed multifocal atrial tachycardia (MAT).

Reasoning: The QRS complexes generally look the same, except for the two that are slightly taller than the surrounding beats. The striking features of the PACs are the irregular R-R intervals and the fluctuating shapes of the P and P' waves. AV conduction is normal and frequent PACs are seen. Multifocal atrial tachycardia is defined as an irregular rhythm with a rate over 100/minute having three or more different P waves. The size of the QRS complexes vary and this is termed *electrical alternans*, which is seen in congestive heart failure and pericardial effusion. Multifocal atrial tachycardia (MAT) is usually found in patients with chronic obstructive pulmonary disease (COPD). MAT, in essence, is a tachycardic rhythm with frequent PACs. MAT develops due to atrial dilatation caused by increased pulmonary resistance in COPD.

FIGURE 26–11

DATA:

- Rate: ventricular: 37/minute; sinus: 74/minute
- Rhythm: regular
- QRS Duration: 0.08 second
- PR Interval: 0.16 second
- AV Conduction Ratio: 2:1
- ST Segment: normal
- Other Findings: twice as many P waves as QRS complexes

Interpretation: Second degree AV heart block with 2:1 AV conduction and a bradycardic ventricular rate at 37/minute

Reasoning: The ventricular rhythm is regular and the QRS complexes have a normal appearance. The atrial rhythm is also regular but occurs twice as fast as the ventricular rate. There are two P waves for each QRS complex because only one of each pair of the P waves is conducted, while the other is blocked. A slow ventricular response of 37 bpm results from the 2:1 AV block.

FIGURE 26–12

DATA:

- Rate: ventricular: 39/minute
- Rhythm: regular
- QRS Duration: 0.12 second
- PR Interval: absent
- AV Conduction Ratio: absent
- ST Segment: 2.5 mm elevation
- Other Findings: many more P waves than QRS complexes

Interpretation: Third degree (complete) AV heart block with a bradycardic ventricular rate of 39/minute

Reasoning: The ventricular rhythm is slow and regular. The distorted QRS complexes are wide and notched. The atrial rhythm is regular and more rapid than the ventricular activity. Because these are an excess of P waves, some type of AV block must be present. In order to identify the specific conduction disorder, the relationship between the P waves and the QRS complexes should be examined. The easiest way is to plot the PR intervals for the P waves that immediately precede each QRS complex. If the PR intervals have a fixed duration, it would be an incomplete block—that is, a second-degree block; Mobitz Type II. If the PR intervals show a progressive increase, then a specific form of second-degree block—Wenckebach—would exist. The P waves appear to "march through" the QRS complexes because AV dissociation exists. Many P waves are scattered among the ST segments and T waves, making them hard to see. An independent escape pacemaker originates within the His-Purkinje system in the ventricular conduction pathway to pace the ventricles.

FIGURE 26–13

DATA:

- Rate: sinus: 70/minute; ventricular: 170/minute
- Rhythm: irregular
- QRS Duration: sinus: 0.12 second; ventricular: 0.20 second
- AV Conduction Ratio: sinus: 1:1
- PR Interval: sinus: 0.16 second
- ST Segment: 2 mm depression

■ Other Findings: short burst of distorted beast

Interpretation: Sinus rhythm with non-sustained-ventricular tachycardia (VT).

Reasoning: There are two types of QRS complexes: a slower, group with narrower complexes and a rapid rhythm with distorted complexes in the center of the ECG strip. The slower beats are preceded by P waves, which have the same appearance. A single wide-complex beat occurs after beat number 3 and this is a PVC. Following the fifth beat, a group of four rapid, wide-complex beats occurs that lack P waves and have T waves, which aim in a direction opposite to the QRS complexes. This is a brief (nonsustained) bout of ventricular tachycardia.

FIGURE 26–14

DATA:

■ Rate: sinus: 110/minute; ventricular: 40/minute

■ Rhythm: irregular

■ QRS Duration: 0.16 second

■ PR Interval: 0.20 second

■ AV Conduction Ratio: variable: 2:1 to 3:1

■ ST Segment: 6 mm elevation

■ Other Findings: more P waves than QRS complexes

Interpretation: High grade, second-degree AV heart block; Mobitz Type II with a bradycardic ventricular rate of 45/minute

Reasoning: The ventricular complexes are wide and irregular. Atrial activity is regular and the P waves are normal. The AV conduction ratio varies. For some groups of QRS complexes, a 2:1 conduction exists, whereas others have a 3:2 AV relationship. A high grade form of second degree AV heart block is present when consecutive P waves are blocked. In the case of Mobitz Type II heart block, a high grade block indicates that there is a more advanced form of conduction disturbance than when only a single P wave is blocked. For instance, when three consecutive P waves are blocked, only one of every four P waves is conducted in a 4:1 AV conduction.

Discussion: There are several ECG findings in this tracing that cause concern about the status of this patient's AV conduction. First, the heart block is a high grade type which is a serious form of heart block. Second, the QRS complexes are wide and distorted, indicating abnormal intraventricular conduction. Also, the ST segments are markedly elevated, pointing toward myocar-

dial ischemia/ injury. The patient's rhythm needs to be monitored very closely for the sudden development of complete AV heart block.

FIGURE 26–15

DATA:

■ Rate: 85/minute

■ Rhythm: regular

■ QRS Duration: 0.24 second

■ PR Interval: 0.20 second

■ AV Conduction Ratio: 1:1

■ ST Segment: 7 mm "scooped out" depressed appearance

Interpretation: Sinus rhythm with an intraventricular conduction delay

Reasoning: The ventricular rhythm is regular but the QRS durations are wider than normal. The atrial rhythm is regular and the P waves are normal. The AV conduction ratio is 1:1 and the rate is within 60 to 100 beats per minute. ST segment depression indicates abnormal ventricular repolarization. There are several reasons why depressed ST segments occur, including ischemia, drugs, such as digitalis, and as a secondary repolarization event that is associated with abnormal depolarization as caused by the large energy flow associated with ventricular hypertrophy.

FIGURE 26–16

DATA:

- Rate: 200/minute

- Rhythm: regular

- QRS Duration: 0.06 second

- PR Interval: absent

- AV Conduction Ratio: absent

- ST Segment: 4 mm depression

- Other Findings: rapid narrow complex tachycardia

Interpretation: **Supraventricular tachycardia (SVT) at 200/minute**

Reasoning: The rapid ventricular rhythm is regular and consists of narrow complexes, indicating that they arose from a supraventricular focus. Atrial activity is missing so an AV relationship is not measurable. This dysrhythmia is a paroxysmal supraventricular tachycardia. As Figure 26–16 ans. shows, the dysrhythmia terminated abruptly when the patient performed a Valsalva maneuver by bearing down and straining against a closed glottis as if having a bowel movement. Valsalva maneuvers increase vagal tone and are sometimes effective in terminating supraventricular reentry tachydysrhythmias.

FIGURE 26–17

DATA:

- Rate: 60/minute

- Rhythm: grossly irregular

- QRS Duration: 0.04 second

- PR Interval: absent

- AV Conduction Ratio: not measurable

- ST Segment: 3 mm elevation

- Other Findings: wavy baseline

Interpretation: **Atrial fibrillation with a controlled ventricular response of 60/minute**

Reasoning: The ventricular rhythm is grossly irregular and the QRS complexes are narrow, indicating that they arose from a supraventricular focus. Regular atrial activity is absent. The atrial activity consists of very rapid waves that have been estimated from electrophysiology studies to range from 350 to 600/minute and cause the baseline to resemble a fine wavy line. Atrial fibrillation with a controlled ventricular response, meaning a rate under 100/minute, only occurs following treatment. Untreated atrial fibrillation has a ventricular rate between 140 and 160/minute.

FIGURE 26–18

DATA:

- Rate: 75/minute

- Rhythm: irregular

- QRS Duration: 0.06 second

- PR Interval: 0.14 second

- AV Conduction Ratio: 3:2

- ST Segment: 2 mm elevation

- Other Findings: grouped beating

Interpretation: **Sinus rhythm with frequent nonconducted PACs and a single aberrantly conducted PAC (beat number 11)**

Reasoning: The ventricular pattern is irregular consisting of two beats separated by pauses. The atrial rhythm is also irregular in a similar manner. The AV conduction ratio is 3:2 for each group where only two QRS complexes are conducted. The clue to the correct interpretation is the peaked T waves occurring immediately before the pauses. The tall, distorted T waves are caused by hidden P′ waves that occur so early during a refractory phase that the P′ waves are not conducted. The last QRS complex in the tracing is a PAC that was aberrantly conducted because the PAC occurs

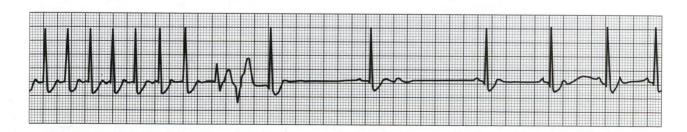

Figure 26-16 Answer

later than the nonconducted P′ waves and encounters a partially repolarized ventricule. The last beat follows a tall, distorted T wave.

FIGURE 26–19

DATA:

- Rate: 230/minute

- Rhythm: irregular

- QRS Duration: 0.20 second

- PR Interval: absent

- AV Conduction Ratio: absent

- ST Segment: merges with QRS complexes

- Other Findings: waxing-waning rhythm and complex sizes

Interpretation: Torsade de Pointes (TdP), which is also known as polymorphic ventricular tachycardia, at a rate of 230/minute

Reasoning: The ventricular complexes appear wide because the ST segments merge into the QRS complexes. This V$_1$ tracing differs from traditional monomorphic ventricular tachycardia, which consists of identically appearing QRS-T complexes. During Torsade de Pointes, in contrast, the ventricular axis continually shifts from positive to negative, causing it to appear as if the axis of the QRS complexes rhythmically swing above and below the ECG baseline.

FIGURE 26–20

DATA:

- Rate: 42/minute

- Rhythm: irregular

- QRS Duration: sinus: 0.10 second; ventricular: 0.18 second

- PR Interval: 0.14 second

- AV Conduction Ratio: 1:1

- ST Segment: 4 mm depression

- Other Findings: both narrow and wide QRS complexes are present

Interpretation: Sinus bradycardia at a rate of 42/minute with escape ventricular complexes

Reasoning: The ventricular activity consists of two types of complexes: narrow and wide QRSs. The narrow-complex QRS beats are preceded by P waves. The wide complex beats (beats number 3 and 6) lack P waves, and are ventricular in origin. They have ST-T complexes opposite in direction to the abnormal QRS deflections. This rhythm is a sinus bradycardia with escape ventricular ectopic complexes.

Discussion: Suppressing ventricular beats with lidocaine in the setting of such a slow sinus rhythm is not indicated. A better approach would be accelerating the sinus rate in a controlled fashion. This can be done by using an external pacemaker if the patient is symptomatic. A faster sinus rate will automatically suppress the ectopic beats.

FIGURE 26–21

DATA:

- Rate: ventricular: 40/minute; atrial: 60/minute

- Rhythm: ventricular: irregular; atrial: regular

- QRS Duration: 0.10 second

- PR Interval: progressive increments: 0.16 second; 0.24 second; then a dropped QRS beat

- AV Conduction Ratio: 3:2 and 5:4

- ST Segment: normal

- Other Findings: grouped beating

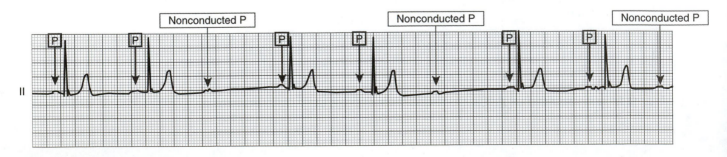

Figure 26-21 Answer

Interpretation: **Sinus rhythm with second-degree AV heart block; Mobitz Type I (Wenckebach) with a variable AV conduction of 3:2 and 2:1 and an average ventricular rate of 45/minute**

Reasoning: The ventricular rhythm shows grouped beating: cycles of two beats separated by a pause. In strip B a group of four P-QRS-T complexes is flanked on either side by pauses. All ventricular complexes have narrow QRS complexes. The atrial activity is regular, signifying normal sinus activity, while some ventricular beats are missing (Figure 26–16 Answer). The PR intervals show a pattern: increasing durations that are followed by a dropped QRS, after which the cycle repeats again. The last P wave of each set of grouped beats is not conducted (see Figure 26–16 Answer). The resulting pause allows the AV node to become fully repolarized and the next arriving P wave is conducted with the shortest PR interval. In strip B, a different conduction cycle of 5:4 follows the 3:2 AV conduction ratio. Conduction of each successive P wave becomes more difficult until the pause from the blocked QRS allows the AV node to recover.

FIGURE 26–22

DATA:

- Rate: (A) 150/minute; (B) 75/minute

- Rhythm: (A) regular; (B) irregular

- QRS Duration: (A) 0.36 second; (B) 0.20 second

- PR Interval: absent

- AV Conduction Ratio: absent

- ST Segment: distorted

- Other Findings: wide, distorted complexes

Interpretation: **Ventricular tachycardia that degenerates into an accelerated idioventricular rhythm after a brief asystolic pause**

Reasoning: Wide and distorted QRS complexes, which lack P waves, indicate that the dysrhythmia originated within the ventricle. In strip A, the rate is so fast that the rhythm looks like a regular sine wave that is termed ventricular flutter. P waves, PR intervals, and AV conduction ratios are absent. In strip B a less organized and slower rhythm follows a brief pause. This rhythm was recorded during a cardiac resuscitation and a short time later. cardiac standstill occurred

FIGURE 26–23

DATA:

- Rate: 45/minute

- Rhythm: irregular

- QRS Duration: 0.10 second

- PR Interval: sinus: 0.20 second

- AV Conduction Ratio: 1:1

- ST Segment: 2 mm depression

- Other Findings: biphasic T waves

Interpretation: **Sinus bradycardia at 45/minute with two consecutive PACs (beats number 4 and 5)**

Reasoning: There are two early beats in the middle of the tracing that disrupt the regular ventricular rhythm. The two early beats look identical to the surrounding P-QRS-T complexes. P waves are seen before every narrow QRS complex, indicating that they are supraventricular impulses. A single P wave precedes every R wave, so 1:1 AV conduction exists. The PR intervals are constant and the P waves are notched. Sinus bradycardia is present because the rate is below 60/minute along with two premature atrial complexes In most cases, the P wave shapes and the PR intervals for the PACs will differ from the sinus beats but that is not the case here.

FIGURE 26–24

DATA:

- Rate: 110/minute

- Rhythm: regular

- QRS Duration: 0.08 second

- PR Interval: 0.16 second

- AV Conduction Ratio: 1:1

- ST Segment: 1 mm elevation

- Other Findings: peaked T and P waves

Interpretation: **Sinus tachycardia at 110/minute**

Reasoning: Each cardiac cycle consists of normal appearing P-QRS-T complexes. The PR intervals and AV conduction ratios are normal. The SA node is discharging faster than 100/minute. In adults, sinus tachycardia occurs between 100 and 150/minute but in certain cases the rate may even rise to 180/minute. In small children and infants who are severely stressed, sinus rates commonly exceed 175/minute. Severely taxed infants can even exceed 200/minute.

FIGURE 26–25

DATA:

- Rate: 75/minute

- Rhythm: regular

- QRS Duration: 0.16 second

- PR Interval: 0.20 second

- AV Conduction Ratio: 1:1

- ST Segment: 5 mm. depression.

- Other Findings: wide QRS complexes

Interpretation: Sinus rhythm with an intraventricular conduction defect (IVCD)

Reasoning: The ventricular rhythm is regular with constant R-R intervals. The QRS complexes are wide but the depressed ST segment makes a precise measurement of the QRS duration difficult. A single P wave occurs before each QRS complex, resulting in a constant 1:1 AV conduction ratio. Sinus rhythm is present even though the QRS complex is abnormal.

The QRS complex is wider than normal so a delay in the depolarization of the ventricles is present. The most common reason for this is due to a depolarization delay in one or both bundle branches. Lead MCL_1 or V_1 must be used to determine whether the block is occurring in the right or left bundle.

FIGURE 26–26

DATA:

- Rate: absent

- Rhythm: absent

- QRS Duration: absent

- PR Interval: absent

- AV Conduction Ratio: absent

- ST Segment: absent

- Other Findings: flat line appearance

Interpretation: Asystole

Reasoning: The total absence of electrical activity is evident by a flat ECG. During an isoelectric phase, current does not flow between heart cells because complete cardiac cycles are missing. The complete lack of electrical activity makes resuscitation very difficult as there is no cell excitability.

FIGURE 26–27

DATA:

- Rate: 170/minute

- Rhythm: regular

- QRS Duration: 0.10 second

- PR Interval: absent

- AV Conduction Ratio: absent

- ST Segment: 3 mm depression

- Other Findings: regular, rapid, narrow QRS complex rhythm

Interpretation: Supraventricular tachycardia (SVT) at 170/minute

Reasoning: The ventricular rhythm is precisely regular and the QRS complexes are narrow. A QRS duration of 0.06 to 0.08 second signifies that the ventricles are being activated normally and that the pacemaker impulse must have arisen from a pacemaker site *above* the bifurcation of the His bundle. Supraventricular sites include sinus, atrial, and junctional pacemakers, which all have narrow QRS complexes. Distinct atrial waves are *not* visible in most SVTs. The upright deflections that are seen between the R waves are actually T waves, although they are commonly mistaken for P waves. Paroxysmal SVT means that the dysrhythmia's start or end is abrupt. PSVT is one form of a larger dysrhythmia group known as SVTs, which are narrow complex, rapid dysrhythmias: atrial fibrillation, junctional tachycardia, atrial flutter, multifocal atrial tachycardia (MAT), and sinus tachycardia.

FIGURE 26–28

DATA:

- Rate: 57/minute
- Rhythm: regular
- QRS Duration: 0.08 second
- PR Interval: 0.36 second
- AV Conduction Ratio: 1:1
- ST Segment: normal
- Other Findings: regular, narrow complex rhythm

Interpretation: Sinus bradycardia with a prolonged PR interval

Reasoning: The regularly occurring QRS complexes are narrow. One P wave precedes each ventricular complex that has a fixed PR interval. The PR interval is prolonged beyond 0.20 second, indicating that a delay occurs before ventricular activation starts. This rhythm is *not* considered to be a first-degree AV block because the sinus rate is less than 60/minute. Transiently prolonged PR intervals commonly accompany bradycardic rates when there is enhanced parasympathetic tone.

FIGURE 26–29

DATA:

- Rate: 90 to 100/minute
- Rhythm: grossly irregular
- QRS Duration: 0.08 second
- PR Interval: absent
- AV Conduction Ratio: 1:1
- ST Segment: 1 mm depression
- Other Findings: grossly irregular pattern

Interpretation: Atrial fibrillation with a controlled ventricular response of 90–100/minute

Reasoning: The R-R intervals are grossly irregular but the ventricular complexes are normal. P waves or other atrial waves are not seen; instead, a flat baseline is present. Fibrillatory (f) waves are not detected in certain leads because the main vector (direction of energy) is oriented perpendicular to the lead's recording electrodes. The waves are so small in this ECG strip that they appear almost flat. The major clue that atrial fibrillation exists is the grossly irregular ventricular activity consisting of narrow QRS complexes.

FIGURE 26–30

DATA:

- Rate: absent
- Rhythm: absent
- QRS Duration: absent
- PR Interval: absent
- AV Conduction Ratio: absent
- ST Segment: absent
- Other Findings: almost flat baseline

Interpretation: Fine amplitude ventricular fibrillation

Reasoning: No ventricular or atrial complexes exist. The wavy baseline consists of very small waves that are no higher than 3 mm. For maximal defibrillation success, the coarseness of the waves need to be increased with epinephrine and CPR.

> ***ECG Interpretation Tip*** *The ECG recorder should be checked to make sure that it is properly calibrated or else the tracing will have an misleading size. For instance, if the standardization control is set on 1/2 standardization, a complex that should yield a 10 mm deflection will appear only half as tall. The rhythm should be checked in other leads because fine amplitude ventricular fibrillation has masqueraded as asystole in leads that record perpendicular to the main energy direction. Full standardization settings should be used and the lead selection should be confirmed in cases of asystole.*

FIGURE 26–31

DATA:

- Rate: 65/minute
- Rhythm: regular
- QRS Duration: 0.08 second
- PR interval: (A) 0.28 second; (B): 0.56 second
- ST Segment: normal
- Other Findings: biphasic T waves

Interpretation: Sinus rhythm with first-degree AV heart block

Reasoning: The ventricular rhythm is regular and the QRS complexes are narrow. Each QRS complex is preceded by a P wave in a 1:1 relationship. The PR intervals are considerably longer than the upper limit of normal. The PR interval in strip A is 0.28 second while in strip B, which was recorded a few minutes later, doubles to 0.56 second. The prolonged PR interval in strip B causes the P waves to merge with the T waves. If only the bottom ECG strip was present, the ECG rhythm could easily have been mistaken for a junctional rhythm with distorted T waves. Following atropine administration, the first degree AV block reversed to NSR.

FIGURE 26–32

DATA:

- Rate: 25/minute
- Rhythm: regular
- QRS Duration: > 0.20 second
- PR Interval: absent
- AV Conduction Ratio: absent
- ST Segment: massively elevated
- Other Findings: slow, bizarrely shaped, large complexes

Interpretation: Sinus block (arrest) with an idioventricular escape rhythm at 25/minute

Reasoning: The ventricular rhythm is regular but the complexes are very wide with a distorted shape that no longer resembles normal QRS-T complexes. The QRS complexes are very large and the ST segments are elevated at least 15 mm. No atrial activity is seen. The term "agonal activity" is commonly used to describe very slow idioventricular rhythms. The rhythm subsequently failed altogether and several agonal idioventricular beats appeared just before death.

FIGURE 26–33

DATA:

- Rate: 150/minute
- Rhythm: regular
- QRS Duration: 0.20 second
- PR Interval: absent
- AV Conduction Ratio: absent
- ST Segment: difficult to measure because of absent isoelectric baseline
- Other Findings: rapid, distorted rhythm

Interpretation: Ventricular tachycardia (VT) at 150/minute

Reasoning: The ventricular activity is rapid and consists of distorted and wide QRS complexes. No P waves are visible. The rhythm looks like a string of rapid PVCs linked together. AV conduction is not present. Sustained episodes of ventricular tachycardia compromise cardiac output, produces severe signs and symptoms, and requires aggressive therapy.

FIGURE 26–34

DATA:

- Rate: 50/minute
- Rhythm: regularly irregular
- QRS Duration: 0.06 second
- PR Interval: 0.16 second
- AV Conduction Ratio: 1:1
- ST Segment: normal
- Other Findings: regularly irregular ventricular pattern

Interpretation: Sinus bradycardia with atrial trigeminy; a PAC occurs following two sinus beats

Reasoning: The ventricular activity is regularly irregular. The QRS complexes, including the early beats, have a normal QRS configuration. Atrial activity, in contrast, consists of different shapes: every third beat has a more rounded appearance than the other P waves. The atrial rhythm has the same rhythm as the ventricles: the third P wave of each cycle is a P´ wave that occurs early during the R-R intervals. The PACs are beats number 3, 6, and 9.

FIGURE 26–35

DATA:

- Rate: 55/minute

- Rhythm: irregular

- QRS Duration: 0.06 second

- PR Interval: 0.2 second

- AV Conduction Ratio: 1:1 for most P waves but some P´ waves are not conducted

- ST Segment: normal

- Other Findings: negative wave after beats number 3 and 7

Interpretation: **Sinus bradycardia at 55/minute with one conducted PAC and two nonconducted PACs**

Reasoning: The ventricular rhythm is irregular but the QRS complexes are normal. The fifth beat is a conducted PAC. The atrial complexes have different P and P wave shapes. The P´ wave of the fifth beat can be seen deforming the T wave of beat number 4. The two inverted round waves, which follow beats number 3 and 7, are nonconducted P´ waves. They could represent junctional beats or atrial beats, but without an associated QRS complex it is not possible to determine. Nonconducted PACs are the most frequent causes of pauses in cardiac activity.

FIGURE 26–36

DATA:

- Rate: ventricular: 30/minute; atrial: 75/minute

- Rhythm: ventricular: regular; atrial: regular

- QRS Duration: 0.10 second

- PR Interval: absent

- AV Conduction Ratio: absent

- ST Segment: normal

- Other Findings: many more P waves than QRS complexes

Interpretation: **Complete AV heart block and a ventricular escape rhythm at 30/minute**

Reasoning: The ventricular rhythm is regular but very slow. The bradycardic QRS complexes look surprisingly narrow. Atrial activity consists of rapid and regular P waves. There is no fixed AV relationship so an AV conduction ratio is absent. Independent atrial and ven-

tricular rhythms are characteristic of complete AV dissociation.

FIGURE 26–37

DATA:

- Rate: 74/minute

- Rhythm: regular

- QRS Duration: 0.14 second

- AV Conduction Ratio: absent

- PR Interval: absent

- ST Segment:

- Other Findings: isolated P waves; small spikes occur before the QRS complexes

Interpretation: **Artificial pacemaker rhythm with 1:1 capture**

Reasoning: The ventricular rhythm is regular with wide and distorted QRS complexes. The initial component of each QRS complex consists of a small pacemaker spike. Scattered P waves can be seen but are not conducted. Each pacemaker spike results in a ventricular depolarization complex, termed 1:1 capture. The patient's underlying rhythm, which can be assessed by observing the many nonconducted P waves is a complete AV heart block.

FIGURE 26–38

DATA:

- Rate: ventricular: 75/minute; atrial: 300/minute

- Rhythm: regular

- QRS Duration: 0.08 second

- AV Conduction Ratio: 4:1

- PR Interval: 0.12 second

- ST Segment: distorted by flutter waves

- Other Findings: "saw-tooth" baseline pattern

Interpretation: **Atrial flutter with 4:1 AV conduction and a ventricular rate of 75/minute**

Reasoning: The ventricular rhythm is regular and the QRS complexes are narrow. Atrial activity consists of sharp waves having a positive and negative component, which gives the appearance of the teeth of a saw blade or the top of a picket fence. There are four flutter (F) waves for each QRS complex yielding a 4:1 conduction ratio and a rate of 75/minute. Most examples of atrial flutter have constant AV conduction ratios yielding a repetitive pattern of beats. In the present case, the conduction ratios change between 3:2 and 2:1. The reason for variable conduction is because therapy was started and the medication is affecting AV conduction. Untreated atrial flutter has a fixed ratio.

FIGURE 26–39

DATA:

- Rate: ventricular: 60/minute; atrial: 75/minute

- Rhythm: ventricular: irregular; atrial: regular

- QRS Duration: 0.08 second

- PR Intervals: varies: 0.22 second; 0.28 second dropped beat

- AV Conduction Ratio: variable: 3:2 and 2:1

- ST Segment: normal

- Other Findings: pauses in cardiac activity

Interpretation: Sinus rhythm with second-degree AV heart block; Mobitz Type I (Wenckebach); variable AV conduction (3:2 and 2:1)

Reasoning: The ventricular activity is composed of normal appearing QRS complexes with an irregular rhythm. Atrial activity consists of regular upright P waves. The key findings that identify this as a Wenckebach form of heart block include:

- regular P-P intervals;

- progressively increasing PR intervals;

- grouped QRS complexes beating; and

- dropped QRS complexes due to nonconducted P waves.

FIGURE 26–40

DATA:

- Rate: 60/minute

- Rhythm: regularly irregular

- QRS Duration: 0.06 second

- PR Interval: 0.18 second

- AV Conduction Ratio: 1:1

- ST Segment: normal

Interpretation: Sinus rhythm with a

sinus dysrhythmia

Reasoning: The ventricular complexes are normal but the rhythm is regularly irregular. Atrial activity consists of normal upright P waves but the rhythm is regularly irregular. The PR intervals are fixed and normal. The AV conduction ratio is 1:1. This ECG tracing differs from NSR only in that the sinus rhythm is irregular. During sinus dysrhythmias the SA node discharges in a *regularly irregular* pattern, which is due to the autonomic changes associated with breathing. During inhalation the heart rate increases as the sinus node discharges faster and the cardiac cycles crowd closer together. Conversely, during exhalation, the sinus node slows and the cardiac complexes spread further apart.

> ***Clinical Note*** *Sinus dysrhythmia is more pronounced in young children and patients with advanced chronic lung disease (COPD). Sinus dysrhythmia is really only a variation of normal sinus rhythm and not a pathologic rhythm disturbance. Considering its benign nature, the only reason to recognize sinus dysrhythmia is to be able to tell it apart from more serious causes of irregular rhythms, such as heart blocks.*

FIGURE 26–41

DATA:

- Rate: sinus: 55/minute; pacer beats: 60/minute

- Rhythm: irregular

- QRS Duration: sinus: 0.08 second; paced beats: 0.20 second

- PR Interval: 0.16 second for sinus beats

- AV Conduction Ratio: 1:1 for sinus beats

- ST Segment: sinus: 1 mm depression; paced beats: 3 mm elevation

- Other Findings: sinus beats have inverted T waves

Interpretation: Sinus bradycardia at 55/minute with artificially paced beats with 1:1 capture

Reasoning: The ventricular rhythm is irregular and the QRS complexes have variable shapes. Beats number 1, 2, and 9 are wide and distorted. They are proceeded by a pacemaker spike and lack P waves: these are artificially paced beats. Beats number 3, 4, 6, and 7 have P waves before the narrow QRS complexes and are sinus beats with a normal PR interval and 1:1 AV conduction. Beats number 5 and 8 have an unusual appearance because they share characteristics of both paced and intrinsic beats: P waves and pacer spike. The 5th and 8th beats are *fusion beats* because the QRS complexes share components from both types of beats. Fusion beats are formed when the sinus impulse and the pacemaker device simultaneously depolarize heart tissue. As a result, fusion beats have both a P wave as well as a pacemaker spike.

This ECG rhythm is a sinus bradycardia because the rate is just below 60 per minute. Artificially paced beats occur when the sinus rate drops below 60/minute. The artificial pacemaker functions similar to an intrinsic escape pacemaker—silent when the sinus rate is faster than the programmed pacer discharge rate and active when the ventricles have not been paced for one or more seconds.

FIGURE 26–42

DATA:

- Rate: (A) ventricular: 30/minute; atrial: 56/minute (B) ventricular: 26/min.; atrial: absent

- Rhythm: ventricular: (A and B) regular; atrial: (A) irregular; (B) absent

- QRS Duration: (A and B) 0.06 second

- PR Interval: (A and B) absent

- AV Conduction Ratio: (A and B) absent

- ST Segment: (A) normal: (B) 4 mm elevation

- Other Findings: unassociated P waves

Interpretation: **Sinus rhythm with a complete AV heart block and an AV junctional escape rhythm at 35/minute in Strip A. Strip B is a sinus block with an extremely slow junctional rhythm at 20/minute.**

Reasoning: In strip A the ventricular rhythm is regular with normal QRS complexes that are not related to regular P waves. The atrial rhythm is irregular, having 56 P waves per minute but they are *not* associated with QRS complexes. One pacemaker controls the atria while another paces the ventricles. Their function is uncoordinated so third-degree AV block is present.

In strip B there are no longer two pacemakers: only a slow, regular QRS rhythm at 26/minute without any P waves. Because P waves are no longer seen in strip B, sinus failure has developed in addition to the complete heart block. The slow rate reflects a passive junctional

escape rhythm because the QRS complex is 0.10 second or less. However, most junctional rhythms discharge between 40 and 60/minute. A short time later the junctional pacemaker also failed and asystole occurred.

FIGURE 26–43

DATA:

- Rate: 75/minute

- Rhythm: regular

- QRS Duration: 0.10 second

- PR Interval: 0.20 second

- AV Conduction Ratio: 1:1

- ST Segment: 5 mm elevation

- Other Findings: biphasic T waves

Interpretation: **Normal sinus rhythm at 75/minute**

Reasoning: The ventricular and atrial activity is normal with a 1:1 AV conduction ratio. No deviations from NSR are found. The ST segments are elevated and the T waves are biphasic. The negative component dips 5 mm below the baseline. No dysrhythmias are present in this tracing.

FIGURE 26–44

DATA:

- Rate: 130/minute

- Rhythm: regular

- QRS Duration: 0.10 second

- PR Interval: absent

- AV Conduction Ratio: absent

- ST Segment: 5 mm depression

- Other Findings: ST segments are distorted by retrograde P waves

Interpretation: **AV junctional form of supraventricular tachcycardia at 130/minute**

Reasoning: The ventricular rhythm is rapid and regular with distorted QRS complexes. Significant abnormalities of the ST-T wave segments do not allow a precise measurement of QRS duration. The atrial activity is regular, but it *follows* the QRS complex rather than preceding it as in NSR. The P waves that follow the QRS complexes are termed *retrograde impulses* because the atria were stimulated by an ectopic impulse that traveled backwards through the AV pathway. Escape junctional pacemakers discharge between 40 and 60/minute. Enhanced automaticity of a junctional focus or the establishment of an AV nodal reentry cycle are the likely causes of the junctional tachycardia.

FIGURE 26–45

DATA:

- Rate: 250 to 300/minute

- Rhythm: grossly irregular

- QRS Duration: between 0.16 and 0.24 second

- PR Interval: absent

- AV Conduction Ratio: absent

- ST Segment: not measurable

- Other Findings: ventricular complex sizes vary greatly

Interpretation: **Torsade De Pointes (TdP) is also known as polymorphic ventricular tachcycardia**

Reasoning: The ventricular complexes rhythmically alter their major axis from a positive to a negative direction. The ventricular rate is extremely fast and the QRS complexes appear to twist about the baseline alternately pointing above and below the ECG baseline. Atrial activity is absent so AV conduction does not occur. This tracing initially looks like the chaotic rhythm that occurs in ventricular fibrillation. However, upon closer inspection, the rhythmic variation in the QRS complex sizes is seen. Electrical cardioversion is indicated to treat both dysrhythmias.

FIGURE 26–46

DATA:

- Rate: 80/minute

- Rhythm: regular

- QRS Duration: 0.12 second

- PR Interval: 0.24 second

- AV Conduction Ratio: 1:1

- ST Segment: normal

- Other Findings: inverted T waves

Interpretation: **Sinus rhythm with a first-degree AV heart block at 80/minute**

Reasoning: The QRS complexes have a regular rhythm and a wide shape of 0.12 second duration. Each QRS is preceded by a single P wave that has a constant PR interval. The atrial rhythm has fixed P-P intervals. The PR duration of 0.24 second indicates a prolonged of conduction time before the ventricles are activated. The delay involved is a first-degree AV block and is localized to the AV node.

FIGURE 26–47

DATA:

- Rate: 160/minute

- Rhythm: regular

- QRS Duration: 0.24 second

- PR Interval: absent

- AV Conduction Ratio: absent

- ST Segment: distorted by the wide QRS-T complex

- Other Findings: wide QRS complex tachycardia

Interpretation: **Ventricular tachycardia (VT) at 160/minute**

Reasoning: The rapid ventricular rhythm resembles a series of rapidly occurring PVCs. The QRS complexes are wide and bizarre without associated atrial activity. P waves are present but are lost within the wide QRS complexes because they lack a fixed relationship to ventricular activity.

FIGURE 26–48

DATA:

- Rate: 70/minute

- Rhythm: regularly irregular

- QRS Duration: sinus: 0.08 second; PVC: 0.20 second

- PR Interval: sinus: 0.18 second; PVC: absent

- AV Conduction Ratio: sinus: 1:1; PVC: absent

- ST Segment: sinus: normal; PVC: elevated and opposite to the PVC's QRS complex

- Other Findings: regular alternating pattern: a narrow QRS complex is followed by a wide QRS complex

Interpretation: **Sinus rhythm with ventricular bigeminy; every other sinus beat is a PVC**

Reasoning: The ventricular rhythm is regularly irregular; the R-R intervals display a repeating short-long/short-long pattern. The QRS complexes have two shapes: narrow with sharp waves and wide with distorted waves. Atrial activity can only be seen before the narrow QRS complexes, indicating a sinus origin. The wide QRS complexes come early, or prematurely, during the R-R interval; therefore every other beat is a PVC. A reentry dysrhythmia mechanism links a PVC with the preceding sinus beat.

FIGURE 26–49

DATA:

- Rate: ventricular: 150/minute

- Rhythm: regular

- QRS Duration: 0.06 second

- PR Intervals: absent

- AV Conduction Ratio: absent

- ST Segment: normal

- Other Findings: narrow complex tachydysrhythmia

Interpretation: Supraventricular tachycardia (SVT) at 150/minute

Reasoning: The ventricular rhythm is regular and occurs well over 100 times per minute. Atrial activity is not detectable. The positive deflection noted between the QRS complexes may be T waves or atrial waves. Because P waves are missing yet the QRS complexes are 0.10 second or less, this dysrhythmia must be a supraventricular tachycardia (SVT). In an effort to further identify the particular form of SVT that is present, diagnostic maneuvers are useful. For instance, digital pressure over only one carotid sinus in the neck (or carotid sinus massage, CSM) was briefly applied. CSM caused a reflex increase in vagal tone, which increased AV nodal refractoriness and resulted in reentry impulse interruption. Flutter waves became visible and the ECG interpretation became clear: atrial flutter with 2:1 AV conduction with a ventricular response of 150/minute.

FIGURE 26–50

DATA:

- Rhythm: (A) ventricular: regular; atrial: regular

- Rate: (A) ventricular: 50/minute; atrial: 120/minute

- QRS Duration: (A) 0.20 second

- PR Interval: absent

- AV Conduction Ratio: absent

- ST Segment: 5 mm elevation

- Other Findings: The ECG recorder computer analyzes the tracing and prints an upward pointing arrow at the bottom of the strip to indicate where the pacer spike occurs. The printer also places an inverted triangle above the sensed intrinsic beats in strip B. Strip A is recorded *without* the external pacemaker activated.

Interpretation: Complete AV heart block is present in strip A. An artificial pacemaker begins to function in strip B and fully captures the heart in strip C.

Reasoning: In strip A the characteristic findings of a third degree AV block are present: regular ventricular rhythm, regular atrial rhythm, but no relationship between them. The QRS complexes occur at a rate below 60/minute and are wide and distorted. In strip B, intrinsic beats are marked by the recorder as an inverted solid triangle, while pacer spikes are marked at the bottom of the tracing by an upright arrow. The pacemaker output was being adjusted during strip B by increasing the pulse generator's power output. Note the mark: "73 mA (milliamp)" at the top of the tracing. In strip C the pacer output has been increased to 111 milliamp, resulting in all pacemaker spikes capturing the ventricle and palpable pulses.

FIGURE 26–51

DATA:

- Rate: ranges from 45 to 70/minute

- Rhythm: irregularly irregular

- QRS Duration: 0.06 second

- PR Interval: absent

- AV Conduction Ratio: absent

- ST Segment: normal

- Other Findings: long ECG pauses

Interpretation: **Atrial fibrillation at a slow rate of approximately 45 to 50/minute**

Reasoning: The ventricular rhythm is irregularly irregular and the QRS complexes are narrow. The ventricular rate is very slow. The atrial activity lacks P waves and is replaced by a fine fibrillatory baseline. There is random AV conduction resulting in the irregular rhythm. Toward the beginning and end of the tracing, the QRS complexes are grouped together. A bradycardic ventricular response in the setting of rapid atrial tachydysrhythmias is usually due to overtreatment with medication that results in a pharmacological AV block. Drugs that are commonly responsible for abnormally slow ventricular rates include diltiazem, beta blockers, and digoxin. When untreated, new-onset atrial fibrillation usually has a ventricular rate in the range of 150/minute. The best treatment for reversing medication overtreatment is to let the drug wear off as it is metabolized. If a more rapid response is required in an unstable patient, the ventricular rate can be increased with an external artificial pacemaker, but this is rarely needed.

FIGURE 26–52

DATA:

- Rate: 40/minute

- Rhythm: regular

- QRS Duration: 0.06 second

- PR Interval: 0.14 second

- AV Conduction Ratio: 1:1

- ST Segment: normal

Interpretation: **Sinus bradycardia at 40/minute**

Reasoning: The ventricular activity is composed of narrow QRS complexes and a regular rhythm. Each regularly occurring P wave is followed by a single QRS complex yielding a 1:1 AV conduction ratio. The PR interval is normal. The sinus rate is 40 per minute, which is much slower than the rate of 60 per minute normally expected for NSR rhythms.

FIGURE 26–53

DATA:

- Rate: ventricular: 35/minute; atrial: 70/minute

- Rhythm: regular

- QRS Duration: 0.12 second

- PR Interval: 0.20 second

- AV Conduction Ratio: 2:1

- ST Segment: 4 mm depression

- Other Findings: twice as many P waves as QRS complexes

Interpretation: **Sinus rhythm with second-degree AV heart block and a 2:1 AV conduction with a ventricular rate of 35/minute**

Reasoning: The ventricular activity is a regular rhythm with wide complexes occurring at a slow rate. There are twice as many P waves as QRS complexes. The PR intervals for the conducted P waves are fixed and the AV conduction ratio is 2:1, which represents a second degree AV heart block. To determine which form of incomplete AV block is present requires inspection of two consecutively conducted P waves for PR interval prolongation. Because every other P wave is dropped, this is not possible in this case.

Discussion: It is possible to make a pretty good guess about whether Mobitz I or II is present by looking at the PR intervals and the QRS durations. This ECG strip shows a *wider than normal* QRS duration, while the PR interval is normal. The abnormal QRS duration points toward an *intraventricular* conduction delay, which is more likely to be associated with a Mobitz Type II because it is an *infra*nodal problem. A Wenckebach block, in contrast, represents a *nodal* delay that would have had a prolonged PR interval—which Figure 26–53 did not have.

FIGURE 26–54

DATA:

- Rate: 85/minute

- Rhythm: irregular at points

- QRS Duration: 0.08 second

- PR Interval: 0.16 second

- AV Conduction Ratio: 1:1

- ST Segment: normal

- Other Findings: tall, pointed P waves.

Interpretation: Sinus rhythm with two PACs (beats number 6 and 11)

Reasoning: The ventricular activity is composed of narrow complexes but there are two differently shaped QRS complexes. The distorted QRS complexes of beats number 6 and 11 occur during the early portion of the R-R interval. Atrial activity consists of tall, pointed P waves. The two early beats lack clear atrial waves which are probably hidden within the preceding T waves. This tracing shows the hallmark findings of a PAC:

- narrow, normally shaped QRS complexes;

- altered P´ waves;

- 1:1 AV conduction; and

- occur early during the R-R interval.

FIGURE 26–55

DATA:

- Rate: ventricular: 60/minute; atrial: 120/minute

- Rhythm: regular

- QRS Duration: 0.12 second

- PR Intervals: 0.14 second

- AV Conduction Ratio: 2:1

- ST Segment: 3 mm elevation

- Other Findings: twice as many P waves as QRS complexes

Interpretation: Sinus rhythm with second-degree AV heart block with a 2:1 AV conduction at a ventricular rate of 60/minute

Reasoning: The ventricular rhythm is regular and the QRS duration is slightly longer than normal. Atrial activity consists of P waves at a rapid rate of 120 per minute, which is twice the ventricular rate and indicates that *every other* P wave is blocked. A 2:1 AV conduction defect is present and this is a second degree AV heart block. Because the QRS complexes are wider than normal and the PR intervals of the conducted beats are normal, the AV block is probably a Mobitz Type II. Wide QRS complexes represent an infranodal block and Mobitz Type II block occurs below the AV node, usually in the bundle branches.

FIGURE 26–56

DATA:

- Rate: 160/minute

- Rhythm: irregular

- QRS Duration: 0.06 second

- PR interval: absent

- AV Conduction Ratio: absent

- ST Segment: normal

- Other Findings: rapid, narrow QRS complex rhythm

Interpretation: Atrial fibrillation with a ventricular rate of 160/minute

Reasoning: The ventricular activity is composed of rapid narrow QRS complexes with an irregular rhythm. At first glance it may be difficult to appreciate the irregular rhythm because the rate is so rapid, but a careful examination will reveal R-R interval variability. P waves are missing and the atrial activity is composed of fibrillatory (f) waves. Again, because the R-R intervals are so short, inspecting the baseline is difficult, but P waves are clearly absent. Narrow QRS complexes mean that the ventricular depolarization must have originated from a supraventricular focus. This narrow QRS complex tachydysrhythmia is atrial fibrillation. The variable R-R intervals are due to random AV conduction of very rapid atrial waves in fibrillation.

FIGURE 26–57

DATA:

- Rate: initial portion of (A) 95/minute; (B) <20/minute

- Rhythm: irregular

- QRS Duration: 0.08 second

- PR Interval: 0.18 second in strip A

- AV Conduction Ratio: 1:1 for early portion of strip A

- ST Segment: 2 mm depression

- Other Findings: absent cardiac complexes in strip C

Interpretation: sinus rhythm with a sinus block and an AV junctional escape beat in strip A. A slow ventricular rhythm occurs in strip B, which is followed by asystole in strip C.

Reasoning: The early portion of strip A shows a NSR

rhythm at 96/minute but midway through the top tracing the rate abruptly slows. The last ventricular complex in strip A is narrow but lacks a P wave so it must be a junctional escape beat. In strip B only two narrow QRS complexes that lack P waves are present, corresponding to a ventricular rate less than 20 per minute. Asystole follows in strip C and resuscitation efforts were not successful. This was an abrupt failure of the entire cardiac conduction system within 30 seconds.

FIGURE 26–58

DATA:

- Rate: ventricular: 42/minute

- Rhythm: regular

- QRS Duration: 0.20 second

- PR Interval: absent

- AV Conduction Ratio: absent

- ST Segment: 4 mm depression

- Other Findings: T waves are deeply inverted

Interpretation: Sinus arrest with an idioventricular escape rhythm at 42/minute

Reasoning: The ventricular activity has wide and bizarrely shaped QRS complexes occurring at a slow rate. Atrial activity is lacking, and a PR interval or AV conduction ratio cannot be determined. The sinus node and AV junction have failed as pacemakers. A slow escape pacemaker develops in the ventricles.

FIGURE 26–59

DATA:

- Rate: 170/minute

- Rhythm: irregular

- QRS Duration: 0.06 second

- PR Interval: for 4 sinus beats: 0.14 second

- AV Conduction Ratio: for sinus beats: 1:1

- ST Segment: 4 mm depression

- Other Findings: rapid, irregular narrow-complex rhythm.

Interpretation: Supraventricular tachycardia with four sinus "capture" beats (beats number 5, 11, 17, and 23).

Reasoning: The ventricular rhythm is irregular and consists of narrow QRS complexes. P waves are only seen in front of four of the QRS complexes. The rate of 170/minute is faster than that seen with sinus rhythms. The lack of P waves during most of the ECG tracing also argues against this being a sinus rhythm. The main rhythm is a supraventricular tachycardia, which is disrupted by several sinus *capture beats* (beats number 5, 11, 17, and 23). The sinus beats "capture" control away from the reentry SVT dysrhythmia because the sinus node discharge finds a polarized AV node that is able to react to the P wave by conducting the impulse.

FIGURE 26–60

DATA:

- Rate: 70/minute

- Rhythm: regularly irregular

- QRS Duration: 0.06 second

- PR Interval: 0.32 second

- AV Conduction Ratio: 1:1

- ST Segment: normal

- Other Findings: waxing-waning rhythm

Interpretation: Sinus dysrhythmia with a first-degree AV block

Reasoning: The ventricular activity is made up of narrow QRS complexes but the rhythm is irregular. The complexes are spaced close together during the initial portion of the tracing but are spread apart toward the end of the strip. Atrial activity has a fixed PR interval that is beyond the normal 0.20 second. Prolonged PR intervals represent a delayed start of ventricular activation and is a first-degree AV block. A sinus dysrhythmia causes the irregular rhythm because the patient's respiratory cycle affects the sinus node's rhythm.

FIGURE 26–61

DATA:

- Rate: ventricular: 40/minute; atrial: 60/minute

- Rhythm: regularly irregular

- QRS Duration: 0.06 second

- PR Interval: 0.24 second; 0.36 second; dropped beat

- AV Conduction Ratio: mainly 3:2, but also 2:1

- ST Segment: 1 mm depression

- Other Findings: grouped beats separated by pauses

Interpretation: **Sinus rhythm with second-degree AV heart block; Mobitz Type I (Wenckebach); 3:2 and 2:1 AV conduction with a ventricular rate of 40/minute**

Reasoning: The ventricular activity is characteristic of an incomplete AV heart block: grouped beating of two QRS complexes separated by a pause containing the nonconducted P wave. The P-P intervals are constant, which indicates a regularly discharging sinus node. Not all of the P waves are followed by QRS complexes—yet all of the QRS complexes are preceded by at least one P wave. The PR intervals show a cyclic variation: 0.24 second, 0.36 second, followed by a dropped beat. The AV conduction ratio for most of the grouped beats shows three P waves for every two QRS complexes, indicating that the third P wave of each group is not conducted. The last group of beats shows a 2:1 AV conduction ratio.

This tracing illustrates a key characteristic of Wenckebach blocks: progressive increase in PR duration coupled with a nonconducted QRS complex. Besides looking at PR intervals to find Wenckebach, consider the *R-R interval* as well. The longest R-R interval in a Wenckebach block will be *less than twice the shortest one*. This occurs because the QRS complexes begin to lag further behind the P waves as the PR intervals lengthen. The longest R-R interval includes the dropped beat and is *less than twice the shortest R-R interval*, because the maximal increase in PR intervals occurs between the first and second cycle. This secondary characteristic is helpful in spotting a Wenckebach block when the PR increase is not so evident.

FIGURE 26–62

DATA:

- Rate: 230/minute
- Rhythm: irregular
- QRS Duration: 0.20 second
- PR Interval: absent
- AV Conduction Ratio: absent
- ST Segment: distorted
- Other Findings: wide-complex tachydysrhythmia

Interpretation: **Sinus tachycardia is disrupted by two bouts of ventricular tachycardia (VI).**

Reasoning: The initial three beats are sinus, but the fourth beat is ventricular and occurs prematurely. The ectopic beat occurs during the vulnerable period of the third sinus complex when the conduction fibers have not all become fully repolarized (Figure 26–62 Answer). The PVC causes a five-beat episode of ventricular tachycardia because of an "R-on-T" phenomenon. The second and longer period of ventricular tachycardia happens during the latter half of the tracing, and is again caused by an "R-on-T" PVC (see Figure 26–62 Ansewr). The first beat after the initial run of ventricular tachycardia subsides is referred to as a sinus "capture beat" (see 26-62 Answer) because it captures the rhythm away from the ventricular focus. Ventricular tachycardia is recognized by its wide and distorted QRS complexes and regular R-R intervals. The ectopic beats lack associated P waves, so there is no AV relationship.

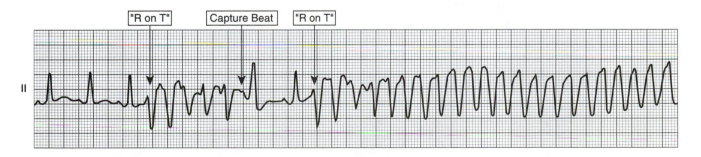

Figure 26-62 Answer

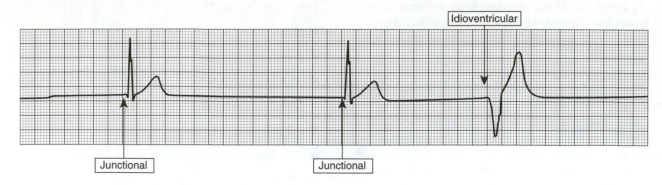

Figure 26-63 Answer

FIGURE 26–63

DATA:

- Rate: A: 90/minute; B-C: 20 to 30/minute

- Rhythm: irregular

- QRS Duration: A: 0.10 second; B: 0.12 second and 0.20 second; C: 0.24 second

- PR Interval: A: 0.16 second; B and C: absent

- AV Conduction Ratio: A: 1:1; B-C: absent

- ST Segment: A-B: normal; C: distorted

- Other Findings: rapid alteration in rhythm and QRS complexes

Interpretation: Sinus arrest with slow AV junctional and idioventricular escape rhythms

Reasoning: In strip A, normal appearing P-QRS-T complexes initially occur but the P waves soon disappear. The new rhythm in strip B is slower but still retains the narrow QRS complexes until the midpoint of strip B. These narrow beats are junctional escape complexes because P waves are not associated with them (Figure 26–63 Answer). The last beat in strip B is different from the narrow complexes and has a wide, distorted QRS complex. This single idioventricular complex (beat number 3 in strip B) lacks a P wave and has a wide and bizarre QRS complex (Figure 26–63 Answer). In strip C, a lone junctional beat is followed by a series of ventricular escape beats. Beats number 2 through 5 in strip C are wide and distorted. Within a minute even these escape rhythms failed and asystole occurred.

FIGURE 26–64

DATA:

- Rate: 66/minute

- Rhythm: irregular

- QRS Duration: 0.08 second

- PR Interval: 0.18 second

- AV Conduction Ratio: 1:1

- ST Segment: normal

- Other Findings: regularly irregular narrow-complex rhythm

Interpretation: Sinus rhythm with frequent PACs and atrial bigeminy

Reasoning: The early part of this tracing shows a regularly irregular pattern: two beats appear close together and are followed by a pause. Each sinus beat is coupled to a PAC yielding long-short cycles. The QRS complexes of the sinus and ectopic atrial beats are identical, indicating that intraventricular conduction is normal. The T waves of the sinus beats—which appear just ahead of the PACs—are distorted by P′ waves.

A reentry mechanism causes the repeating pattern of a sinus beat coupled to a PAC. This pattern is similar to a ventricular bigeminy except for the site of reentry. Atrial bigeminy occurs much less frequently than ventricular bigeminy cycles occur.

FIGURE 26–65

DATA:

- Rate: 210/minute
- Rhythm: regular
- QRS Duration: 0.10 second
- PR Interval: absent
- AV Conduction Ratio: absent
- ST Segment: 3 mm depression
- Other Findings: narrow-complex tachycardia

Interpretation: Supraventricular tachycardia (SVT) at 210/minute

Reasoning: The QRS complexes are normal in shape and duration, indicating conduction from a *supraventricular* focus. The R-R intervals are precisely regular. Distinct atrial activity, that is, P, P´, flutter or fibrillatory waves are not seen. Based on the findings of a narrow-complex tachycardic rhythm with a rate in excess of 200 per minute, the dysrhythmia is most likely to be a paroxysmal form of supraventricular tachycardia—a PSVT. Several minutes later NSR suddenly resumed after treatment with adenosine.

FIGURE 26–66

DATA:

- Rate: 160/minute
- Rhythm: regular
- QRS Duration: 0.20 second
- PR Interval: absent
- AV Conduction Ratio: absent
- ST Segment: distorted and opposite to the QRS main deflection
- Other Findings: isoelectric baseline is not visible

Interpretation: Ventricular tachycardia (VT) at 160/minute

Reasoning: The ventricular rhythm is rapid with wide and bizarre QRS complexes. Atrial activity is not associated within the QRS complexes, so an AV conduction ratio is absent. This dysrhythmia resembles a series of rapid consecutive PVCs.

> **Clinical Note** Wide QRS complexes should be considered to be ventricular tachycardias until proven otherwise. This is especially true when the patient is hypotensive, has a history opf a past MI showing symptoms and signs of shock, or having ischemic chest pain. In such cases, wide-complex tachydysrhythmias need to be electrically cardioverted as soon as possible because they can degenerate into ventricular fibrillation.

FIGURE 26–67

DATA:

- Rate: ventricular: 37/minute; atrial: 75/minute
- Rhythm: regular QRS complexes and P waves
- QRS Duration: 0.12 second
- PR Interval: absent
- AV Conduction Ratio: absent
- ST Segment: normal
- Other Findings: many more P waves than QRS complexes; some T waves are distorted because they contain nonconducted P waves

Interpretation: Third-degree (complete) AV heart block with a ventricular escape rhythm at

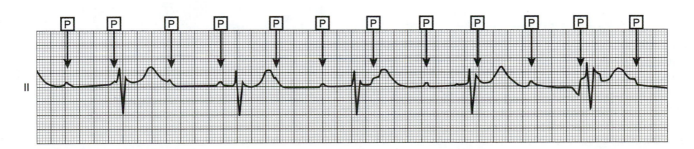

Figure 26-67 Answer

35/minute

Reasoning: The QRS complexes are slow and wide. Regular atrial activity is noted, but complete AV dissociation exists because the P waves are not related to the QRS complexes. Some of the P waves distort the ST segments and T waves (Figure 26–27 Answer). P waves appear to "march through" the QRS complexes because there are independent atrial and ventricular pacemakers.

FIGURE 26–68

DATA:

■ Rate: 60/minute

■ Rhythm: regular

■ QRS Duration: 0.20 second

■ PR Interval: 0.40 second

■ AV Conduction Ratio: 1:1

■ ST Segment: 1 mm depression

■ Other Findings: distorted QRS complexes and notched P waves

Interpretation: Sinus rhythm with first degree AV heart block and an intraventricular conduction defect (bundle branch block)

Reasoning: The ventricular complexes are distorted and wide due to an intraventricular conduction abnormality. The ventricles are depolarized *sequentially rather than simultaneously*, as normally occurs in NSR. Sequential chamber activation causes two separate portions of the QRS complex to appear: an initial R and subsequent r´ wave. As a result, there is slowed and asynchronous activation of each ventricle.

Every QRS complex is preceded by a single P wave. The P-P intervals and PR intervals are fixed. The P waves are notched and this indicates sequential activation rather than simultaneous discharge. This does not effect cardiac output. The PR interval is 0.40 second, which is considerably longer than normal. The prolonged PR interval represents a delay before the ventricles are depolarized. The notched P waves, prolonged PR intervals, and delayed QRS duration indicate a slowed conduction velocity.

Discussion: Slowed conduction velocity can be caused by enhanced vagal tone, or generalized myocardial ischemia, as well as medication such as procainamide. Sequential activation of the atria usually happens because one or both of the atria become larger and thicker (hypertrophied) after experiencing chronic volume or pressure overload. As the atria enlarge, they

take slightly longer to be activated.

FIGURE 26–69

DATA:

■ Rate: 67/minute

■ Rhythm: irregular

■ QRS Duration: sinus: 0.6 second; PVC: 0.20 second

■ PR Interval: 0.16 second

■ AV Conduction Ratio: 1:1

■ ST Segment: normal for sinus beats; elevated and opposite the QRS deflection for the PVCs

■ Other Findings: T waves are as tall as the QRS complexes

Interpretation: Sinus rhythm with two unifocal (uniformed) PVCs

Reasoning: The ventricular rhythm is irregular because two beats (beats number 4 and 9) occur early during the R-R cycles. Because the premature complexes have wide QRS complexes, lack P waves, and are followed by compensatory pauses, they must be ectopic ventricular beats. The sinus complexes have normal P-QRS-T waves. The coupling intervals of the PVCs to the previous sinus beats are constant.

Clinical Note Tall T waves will cause the ECG monitor's automatic rate detector to count the T waves in addition to the R waves, resulting in double the actual cardiac rate. T waves that are taller than R waves also present a problem when trying to perform synchronized cardioversion, because the QRS detector may focus on the T wave and deliver a shock during the vulnerable phase of the cycle. Both problems can be remedied by selecting a different monitoring lead that displays R waves that are taller than the T waves.

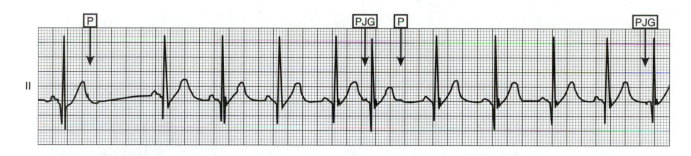

Figure 26-70 Answer

FIGURE 26–70

DATA:

- Rate: 75/minute

- Rhythm: irregular

- QRS Duration: 0.10 second

- PR Interval: 0.12 second

- AV Conduction Ratio: 1:1 except for the nonconducted PAC

- ST Segment: normal

- Other Findings: short pause after the second beat

Interpretation: Sinus rhythm with conducted and nonconducted premature atrial complexes (PALS)

Reasoning: The ventricular rhythm is irregular because PACs disrupt the sinus node function. The QRS complexes of the sinus and atrial beats show the same narrow shape, indicating that they both have a supraventricular origin. The pause involving the long R-R interval occurs just after the distorted downslope of beat number 1's T wave—which is caused by a *nonconducted P′ wave* (Figure 26–70 Answer). Beats number 6 and 11 are *conducted* premature atrial complexes because their P′ waves and PR intervals differ from the sinus beats. The AV conduction ratio is 1:1 except for the nonconducted PAC, where it is 2:1 for a single cycle.

FIGURE 26–71

DATA:

- Rate: (A) 50/minute; (B) 120/minute

- Rhythm: (A and B) irregular

- QRS Duration: (A) 0.30 second; (B) 0.24 second

- PR Interval: (A) 0.40 second; (B) absent

- AV Conduction Ratio: (A) 1:1; (B) absent

- ST Segment: 7 mm elevation

- Other Findings: very irregular rhythm with distorted QRS complexes

Interpretation: Sinus bradycardia at 50/minute with a prolonged PR interval and a nonconducted PAC in strip A. The rhythm degenerates into ventricular tachycardia in strip B.

Reasoning: The QRS complexes are extremely wide and distorted, while the rhythm is slow and irregular in strip A. While each QRS in strip A is preceded by a P wave, a noticeable pause in activity occurs after beat number 4, which is caused by a blocked premature P′ wave. The nonconducted P′ wave can be seen in beat number 4's ST-T wave segment. In strip B, a rapid ventricular rhythm occurs. Toward the end of tracing B, the rhythm becomes more irregular and the QRS complexes become more distorted. The pacemaker is not dependable and the patient subsequently had an asystolic cardiac arrest.

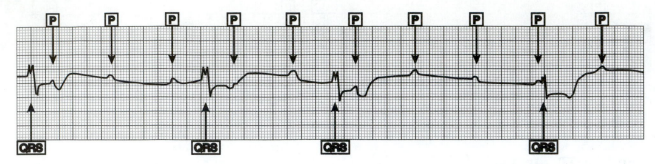

Figure 26-72 Answer

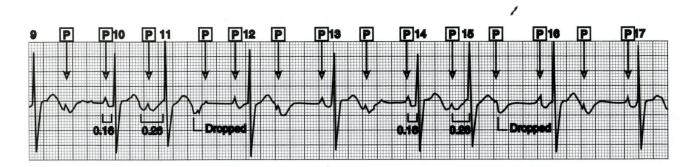

Figure 26-73 Answer

FIGURE 26–72

DATA:

- Rate: ventricular: 30/minute; atrial: 70/minute

- Rhythm: ventricular: irregular; atrial: regular

- QRS Duration: 0.20 second

- PR Interval: absent

- AV Conduction Ratio: absent

- ST Segment: 5 mm depression

- Other Findings: many more P waves than QRS complexes

Interpretation: Third-degree (complete) AV heart block and a ventricular escape rhythm at 30/minute

Reasoning: The ventricular rhythm is slightly irregular and the QRS complexes are wide and notched. Atrial activity consists of normal appearing P waves but they occur much faster than ventricular activity (Figure 26–72 Answer). No set AV relationship exists as there is a complete interruption of AV conduction. The pronounced ST segment depression points to myocardial ischemia.

FIGURE 26–73

DATA:

- Rate: ventricular: 55/minute; atrial: 100/minute

- Rhythm: irregular

- QRS Duration: 0.12 second

- PR Interval: 0.16 second; 0.24 second

- AV Conduction Ratio: 2:1; 3:2

- ST Segment: normal

- Other Findings: irregular rhythm with more P waves than QRS complexes

Interpretation: Sinus rhythm with second-degree AV heart block; Mobitz Type I (Wenckebach) with variable AV conduction and a ventricular rate of 60/minute

Reasoning: Each QRS complex is normal and has a consistent shape and duration. The ventricular rhythm is irregular. The sixth QRS complex in strip A and beats number 3 and 7 in strip B have *shorter R-R intervals* than other beats (Figure 26–73 Answer). Atrial activity occurs regularly and has constant P-P intervals. Each P wave has a normal, upright, and consistent shape. The AV relationship is clearly abnormal because P waves appear without ventricular activity. The AV conduction ratio varies from 2:1 to 3:2 conduction. Most of the QRS complexes have *more than one P wave* associated with them and form a 2:1 conduction ratio. As a result, every other or every third P wave is not conducted and the QRS complex is "dropped". Since the sinus rate is 100/minute the ventricular rate is just below 60/minute despite the dropped QRS complexes.

FIGURE 26–74

DATA:

- Rate: 160/minute

- Rhythm: irregular

- QRS Duration: 0.08 second

- PR Interval: absent

- AV Conduction Ratio: not measurable

- ST Segment: variable depression; from 4 to 8 mm depression

- Other Findings: irregular, narrow-complex tachydysrhythmia

Interpretation: **Atrial fibrillation with a tachycardic ventricular response of 160/minute**

Reasoning: The ventricular complexes appear narrow and normal. The rhythm of the QRS complexes is grossly irregular due to the slight beat-to-beat variability. The variability is hard to appreciate because the rapid ventricular rate crowds the QRS complexes close together. A normal QRS duration indicates a *supra*ventricular origin, yet P waves are absent so the rhythm cannot be sinus. Based on the following findings: narrow QRS complexes, irregular ventricular activity, and missing P waves, this dysrhythmia is atrial fibrillation. Even without being able to see the characteristic fibrillatory ("f") waves, the irregularly irregular pattern confirms AF.

FIGURE 26–75

DATA:

- Rate: ventricular: 50/minute; atrial: 70/minute

- Rhythm: regularly irregular

- QRS Duration: 0.20 second

- PR Interval: 0.26 second; 0.52 second; dropped beat; cycle repeats

- AV Conduction Ratio: 3:2

- ST Segment: normal

- Other Findings: grouped beating

Interpretation: **Sinus rhythm with second-degree AV heart block; Mobitz Type I (Wenckebach); 3:2 AV conduction and a ventricular rate of 50/minute**

Reasoning: The ventricular rhythm consists of irregular beats with QRS complexes that are wider than normal. Each QRS complex is preceded by a P wave; *however, not every P wave is followed by a QRS complex.* This indicates that an AV block or conduction failure is present. The atrial rhythm is regular but the third P wave of each cycle is hidden by the QRS complex (Figure 26–75 Answer). The third P wave of each group is not conducted, yielding a 3:2 AV conduction. PR intervals show a progressive increase as expected for Wenckebach. The QRS complexes appear to fall further behind the P waves as the cycles advance, until a P wave is not conducted. The cycle starts over with progressive PR intervals until there is a dropped QRS complex.

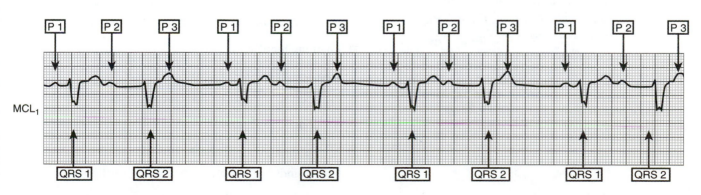

Figure 26-75 Answer

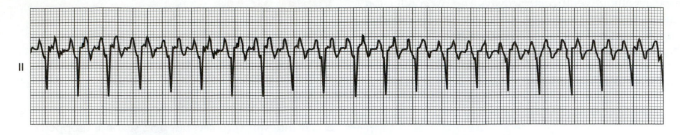

Figure 26-76 Answer

FIGURE 26–76

DATA:

- Rate: ventricular: 150/minute; atrial: 300/minute
- Rhythm: regular
- QRS Duration: 0.10 second
- PR Interval: not measurable
- AV Conduction Ratio: 2:1
- ST Segment: difficult to evaluate due to the flutter waves
- Other Findings: atrial waves form a "picket-fence" appearance

Interpretation: Atrial flutter with 2:1 AV conduction and a ventricular rate of 150/minute

Reasoning: The ventricular rate is very rapid and each P´ wave ("F" or flutter wave) has a positive and negative component. The atrial rate is twice that of the ventricles. The atrial rate is 300/minute and there is one large ECG box between two flutter waves. AV conduction consists of two flutter waves for each QRS complex, yielding a 2:1 conduction.

> ***ECG Interpretation Tip*** *An easy way to appreciate the flutter wave appearance is to invert the strip (Figure 26–76 Answer). This brings the area of interest—the flutter waves that distort the baseline—into view. Viewing the atrial baseline upside-down makes it easy to concentrate on the flutter wave appearance which is likened to a picket-fence or saw-tooth pattern.*

FIGURE 26–77

DATA:

- Rate: 50/minute
- Rhythm: irregular
- QRS Duration: 0.10 second
- PR Interval: 0.20 second
- AV Conduction Ratio: 1:1
- ST Segment: 13 mm elevation
- Other Findings: distorted ST segment

Interpretation: Sinus bradycardia at a rate of 50/minute with a PAC and significantly elevated ST segments

Reasoning: The QRS complexes are narrow but due to the significantly elevated ST segments appear wide. The ventricular rhythm is irregular beginning just after the first beat. The atrial rhythm is also irregular. Atrial activity consists of normal P waves for most QRS complexes but beat number 2 has a tall pointed P´ wave (where the early beat develops). AV conduction is normal. The rate is less than 60/minute

FIGURE 26–78

DATA:

- Rate: (A) 90/minute; (B and C) 25-30/minute
- Rhythm: regular
- QRS Duration: 0.06 second
- PR Interval: (A and B) 0.18 sec.; (C) absent
- AV Conduction: absent
- ST Segment: (C) 1 mm elevation
- Other Findings: progressive slowing of the rate

Interpretation: An accelerated supraventricular

rhythm abruptly degenerates into a low atrial and a slow AV junctional escape rhythm at 25/minute

Reasoning: The ventricular complexes are the same in all three tracings; however the rate dramatically slows after strip A. In strip B atrial activity can be seen just ahead of the QRS complexes. Atrial waves are not present in strip C. Strip C shows a slow junctional rhythm in the face of sinus node failure. The sequence of tracings shows a progressive failure of impulse formation and the conduction system in a dying heart.

FIGURE 26–79

DATA:

- Rate: 90/minute

- Rhythm: regular

- QRS Duration: 0.12 second

- PR Interval: 0.32 second

- S-T Segment: normal

- Other Findings: notched P waves and distorted QRS complexes

Interpretation: Sinus rhythm with a first-degree AV heart block and an intraventricular conduction defect (IVCD)

Reasoning: The ventricular rhythm is regular but the QRS complexes are wider than in NSR. The atrial rhythm is regular but the P waves are notched, indicating delayed and sequential atrial activation. There is a single P wave for every QRS complex but the PR intervals are considerably prolonged beyond 0.20 second. A delay occurs before ventricular activation occurs.

FIGURE 26–80

DATA:

- Rate: considerable variation between bradycardia (40/minute) and tachycardia (150/minute)

- Rhythm: irregular

- QRS Duration: 0.06 second

- PR Interval: absent

- AV Conduction Ratio: not detectable

- ST Segment: variable; ranges from isoelectric baseline to 3 mm depression

- Other Findings: alternating fast and slow narrow complex rhythm

Interpretation: Tachycardiac-bradycardia syndrome; atrial fibrillation with alternating bradycardia and tachycardia ventricular responses

Reasoning: The ventricular complexes are narrow. The rate varies greatly from very fast to very slow. Atrial activity cannot be seen. The narrow QRS complex rhythm indicates a supraventricular rhythm. The grossly irregular rhythm with normal QRS duration points toward atrial fibrillation. The term "tachy-brady" syndrome is a general description applied to a dysrhythmia when there are wide swings in the ventricular rate. The rhythm in a tachy-brady syndrome is unreliable because patients may become symptomatic from too fast or too slow a rate.

CONCLUSION

Congratulations on completing the final self-assessment exercise! The ECG tracings contained some difficult dysrhythmias that are typical of those encountered in daily clinical practice. You have mastered the essentials of dysrhythmia interpretation.

Index